CW00971783

THE TEACHING HOSPITAL

Brigham and Women's Hospital and the Evolution of Academic Medicine

Peter V. Tishler, MD
Physician, Department of Medicine and Genetics Division
Brigham and Women's Hospital
Associate Professor of Medicine
Harvard Medical School
Boston, Massachusetts

Christine Wenc
Editor, Department of Medicine
Brigham and Women's Hospital
Boston, Massachusetts

Joseph Loscalzo, MD, PhD
Chairman, Department of Medicine
Physician-in-Chief
Brigham and Women's Hospital
Hersey Professor of the Theory and Practice of Physic
Harvard Medical School
Boston, Massachusetts

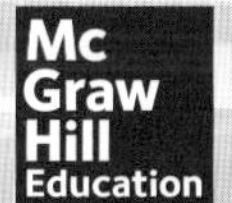

Medical

New York Chicago San Francisco Athens London Madrid Mexico City
Milan New Delhi Singapore Sydney Toronto

The Teaching Hospital

1 2 3 4 5 6 7 8 9 0 CTP/CTP 18 17 16 15 14

ISBN 978-0-07-178401-6
MHID 0-07-178401-2

This book was set in Mercury Text G2 by Cenveo® Publisher Services.
The editors were James F. Shanahan and Regina Y. Brown.
The production supervisor was Catherine H. Saggese.
Project management was provided by Nidhi Chopra, Cenveo Publisher Services.
The text designer was Tina Henderson. The cover designer was Joanne Lee.
China Translation & Printing Services, Inc. was printer and binder.

This book was printed on acid-free paper.

Library of Congress Cataloging-in-Publication Data

The teaching hospital : Brigham and Women's Hospital and the evolution of academic medicine / [edited] by Peter V. Tishler, Christine Wenc, Joseph Loscalzo.
p. ; cm.
Brigham and Women's Hospital and the evolution of academic medicine
Includes bibliographical references and index.
ISBN 978-0-07-178401-6 (hardcover : alk. paper)—ISBN 0-07-178401-2 (hardcover : alk. paper)
I. Tishler, Peter V., editor of compilation. II. Wenc, Christine, editor of compilation. III. Loscalzo, Joseph, editor of compilation. IV. Title: Brigham and Women's Hospital and the evolution of academic medicine.
[DNLM: 1. Peter Bent Brigham Hospital. 2. Affiliated Hospitals Center (Boston, Mass.) 3. Brigham and Women's Hospital. 4. Hospitals, Teaching—history—Massachusetts. 5. History, 20th Century—Massachusetts. 6. History, 21st Century—Massachusetts. WX 28 AM4]
RA982.B72
362.1109744'61—dc23

2013043239

ADVANCE PRAISE FOR THE TEACHING HOSPITAL

Very few institutions have had a greater impact on the science and practice of medicine than Boston's Peter Bent Brigham Hospital. This well-documented and extensively illustrated book is a welcome addition to the literature of the history of medicine. Dozens of authors have created a colorful mosaic of the careers and contributions of many individuals who have contributed to the development of a world-class academic medical center.

W. Bruce Fye, Professor of Medicine and the History of Medicine, Mayo Clinic

Readers get a panoramic view of 20th- and 21st-century American medical education, research, and healthcare delivery through the lens of a single institution, Brigham and Women's Hospital. Anchored as a narrative in national historical context by clinician-historians Scott Podolsky and Jeremy Greene's overview, this multilevel history encapsulates the complex trends and contradictory movements of American medicine. The highly readable, illustrated contributions cover a range of landmark issues from hospital architecture, medical leadership, and biomedical innovation, the perspective of participants in the hospital enterprise from orderlies to residents to CEOs, the creation of large healthcare systems, the impact of government health and urban policies, and the negotiation with local and global communities over the teaching hospital's mortar and mission across periods of intense social and political change.

Jennifer Gunn, Associate Professor and Director Program in the History of Medicine, University of Minnesota

This wonderful collection of essays places the Brigham and Women's Hospital into a deep historical, cultural, and scientific perspective. The Brigham's remarkable history—integrating patient care, teaching, and cutting edge research—has crucial implications for health care in the 21st century. The Teaching Hospital will be widely read by patients and professionals alike, seeking to understand how history can be utilized to illuminate the present and guide the future.

Allan M. Brandt, Amalie Moses Kass Professor of the History of Medicine, Harvard University

CONTENTS

PART 2: EVOLUTION OF CLINICAL CARE

FOREWORD

Kenneth M. Ludmerer

The surgeon Thomas E. Starzl once wrote, "If gold medals and prizes were awarded to institutions instead of individuals, the Peter Bent Brigham Hospital . . . would have qualified."[1] I agree with Starzl. In my own journey in medical education, I have come to regard the Brigham, along with the Johns Hopkins Hospital and Medical School, as one of the two most important shapers of American medical education. The story of the Brigham is an inspiring one, and the writers and editors of this book have provided a great service by recording its history in a fashion that is at once comprehensive and scholarly as well as lively and engaging.

What accounts for the Brigham's historical importance? The answers to this question are found herein. The Johns Hopkins Hospital (founded 1889) and Medical School (founded 1893) provided a model for medical education that eventually became universally adopted in America. However, progress in the implementation of the model was frustratingly slow until the opening of the Peter Bent Brigham Hospital in 1913. The Brigham from the start allowed medical students to work as clinical clerks and sponsored a modern residency program in several specialties. In both activities, it was the first hospital since the Johns Hopkins Hospital to do so. The Brigham also engaged from the start in a close partnership with Harvard Medical School, employed a "full-time" system of clinical appointments, and became a major innovator in clinical research. In these regards the Brigham approximated Abraham Flexner's model of a true university hospital perhaps more closely than any other American hospital. The success of the Brigham in implementing the new educational model inspired other hospitals to do so, including the much older and larger Massachusetts General Hospital. As Johns Hopkins was the pioneer of modern medical education in America, the Brigham was the catalyst in enabling the model to spread and become widely implemented.

The splendid scholars who have contributed to this volume have produced a history worthy of the institution. They provide a rich account of the evolution of the Brigham in all its dimensions: as an educational and clinical innovator, its role in fostering groundbreaking biomedical research, the expansion of its ties to the local community as well as to the nation and world, the financial and administrative growth of the Brigham as an institution, the personalities who have made the Brigham the Brigham, and the culture and inner life of the hospital. The chapters are replete not only with information and stories, but also with critical analysis—examining the problems of the hospital as well as its many achievements and placing the evolution of the Brigham in a broad medical and cultural context.

One of the themes in the book is the presence of both continuity and change in the evolution of the Brigham. In recent decades, the Brigham has experienced enormous expansion in size, budget, staffing, mission, and the scope of problems requiring its critical gaze. It has become a massive, complex health system employing futuristic clinical technologies, studying problems from molecules to populations, and addressing many of the thorniest moral and social dilemmas of our age. It is safe to say that those present at the hospital's founding a century ago would not recognize today's Brigham. Yet, throughout this evolution there have been fundamental continuities: the Brigham's creativity, its courage to examine critically every presumed fact and certainty, its engagement with not only the scientific dimension of medical care but with the human and moral dimensions as well, and its commitment not just to excellence but to leadership. These qualities represented the essence of the Brigham from the beginning, and they characterize the Brigham today.

This book appears at a propitious moment. The American medical system is under constant criticism for its well-known shortcomings: excessive costs, inconsistent quality, inadequate access, and poor results in public health. We live in a cynical age—an age of debunking and deconstruction—and our healthcare system has understandably experienced its share of attack. Yet, the great strength of the Brigham has always been its ability and willingness to examine shortcomings directly—its own and those of American medicine more broadly. In keeping with that tradition, the essays in the book examine problems that remain to be solved. However, in so doing, the essays also reveal a glorious observation that deserves to be celebrated: the commitment of the Brigham not just to mere excellence but rather to the effort to approximate perfection. In this, the Brigham offers the inspiration and confidence that medical education, patient care, and healthcare delivery in America might get better, and in telling the story, this book serves the future as well as the past.

NOTES

1. Starzl TE. The landmark identical twin case. J Am Med Assoc 1984;252:2573

PEOPLE FIRST: A PERSONAL VIEW FROM THE PRESIDENT

Elizabeth G. Nabel

This year we celebrate the history of the Brigham and Women's Hospital—a world-class medical institution dedicated to putting people first. Through a continued commitment to rigorous science, innovative education, and compassionate care, our hospital has changed the face of academic medicine. In the next century, we aspire to a greater leadership role in transforming science-driven health care.

In many ways, today we stand at a similar crossroads as did the founders of the Peter Bent Brigham Hospital at the beginning of the twentieth century. Abraham Flexner's call for revamping medical education in 1910 set into motion sweeping reforms that invited the establishment of the Peter Bent Brigham in 1913. Almost immediately, this institution became emblematic of the central and vital role of academic medical centers in training new physicians. At the same time, the societal climate of turn-of-the-century urban America defined the need to provide health care to all. The seeds of a new and transformative era were sown. Beginning with the use of chemicals to fight infectious disease, which was rampant in impoverished and overcrowded areas, the American populace grew to appreciate the extraordinary value science could play in helping people. Brigham and Women's Hospital, the result of a merger between the Boston Hospital for Women, the Robert Breck Brigham Hospital, and the Peter Bent Brigham Hospital, has long led the nation as a top academic medical center. We are the home of the nation's first maternity ward, New England's first coronary care unit, the first successful human organ transplant, and most recently, the first human full-face transplant. We have made our name in several clinical specialties, such as transplant medicine, kidney disease, heart disease, and rheumatology, as well as in cutting-edge areas of research such as stem cells, systems biology, bioengineering, and personalized medicine.

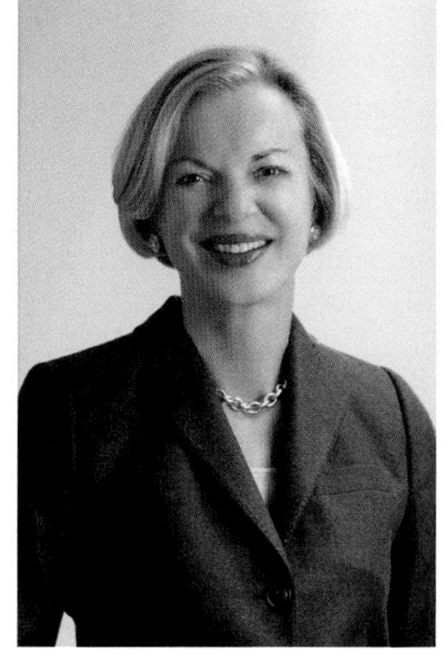

It was the Brigham's innovative spirit and tradition of accomplishment—and its dedication to excellence and spark of promise—that drew me here in 1982. Freshly inducted into the world of medicine, as a new intern, I was full of dreams. I was ready to care, ready to learn, ready to be an instrument of change as a twentieth-century doctor. Although I did not know or expect it, I was also ready to begin an immensely satisfying personal journey with the man who would soon become my husband. With Gary, I would share my dreams, work together on scientific problems, and raise three children. The first, our son Christopher, began his life right here at the Brigham on a frigid yet brilliantly sunny January morning in 1986. Throughout my career, I have spent time away from Francis Street, yet its impact never left me. In 2010, I returned to this wonderful institution, having made a circuitous route from resident to president. This is a role that I cherish and respect, since I now have the opportunity to nurture and challenge the Brigham the same way it nurtured and challenged me. I know from conversations that I have had with many others here that I am not unique in this way.

Belonging to a generation that crosses the threshold of a new century offers me the chance to reflect on the past and look toward the future in distinctive ways. In doing so, I know the path must be defined by clear vision. The twenty-first-century Brigham is and will continue to be an environment of patient-centered care that puts people first by being seamless, participatory, comprehensive, cost-effective, and compassionate.

Today, a new and different—but equally significant—revolution is underway. The nation's investment in biomedical research, in which the Brigham maintains a leading position, has been a wellspring of knowledge about the human condition and how it fails in disease. The human genome, the genetic script that defines our species, has been deciphered. An array of amazing technologies enables us to view disease processes in real time, noninvasively. Today's call to action is convergence—bringing together the strengths of the programs we have built, and cross-fertilizing them with the seeds that will grow into new fields of inquiry. A perfect example is the OurGenes, OurHealth, OurCommunities project, which will gather comprehensive information from 100,000 patients—genetic, environmental, family medical history, and medical records—with the vision that the data can drive future understanding and treatment of disease. The promising field of regenerative medicine offers genuine hope that regrowing injured and damaged organs will also be part of routine care in the next century. The Brigham will continue to be a leading presence in the nation's hotbed of scientific inquiry.

By embracing innovation in everything we do, the Brigham has a tremendous opportunity to find new paths toward achieving our mission: transforming health care through science, education, and compassionate care, both locally and globally. Our vision applies to everyone we serve, from the twenty-year-young man with leukemia to his eighty-year-old grandmother with diabetes and high blood pressure, and from the new interns we coach in the ways of the hospital to the healthcare volunteers who give their time and talents to help patients living with chronic disease.

How will the Brigham's clinical mission and vision evolve in the twenty-first century? By establishing a seamless, family-centered care system, we will provide a reliably excellent experience for patients, families, and their providers. By pursuing cutting-edge innovation and discovery, we will strengthen our leadership position in translational research and realize the goal of personalized medicine. By augmenting our leadership in education, we will continue our tradition of lifelong learning, through attracting and keeping the best faculty, students, and healthcare providers. By engaging our multifaceted workforce, we will build and sustain a culture of wellness, high performance, and service excellence. Striving for health equity, we will deliver high-quality culturally and linguistically appropriate health care. We will provide affordable care through the most efficient and effective use of all of our resources. We will expand our local and global alliances—the Student Success Jobs Program, Partners In Health, the Brigham Outreach Program to the Indian Health Service, and others. These synergies have introduced new thoughts and strategies, melded resources and talents, and broadened our reach to patients in the vast diversity of Boston's neighborhoods and beyond. Above all, we will achieve excellence in all we do: in patient care, in research, and in community engagement.

The Brigham's next hundred years will catalyze a transformation in science-driven health care. We will embrace a holistic view of care that empowers patients to maintain health throughout life and avoid costly readmissions. We will join our talents to put patients first by sharing responsibility through team-based care. We will dissolve the scientific and medical boundaries that no longer fit, making way for new knowledge and new structures of thought and practice. We will remain committed to nurturing the individual creative minds who lead the transformation of discovery to health. We will redefine the meaning of community to encompass the needs of the local, national, and global neighborhoods we serve through research, education, and patient care.

Just as I arrived at the Brigham many years ago eager and proud to learn from the masters of the day, current students, residents, fellows, and faculty come here for the same reason. They know that their dreams will find fertile ground in this special place, and I have no doubt that today's young investigators who come here to explore will make the breakthroughs of tomorrow.

Throughout the years, I have played several different roles here at the Brigham, ranging from new doctor to new patient to new leader. I have been so fortunate to benefit from the gifts of this fine institution. My own journey is emblematic of the vision and values held by our founders. As I lead this institution across the threshold of a new era, I am committed to being equally bold and compassionate, as well as to the belief that intertwined research and patient care always put people first. That is the Brigham way.

UNEQUALLED STRENGTH THROUGH MISSION, PEOPLE, AND PARTNERSHIPS

Gary L. Gottlieb

The Brigham's first decade of the twenty-first century was built on the foundation of partnerships developed over the prior twenty years. While we celebrate the richness of a history with roots 180 years old, the Brigham and Women's Hospital (BWH) of the twenty-first century is a relatively young organization. Its remarkable achievements are derived from its breathtaking mission and its consistently outstanding talent. However, the Brigham's star shines even more brightly because of carefully crafted partnerships that consistently make the whole even more special than the sum of the extraordinary parts.

The BWH was created in 1980 by the merger of the Peter Bent Brigham and Robert Breck Brigham Hospitals and the Boston Hospital for Women, each of which was an important member of the Harvard Medical School community. Under the leadership of H. Richard Nesson, the new organization thrived and further developed into a clinical and academic powerhouse. Nesson's visionary stewardship fostered a long-standing relationship with Harvard Community Health Plan, the predecessor of Harvard Vanguard Medical Associates. He drove pioneering investments in information technology as a tool to improve patient safety, care quality, and management efficiency, and he was an outspoken advocate for provision of the best possible care to those in need in the local community. As a magnificent leader who presided over a remarkably successful merger, Nesson was a natural founding architect of the Brigham's agreement to merge with the Massachusetts General Hospital (MGH) to create the Partners HealthCare system in 1993. When Nesson became Partners' founding chief executive officer (CEO) in 1994, Jeff Otten, BWH president, continued diligently to foster key community relationships and strengthen the bonds of the Harvard medical community while building a partnership with MGH.

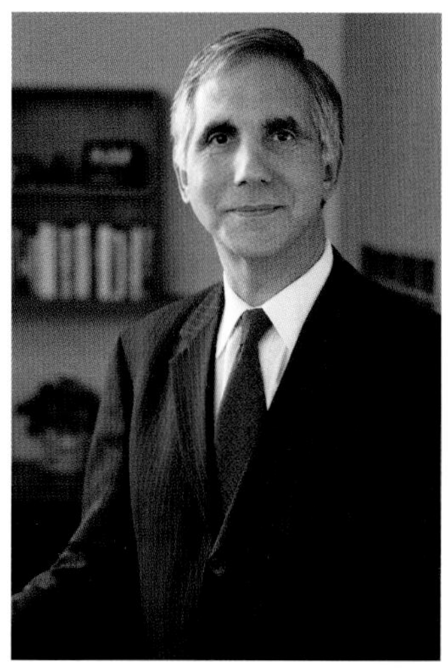

Partners' alliance with Dana-Farber Cancer Institute (DFCI) and the formation of Dana-Farber Partners Cancer Care in 1996 was a catalyst in Otten's efforts to forge closer clinical ties with the DFCI. Shortly thereafter, DFCI's inpatient beds moved into the Brigham's patient bed tower, and the Brigham's Medical Oncology services moved to DFCI. This was synergistic with the official opening of the Dana-Farber/Brigham and Women's Cancer Center in 2000, allying HMS and the Harvard School of Public Health with all of their teaching hospitals to form the largest of the National Cancer Institute's comprehensive Cancer Centers.

In the late 1990s, in the context of increasing penetration of managed care and downward pressure on costs, the Brigham focused intensely on improving its efficiency and on using its resources most effectively to serve a growing patient population. Inspired by the notion across Partners of "getting the right care in the right place," Faulkner Hospital became a member of the Brigham family in 1998, launching a set of efforts to move ambulatory and secondary care closer to people's homes and concentrate higher intensity services at the Brigham. As the

Brigham moved forward with these and other efforts, spurred by an evolving payment environment, the hospital worked with its physician groups and storied academic departments to form the Brigham and Women's Physician Organization (BWPO) in 2001. The development of the BWPO was the foundation for a string of collaborations between the hospital and its departments and among the physicians at the BWH, MGH, and across the Partners network to improve the quality and safety of patient care and to face the marketplace collectively. Finally, in the capstone of his tenure, Otten worked closely with the Brigham's friends and neighbors in Mission Hill and with the Roxbury Tenants of Harvard to create the real estate that would allow expansion of the campus across Huntington Avenue and Francis Street.

It was on this platform of partnerships and this vision that I had the privilege of becoming the president of the Brigham in 2002. For every moment of the following eight years, the beacon of the Brigham's mission and the brilliance and commitment of its people embraced a course that enabled innovation, collaboration, and growth.

At Partners, CEO James J. Mongan inspired us with a strategy of uniform quality and safety, launching High Performance Medicine and playing to the Brigham's sweet spot of performance improvement informed by science and facilitated by technology. A wave of efforts including the development of electronic medication administration and bar coding, patient safety walk rounds, and an automated balanced scorecard reflected the translation of world-leading research in patient safety into effective management tactics. The development of the Center for Clinical Excellence became a source of truth in measurement and in further embedding quality, safety, and patient satisfaction in the operations and culture of the hospital. These efforts were reinforced by first-class trustee leadership under Brigham Board Chair G. Marshall Moriarty and the Board's Clinical Improvement Committee, earning national recognition for the hospital.

The building blocks established in the late 1990s allowed the Brigham to reimagine its footprint, establishing a "distributed main campus:" the highest intensity services, obstetrics and gynecology, and care for the local community, as well as the core of biomedical sciences, would be sited at the Brigham's main campus and its community health centers; procedure-based ambulatory care and secondary and light tertiary care would migrate to Faulkner; and a broad base of outpatient services would move to an expanded ambulatory care center in nearby Brookline. This allowed planning to expand and renew the Brigham's main campus, with the addition of the Carl J. and Ruth Shapiro Cardiovascular Center, expansion of the Intensive Care Unit capacity, and the complement of private rooms in the tower, all juxtaposed with expanded basic research space in Longwood.

DFCI CEO Edward J. Benz and his team helped us to transform an affiliation into a vital and dynamic partnership providing seamless care in settings that could accelerate the translation of great science into cures for cancers. The Dana-Farber/Brigham and Women's Cancer Center (DF/BWECC) was launched officially in 1997. It was defined by interdisciplinary disease centers across cancer subspecialties. Each was co-led and designed to provide cutting-edge patient- and family-centered care that married the deepest resources in both institutions. These efforts were supported by grand investments in molecular diagnostics and innovative science. The DF/BWCC worked to bring these services into the community, establishing ambulatory centers at the Faulkner, South Shore, and Milford-Whitinsville Hospitals.

At South Shore Hospital, the DF/BWCC facility helped to reinforce and cement a blossoming partnership in a broad array of clinical services. We also fortified our community investments by developing a freestanding ambulatory care center in Foxboro with the MGH, bringing urgent and primary care as well as specialty and procedural medicine right to our patients' doorsteps.

The heart of our community, the neighborhoods right around the Brigham, Faulkner, and our community health centers became critical partners in our efforts to eliminate intolerable disparities in healthcare access and outcomes. Through investments in our schools, workforce development, our own and partnering health centers, and together with public agencies, the Brigham's revitalized Center for Community Health Equity became a centerpiece of sustaining strategic and operational efforts to truly improve the health and health care of those at greatest need. And the focus on global health-care equity intensified as well, with growth in the Brigham's presence in Haiti, Peru, Rwanda, Lesotho, and Malawi through the Department of Medicine's Division of Global Health Equity and Partners in Health. The Brigham also played a seminal role in the development and growth of the Harvard Humanitarian Initiative.

Through the magnificent leadership of the hospital's chiefs, the Brigham's signature research enterprise grew enormously, abetted by the creation of the Biomedical Research Institute (BRI). Through the BRI and its centers of excellence, cross-institutional collaboration and focused strategic investment in science created the potential to imbed the scientific mission in every element of the hospital's activities. Together with continued nurturance of the nation's leading training programs, the growth of scientific excellence perpetuated the Brigham's magnetic force that attracted the world's most extraordinary young people to dedicate themselves to improve the human condition.

I was humbled by the opportunity to facilitate the great works of the people of the BWH and to help to strengthen its foundations and build on the partnerships that allow it to deliver on its mission.

INTRODUCTION AND ACKNOWLEDGEMENTS

Peter V. Tishler

While leaving Medical Grand Rounds in the fall of 2010, Chief of Medicine Joseph Loscalzo asked me a question that ultimately directed my professional life. "We are approaching the 100th anniversary of the Brigham. Would you write a book on the history of our hospital?" I was surprised by this request, considered it for a few milliseconds, and then accepted it with enthusiasm. Since then, as we have enlisted the help of many Brigham staff and delved into the history and the workings of this hospital, I have been happy with this assignment. The Brigham is a truly wonderful hospital, and celebrating its birthday is an equally inspiring event.

I came to the Brigham in 1977, from the Harvard Medical Unit at the Boston City Hospital (BCH), where I trained in internal medicine and spent many research and clinical years. I did not arrive alone. Boston University had been officially awarded sole administrative and clinical responsibility for the BCH, and thus all members of the Harvard Medical Unit departed. One group, including the Channing Laboratory of which I was a member, affiliated with the Brigham. We were not the first BCHers to interact in a major way with the Brigham. Francis Weld Peabody, the first director of the Harvard Medical Unit at the BCH in the 1920s, was an early and charismatic leader at the new Brigham from its opening in 1913. Soma Weiss, a protégé of Peabody and a major medical innovator (I call him "the Osler of his day"), came from the BCH to the Brigham as the second physician-in-chief. He brought with him from the BCH innovative physicians, including Lewis Dexter, John Romano, Eugene A. Stead, Jr., and Charles A. Janeway, and hired Paul B. Beeson, my mentor and friend from medical school. All enriched the Brigham staff. Other physicians visited the Brigham periodically in a professional capacity, including BCH Chief of Neurology Derek E. Denny-Brown, who evaluated patients with neurological disease prior to the Brigham's initial hiring of full-time neurologists (Denny-Brown's trainees H. Richard Tyler and David M. Dawson). As a historian of the Harvard Medical Unit at the BCH, I was aware of the profound, formative Brigham activities of these individuals. In addition, my BCH friends, including physicians Martin A. Samuels in neurology and H. Franklin Bunn in hematology, were also ensconced at the Brigham when I arrived. Stimulated by these individuals, my personal interest and enthusiasm for the Brigham then and subsequently was and remains great. My being asked to chaperone a book about the hospital and its people was profoundly pleasing.

In the preparation of this book, I have had wonderful interactions with individuals who are universally revered. Eugene Braunwald has been characterized by many people as their major mentor and champion as they developed their leadership capabilities. The physicians who created independent departments from their former divisions in the Department of Medicine (Jonathan F. Borus in psychiatry, Thomas S. Kupper in dermatology, and Martin Samuels in neurology) expressed their gratitude to Braunwald in the highest of terms. Nicholas L. Tilney, a senior member of the Department of Surgery, exploited both his knowledge of the history of medicine and his very creative writing skills to provide so much for the book. Andrew G. Jessiman impressed many of us with his leadership in developing community outreach for the Brigham. Bernard Lown, a major innovator of care for Brigham patients with heart disease since 1950, parleyed his intense dedication to health and peace to form the Nobel Prize–winning Physicians for Social Responsibility and still writes regularly about the inequities of medicine and medical care. Marshall A. Wolf, an outstanding physician, is a leader in medical residency training and a personal mentor for many young people and associates at this institution. I must also mention two physicians among the many whom I did not know, Henry A. Christian and Harvey W. Cushing, by far the major leaders and innovators at the Brigham at its inception.

A group of dedicated, talented writers has taken charge of the preparation of this book. Joseph Loscalzo initiated this effort and is actively involved in its structure and input. Christine Wenc, the managing editor, has worked tirelessly to create the book and assist many individuals in their writing. Her dedication to this task has been invaluable. The stellar input of Scott H. Podolsky and Jeremy A. Greene, historians as well as physicians, is really a day's work for them. Joel T. Katz has led the medical residency training program at the Brigham for many years, and his writing is a reflection of the educational excellence that he has created. The assistance from Catherine M. Pate, the Brigham archivist, has been generous. I personally am indebted to her for her help as I write about the history of the Brigham.

This is a work of faith and dedication. I have been so happy to do it!

ACKNOWLEDGMENTS

Christine Wenc

Many people made invaluable contributions to this book. I first want to thank Cathy Pate, the Brigham and Women's Hospital (BWH) archivist, who worked innumerable hours on this project and fielded many questions. We are grateful for her knowledge and dedication. I also want to praise the work of our photo researcher/editor, Sarah Morris, for her superb research skills and knowledge of both the BWH archives and of digital photography. Sarah's amazing organizational abilities made the formidable task of image selection and processing possible. Ann Conway, whose work became known to me when I discovered her sociology PhD thesis on the early organization of the Peter Bent Brigham Hospital, took on the complex concept of "community" and made a major contribution to this book. Linda Smith transcribed a huge number of research and video interviews with efficiency and good humor, and probably knows more about the hospital than anyone now. David McCready gave wonderful advice and support throughout the project, and Lee Riley was my model manager. Peter Tishler provided his editorial expertise and impressive knowledge of the hospital at every turn. The other members of the BWH history book committee—Joseph Loscalzo, Jeremy Greene, Scott Podolsky, and Joel Katz—were also a pleasure to work with and made this project fascinating. It was deeply rewarding for me to collaborate with these physicians. I would also like to remember and recognize Nicholas L. Tilney, who generously contributed several essays to this book and advised with similar generosity on other chapters before his death in March 2013. He will be missed. Our editors at McGraw-Hill, Jim Shanahan and Regina Brown, were helpful and patient as we sorted out the components of this very large undertaking. On a personal note, I want to thank my family for their love, support, and patience as I made my way through a project that probably seemed to them would never end. I could not have done it without you. I hope that the result may be a valuable contribution to the history of twentieth and twenty-first-century medicine.

TIMELINE

1832-1912	
Boston Lying-In Hospital (BLI)	1832
Anesthesia in childbirth (BLI)	1847
Free Hospital for Women	1875
Antiseptic techniques (BLI)	1883

1913-1939	
Carrie M. Hall, Nursing Superintendent	1912
Peter Bent Brigham Hospital	1913
Henry A. Christian, Physician-in-Chief	1913
Harvey W. Cushing, Surgeon-in-Chief	1913
William T. Councilman, Pathologist-in-Chief	1913
Robert Breck Brigham Hospital (RBBH)	1914
Pernicious anemia treatment	1926
Elliott C. Cutler, Surgeon-in-Chief	1932
Nobel Prize in Medicine to G. Minot, W. Murphy	1934
25th reunion	1938
Soma Weiss, Physician-in-Chief	1939
Charles Janeway, John Romano, Eugene A. Stead arrive with Weiss	1939

1940-1959	
Albumin treatment of blood loss	1941
Sudden death of Soma Weiss	1942
George W. Thorn, Physician-in-Chief	1942
Blood bank	1942
Hemodialysis	1947
Francis D. Moore, Surgeon-in-Chief	1948
Human ovum fertilized in vitro	1944
Cortisone therapy	1949
First female Harvard Medical School graduate	1951
Veterans Administration affiliation	1953
Twin renal transplant	1954

1960-1969	
Surgical Intensive Care Unit	1960
Peritoneal dialysis	1960-1962
Clinical Research Center	1961
DC defibrillator	1962
Robert J. Glaser, President Affiliated Hospitals Center	1963-1965
Blood Center dedication	1963
Samuel A. Levine Coronary Care Unit	1963
50th reunion	1963
50th reunion history book	1963
K. Frank Austen, Physician-in-Chief, RBBH	1965
Death of Samuel A. Levine, MD	1966
Boston Hospital for Women (BHW)	1966
Harvard Community Health Plan	1969
Anesthesiology Department	1969

1970-1979	
Harvard-MIT Health Sciences and Technology affiliation	1970
Orthopedics Department	1971
Eugene Braunwald, Physician-in-Chief	1972
Fetal heart monitoring	1973
Brookside Park Family Life Center affiliation	1974
Affiliated Hospitals Center	1975
John A. Mannick, Surgeon-in-Chief	1976
Nurses' Health Study	1976
Channing Laboratory arrives	1977
Cyclosporin-A treatment of renal transplant patients	1979

1980-1989	
Renamed Brigham & Women's Hospital	1980
New building—Tower	1980
H. Richard Nesson, President	1982
First heart transplant in NE	1984
TIMI Study Group	1984
Joseph Loscalzo, Medical Chief Resident	1983-1984
Thorn Research Building	1984
Nobel Peace Prize to IPPNW, B. Lown	1985
PBBH Nursing School Closes	1985
Nesson Ambulatory Building	1986
Partners in Health	1987
75th anniversary/celebration	1989

1990-1999

Nobel Prize in Medicine to J. Murray	1990
First heart-lung transplant in MA	1992
Intraoperative magnetic resonance imaging	1994
Center for Women & Children	1994
Partners HealthCare	1994
Triple organ transplant	1995
Neurology Department	1995
Minimally invasive aortic surgery	1996
Dana-Farber Cancer Institute joins	1997
Jeffrey R. Otten, President	1997
Faulkner Hospital affiliation	1998
Psychiatry Department	1999

2000-2009

Quadruple organ transplant	2000
Dermatology Department	2000
Robotic pulmonary lobectomy	2000
Neurosurgery Department	2001
Radiation Therapy Department	2001
Gary L. Gottlieb, President	2002
Dual chamber ICD inserted	2004
Five lung transplants/36 hours	2004
Wrist replacement	~2004
Biomedical Research Institute	2005
500th heart transplant	2005
1,000th intraoperative MR-guided craniotomy for brain tumor	2006
Carl J. & Ruth Shapiro building	2008
Aqualine One 320 slice CT scanner	2008
Partial face transplant	2009

2010-2013

Elizabeth G. Nabel, President	2010
Response to Haitian earthquake	2010
Laying cornerstone, Mirebalais Hospital, Haiti	2010
Phyllis Jen Center dedicated	2010
Lung stem cells reported	2010
OurGenes, OurHealth, OurCommunity	2010
Advanced Multimodality Image Guided OR (AMIGO)	2011
Personalized Cancer Medicine Partnership of BWH, DFCI	2011
Full face transplant	2011
Bilateral hand transplant	2011
First Brigham Research Institute Research Day	2012
First temporary artificial heart implant in New England	2012
20 years on *US News and World Report* Honor Roll	2012

CONTRIBUTORS

Janet L. Abrahm, MD, Chief, Division of Adult Palliative Care, Brigham and Women's Hospital and Dana-Farber Cancer Institute; Professor of Medicine, Harvard Medical School

Ronald J. Anderson, MD, Division of Rheumatology, Immunology and Allergy, and former Director of Clinical Training Programs in Rheumatology, Department of Medicine, Brigham and Women's Hospital; Associate Professor of Medicine, Harvard Medical School

Stanley W. Ashley, MD, Chief Medical Officer, Brigham and Women's Hospital; Frank Sawyer Professor of Surgery, Harvard Medical School

K. Frank Austen, MD, Senior Physician, Division of Rheumatology, Immunology and Allergy, Department of Medicine, Brigham and Women's Hospital; AstraZeneca Professor of Respiratory and Inflammatory Diseases, Harvard Medical School

David W. Bates, MD, MSc, Senior Vice President for Quality and Safety, Chief Quality Officer, Brigham and Women's Hospital and Brigham and Women's Physicians Organization, Division of General Internal Medicine and Primary Care, Brigham and Women's Hospital; Professor of Medicine, Harvard Medical School; Professor of Health Policy and Management, Harvard School of Public Health

Margaret Bernazzani, BSN, RN, Department of Nursing, Brigham and Women's Hospital

Barbara E. Bierer, MD Professor of Medicine (Pediatrics) Harvard Medical School; Senior Vice President, Research, Department of Medicine, Brigham and Women's Hospital

Peter McL. Black, MD, PhD, Founding Chair, Department of Neurosurgery, Brigham and Women's Hospital; Franc D. Ingraham Professor of Neurosurgery, Harvard Medical School

Roger Blanza, BSN, RN, Department of Nursing, Brigham and Women's Hospital

J. Stephen Bohan, MD, MS, Director of Clinical Operations, Executive Vice Chair, Department of Emergency Medicine, Brigham and Women's Hospital; Assistant Professor of Medicine, Harvard Medical School

Joseph V. Bonventre, MD, PhD, Chief, Renal Division, Director, Health Science and Technology Center for Biomedical Engineering, and Co-Director, Stem Cell, Regenerative Medicine and Tissue Engineering Center, Brigham and Women's Hospital; Samuel A. Levine Professor of Medicine, Harvard Medical School

Eugene Braunwald, MD, Physician-in-Chief and Chair, Department of Medicine, Brigham and Women's Hospital, 1972-1996; Distinguished Hersey Professor of the Theory and Practice of Medicine, Harvard Medical School

Mark E. Brezinski, MD, PhD, Director of Center for Optical Coherence Tomography and Modern Physics, Department of Orthopedic Surgery, Brigham and Women's Hospital; Associate Professor of Orthopedics, Harvard Medical School

H. Franklin Bunn, MD, Physician, Brigham and Women's Hospital; Professor of Medicine, Harvard Medical School

David E. Clapham, MD, PhD, Aldo R. Castañeda Professor of Cardiovascular Research and Professor of Neurobiology, Harvard Medical School

Lawrence H. Cohn, MD, Division of Cardiac Surgery, Brigham and Women's Hospital; Hubbard Professor of Cardiac Surgery, Harvard Medical School

Ann Conway, PhD, medical sociologist, independent research and writing professional to health and nonprofit organizations, and former BWH archives director

David M. Dawson, MD, Physician, Department of Neurology, Brigham and Women's Hospital; Professor of Neurology, Harvard Medical School

James B. Dealy, Jr., MD, Chief, Department of Radiology, Brigham and Women's Hospital, 1957-1965; Associate Clinical Professor of Radiology, Harvard Medical School (deceased)

Daniel F. Dedrick, MD, Staff Anesthesiologist, Brigham and Women's Hospital; Assistant Professor of Anesthesia, Harvard Medical School

Kristin DeJohn, BA, Boston-based freelance writer and television producer; contributing writer for *Brigham and Women's Magazine*

Sukumar P. Desai, MD, MS, MBA, Staff Anesthesiologist, Brigham and Women's Hospital; Assistant Professor of Anesthesia, Harvard Medical School

Joseph L. Dorsey, MD, Emeritus Chief, Division of HVMA Medicine, Brigham and Women's Hospital; Clinical Professor of Medicine, Harvard Medical School

Division of Global Health Equity administrative staff, Brigham and Women's Hospital

Sasha Dubois, BSN, RN, Department of Nursing, Brigham and Women's Hospital

Patricia Dykes, RN, DNSc, Senior Nurse Scientist, Center for Nursing Excellence, Brigham and Women's Hospital

Arnold M. Epstein, MD, Division of General Internal Medicine, Brigham and Women's Hospital; Professor of Medicine and Health Care Policy, Harvard Medical School; John H. Foster Professor and Chair, Department of Health Policy and Management, Harvard School of Public Health

Mary Lou Etheredge, RN, MS, Executive Director Nursing Practice Development, Brigham and Women's Hospital

Maureen B. Fagan, DNP, Executive Director, Center for Patients and Families, Brigham and Women's Hospital

Jeffrey S. Flier, MD, Dean and Caroline Shields Walker Professor of Medicine, Harvard Medical School

John A. Fox, MD, Staff Anesthesiologist and Assistant Director of Cardiac Anesthesiology, Brigham and Women's Hospital; Assistant Professor of Anesthesia, Harvard Medical School

Lara Freidenfelds, PhD, independent historian of women's health, medicine and the body in America

Kathleen Gallivan, PhD, Director, Chaplaincy Services Department, Brigham and Women's Hospital

Tejal Gandhi, MD, Division of General Internal Medicine, Brigham and Women's Hospital; Associate Professor of Medicine, Harvard Medical School

Tina Gellsomino, MSW, LCSW, Administrative Director, Office for Women's Careers, Center for Faculty Development and Diversity, Brigham and Women's Hospital

Michael A. Gimbrone, Jr., MD, Emeritus Chair of Pathology, Brigham and Women's Hospital; Director, Center for Excellence in Vascular Biology, Brigham and Women's Hospital; Distinguished Ramzi S. Cotran Professor of Pathology, Harvard Medical School

Donald Peter Goldstein, MD, Senior Scientist and Attending Gynecologist, Division of Gynecologic Oncology, Department of Obstetrics and Gynecology, Brigham and Women's Hospital; Professor of Obstetrics, Gynecology and Reproductive Biology, Harvard Medical School

Gary L. Gottlieb, MD, MBA, President and Chief Executive Officer, Partners HealthCare System, Inc; Professor of Psychiatry, Harvard Medical School

Jeremy A. Greene, MD, PhD, Associate Professor, Elizabeth Treide and A. McGehee Harvey Professorship in the History of Medicine, Institute of the History of Medicine, The Johns Hopkins University

Robert I. Handin, MD, Division of Hematology, Brigham and Women's Hospital; Professor of Medicine, Harvard Medical School

James H. Herndon, MD, orthopaedic Surgeon, Brigham and Women's Hospital and Massachusetts General Hospital; Chair Emeritus, Partners Department of Orthopaedic Surgery; William H. and Johanna A. Harris Professor of Orthopaedic Surgery, Harvard Medical School

Susan R. Holman, PhD, Senior Writer, Harvard Global Health Institute; visiting adjunct faculty member, Episcopal Divinity School

Andrew G. Jessiman, MD, Vice-President, Professional Services, Brigham and Women's Hospital (retired); Lecturer in Medicine, Harvard Medical School (retired)

Ferenc A. Jolesz, MD, Director, Division of MRI and National Center for Image Guided Therapy, Brigham and Women's Hospital; B. Leonard Holman Professor of Radiology, Harvard Medical School

Elizabeth W. Karlson, MD, Director of Rheumatic Disease Epidemiology, and co-chair, Center for Human Genetics at the Biomedical Research Institute, Brigham and Women's Hospital; Associate Professor of Medicine, Harvard Medical School

Dennis L Kasper, MD Channing Professor of Medicine and Professor of Microbiology and Immunobiology Harvard Medical School

Amalie M. Kass, MEd, Lecturer in the History of Medicine, Harvard Medical School

Joel T. Katz, MD, Associate Physician and Director, Internal Medicine Residency Program, Brigham and Women's Hospital; Associate Professor of Medicine, Harvard Medical School

Marilyn Givens King, Associate Director, MSN programs, WellStar School of Nursing of the Kennesaw State University

Thomas S. Kupper, MD, Chair, Department of Dermatology, Brigham and Women's Hospital; Thomas B. Fitzpatrick Professor of Dermatology, Harvard Medical School

Edward R. Laws, Jr., MD, Director, Pituitary/Neuroendocrine Program, Department of Neurosurgery, Brigham and Women's Hospital; Professor of Surgery, Harvard Medical School

Thomas H. Lee, Jr., MD, Network President, Partners HealthCare System; Professor of Medicine, Harvard Medical School

Robert W. Lekowski, MD, MPH, Director of Residency Program, Department of Anesthesiology, Perioperative and Pain Medicine, Brigham and Women's Hospital. Assistant Professor of Anesthesia, Harvard Medical School

Peter Libby, MD, Chief, Cardiovascular Medicine, Brigham and Women's Hospital; Mallinckrodt Professor of Medicine, Harvard Medical School

Joseph Loscalzo, MD, PhD, Chairman, Department of Medicine, Physician-in-Chief, Brigham and Women's Hospital; Hersey Professor of the Theory and Practice of Physic, Harvard Medical School, Boston, Massachusetts

Bernard Lown, MD, Senior Physician Emeritus, Brigham and Women's Hospital; Professor, Harvard School of Public Health; Nobel Peace Prize Co-recipient, 1985

Kenneth Ludmerer, MD, Mabel Dorn Reeder Distinguished Professor in the History of Medicine, Washington University

Yilu Ma, MS, Director, Interpreter Services Department, Brigham and Women's Hospital

JoAnn E. Manson, MD, DrPH, Chief, Division of Preventive Medicine, Brigham and Women's Hospital; Professor of Medicine and the Michael and Lee Bell Professor of Women's Health, Harvard Medical School

Cara Marcus, MSLIS, Director of Library Services, Brigham and Women's Faulkner Hospital

Margaret Marsh PhD, Distinguished Professor of History and University Professor, Rutgers University

Ramon F. Martin, MD, PhD, Staff Anesthesiologist and Director, Out of OR Anesthesia, Brigham and Woman's Hospital; Assistant Professor of Anesthesia, Harvard Medical School

Nicole L. Mayard, MPH, Senior Research Assistant, OurGenes, OurHealth, OurCommunity Project at the Biomedical Research Institute, Brigham and Women's Hospital

Julie B. McCoy, BA, Senior Editor, Harvard Medical School

Thomas M. Michel, MD, PhD, Senior Physician in Cardiovascular Medicine, Brigham and Women's Hospital; Professor of Medicine and Biochemistry, Harvard Medical School

Andrew D. Miller, MD, Staff Anesthesiologist, Brigham and Women's Hospital; Instructor in Anesthesia, Harvard Medical School

Sarah Morris, AB, photo editor, *The Teaching Hospital*; independent researcher, editor, writer, and exhibit developer

Bryan Murphy, MD, Communications Specialist, Department of Radiology, Brigham and Women's Hospital

Elizabeth G. Nabel, MD, President, Brigham and Women's Hospital; Professor of Medicine, Harvard Medical School

Carol C. Nadelson, MD, Senior Advisor, Center for Faculty Development and Diversity, Brigham and Women's Hospital; Professor of Psychiatry, Harvard Medical School

Patrice Nicholas, RN, MPH, DNSc, Director, Global Health and Academic Partnerships, Center for Nursing Excellence, Brigham and Women's Hospital

Nawal Nour, MD, MPH, Director, Global Ob/Gyn and African Women's Health Center; Director, Ambulatory Obstetrics at BWH; Associate Professor, Harvard Medical School

Nicholas E. O'Connor, MD, Surgeon, Brigham and Women's Hospital; Assistant Professor of Surgery, Harvard Medical School

Scott Podolsky, MD, Associate Professor of Global Health and Social Medicine and Director of the Center for the History of Medicine, Countway Medical Library, Harvard Medical School

Curtis Prout, MD (deceased), Chief of Medicine and Associate Director at Harvard University Health Services (1961-1972); Physician, Brigham and Women's Hospital, (1947-2010); Assistant Dean for Student Affairs, Harvard Medical School

Martin A. Samuels, MD, Chair, Department of Neurology Brigham and Women's Hospital; Professor of Neurology, Harvard Medical School

Monica M. Sa Rego, MD, Clinical Director, Department of Anesthesiology, Perioperative and Pain Medicine, Brigham and Women's Hospital; Instructor in Anesthesia, Harvard Medical School

Arthur A. Sasahara, MD, Professor of Medicine Emeritus, Harvard Medical School; Senior Physician, Cardiovascular Medicine, Brigham and Women's Hospital

Paul E. Sax, MD, Clinical Director, Division of Infectious Diseases, Brigham and Women's Hospital; Professor of Medicine, Harvard Medical School

Frederick J. Schoen, MD, PhD, Executive Vice Chair, Department of Pathology, Brigham and Women's Hospital; Professor of Pathology and Health Sciences and Technology, Harvard Medical School

Christine E. Seidman, MD, Director, Cardiovascular Genetics Center, Brigham and Women's Hospital; Thomas W. Smith Professor of Medicine and Genetics, Harvard Medical School

Julian L. Seifter, MD, Renal Division, Brigham and Women's Hospital; Associate Professor of Medicine, Harvard Medical School

Steven E. Seltzer, MD, Chair, Department of Radiology, Brigham and Women's Hospital; Cook Professor of Radiology, Harvard Medical School

Lawrence N. Shulman, MD, Chief Medical Officer and Vice President for Medical Affairs, Dana-Farber Cancer Institute; Associate Professor of Medicine, Harvard Medical School

David A. Silbersweig, MD, Chair, Department of Psychiatry, Brigham and Women's Hospital; Stanley Cobb Professor of Psychiatry, Harvard Medical School

Bernice J. Sinclair, RN, (deceased) formerly Instructor in Nursing, Peter Bent Brigham Hospital School of Nursing

Jacqueline Slavik, PhD, Executive Director, Biomedical Research Institute, Brigham and Women's Hospital

Jackie Somerville, RN, PhD, Chief Nursing Officer and Senior Vice President for Patient Care Services, Brigham and Women's Hospital

Frank E. Speizer, MD, Channing Laboratory and Department of Medicine, Brigham and Women's Hospital; Edward H. Kass Distinguished Professor of Medicine, Harvard Medical School

Paul Thayer, DMin, Associate Professor of Education and Child Life; Chair, Department of Child Life and Family Studies, Wheelock College

Nicholas L. Tilney, MD, (deceased) Department of Surgery, Brigham and Women's Hospital; Francis D. Moore Distinguished Professor of Surgery, Harvard Medical School

Lori Wiviott Tishler, MD, Medical Director, Phyllis Jen Center for Primary Care, Brigham and Women's Hospital; Assistant Professor of Medicine, Harvard Medical School

Peter Tishler, MD, Physician, Department of Medicine and Genetics Division, Brigham and Women's Hospital; Associate Professor of Medicine, Harvard Medical School

Sigrid L. Tishler, MD, Physician, Brigham and Women's Hospital; Founding Physician, Oncology Department, Harvard Vanguard Medical Associates; Assistant Professor of Medicine, Harvard Medical School (retired)

Jerry S. Trier, MD, Division of Gastroenterology, Hepatology and Endoscopy, Brigham and Women's Hospital; Professor of Medicine emeritus, Harvard Medical School

Katherine Wai, BS, Research Assistant, Department of Emergency Medicine, Brigham and Women's Hospital

Christine Wenc, MA, AM, Editor, Department of Medicine, Brigham and Women's Hospital; managing editor, *The Teaching Hospital*. Editor, writer, and consultant for history of medicine, publishing and public history projects

Anthony D. Whittemore, MD, Chief Medical Officer, Emeritus, Brigham and Women's Hospital; Professor of Surgery, Harvard Medical School

Gordon H. Williams, MD, Director, Center of Clinical Investigation, Brigham and Women's Hospital; Professor of Medicine, Harvard Medical School

Saul E. Wisnia, BA, Senior Public Editor and Writer, Dana-Farber Cancer Institute

Michael J. Zinner, MD, Surgeon-in-Chief, Brigham and Women's Hospital; Clinical Director, Dana-Farber/Brigham and Women's Hospital Cancer Center; Mosley Professor of Surgery, Harvard Medical School

James E. Zuckerman, MD, Department of Obstetrics and Gynecology, Brigham and Women's Hospital; Assistant Clinical Professor, Department of Obstetrics, Gynecology and Reproductive Biology, Harvard Medical School

DEPARTMENT CHAIRS, 1913–2012

ANESTHESIOLOGY, PERIOPERATIVE AND PAIN MEDICINE

William S. Derrick, 1947-1954 (Div Chf)
Leroy D. Vandam, 1954-1970 (Div Chf)
Lleroy D. Vandam, 1970-1979
Benjamin G. Covino, 1979-1991
Gerald W. Ostheimer, 1991 (acting)
Simon Gelman, 1992-2002
Charles A. Vacanti, 2002-

DERMATOLOGY

Harley A. Haynes, 1976-1998 (Div Chf)
Thomas S. Kupper, 1998-2000 (Div Chf)
Thomas S. Kupper, 2000-

EMERGENCY MEDICINE

Ron M. Walls, 1994-

MEDICINE

Henry A. Christian, 1913-1938
Soma Weiss, 1939-1942
George W. Thorn, 1942-1972
Eugene Braunwald, 1972-1996
Victor J. Dzau, 1996-2004
Joseph Loscalzo, 2005-

NEONATOLOGY/NEWBORN MEDICINE

H. William Taeusch, 1974-1981
Barry T. Smith, 1981-1986
Michael F. Epstein, 1986-1989 (acting)
Merton R. Bernfield, 1989-1998
Steven A. Ringer, 1998-2004 (dir nb med)*
Steven A. Ringer, 2004- *

(*overall Chair, Newborn Medicine, HMS (inc. BWH) Gary Silverman (1998-2003), Stella Kourembanas (2004-)

NEUROLOGY

H. Richard Tyler, 1956-1988 (Div Chf)
Martin A. Samuels, 1988-1995 (Div Chf)
Martin A. Samuels, 1995-

NEUROSURGERY

Harvey Cushing, 1913-1932 (Chair, Surgery)
Franc D. Ingraham, 1944-1965 (Div Chf)
Donald D. Matson, 1965-1968 (Div Chf)
John Shillitro Jr., 1968-1971 (Acting Div Chf)
Keasley Welch, 1971-1987 (Div Chf)
Peter M. Black, 1987-2001 (Div Chf)
Peter M. Black, 2001-2006
Arthur Day, 2007-2009
A. John Popp, 2009-2012
E. Antonio Chiocca, 2012-

OBSTETRICS AND GYNECOLOGY

Kenneth J. Ryan, 1973-1993
Robert L. Barbieri, 1993-

ORTHOPEDIC SURGERY

Clement Sledge, 1971-1996
Thomas S. Thornhill, 1997-

PATHOLOGY

William T. Councilman, 1912-1916
S. Burt Wolbach, 1916-1947
Alan R. Moritz, 1947-1949
Samuel P. Hicks, 1950-1951
Clinton Van Z. Hawn, 1951-1952
Gustave J. Dammin, 1952-1972
Ramzi S. Cotran, 1972
Michael A. Gimbrone, 2001-2011
Jeffrey A. Golden, 2012-

PSYCHIATRY

Peter Reich (Div Chf)
Jonathan F. Borus, 1990-1999 (Div Chf)
Jonathan F. Borus, 1999-2008
David A. Silbersweig, 2008-

RADIATION THERAPY/ONCOLOGY

Samuel Hellman, 1968-1983
C. Norman Coleman, 1985-1999 (Dir., JCRT; Div Chf)
Jay Harris, 1999-2001 (Div. Chf)
Jay Harris, 2001-

RADIOLOGY

Lawrence Reynolds, 1919-1920
Merrill C. Sosman, 1922-1956
James B. Dealy, 1956-1957 (acting)
James B. Dealy, 1957-1965
Lloyd Hawes, 1965-1967 (acting)
Herbert L. Abrams, 1967-1984
David C Levin, 1985-1986 (acting)
B. Leonard Holman, 1986-1988 (acting)
B. Leonard Holman, 1988-1997
Steven Seltzer, 1997-

SURGERY

Harvey Cushing, 1912-1932
Elliott C. Cutler, 1932-1947
Francis D. Moore, 1948-1976
John A. Mannick, 1976-1994
Michael J. Zinner, 1994-

EXECUTIVE MANAGERS, 1908-2012

SUPERINTENDENT

Herbert B. Howard, MD, 1908-1919
Joseph B. Howland, MD, 1919-1938
Norbert A. Wilhelm, MD, 1938-1943

DIRECTORS

Norbert A. Wilhelm, MD, 1944-1957
Victoria M. Cass, MD, 1957 (acting)
F. Lloyd Mussells, MD, 1958-1967
William E. Hassan, Jr, PhD, 1967-1977

EXECUTIVE VICE PRESIDENT/CHIEF OPERATING OFFICER

William E. Hassan, Jr. PhD, 1977-1983
L. James Wiczai, ?1981-1989
Elaine R. Smith, 1990-
Jeffry R. Otten, 1993-1997, Chief Executive Officer
Kate Walsh, MPH, 2004-2010
Mairead Hickey, RN, PhD, 2010-

HONORS AND AWARDS

Nobel Prize Recipients

George R. Minot, William P. Murphy	1934	IPPNW: Bernard Lown, Herbert L. Abrams, James E. Muller	1985
Baruj Benacerraf	1980	Joseph E. Murray, E. Donnall Thomas	1990

MacArthur Fellows

Atul Gawande	2006	Vamsi Mootha	2004
Jim Y. Kim	2003	Nawal M. Nour	2003
Paul E. Farmer	1993		

Member, National Academy of Sciences

Deceased

William T. Councilman	1854-1933	Ruth Sager	1918-1997
Otto Folin	1867–1934	Bert L. Vallee	1919-2010
Harvey W. Cushing	1869-1939	Joseph E. Murray	1919-2012
Hans Zinsser	1878-1940	Baruj Benacerraf	1920-2011
George R. Minot	1885-1950	E. Donnell Thomas	1920-2012
Francis G. Blake	1887-1952	Donald S. Fredrickson	1924-2002
Robert E. Gross	1905-1988	Eva J. Neer	1937-2000
Paul B. Beeson	1908-2006	Bernard N. Fields	1938-1995
Edwin B. Astwood	1909-1976	Steven C. Hebert	1946-2008

Living

Irving M. London	1971	Richard P. Lifton	2001
K. Frank Austen	1974	Bruce M. Spiegelman	2002
Eugene Braunwald	1974	Laurie H. Glimcher	2002
Stuart F. Schlossman	1992	Christine E. Seidman	2005
Elliot D. Kieff	1996	Michael B. Brenner	2007
Thomas P. Stossel	1997	Jonathan G. Seidman	2007
Michael A. Gimbrone	1997	William G. Kaelin	2010
		Donald E. Ganem	2010

Single date = date of appointment; dual dates = dates of birth and death. This list may not be complete.

Members, Institute of Medicine, National Academy of Sciences

Name	Date Elected	Name	Date Elected
Paul B. Beeson	1970†	Kenneth J. Ryan	1971
Eugene A. Stead	1970†	Jack D. Myers	1977†
James V. Warren	1971†	Eugene Braunwald	1974
Howard H. Hiatt	1971	Arnold S. Relman	1978

Name	Date Elected
Curtis Prout	1980†
Herbert Abrams	1980
Daniel D. Federman	1981
John Romano	1982†
Baruj Benacerraf	1982†
Barbara J. McNeil	1982
George L. Engel	1983†
S. James Adelstein	1985
Edward H. Kass	1986†
Ramzi S. Cotran	1986†
Samuel Hellman	1987
Steven A. Rosenberg	1987
Bernard Lown	1988
Bernard N. Fields	1988†
David G. Nathan	1989
David M. Livingston	1990
K. Frank Austen	1991
Clement B. Sledge	1992
Stuart F. Schlossman	1993
Francis D. Moore	1993†
Glenn D. Steele	1993
Joseph E. Murray	1994†
Ferenc A. Jolesz	1995
Murray F. Brennan	1995
Merton R. Bernfield	1996†
Risa Lavisso-Mourey	1997
Jonathan M. Samet	1997
Eva J. Neer	1998†
Edward J. Benz, Jr	1998
Laurie H. Glimcher	1998
Thomas P. Stossel	1998
Walter C. Willett	1998
Victor J. Dzau	1998
Elizabeth G. Nabel	1998
Michael A. Gimbrone	1999
Christine E. Seidman	1999
Robert A. Greenes	1999

Name	Date Elected
David Ginsburg	1999
Arnold M. Epstein	2000
Frank E. Speizer	2000
Elliott D. Kieff	2001
Dennis L. Kasper	2001
Craig B. Thompson	2002
Richard P. Lifton	2002
Donald E. Ganem	2003
Paul E. Farmer	2003
Jeffrey S. Flier	2003
Jeffrey M. Drazen	2003
Jim Y. Kim	2004
Timothy J. Eberlein	2004
Ronald A. DePinho	2004
Edward R. Laws, Jr.	2004
Troyen A. Brennan	2005
David W. Bates	2005
Dennis J. Selkoe	2005
Mitchell A. Lazar	2006
Joseph Loscalzo	2006
Graham A. Colditz	2006
Elazer R. Edelman	2006
Christopher J. L. Murray	2007
William G. Kaelin	2007
Jonathan G. Seidman	2007
Emery N. Brown	2007
Gary H. Gibbons	2007
Raju S. Kucherlapati	2008
Kenneth C. Anderson	2010
Charles A. Czeisler	2010
John Z. Ayanian	2010
Nancy Berliner	2010
Gary L. Gottlieb	2010
George E. Thibault	2010
Karen H. Antman	2011
JoAnn E. Manson	2011
Atul Gawande	2011
Andrew L. Schafer	2012

(† = deceased)
This list may not be complete. Any omissions are the fault of the editors.

PRESIDENTS, PETER BENT BRIGHAM HOSPITAL, AFFILIATED HOSPITALS CENTER, BRIGHAM AND WOMEN'S HOSPITAL, 1902-2012

Peter Bent Brigham Hospital		Affiliated Hospitals Center		Brigham and Women's Hospital	
Alexander Cochrane	1902-1915				
Charles P. Curtis	1915-1936				
Walter Hunnewell Pro tem	1917-1918				
William Amory	1936-1942				
Charles S. Pierce	1942-1949				
Robert Cutler	1949-1955				
Charles B. Barnes	1955-1962				
Alan Steinert	1962-1969	Robert J. Glaser	1963-1965		
Sims McGrath	1969-1972/3	F. Stanton Deland Jr.	1966-1977		
Alan Steinert Jr	1973-1978				
		F. Stanton Deland Jr.	1977-1979		
		Robert G. Petersdorf	1979-1981	H. Richard Nesson	1982-1997
				Jeffrey R. Otten	1997-2002
				Gary Gottlieb	2002-2010
				Elizabeth Nabel	2010-

CREDITS

Title page image
David J. Goldberg

Chapter 1
Figure 1-0, Brigham and Women's Hospital Archives; Figure 1-1, History of the Brigham Family by W. I. Tyler Brigham: Grafton Press, New York, 1907. Page 296; Figure 1-2, Harvard Medical Library in the Francis A. Countway Library of Medicine; Figure 1-3, City of Boston Archives; Figure 1-4, Harvard Medical Library in the Francis A. Countway Library of Medicine; Figure 1-5, Brigham and Women's Hospital Archives; Figure 1-6, Brigham and Women's Hospital Archives; Figure 1-7, Brigham and Women's Hospital Archives; Figure 1-8, Brigham and Women's Hospital Archives; Figure 1-9, Brigham and Women's Hospital Archives; Figure 1-10, Harvard Medical Library in the Francis A. Countway Library of Medicine; Figure 1-11, Brigham and Women's Hospital Archives; Figure 1-12, Harvard Medical Library in the Francis A. Countway Library of Medicine; Figure 1-13, Brigham and Women's Hospital Archives; Figure 1-14, Yale University, Harvey Cushing/John Hay Whitney Medical Library; Figure 1-15, Brigham and Women's Hospital Archives; Figure 1-16, Brigham and Women's Hospital Archives, photo by Russell B. Harding; Figure 1-17, McGraw-Hill Education; Figure 1-18, Brigham and Women's Hospital Archives; Figure 1-19, Harvard Medical Library in the Francis A. Countway Library of Medicine; Figure 1-20, Brigham and Women's Hospital Archives; Figure 1-21, Yousuf Karash; Figure 1-22, Brigham and Women's Hospital Archives; Figure 1-23, Brigham and Women's Hospital Archives; Figure 1-24, From *Time Magazine*, May 3, 1963. (C) 1963 Time Inc. Used under license.; Figure 1-25, Brigham and Women's Hospital Archives; Figure 1-26, Brigham and Women's Hospital Archives; Figure 1-27, Brigham and Women's Hospital Archives; Figure 1-28, Brigham and Women's Hospital Archives; Figure 1-29, Brigham and Women's Hospital Archives; Figure 1-30, Bertrand Goldberg Archive, Ryerson and Burnham Archives, The Art Institute of Chicago; Figure 1-31, Brigham and Women's Hospital Archive, photo by Daniel Bernstein Photography; Figure 1-32, Brigham and Women's Hospital Archives; Figure 1-33, Brigham and Women's Hospital; Figure 1-34, Brigham and Women's Hospital Archives; Figure 1-35, Brigham and Women's Hospital Archives; Figure 1-36, Brigham and Women's Hospital Archives; Figure 1-37, Brigham and Women's Hospital Archives; Figure 1-38, Brigham and Women's Hospital; Figure 1-39, Mainframe Photographics, Inc.; Figure 1-40, Courtesy of Joseph Loscalzo, MD PhD.

Chapter 2
Figure 2-0, Brigham and Women's Hospital; Figure 2-1, Harvard University Archives, HUP Eliot, Charles W. (38b); Figure 2-2, Harvard Medical Library in the Francis A. Countway Library of Medicine; Figure 2-3, Yale University, Harvey Cushing/ John Hay Whitney Medical Library; Figure 2-4, Brigham and Women's Hospital Archives; Figure 2-5, *The Medical World;* IC 77; John P. McGovern Historical Collections and Research Center, Houston Academy of Medicine-Texas Medical Center Library; Figure 2-6, Brigham and Women's Hospital Archives; Figure 2-7, Brigham and Women's Hospital Archives; Figure 2-8, Brigham and Women's Hospital Archives; Figure 2-9, Courtesy Trustees of the Boston Public Library; Figure 2-10, Brigham and Women's Hospital Archives; Figure 2-11, Brigham and Women's

Hospital Archives; Figure 2-12, Brigham and Women's Hospital Archives; Figure 2-13, Bradford F. Herzog; Figure 2-14, Brigham and Women's Hospital Archives; Figure 2-15, Brigham and Women's Hospital; Figure 2-16, Brigham and Women's Hospital Archives; Figure 2-17, Brigham and Women's Hospital Archives; Figure 2-18, Stu Rosner; Figure 2-19, Brigham and Women's Hospital; Figure 2-20, Tony Rinaldo; Figure 2-21, Brigham and Women's Hospital Archives; Figure 2-22, Brigham and Women's Hospital, photo by Russell B. Harding; Figure 2-23, Brigham and Women's Hospital Archives; Figure 2-24, Harvard Medical Library in the Francis A. Countway Library of Medicine.

Chapter 3

Figure 3-0, Brigham and Women's Hospital Archives; Figure 3-1, Brigham and Women's Hospital Archives; Figure 3-2, Brigham and Women's Hospital Archives, photo by John E. Withee; Figure 3-3, FrankSiteman.com; Figure 3-4, FrankSiteman.com; Figure 3-5, Stu Rosner; Figure 3-6, Brigham and Women's Hospital; Figure 3-7, Brigham and Women's Hospital Archives; Figure 3-8, Harvard Medical Library in the Francis A. Countway Library of Medicine, photo by Barbara Steiner; Figure 3-9, Brigham and Women's Hospital; Figure 3-10, AP Photo/Mike Kullen; Figure 3-11, Brigham and Women's Hospital Archives; Figure 3-12, Brigham and Women's Hospital Archives; Figure 3-13, Bradford F. Herzog; Figure 3-14, Jason Grow; Figure 3-15, Harvard Medical Library in the Francis A. Countway Library of Medicine; Figure 3-16, Harvard Medical Library in the Francis A. Countway Library of Medicine; Figure 3-17, Brigham and Women's Hospital Archives; Figure 3-18, Brigham and Women's Hospital Archives; Figure 3-19, Courtesy of Jodi Hartley; Figure 3-20, Bradford F. Herzog; Figure 3-21, Lightchaser Photography; Figure 3-22, LarryMaglott.com; Figure 3-23, Edward G. Miner Library, University of Rochester Medical Center; Figure 3-24, Brigham and Women's Hospital; Figure 3-25, Tilney, Nicolas L., MD. *A Perfectly Striking Departure: Surgeons and Surgery At The Peter Bent Brigham Hospital 1912-1980* . Sagamore Beach, MA: Science History Publications/USA, 2006; 128.; Figure 3-26, Photo Researchers, Inc.; Figure 3-27, Minot GR, Cohn EJ, Murphy WP, Lawson HA. "Treatment of pernicious anemia with liver extract: effects upon the production of immature and mature red blood cells." *American Journal of the Medical Sciences,*1928;175:599-621.; Figure 3-28, Brigham and Women's Hospital Archives, photo by Daniel Bernstein; Figure 3-29, Brigham and Women's Hospital; Figure 3-30, Brigham and Women's Hospital; Figure 3-31, Lee Pellegrini, Boston College; Figure 3-32, Brigham and Women's Hospital Archives; Figure 3-33, FrankSiteman.com; Figure 3-34, LarryMaglott.com; Figure 3-35, Mark Ostow; Figure 3-36, Brigham and Women's Hospital Archive; Figure 3-37, Brigham and Women's Hospital Archive, photo by George Miles Ryan Studio; Figure 3-38, Tilney, Nicolas L., MD. *A Perfectly Striking Departure: Surgeons And Surgery At The Peter Bent Brigham Hospital 1912-1980*. Sagamore Beach, MA: Science History Publications/USA, 2006; 206.; Figure 3-39, LarryMaglott.com; Figure 3-40, Brigham and Women's Hospital, photo by Mark Genero, PA-C; Figure 3-41, Ted Polumbaum/Newseum collection; Figure 3-42, Yale University, Harvey Cushing/John Hay Whitney Medical Library; Figure 3-43, Brigham and Women's Hospital Archives; Figure 3-44, Harvard Medical Library in the Francis A. Countway Library of Medicine, photo by White Star IDP; Figure 3-45, Steven C. Borack.

Chapter 4

Figure 4-0, Brigham and Women's Hospital Archives; Figure 4-1, Brigham and Women's Hospital Archives; Figure 4-2, Brigham and Women's Hospital Archives; Figure 4-3, Brigham and Women's Hospital; Figure 4-4, Brigham and Women's Hospital; Figure 4-5, Brigham and Women's Hospital Archives; Figure 4-6, Brigham and Women's Hospital; Figure 4-7, Harvard Medical Library in the Francis A. Countway Library of Medicine, photo by Bradford F. Herzog; Figure 4-8, Brigham and Women's Hospital; Figure 4-9, Brigham and Women's Hospital; Figure 4-10, Brigham and Women's Hospital Archives; Figure 4-11, Getty Images, photo taken by Hansel Mieth for *Life* (March 13, 1939); Figure 4-12, Brigham and Women's Hospital Archives; Figure 4-13, Brigham and Women's Hospital Archives; Figure 4-14, Brigham and Women's Hospital Archives; Figure 4-15,

Brigham and Women's Hospital Archives; Figure 4-16, McCardinal Photo; Figure 4-17, Bradford F. Herzog; Figure 4-18, Kirkwood, Samuel B., and Madelen Pollock. "Health During Pregnancy." Boston: Department of Child Hygiene, Harvard School of Public Health and Boston Lying-In Hospital, 1941.; Figure 4-19, Jeffrey A. Michael; Figure 4-20, Lightchaser Photography; Figure 4-21, Harvard Medical Library in the Francis A. Countway Library of Medicine; Figure 4-22, Brigham and Women's Hospital.

Chapter 5

Figure 5-0, Brigham and Women's Hospital Archives; Figure 5-1, McCardinal Photo; Figure 5-2, McCardinal Photo; Figure 5-3, Harvard Medical Library in the Francis A. Countway Library of Medicine; Figure 5-4, Fay Foto; Figure 5-5, Getty Images, photo taken by Hansel Mieth for *Life* (March 13, 1939); Figure 5-6, Brigham and Women's Hospital; Figure 5-7, LarryMaglott.com; Figure 5-8, John Gillooly for Boston College; Figure 5-9, Brigham and Women's Hospital; Figure 5-10, Courtesy of Christian Arbelaez, MD, MPH; Figure 5-11, LarryMaglott.com; Figure 5-12, Susan R. Symonds for Infinity Portrait Design, Mainframe Photographics, Inc.; Figure 5-13, Brigham and Women's Hospital; Figure 5-14, Brigham and Women's Hospital, Department of Nutrition; Figure 5-15, Brigham and Women's Hospital Archives; Figure 5-16, Brigham and Women's Hospital Chaplaincy, photo by Laurie Bittman; Figure 5-17, Brigham and Women's Hospital; Figure 5-18, McCardinal Photo; Figure 5-19, McCardinal Photo; Figure 5-20, Lightchaser Photography; Figure 5-21, Brigham and Women's Hospital Archives; Figure 5-22, Brigham and Women's Hospital Archives; Figure 5-23, McCardinal Photo; Figure 5-24, McCardinal Photo; Figure 5-25, Sam Ogden, Dana-Farber Cancer Institute; Figure 5-26, Mainframe Photographics, Inc.; Figure 5-27, Brigham and Women's Hospital Archives; Figure 5-28, McCardinal Photo; Figure 5-29, Lightchaser Photography; Figure 5-30, McCardinal Photo.

Chapter 6

Figure 6-0, David J. Goldberg; Figure 6-1, LarryMaglott.com; Figure 6-2, Brigham and Women's Hospital Archives; Figure 6-3, Courtesy Trustees of the Boston Public Library; Figure 6-4, "Walter Channing" by Joseph Alexander Ames.; Figure 6-5, "An Irish family coming off a boat, being greeted by a young couple" by Winslow Homer. Originally published in *Ballou's Pictorial and Drawing Room Companion*, 1857. Reprinted with permission from Schlesinger Library, Radcliffe Institute, Harvard University; Figure 6-6, Brigham and Women's Hospital Archives; Figure 6-7, Brigham and Women's Hospital Archives; Figure 6-8, Brigham and Women's Hospital Archives; Figure 6-9, Brigham and Women's Hospital Archives; Figure 6-10, Brigham and Women's Hospital Archives; Figure 6-11, *History of the Brigham Family* by W. I. Tyler Brigham: Grafton Press, New York, 1907. Page 402.; Figure 6-12, Unknown, "Elizabeth Fay Brigham." Photo by Mainframe Photographics, Inc.; Figure 6-13, Brigham and Women's Hospital Archives; Figure 6-14, Brigham and Women's Hospital Archives; Figure 6-15, Franklin Hospital Archives, photo courtesy of Jonathan Hubbard; Figure 6-16, Franklin Hospital Archives; Figure 6-17, David J. Goldberg; Figure 6-18, LarryMaglott.com; Figure 6-19, Courtesy Trustees of the Boston Public Library; Figure 6-20, Courtesy Trustees of the Boston Public Library; Figure 6-21, Courtesy Trustees of the Boston Public Library; Figure 6-22, Brigham and Women's Hospital Archives; Figure 6-23, Brigham and Women's Hospital Archives; Figure 6-24, Brigham and Women's Hospital Archives; Figure 6-25, Brigham and Women's Hospital Archives; Figure 6-26, Brigham and Women's Hospital Archives; Figure 6-27, Brigham and Women's Hospital Archives; Figure 6-28, Brigham and Women's Hospital Archives, photo by Jim Phelan; Figure 6-29, Harvard Medical Library in the Francis A. Countway Library of Medicine; Figure 6-30, Photo by Alfred Brown. Originally published in the *Harvard Alumni Bulletin* Volume 44 April 25, 1942 Number 13, page 447.; Figure 6-31, Brigham and Women's Hospital Archives; Figure 6-32, Brigham and Women's Hospital Archives; Figure 6-33, Courtesy *Cocheco Times* (Weirs, NH); Figure 6-34, Brigham and Women's Hospital Archives; Figure 6-35, Brigham and Women's Hospital Archives; Figure 6-36, Brigham and Women's Hospital Archives; Figure 6-37, LarryMaglott.com;

Figure 6-38, Brigham and Women's Hospital; Figure 6-39, Brigham and Women's Hospital Archives; Figure 6-40, LarryMaglott.com; Figure 6-41, Brigham and Women's Hospital Archives, photo by Melvin F. Hookailo; Figure 6-42, Jeff Thiebauth; Figure 6-43, Lightchaser Photography; Figure 6-44, LarryMaglott.com; Figure 6-45, McCardinal Photo; Figure 6-46, Brigham and Women's Hospital; Figure 6-47, Brigham and Women's Hospital; Figure 6-48, Bradford F. Herzog; Figure 6-49, Dana-Farber Cancer Institute; Figure 6-50, Sam Ogden, Dana-Farber Cancer Institute; Figure 6-51, Sam Ogden, Dana-Farber Cancer Institute; Figure 6-52, Justin Ide/Harvard University; Figure 6-53, Brigham and Women's Hospital; Figure 6-54, Mark Ostow; Figure 6-55, Mark Rosenberg for Partners In Health; Figure 6-56, Justin Ide/Harvard University; Figure 6-57, Mark Rosenberg for Partners In Health; Figure 6-58, LarryMaglott.com.

THE TEACHING HOSPITAL

BRIGHAM AND WOMEN'S
Faulkner Hospital

CHAPTER 1

THE TEACHING HOSPITAL

THE TEACHING HOSPITAL

Jeremy A. Greene and Scott H. Podalsky

Histories of Brigham and Women's Hospital generally begin with Peter Bent Brigham himself, restauranteur, real estate developer, and opponent of slavery.[1] Brigham never saw the hospital; he died in 1877 at the age of seventy, bequeathing a legacy "for the purpose of founding a hospital in said Boston, to be called the Brigham Hospital, for the care of sick persons in indigent circumstances, residing in the said County of Suffolk."[2]

The hospital described by Brigham's bequest was rather generic: many hospitals in the late nineteenth century were charitable institutions for the suffering poor.[3] Yet Brigham's bequest would become activated at a moment of educational reform both at Harvard and in American medicine more broadly. In time, the founding of the Peter Bent Brigham Hospital (PBBH) and its subsequent development would embody the aspirations, triumphs, and challenges involved in the evolution of the academic medical hospital in twentieth and twenty-first century American medicine.

American medical education for the majority of the nineteenth century was generally a sorry affair and had very little to do with hospitals. As late as 1900, an American physician might complete training and licensing and set up practice without ever setting foot in a hospital. Medical schools were for-profit affairs, with teachers and institutions given strong incentive to pass their paying students and award their diplomas after attendance at a series of lectures, with minimal emphasis on clinical instruction.[4] These "diploma mills," which flooded the marketplace with poorly trained practitioners, had become widespread by the end of the nineteenth century. For-profit hospitals, in turn, had by the last quarter

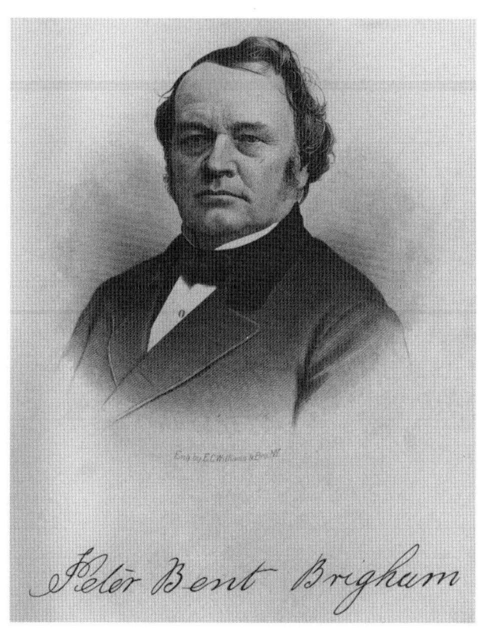

FIGURE 1-1 Portrait of Peter Bent Brigham.

of the nineteenth century likewise begun to proliferate across the country in the wake of the advent of aseptic surgery and the ability to attract paying patients.[5]

How did the modern teaching hospital emerge from the chaos of the late nineteenth century? The answer most often given is the publication of a book: Abraham Flexner's report on *Medical Education in the United States and Canada*, released three years prior to the opening of the PBBH. Indeed, the publication of Flexner's report was a pivotal event, which rechanneled extensive funding from the Rockefeller and Carnegie Foundations toward a standardized vision of medical education that revolved around the teaching hospital. Flexner emphasized learning by doing, rather than learning via rote didactic lectures and memorization.[6] He called for the elimination of the "proprietary" schools and for replacing them with university-affiliated—and hospital-affiliated—medical schools ensuring education from qualified, full-time teachers who instructed their students in the ongoing process of experimentation and calculated reasoning.

Flexner's report, however, did not single-handedly create new spaces for medical education. The modern teaching hospital was built not on ideals alone but also on bricks and mortar, emerging at the intersection of institutional inertia and reforming vision, of hard-nosed pragmatism and philanthropic virtue. When its doors opened just three years after Flexner's report, the Peter Bent Brigham Hospital represented one of the first physical artifacts of a Flexnerian view of medical education: an academic teaching hospital, built precisely for the conjoined purposes of clinical care, biomedical research, and medical education, its doors facing the community of Roxbury on one side and the newly built marble edifices of Harvard Medical School on the other. The history of the Brigham—from conception, to realization, to reconception over the twentieth and twenty-first centuries—documents the challenges of creating and maintaining spaces for academic medicine to flourish. In the following pages, we sketch out—using the *Annual Reports* of the hospital alongside other archival and periodical materials—the challenges entailed in building and maintaining these spaces of clinical care, research, and learning.

IMAGINING THE TEACHING HOSPITAL

As historians of medicine such as Ken Ludmerer and Thomas Neville Bonner have demonstrated, the Flexner report was not so much a revolutionary document as it was the culmination and consolidation of four decades of educational reform.[7] Harvard Medical School (HMS), from the time of University President Charles Eliot's efforts beginning in 1869 onward, had served at the forefront of such reform, mandating an expanded (eventually four-year) curriculum and rigorous preclinical laboratory training. Such efforts, however, were overshadowed after the Johns Hopkins School of Medicine opened in 1893 as an explicit and self-conscious experiment to emulate German medicine with a co-affiliated hospital, medical school, and university to form what has been referred to as the country's "first modern medical school."[8] The medical school at Johns Hopkins opened only *after* a dedicated teaching hospital had been built and would be led by such luminaries as William Osler, William Welch, William Halsted, Howard Kelly, and Franklin Mall, recruited to Baltimore from far and wide to realize a school built on the highest principles possible.[9]

HMS, in contrast, was forced to confront an existing, and highly decentralized, hospital system, whose principal institutions—Massachusetts General Hospital (MGH), McLean Hospital, Boston City Hospital, and Children's Hospital, among them—had been founded independently of any unified academic mission. Yet a few reformers at HMS saw an opportunity in the Brigham bequest to realize closer connections between the medical school and an affiliated hospital of its own. By the 1890s, the school had seemingly outgrown its small physical plant on Boylston Street, and such leaders at HMS as physiologist Henry Bowditch and surgeon J.C. ("Coll") Warren began to plan for a relocation to the Longwood Area, with knowledge of the Brigham bequest in hand.[10]

The formation of the HMS Longwood medical quadrangle required significant bequests from J.P. Morgan and John D. Rockefeller. Rockefeller had sent his personal lawyer, Starr Murphy, to "make a thorough inquiry and report" of HMS in 1901, before Rockefeller would consider such a donation.[11] Murphy's report is telling of contemporary aspirations and anticipates Flexner's general differentiation of the envisioned elite medical schools from the proprietary schools:

> *Medical teaching must be carried on in large establishments. So long as the old method obtained, of teaching by lectures, with only a very little laboratory work, it was possible to establish a medical school almost anywhere, and on an independent basis, as the medical schools of the earlier days were money-making concerns. This, however, was a bad thing for the country, as these schools were able to give degrees, and resulted in turning out a vast horde of wretchedly educated practitioners. The improved method will tend in a large measure to do away with this abuse, as the small schools can no longer furnish the instruction which modern methods require.*[12]

The creation of a *new space for clinical education*—the dedicated teaching hospital—would be key to Harvard's claim to be able to provide a superior environment for medical education. As Murphy continued, Harvard's leaders "hope to be able to erect a hospital which will be so nearly affiliated with the Medical School as to give the officers of the School the power to make appointments to the hospital."[13] Although Murphy noted that relations with MGH and other hospitals already provided extensive "clinical material" to HMS's students, he concluded that the best clinical teachers from afar would only be recruited to a dedicated teaching hospital. "[I]f the plans of the Medical School can be carried out in their entirety, and if the alliance with the hospital can be secured," he concluded, "it will make one of the finest plants for medical education in the world."[14]

As the funding poured in and the marble quadrangle of HMS was erected, however, the ongoing lack of this dedicated teaching hospital became a continued source of irritation and concern. In 1906, pathologist Frank B. Mallory, speaking before the Harvard Medical Alumni Association in the wake of the opening of

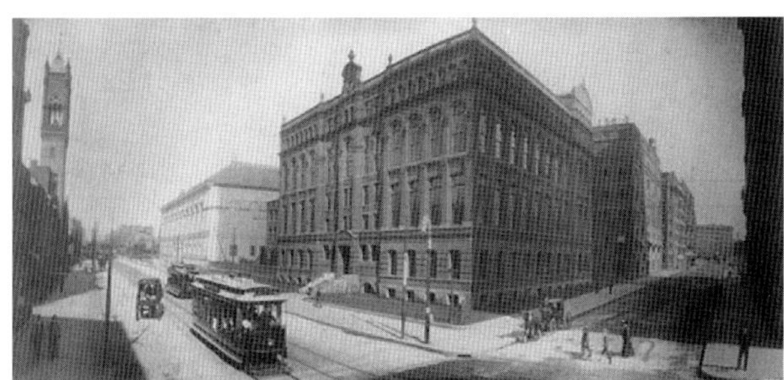

FIGURE 1-2 Harvard Medical School, 1883-1906.

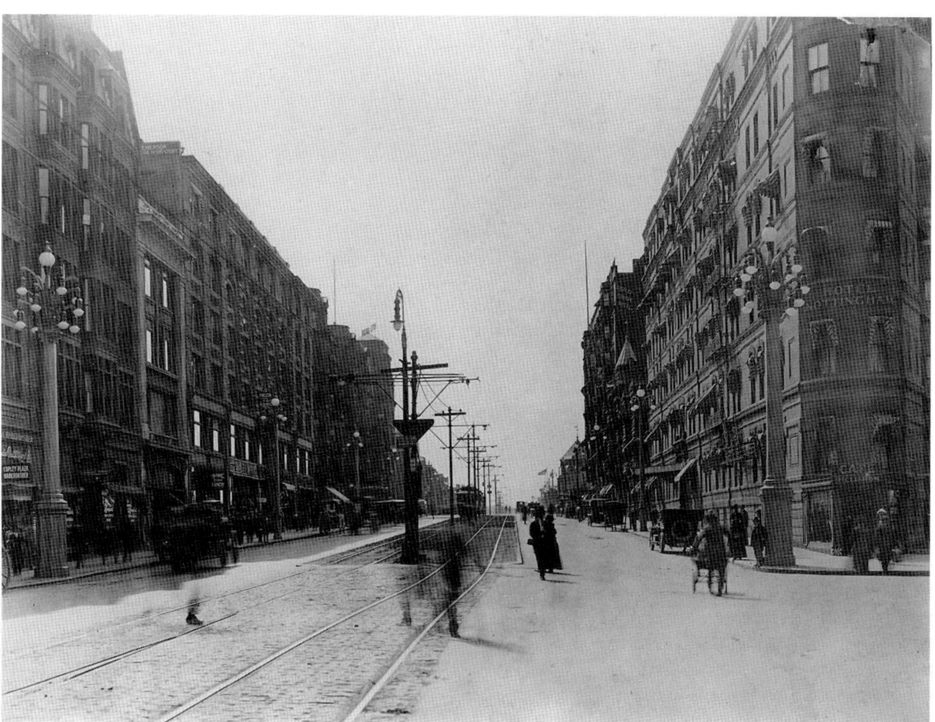

FIGURE 1-3 Huntington Avenue, circa 1910.

the "spacious and well-lighted laboratories" of the Longwood campus, reminded his audience that the primary function of the medical school was still to turn out well-trained clinicians, and that this could not be assured if HMS did not control appointments at the hospitals at which its students trained. Anxiously, he warned his fellow alumni:

If the Harvard Medical School does not adopt some such policy it will not be able to hold a leading position in this country like the other departments of the university, but will remain a local institution, and we shall continue to hear, as often in the past, the fatal excuse of expediency instead of commanding ability urged in behalf of a clinical man's appointment.[15]

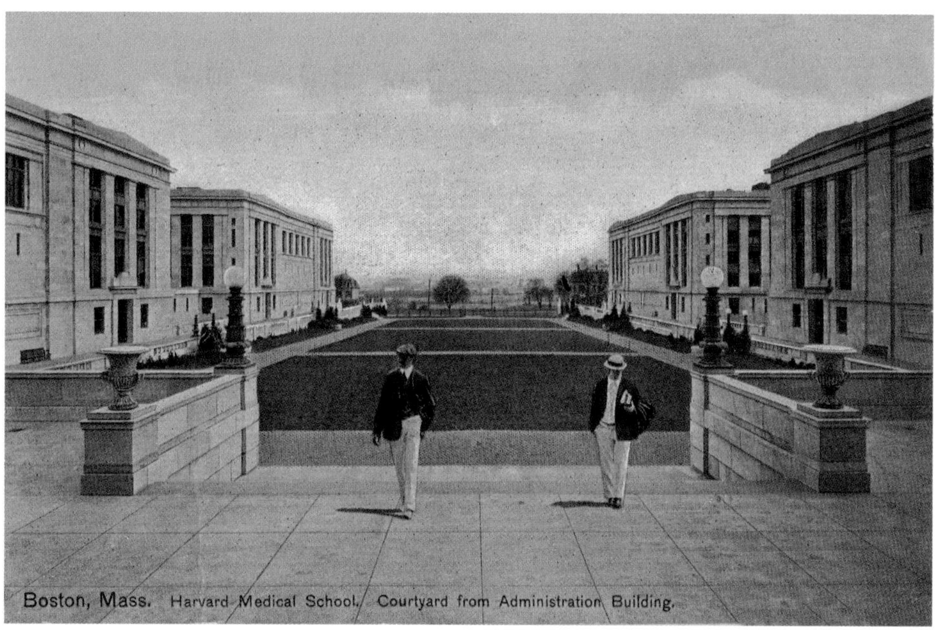

FIGURE 1-4 Vintage postcard of the new Harvard Medical School campus built in 1906.

The editors of the *Boston Medical and Surgical Journal* echoed such a view, hoping that "a university hospital will rise to adorn the knoll back of the new administrative building and furnish such facilities for clinical teaching" within the next five years. "Then and only then," they echoed, "can the active competition of the other medical schools of the country be actively met."[16]

By 1910, such ideas concerning the relationship between the medical school and hospital would be further buttressed by the publication of Flexner's report on *Medical Education in the United States and Canada*. And although Flexner's report is remembered most for its examination of the preclinical years of medical training, he devoted two entire chapters of the report to the relationship between the hospital and the medical school during the third and fourth years of education. Describing the equal applicability of the scientific method to both the preclinical and clinical years, Flexner remarked that "the practicing physician and the 'theoretical' scientist are thus engaged in doing the same sort of thing, even while one is seeking to correct Mr. Smith's digestive aberration and the other to localize the cerebral functions of the frog."[17] The hypothetical Mr. Smith was not to be "corrected" by the student in the trial-and-error world of the poorly supervised apprenticeship—let alone by that student-turned-physician once unleashed upon the medical marketplace—but rather under the watchful eyes of more senior teachers selected for their demonstrated excellence as clinical educators.

For teaching hospitals to be able to provide such worthy teachers, rather than be subjected to the vagaries of chance regarding whether an established hospital physician was actually an effective educator, teaching hospital appointments had to be under the control of the medical school (if not the larger university) itself. HMS, Flexner admitted (echoing Murphy), did not lack for "clinical material" amidst the preponderance of Boston hospitals; but like other medical schools in Boston, Chicago, and New York, its inability to control such appointments was "alike fatal to freedom and continuity of pedagogic policy."[18]

When the Brigham bequest was freed for use the following year, the titular members of the Brigham Corporation likewise felt that their envisioned hospital should be linked to the medical school, although the relationship was cemented by a "gentleman's agreement" rather than a "formal contract."[19] Despite such distinctly Boston flavoring, the founders of the PBBH

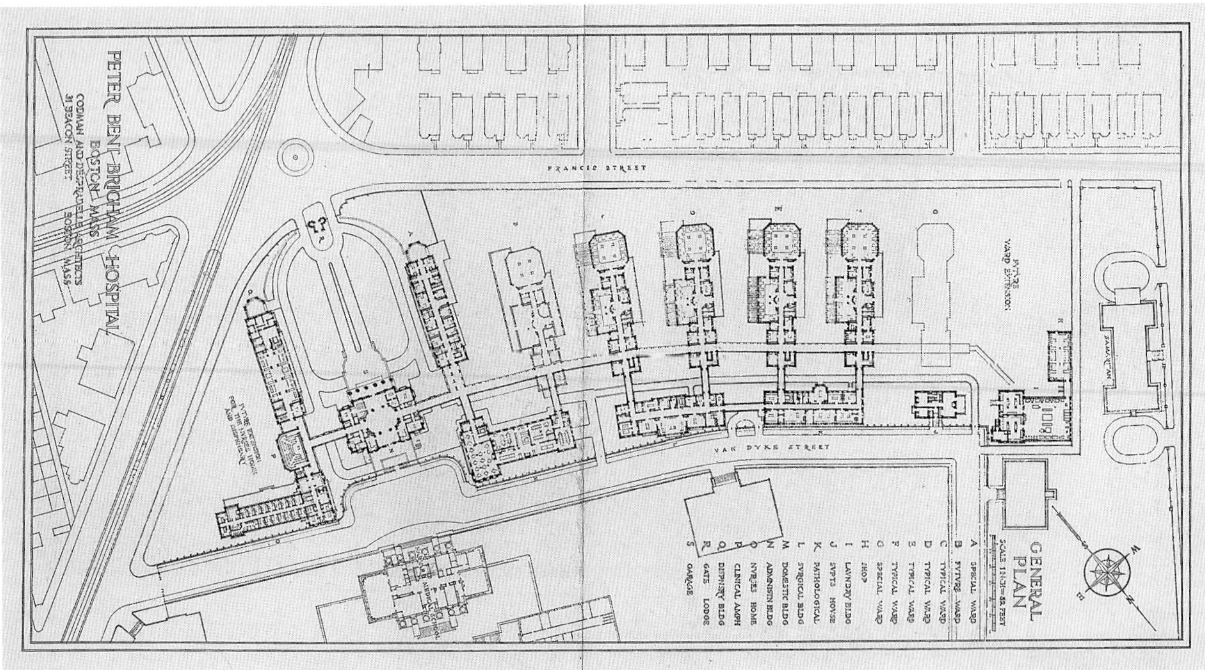

FIGURE 1-5 Peter Bent Brigham Hospital Campus Plan, circa 1914.

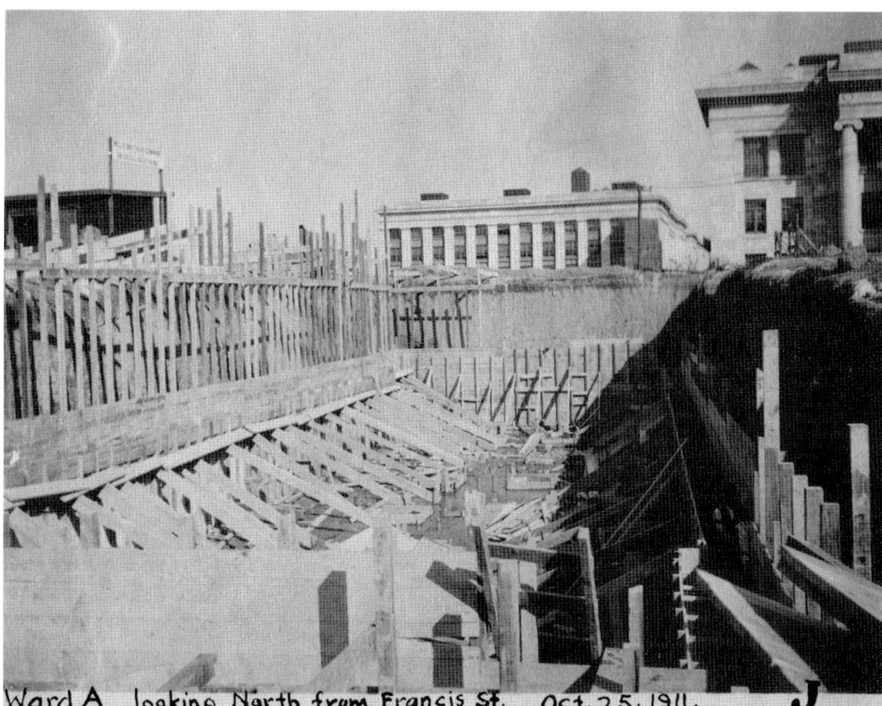

FIGURE 1-6 The construction of Ward A, with Harvard Medical School in the background.

looked to the Johns Hopkins University Hospital as a model, both materially and conceptually. The physician polymath John Shaw Billings, who had designed the Johns Hopkins Hospital (as well as the New York Public Library), was called in to help with the design of the PBBH.[20] The Brigham would be built on the "pavilion" model favored at Hopkins, attempting to maximize the surface area and ventilation available to every patient. Indeed, fifteen years after its opening, it would be said of the Brigham: "Perhaps no hospital in America has had more study and thought put into it than has this institution, and the plan is worthy of much study. Under the guidance of the superintendent, H.B. Howard, the architects and engineers have developed a comprehensive plan which gives the patient every advantage of open air, sunlight, and quick and quiet service."[21] To adapt the Hopkins model to the more severe turns of New England weather, a roof was put over the pathway connecting the pavilions (which would later become known as "the Pike").

Many personal trajectories connected the young PBBH to the Johns Hopkins Hospital as well. As Morris Vogel has related, pathologist William Councilman, who had come to Harvard from Johns Hopkins in 1892,

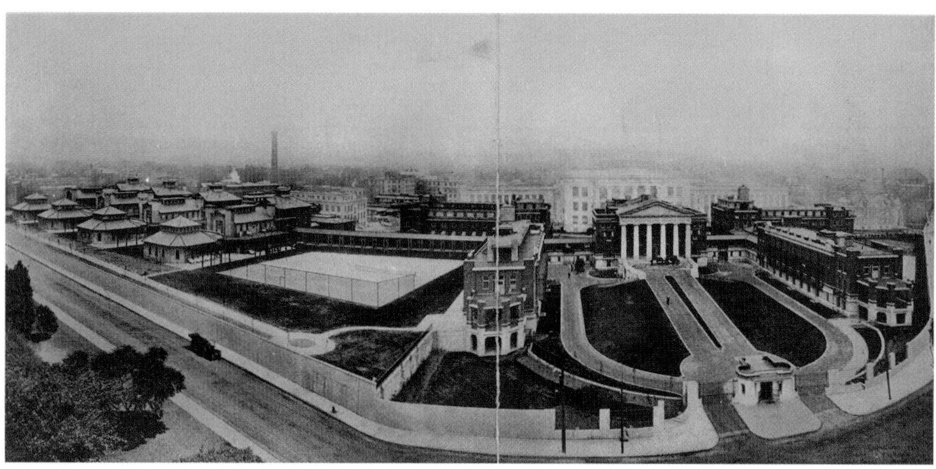

FIGURE 1-7 PBBH campus, circa 1914.

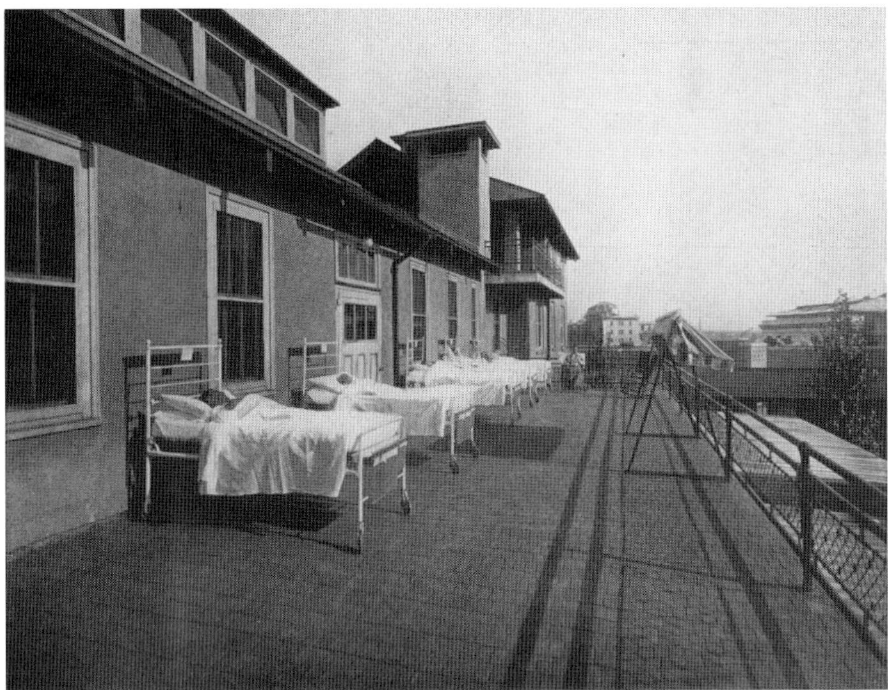

FIGURE 1-8 Pavilion C Terrace, circa 1914.

was instrumental in recruiting to HMS the clinical and pedagogical architects of the Brigham system—founding Physician-in-Chief Henry Christian and founding Surgeon-in-Chief Harvey Cushing—who had both spent formative years at Johns Hopkins under the mentorship of such luminaries as Halsted, Osler, and Welch.[22]

Christian and his first "Resident Physician," Francis Peabody, as well as Channing Frothingham, Reginald

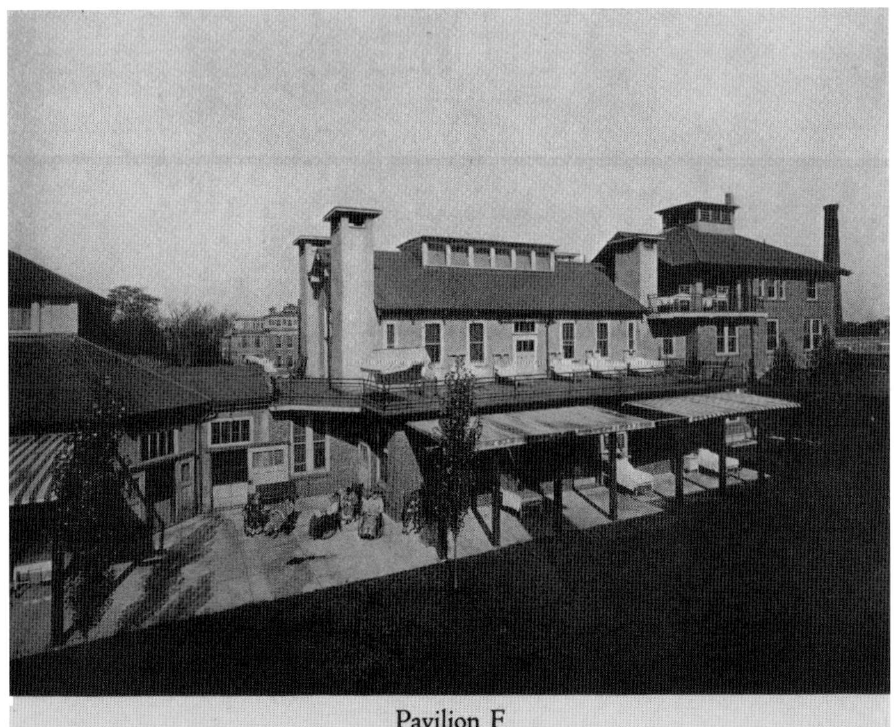

FIGURE 1-9 Pavilion F, circa 1914.

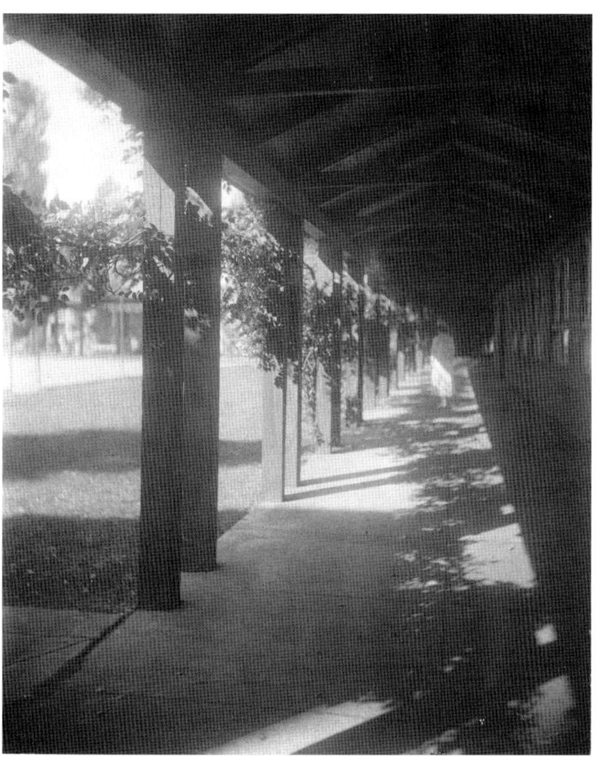

FIGURE 1-10 Nurse on the open-air Pike, circa 1930s.

Fitz, and I. Chandler Walker also attempted to look beyond Baltimore for models by taking an extensive tour of European hospitals and clinics during the summer of 1912. They ranged from Edinburgh (where they commented on the "spirit of cooperation amongst the various physicians") to Hamburg (where they noted that the chief internist insisted on performing his own thoracic surgical procedures), from Naples to St. Petersburg, and seemingly everywhere in between.[23] Returning, the spirit of Johns Hopkins continued to infuse the young hospital. Sir William Osler delivered an impromptu address within months of the hospital's admission of its first patients in early 1913, remarking on the tripartite role of the hospital in providing patient care, clinical research, and medical education.[24] William Welch delivered the official Founders' Day address a year later, speaking of a place "where students actually become a part of the working force of the ward and perform such duties as the taking of histories and examining the blood and secretions, which have to be done in any case—becoming, as Osler has expressed it, a part of the working machinery of the hospital itself."[25]

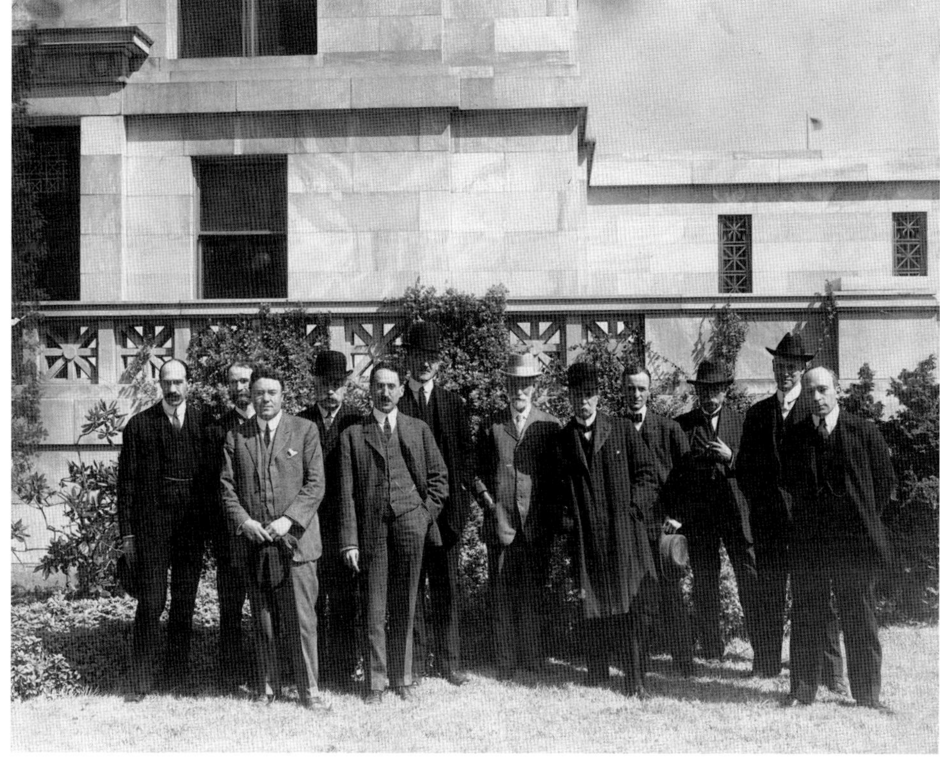

FIGURE 1-11 Sir William Osler visits the Peter Bent Brigham Hospital, April 30, 1913. Photographed against the west wall of the Harvard Medical School administration building (now Gordon Hall). From left to right: John Bremer, Theobald Smith, Walter Cannon, J. Collins Warren, Milton Rosenau, David Edsall, Charles S. Minot, William Osler, Harvey Cushing, William T. Councilman, Henry Christian, S. Burt Wolbach.

BIOGRAPHY

HENRY A. CHRISTIAN, 1876-1951

Peter V. Tishler

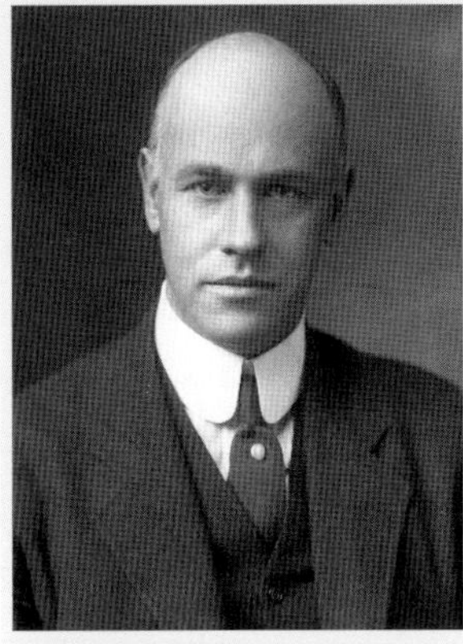

FIGURE 1-12 Henry Christian.

Henry Christian began his mission at the Peter Bent Brigham Hospital in 1908 as a thirty-two-year-old "Boy Dean" and Hersey Professor of the Theory and Practice of Physic at Harvard Medical School (HMS), during which he spent much of his administrative time designing the hospital, supervising its construction, and creating the rules and regulations for the full-time paid Brigham medical staff. When the new Brigham was nearly ready for patients, in 1912, he left the deanship to become physician-in-chief. This was his calling until his retirement in 1939.

What Henry Christian did in his tenure as Chief was extraordinary. He implemented a clinical clerkship for students at HMS, based on an elective program at the Massachusetts General Hospital and clerkships established by William Osler at Johns Hopkins, Christian's alma mater. The Brigham clerkship was the first obligatory clerkship in Boston, implying that its proximity to HMS made the Brigham the major Harvard teaching hospital. He created a housestaff training program, the forerunner of modern-day residency programs, and he hired Francis Weld Peabody, also a legend, as his first medical chief resident to run the program. One of his outstanding teaching innovations was the creation of the annual visiting physician-in-chief *pro tempore*, an event that is just as exciting today as it was in 1913. He insisted that the study of the patient's illness be meticulous and that staff and students "observe, record, tabulate, communicate." He brought about close collaboration between the wards and the laboratories, mandating that much of the laboratory work be done by the house officers. As a clinical caregiver and researcher, Henry Christian was a generalist. His research and clinical investigation, primarily descriptive in nature, established the details and natural histories of varied syndromes, some of which bear his name. He encouraged members of his staff to observe and care for patients in either the "outdoor clinic," which he created, or on the wards, and also employed clinician scientists, such as Peabody, who began the studies of normal physiology and the pathophysiology of disease.

Henry Christian's human qualities were also exemplary. He had a long, mentoring correspondence with a local African-American physician, advising him on training and job opportunities in Massachusetts. In a letter about Soma Weiss to Harvard President James Bryant Conant in 1938, Henry admitted, "I was prejudiced against him in his early days in Boston [the late 1920s and early 1930s] on the basis of his nationality and religious persuasion. When I had the opportunity to know him well and see him often, I realized that my prejudice was unreasonable . . . A few years ago I went to him, told him of my early prejudice, [and] stated that I had misjudged him . . . I told him that he had won my admiration, respect and esteem . . . I will welcome him as my successor with great enthusiasm and cordiality."[26]

Hundreds of letters from trainees and associates are uniformly reverent. Typically, the writers addressed Henry and his wife Elizabeth as "Uncle Henry and Aunt Bessie," and they were lavish in their affection for Henry. Herrman L. Blumgart, a former Brigham House Officer in Medicine, wrote, in 1935,

> *I have had few greater satisfactions than your continued interest and confidence in me throughout the years, and I appreciate more than I can possibly say your kindness and generosity of spirit.*[27]

Maurice A. Schnitker, also a former house officer, expressed his feelings to his former boss in many letters, including one in 1938:

> *I shall bend every effort through the remainder of my life to carry on the very highest standards, and to help to promote those principles, in your name, that you have taught me. I can truthfully say that my seven years at the Brigham have been the happiest years of my life.*[28]

Truly his logical, lively approach to problems, his clinical astuteness, his preoccupation with the educational process, his scholarliness, his kindliness, and his affection for people combined to make Henry Christian one of the master physicians of his time.[29]

BUILDING THE TEACHING HOSPITAL

On January 27, 1913, the hospital admitted its first surgical patient, Mary Agnes Turner, for varicose vein surgery that would keep her at the hospital for ten days.[30] On March 31, 1913, the hospital admitted its first medical patient, with a "renal hypernephroma" that "necessitated his subsequent transfer to the surgical service for a nephrectomy."[31] Things picked up quickly, however. In its first 21 months, the medical service would admit 2,110 patients, with the 438 "readmissions" for salvarsan administration for syphilis the leading inpatient diagnosis, 26 patients admitted with neurasthenia, 14 with hysteria, 1 with "hysterical" hiccoughs, and 20 with pernicious anemia.[32] The surgical service would admit 2,284 patients, with bread-and-butter tonsillectomies and inguinal hernia repairs barely outpacing Cushing's specialized procedures for the treatment of trigeminal neuralgia.[33] Over its first three decades, the hospital and its leaders would redefine the interrelatedness of Sir William Osler's stated tripartite functions. With respect to patient care, the PBBH praised efficiency but remained suspicious of the pursuit of efficiency as its own virtue, criticizing "hospitals in which patients, with the least possible loss of time, properly ticketed and labeled, are shot between admission and discharge, all the principles of piece-work and the labor-saving devices known to Armour and Co. and the Ford automobile factory meanwhile being employed."[34] In this respect, Francis Peabody, whose 1927 lecture *The Care of the Patient* famously concluded that "the secret of the care of the patient is in caring for the patient"—had seemingly set the tone.[35] As Christian reflected, in the wake of Peabody's premature death in 1927: "The early patients received his considerate care; to him they were human fellowships; his attitude towards patients established for us a tradition that is often expressed by our patients in saying everybody at the Brigham is interested in us and so friendly."[36]

At the same time, Christian continued, Peabody's "attitude towards investigation was critical and thoroughly scientific. In other words, from those early days on with patients, he was a physician, a counselor, and friend, with investigation a scientist, coolly critical."[37] And for Christian, Peabody, and their colleagues, such approaches were to be complementary, rather than mutually exclusive. As Christian related in 1922:

> *There is a curious feeling extant that a hospital in which scientific work is going on is one in which the human element is largely left out. This is a feeling very contrary to the fact. The more diligently a disease is studied and the greater the interest in the patient suffering it, the more eager becomes the physician to be able to help the patient.*[38]

The PBBH would be the site of remarkable clinical investigation during its first decades, including

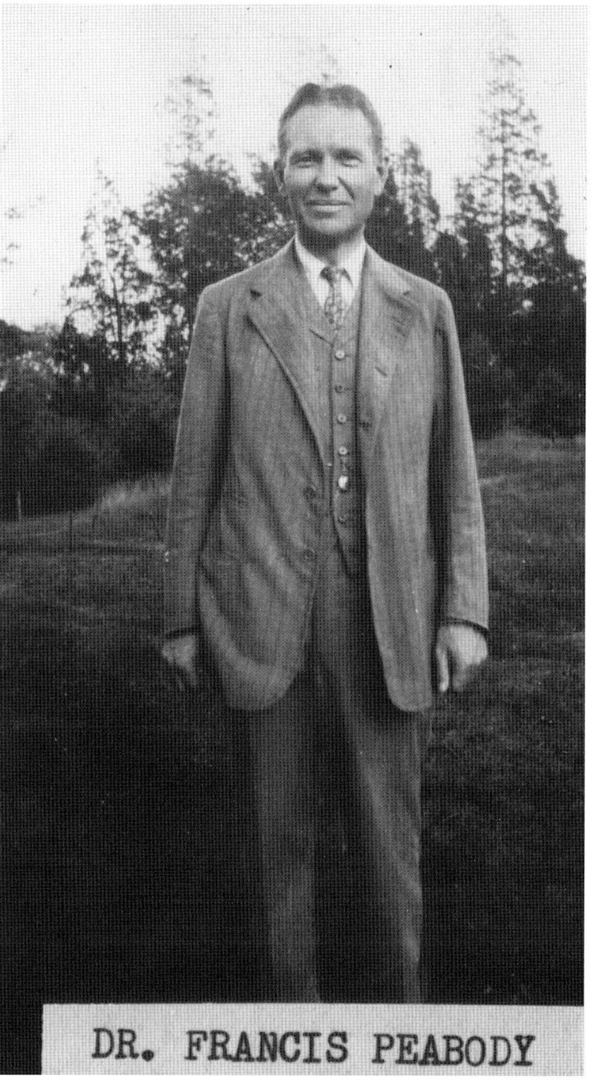

FIGURE 1-13 Francis Peabody.

the testing of liver extract for pernicious anemia (of which Peter Bent Brigham himself is thought to have died), for which George R. Minot and William Murphy would garner the Nobel Prize in Medicine or Physiology in 1934. By 1938, Christian could report that 1,029 papers had been produced over the first quarter-century of investigation by the PBBH's department of medicine, with, for instance, "cardiac infarction . . . the subject of numerous studies, some of which have been influential in increasing the early and more general recognition of this highly important heart disease on the part of practitioners."[39]

Education, finally, remained fundamental to both the mission and structure of the hospital. Harvey Cushing united patient care with his own endocrinological and neurosurgical research, but also emphasized the special character that "the elbow-to-elbow teaching of medical students in the wards, outpatient departments and autopsy rooms" imparted on the organization of hospital life and the nature of medical education.[40] Cushing claimed a direct correlation between the Brigham's evolution and HMS's rise from a provincial to a national institution; in 1901-1902, 93% of the school's students had hailed from New England; by 1924-1925, this figure had been reduced to 35%.[41]

Nevertheless, the construction and maintenance of the specialized geography of the teaching hospital was not without friction, constraint, or "growing pains." The PBBH would be justly famed for being "small and compact and intimate" and for having fostered close relationships among its various departments.[42] Yet, the self-reflective reports of Christian, Cushing, and Chief of Radiology Merrill Sosman—clearly written with an eye to both contemporary audiences *and* posterity—represent an ongoing lament of the need for increasing funding, coordination, staff, space, and laboratories. As the medical housestaff and nurses sang in 1938 at the Brigham's Silver Anniversary play, "Growing Pains, or 'You Can't Run the Brigham Without Any Dough' ":

Some people know it's an easy affair
To make the Brig. go, from a front office chair
You just issue orders with a wave of the hand,
And soak all the boarders as much as you can.
But no matter how fast, no matter how slow,
You can't run the Brigham without any dough.[43]

BIOGRAPHY

HARVEY W. CUSHING (1869-1939) AND THE FOUNDING OF NEUROSURGERY

Peter McL. Black

When the Peter Bent Brigham Hospital was being built in 1911, there was no question regarding who President Eliot of Harvard University wanted to be as its first surgeon-in-chief and Moseley Professor of Surgery. Harvey Williams Cushing, born on April 8, 1869, in Cleveland, Ohio, had attended Yale University and then Harvard Medical School, completed his surgical internship at Massachusetts General Hospital, and trained in general surgery at the Johns Hopkins Hospital in Baltimore. In 1912, he was recruited to the Brigham, President Eliot's great achievement. From then until 1932, he virtually created the field of modern neurosurgery and made the Peter Bent Brigham the leading surgical center in the world. Michael Bliss, a recent biographer, claims that he reversed almost single-handedly the dominance of Europe in international surgery. Previously, aspiring young surgeons typically spent time visiting centers "on the continent." By the end of Cushing's time at the Brigham, the opposite was the rule—aspiring surgeons from around the world visited him to learn. With his good friend, Sir William Osler, he defined the model of the medical academic that has persisted in the United States and world for the last century. He was a quadruple medical threat—surgeon, scientist, teacher, and administrator. He was also an artist and book collector.

As a surgeon, he devoted himself primarily to brain tumor surgery, doing more than 2,000 brain tumor operations during his tenure at the Brigham. His monographs on meningiomas, pituitary tumors, vestibular schwannomas, hemangioblastomas, and general outcomes in brain tumor surgery are classics even today. His meticulous surgical technique involved gentle handling of tissue and careful hemostasis. He showed that brain surgery was feasible, reducing surgical mortality from 80% to 8% and the infection rate to 0.3%.[44] His contributions to neurosurgery included staged surgery for large tumors, closure of the galea to prevent cerebral herniation, safe approach to the posterior fossa, the transsphenoidal approach for pituitary tumors, the first use of electrocautery, and the use of radiographic imaging to guide neurosurgical procedures.[45,46] His operations were carefully documented by his own sketches. His hospital records included visual field tests, letters of referral and follow-up, pathological results, and other relevant data. He cared deeply about his patients, frequently establishing close personal relationships with them. As a result of his careful follow-up, he could write definitive volumes on the diseases he treated.

As a scientist, he made major contributions to neuroscience and neuropathology. Among his accomplishments, he described many phenomena: the Cushing reflex, whereby high intracranial pressure leads to slowing of pulse; Cushing disease, a clinical condition associated "basophil adenomas of the pituitary body and their clinical manifestations"[47]; with Lewis Weed, the circulation of cerebrospinal fluid; glioma classification, based on embryology; and the natural history and treatment of meningiomas. He created a comprehensive tissue bank and registry, with microscopic sections and original specimens of most of the brain tumors on which he operated and follow-up reports on patients' quality of life and survival. Cushing was a prolific contributor to the scientific literature, including more than 300 publications and 13 books related to neurosurgery. His biography of Sir William Osler won the Pulitzer Prize in 1926.

Cushing was an inspiring teacher. He convinced his secretary Louise Eisenhardt to attend medical school; she became not only a major associate but the first editor of the *Journal of Neurosurgery*. Physicians worldwide trained with him at the Brigham, many becoming world-famous neurosurgeons: for example, Franc D. Ingraham, the founder of pediatric neurosurgery and first neurosurgeon-in-chief at the Children's Hospital; Kenneth McKenzie and Wilder Penfield of Canada; Norman Dott and Jeffrey Jefferson of Scotland and England, respectively; Sir Hugh Cairns from Australia; and Dmitri Bagdasar of Romania.

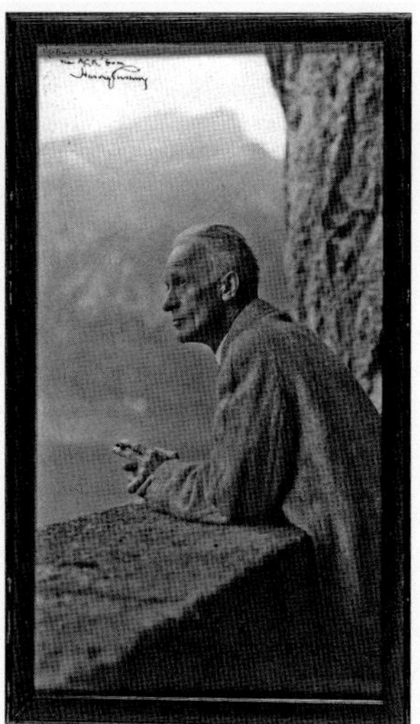

FIGURE 1-14 Harvey Cushing.

Finally, again defining the successful academic surgeon, Cushing encouraged cooperation in neurosurgery on both national and international levels. He promoted establishing neurosurgical societies in which neurosurgeons could meet regularly and learn from each other's successes and failures. He was a member and president of many medical and surgical societies. The Harvey Cushing Society (which later became the American Association of Neurological Surgeons) was founded in his honor. In 1927, he received both an honorary fellowship in the Royal Society of Medicine and membership in the Society of British Neurological Surgeons. He received honorary degrees from various universities, including Harvard, Yale, Oxford, and Cambridge.

Sadly, the Peter Bent Brigham Hospital and Harvard did not treat Cushing well on his retirement in 1932. He returned to Yale University, appointed as the Sterling Professor of Neurology. In addition to his medical career, he founded the Historical Library at the Yale Medical Library with his extensive collection of historic medical books and manuscripts. The Historical Library, which was named for him, has been a beautiful and comfortable environment for generations of students and researchers.

Cushing died on October 7, 1939. During his lifetime, he had been honored and recognized as the founder of neurosurgery, as well as an inspiring teacher and a compassionate surgeon. In the year 2000, he was named the Neurosurgeon of the Century by the journal *Neurosurgery*. He remains a beacon for all academic medicine and was one of the most significant physicians the Brigham has ever produced.

Despite the ongoing efforts of Christian and Cushing to coordinate the efforts of their departments, the nature of the relationship between medicine and surgery would be subject to ongoing internal scrutiny and at times comparison with seemingly more integrated and scientifically managed institutions, such as the emerging Mayo Clinic.[48] Other hospitals were larger, other hospitals had more room for staff, and other hospitals had more modern laboratories, operating rooms, and radiological suites. In 1927, Cushing compared the physical development of "Peter"—as he called the hospital—with the progress of a growing child:

> *With some naivete it was decided [in a prior annual report] that Peter was just the right size for domestic peace and comfort. But he insists on growing, requires an ever-increasing number of attendants, wants more elbow room and in place of his former toys demands complicated forms of apparatus to play with.*[49]

Cushing suggested that "Peter's" growing pains could be compared with other developmental or endocrinological processes. As he continued, some hospitals "start out with unmistakable evidences of gigantism; some later on acquire an acromegalic unwieldiness;

BIOGRAPHY

ADOLPH WATZKA, d. 1956

Christine Wenc

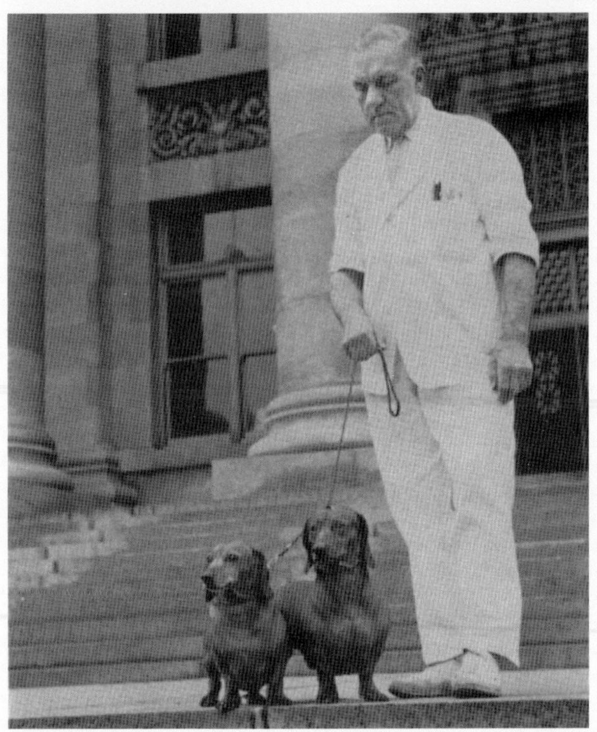

FIGURE 1-15 Fritz, Heidi, and Adolph Watzka.

Bohemian immigrant Adolph Waztka was Harvey Cushing's legendary surgical assistant and all-around operating room helper extraordinaire at the Peter Bent Brigham Hospital for nearly forty years, from 1917 until Watzka's sudden death in 1956. Known simply as "Adolph," he worked with three different chiefs of surgery and was held in high esteem for his remarkable talent in the operating room, talent that included inventing and improving surgical instruments, moving and arranging patients in precisely the right way on the operating table, and wiping Cushing's brow without smudging his eyeglasses.[50,51] Reportedly, he worked without a mask, promising the surgeons that he wouldn't cough or breathe too hard on anyone, and struck fear into the hearts of interns and nurses, although one suspects that the operating room nurses—some of whom may have been World War I and World War II veterans—were probably not the fragile flowers the Adolph legends occasionally make them out to be.

Operating Room Supervisor Katherine Madden, trained at Johns Hopkins, discovered Adolph and brought his skills to the attention of Cushing. Adolph had originally arrived in the United States in 1912 to work for his uncle, a steamfitter and plumber, in New Hampshire. Things didn't work out for Adolph there, however, as his uncle was apparently shorting his paycheck, so he came to Boston to seek his fortune instead. Here Adolph worked in a shoe factory, as a freight handler in the railroad yards, and finally at the harbor as a longshoreman.

As the story goes, in May, 1917—the same month Harvey Cushing sailed for Europe and service in World War I—a federal regulation prohibited subjects of Germany or its allies from going within 300 feet of the shore in Boston.[52] This presented problems for Adolph and his job as a longshoreman, as he was not yet a U.S. citizen, and he ended up in a scuffle with police who were in search of "enemy aliens." He landed in jail and, after being bailed out by a cousin in Stoneham, went in search of new employment and found a job as an orderly at the new Peter Bent Brigham Hospital.[53]

The job did not pay nearly as well as his work on the waterfront, nor was it especially interesting, but it seems that Adolph made himself so useful that he was able to improve his lot substantially. Madden noticed his skills right away and within a month of his hire got him a raise to $12 per week and assigned to surgery. In 1919 she recommended him to Cushing, who had recently returned from the war. Adolph apparently made innovative suggestions to Cushing from the start, advising him to change the shape of his scalpel blade after their first surgery together. Cushing had worked with artisans to develop surgical tools before but had often been frustrated; now, "he had the person he had looked for but had scarcely been able to find."[54] Cushing trained Adolph for twenty years and gave him "extraordinary authority" in the operating room.[55]

Along with his engineering skills, Adolph also was good with patients. As Francis Moore put it:

> *For many patients who only saw him during a few moments of anxiety or apprehension as they were being moved from their bed to the operating table, he was a big, heavyboned, homely man who with great strength achieved complete gentleness, telling the patient exactly what to do to avoid pain or discomfort and with a comforting word.*[56]

In his farewell message in the PBBH 1931 annual report, Cushing remarked: "I roughly calculate that during these past fifteen years he has lifted from stretcher to operating table and back five thousand tons of humanity."[57] Adolph not only repositioned patients, developed operating table maneuvers, and designed instruments still in use in 1951 (years after Cushing's departure), but he also gave ergonomic advice to Brigham surgeons and anesthesiologists to relieve cramping and fatigue. A surgeon from Massachusetts General Hospital asked Adolph to "look over" his operating room, and Adolph made several improvements there as well. Although surgeons from other hospitals wanted to send assistants to the Brigham to be trained in Adolph's techniques, he apparently refused to teach, telling a Collier's reporter for an article published in 1951:

> *There are men—orderlies and male nurses—who could be taught by the surgeons in their own hospitals. If the surgeons come to the Peter Bent, they will discover the knacks and tricks; but I think the chief thing they would take away is a disposition to give the man they select the same freedom, the same encouragement and finally the same authority as surgeons in chief have given me—and, incidentally, to pay such men enough to keep them interested.*[58]

Francis Moore noted in a 1956 eulogy to Adolph that the Brigham "has always been noted for the perfection of surgical technique."[59] It is a tribute to the first four decades of Brigham surgery that a man without formal credentials but with great innate talent was given the opportunity to participate in this "perfection." In a memoir, Charles Hatcher wrote:

> *He was very dedicated, and he had Dr. Moore's ear on a number of important matters. Adolph would roam around the ward, watching everybody operate, and if he thought you were a good surgeon he would begin to polish your operating shoes each night. The next morning they would be back in the rack, clean and gleaming. It was so well known that this was his way of evaluating people that Dr. Moore would ask about someone who was questionable for a promotion, 'Has Adolph shined his shoes yet?'*[60]

Adolph worked for Cushing for twenty years and continued to work at the hospital operating room for other surgeons until his own death in 1956. The 1951 Collier's profile describes a typical operating room scene:

> *By the time the patient comes into the surgeon's view, Watzka is already there and everything is ready. Gently he lifts the prone body from bed to operating table and positions it for the surgeon. There is a knack to hefting the dead weight of an unconscious person; there is an even greater one to doing it without disturbing broken bones or opening incisions. Adolph has both knacks to an extraordinary degree . . . As the incision is made, the room is so quiet that*

the patient's breathing can be heard by every intern, student, visiting doctor and observer in the last row of the balcony. In the silence, they look down at these tense men and women working swiftly against time. Occasionally the soft-spoken words echo: "Up, Adolph!" and "Over, Adolph!", a breath-holding experience until the final: "That does it!"[61]

Adolph never married and lived in a room over the Brigham laundry; in his off hours he was known for how he tended his old Rickenbacker automobile (his mechanical skills apparently extended to cars as well) and his habit of "exercising his brace of dachshunds up and down Shattuck Street."[62] After supervising "literally tens of thousands" of operations at the Brigham, one day Adolph died suddenly of a heart attack at the hospital, falling "right into" the arms of Hatcher as he scrubbed in for surgery.

On the day of his funeral the operating room went dark. Adolph Waztka, without the benefit of a day of formal training, had won such respect and admiration within the hospital that when his coffin was carried out, all of the pallbearers were full professors at Harvard Medical School.[63]

George Thorn, physician-in-chief at the time, wrote: "Adolph was not an employee of the Peter Bent Brigham Hospital; he was the Brigham! Devoted service of this magnitude is both an example and a challenge to all of us, and provides at once the key to that mysterious influence recognized by all as the Brigham spirit."[64] Moore put it this way: "Thus passed from the scene a man who made a humble chore into a fine profession, and in so doing taught an important lesson to hundreds of young doctors who must also find devoted service in what often is a humble role in the care of the sick."[65]

---

and some, which is still worse, give early signs of progeric senility."[66] The PBBH seemed to require a later growth spurt to catch up with such evolving clinical, research, and educational activities.

Nevertheless, in its first quarter-century of growth, its supporters continued to claim that the Brigham embodied the realization of Flexner's ideals more than any other hospital. And on recovering from the PBBH's tenuous financial position of the 1930s, Christian could report in 1937 on the many "pioneer" aspects of the hospital's development. Such innovations included its "graded" medical house officer service (with escalating responsibility assigned as house staff progressed), an "all-day service" ambulatory outpatient department largely staffed by house officers, the initiation of annual physician and surgeon *pro tempore* positions (reflecting an ongoing effort to benefit from the input of those at other institutions), and a focus on the long-term utility and repurposing of medical records, with Christian himself demanding from the hospital's earliest years that they be typed, rather than handwritten.[67] The hospital's evolution had likewise been propelled by a parallel revolution at the PBBH in nursing education and nursing professionalization, as led by the director of nursing, Carrie Hall, and as detailed in Chapter 2 in this volume by Marilyn King.[68]

Cushing stepped down in 1932, at the age of sixty-two, to be replaced by Eliot Cutler, "the first in the United States to describe the threat of pulmonary embolism as a postoperative complication," and who coauthored, with Robert Zollinger, the landmark *Atlas of Surgical Operations*, illustrated by Mildred Codding.[69] Christian stepped down in 1938, to be replaced by the remarkable Soma Weiss, whose tragic early death was much lamented (he diagnosed his own fatal subarachnoid hemorrhage in 1942).[70] As Weiss's successor, George Thorn, looked back in 1943 on the three decades that had passed since the hospital first opened its doors, he noted the "striking" changes in diagnoses on admission. Typhoid fever, a leading reason for admission in 1913, had entirely disappeared. Tonsillitis had been reduced eight-fold and acute rheumatic fever four-fold. Diabetes was on the increase, but so too were admissions for Addison disease, likely reflecting the evolution of the Brigham's reputation as a tertiary care institution more than the underlying burden of disease.[71]

BIOGRAPHY

MILDRED CODDING, 1902-1991, AND THE ART OF MEDICINE

Ann Conway

Mildred Codding, who worked closely with Harvey Cushing as his medical illustrator, is one of a select coterie who portray the "soul" of the early Brigham. Like Cushing, Codding was a disciple and student of the pioneering medical illustrator Max Brödel at Johns Hopkins. Brödel had emigrated from Germany and came to Hopkins in the 1890s, where he worked with Cushing, William Halsted, Howard Kelly, Thomas Cullen, and others, and in doing so defined the new field of medical illustration.

Brödel's dictum was that that medical illustration was far more than photography. "Copying is not medical illustrating," he said. "In a medical drawing, full comprehension must precede execution."[72] Brödel's traditional German upbringing led to a self-acknowledged "reluctance to teach women." However, his experience with Mildred Codding and a few other exceptional women of art and science, who "had long, productive careers in the field and were held in high esteem by their peers," convincingly reversed his bias and thereby the field of medical illustration.[73]

Codding, a 1926 Wellesley College graduate, also earned a master's degree in genetics and zoology from Columbia. Always interested in art, Codding then studied in Brödel's two-year program at Hopkins, which emphasized a thorough knowledge of anatomy as well as artistic skill. Cushing had studied with Brödel twenty years earlier, and they were both colleagues on the Hopkins faculty and close personal friends, which was how Codding learned of the opportunity at Peter Bent Brigham Hospital. After her first year at Hopkins, Codding spent her summer vacation studying at the Brigham. She then devoted her last year of training to study of the nervous system and began working at the Brigham in 1930.

Cushing "was not easy to illustrate for," noted Codding, perhaps because he was a talented artist in his own right. In a 1991 account, she remembered one incident:

> *While she strained, leaning forward from a stool at his back, he'd say, "Do you see this?" Mildred said, "Yes, I see it," to which Cushing said, "Don't mumble, speak up!" Then, during the next case, he'd ask her again if she saw something and this time she spoke up in a clear, confident voice only to hear him say, "Don't talk so much!"*[74]
>
> *Perhaps because of his own expertise, Cushing felt that "the illustrator's role was to elaborate and clarify surgical illustrations for publication." Thus, he made rough sketches immediately following operations, using "a fresh legal-sized blue operative report sheet for each drawing, initially penciling the field starting above at the "PBBH" heading and later adding India ink.*[75]

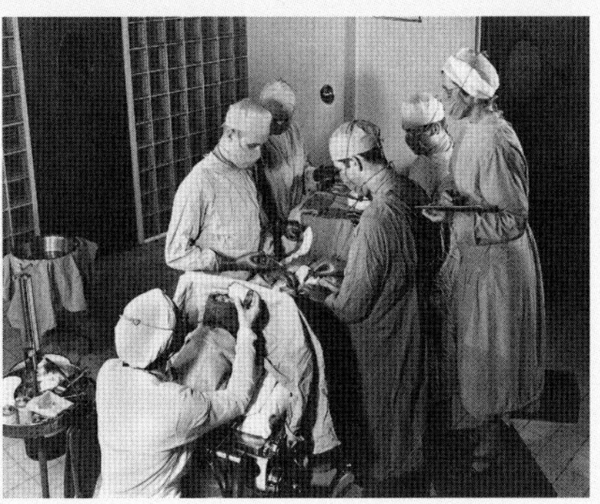

FIGURE 1-16 Mildred Codding, standing at right with drawing materials, 1950s.

Codding's style was more polished than Cushing's, using a "half tone technique" that she described as "more realistic, very smooth, and trompe l'oeil." Often after operations on the second floor, Codding joined Cushing in a walk downstairs:

> *Frequently, after surgery, Cushing would take the stairway down from the second floor operating rooms and have tea with Dr. Eisenhardt, whose office was across the hall from Miss Codding's. They would all sit together among the pathology specimens, plaster casts of acromegalics, and patient photographs—sometimes with Cushing still in his bloody gown—sipping tea.*[76]

Codding stayed at the hospital until 1960. During her career, she provided illustrations for many important surgical atlases and other works, working with Somers Sturgis and Joseph Meigs of Massachusetts General Hospital on an atlas of gynecological operations and, later, a surgical atlas of tumor operations. She illustrated Elliott Cutler and Robert Zollinger's *Atlas of Surgery*, which was the preeminent textbook of its era. She also collaborated with Donald Matson and John Shillito on their atlas of pediatric neurosurgical operations. When Cushing died in 1939, seven years after leaving the Brigham, she was named as one of his survivors.

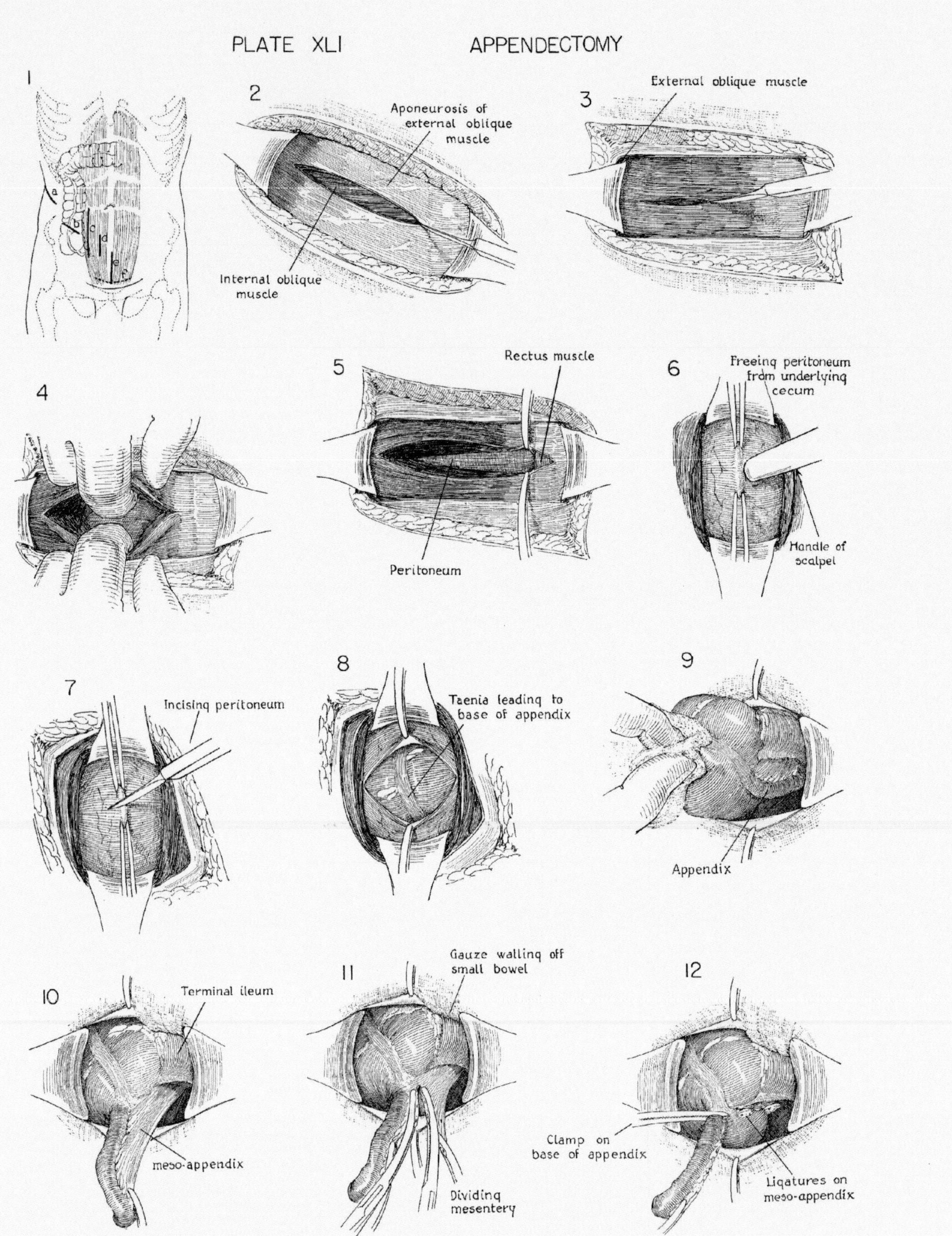

FIGURE 1-17 Illustration by Mildred Codding from the Atlas of Surgery, Elliot C. Cutler and Robert Zollinger, New York: MacMillan, 1939.

BIOGRAPHY

ELLIOT C. CUTLER, 1888-1947

Nicholas L. Tilney

Eliot C. Cutler was named surgeon-in-chief at the Peter Bent Brigham Hospital in 1932, on the retirement of Harvey Cushing. The transition from his dour, compulsive, and intensely focused predecessor was a revelation to his colleagues. Cutler, an ex-Harvard crew captain, was ebullient, enthusiastic, highly visible, and interested in all aspects of surgery and surgical education. A consummate teacher, he instilled students, residents, and faculty alike with new concepts, new ideas, and a new spirit of inquiry. A master surgeon and vocal proponent of Halsted's tenets of careful hemostasis and the gentle handling of tissues, he believed and taught that the well-trained surgeon should feel at home in all areas of the body and be equally facile with operations on the brain, chest, abdomen, and extremities. In addition, he stressed that responsibility of the surgeon toward his patient should extend well beyond the operative period. Spending much time with the residents and students in the surgical laboratory, where he continued Cushing's successful course in aseptic technique, he stressed independent thinking, scientifically controlled research in relevant animal models, and clear communication of experimental findings to diverse audiences.

However, many aspects of the professorial transition had been difficult. The physical plant was growing tired and run down, with much of the original infrastructure being outmoded and extraneous. Finances were inadequate; in practical terms, there was not even enough money to buy new instruments and new equipment. Impoverished by the Great Depression and overburdened by indigent patients, the hospital was under consideration for closure. Cutler even had to face the fact that Cushing would not leave despite agreeing on a retirement date. Indeed, while Cushing was in Europe, Cutler had to empty the contents of Cushing's office into a truck before moving in.

Born in Maine, Cutler graduated from Harvard College in 1909 and from its medical school, first in his class, four years later. His excellent academic record allowed him to gain pathology fellowships in Boston, Heidelberg, and eventually the Rockefeller Institute. Accepted as a house officer by Cushing, he followed his chief to France in 1915 to care for the war wounded,

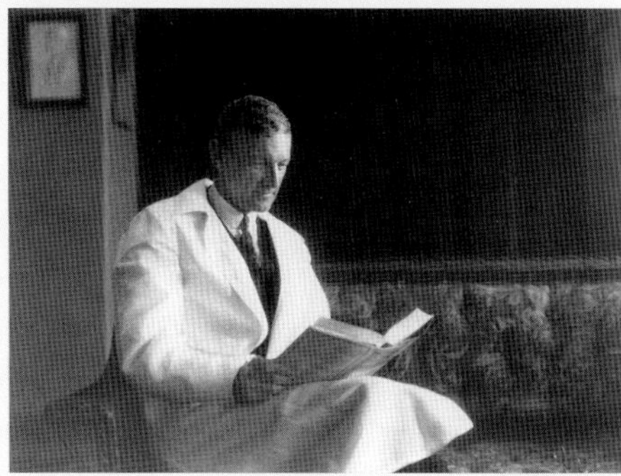

FIGURE 1-18 Eliot Cutler.

repeating the experience two years later after additional experience in surgery and research at the Brigham. Completing his training at the Brigham, he became professor of surgery at Western Reserve in Cleveland in 1924, dedicating many of his energies toward the education of young surgeons, before returning to the Brigham in 1932.

Stressing education throughout his career, he collected a coterie of talented and like-minded followers, including physicians Robert M. Zollinger, J. Engelbert Dunphy, Claude S. Beck, Robert E. Gross, Charles, A. Hufnagel, and David M. Hume. Many members of his inner circle went on to assume important leadership roles in surgical departments throughout the United States.

Cutler's concept of the "compleat" surgeon was mirrored in his own accomplishments. Bucking the prevailing antipathy of powerful colleagues in the surgical literature and at national meetings, he was the first in the country to describe the threat of pulmonary embolism as a postoperative complication. Buoyed by several pulmonary embolectomies in Europe after World War II, one of Cutler's young faculty members, Richard Warren, took his mentor's teachings to heart and successfully carried out the first such procedure in the United States in 1952.

Perhaps enthused by Cushing's initial work on heart surgery in dogs at Johns Hopkins, Cutler was also ahead of his time in believing that mechanical disorders of the heart might be relieved surgically. As mitral stenosis secondary to rheumatic fever was all too prevalent before the advent of penicillin, Cutler and his research fellows created mitral stenosis in dogs in the surgical laboratory, then designed a valvulotome to open the fused and calcified valves. He used the device on a patient in 1923. The young girl improved markedly and lived uneventfully for four and a half years before dying of recurrent stenosis. Attempts on three subsequent patients were unsuccessful, however. He continued his interest in heart surgery throughout the next decade, with an extensive series of canine and human experiments designed to relieve angina pectoris. These remained relatively unsuccessful until the advent of coronary artery bypass operations many years later. However, Cutler's efforts acted as a stimulus for subsequent Brigham accomplishments and innovations, both medical and surgical, in the treatment of a spectrum of cardiac abnormalities.

One of Cutler's principal contributions to improving the care and safety of the surgical patient was his publication of *The Atlas of Surgical Operations*, coauthored with his Brigham colleague, Robert M. Zollinger. Each procedure was shown in a step-by-step fashion, describing well-considered, effective, and standardized operative techniques via clear and accurate pen-and-ink drawings by Mildred Codding, who spent three years on the project. On the opposite page was a concise annotation of each figure, with a brief discussion of indications and preoperative preparation. It went through many editions and was an enduring *vade mecum* for generations of young surgeons.

Cutler served in World War II from 1942 to 1945 as chief consultant in surgery in the European Theater of Operations. Returning to the United States as a brigadier general, he had been highly decorated for his efforts, receiving two distinguished service medals (one in each world war), the United States Legion of Merit, the Order of the British Empire, and the Croix de Guerre, among other honors. In his later years, he was recognized by prestigious professional organizations and served in several important leadership positions. Unfortunately, he had developed widespread prostate cancer while in Europe, but managed to continue lecturing, teaching, and following progress in research until his death at age fifty-nine in 1947. He remains a seminal and high-profile figure in the evolution of modern surgery.

THE GROWTH OF THE TEACHING HOSPITAL: THE THORN/MOORE YEARS

By the early 1940s, the small hospital crafted by Christian, Cushing, Sosman, Weiss, and Cutler, as well as by Carrie Hall and so many others, had found itself upended by World War II. Long-time chronicler of the institution and roentgenologist, Merrill C. Sosman, recorded the mood of the hospital in his annual report of 1943:

> *The year 1943 has not been a real year. It has not been a pleasant progression of seasons, nor an orderly succession of 12 months, nor even a regular sequence of 52 weeks. It has been only an endless succession of days, each day crowded with work and vexations, sandwiched in between the War News in the morning paper and [radio broadcast journalist] Raymond Gram Swing at ten P.M., when all good Roentgenologists go to bed.*[77]

In the midst of and shortly after these dark times, as Sosman would later narrate, the hospital appointed two bright, charismatic department heads to rebuild the institution: the Buffalo-born endocrinologist George Thorn, who became physician-in-chief in 1942, and the surgeon Francis Moore, who became surgeon-in-chief in 1948. Both assumed leadership positions while still in their thirties, and both would have long tenures, stretching to the 1970s. The three decades in which they jointly led the hospital would produce remarkable growth and change in the "small" hospital the Brigham—and in the broader field of academic medicine.

Thorn took the helm of a wartime department of medicine so depleted of faculty and finances that it was barely a department. Yet, looking back to the therapeutic landscape of the 1913 Brigham of Christian's first report, he took heart in the expansion of therapeutics that had, by 1943, already dramatically transformed the landscape of clinical care. He noted that the kinds of collaborations

BIOGRAPHY

SOMA WEISS, 1899-1942

Peter V. Tishler and Joel T. Katz

Soma Weiss (physician-in-chief, 1939-1942), the second chair of medicine at Peter Bent Brigham Hospital, was a revered and charismatic teacher who stood out in this regard even compared with many other giants. In 1931, while a physician and faculty member at Harvard Medical School, Weiss cared for Alfred S. Reinhart, a Harvard medical student who was stricken with an untreatable, fatal heart infection. Weiss took on the care of this "young man of exceptional ability" so that he could comfort him and help him make peace with his mortality. Weiss encouraged the student to record his manifestations of the disease and reactions to its adverse events. With Weiss's counsel, Alfred realized that he would make a contribution to medicine for which he would be remembered, and this was very helpful as he coped with his illness.

Years later, Weiss published the student's memoir, introducing it by asserting: "To understand and relieve the symptoms is still the main labor of the physician in the management of patients during the long and usually hopeless course of [this disease]."[78] This sympathy and caring epitomized Soma Weiss during his brief but exceptionally productive life, which included sixteen years at Harvard Medical School and three years at the Peter Bent Brigham Hospital. His charisma, sensitivity, ebullience, and flair for the art and science of medicine were key characteristics of his leadership, whether in training talented physicians who became academic leaders, caring for individual patients, changing the face of medical care, or conducting incisive medical research.

Soma Weiss arrived in New York from Hungary in 1920, driven from his country by political and social unrest. He brought with him outstanding academic performance, an introduction to scientists and educators, and probably sufficient funds so that he rapidly obtained his B.S. from Columbia (1921) and MD from Cornell Medical School (1923). While he was at Cornell and Bellevue Hospital, his supervisor noted that "he was our most brilliant student" who

> *knew his patients thoroughly and was so accurate in his diagnoses that it would have been embarrassing for the attending staff had it not been for his great tact and tolerance . . . There came to the wards of Bellevue all sorts and conditions of men . . . He treated them all with equal kindness and they all trusted him.*[79]

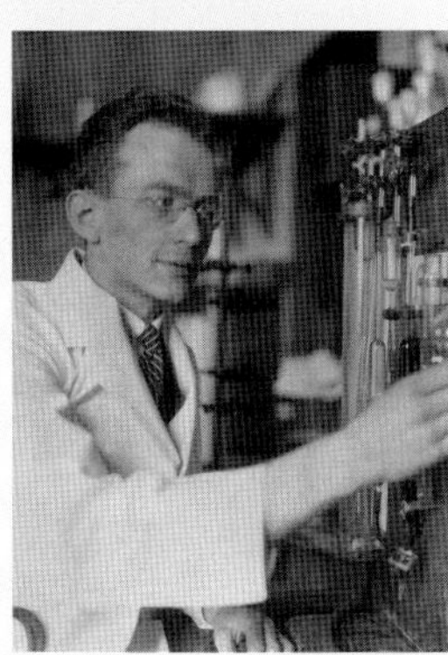

FIGURE 1-19 Soma Weiss.

Recruited in 1925 to the Thorndike Memorial Laboratory at the Boston City Hospital, he quickly became a leader. He was omnipresent on the wards, caring for patients and nurturing and educating young medical residents and students. Weiss achieved true eminence for his widely celebrated weekly bedside teaching rounds, initially at Boston City Hospital and then at Peter Bent Brigham Hospital, which attracted students from all of the Boston medical schools and residents in various disciplines.[80] "He loved being called in from home for consultations at night. Even in the wee hours, he would bring enthusiasm and fresh insight to a case and discuss every detail with the house officers and students."[81] Simultaneously, he carried out and published prolific research with trainees (fellows) in groundbreaking areas of cardiovascular pathophysiology, drug therapy, and vitamin deficiency. His presence was a major reason why the Harvard Medical Services at Boston City Hospital attracted the best and the brightest medical graduates for postgraduate training.

In 1939, after seven years as clinical director of the Harvard Medical Services at Boston City Hospital, Weiss became the physician-in-chief of the Peter Bent Brigham Hospital and the Hersey Professor of the Theory and Practice of Physic at Harvard Medical School. His appointment was unusual, because anti-Semitism limited access to leadership positions at that time. He brought to the Brigham his indomitable enthusiasm, energy, and good humor. He created a new excitement: Change was in the air! Some changes Weiss made early on were symbolic of his protean interests—for example, his hanging reproductions of rare works of art provided by his father-in-law Paul

Sachs of the Fogg Art Museum. He introduced new (for the Brigham) concepts of studying health and disease: the exploration of physiology and pathophysiology, gleaned from his experiences at Boston City Hospital and Cornell. By fostering this approach—replacing the prevalent question "What happens?" with "Why does this happen?"—he led in perpetuating this philosophy of medical research worldwide.[82] He attracted a cadre of bright young staff physicians and residents to extend his medical reach and established teaching conferences that were exceptionally popular. His sunny good nature and mild humor helped create an atmosphere for learning. Weiss's teaching was particularly effective because he avoided adherence to hierarchy. "A professor or a student . . . might have an equally good contribution to make to understanding a patient."[83]

Thanks in part to his experiences with Alfred Reinhart, Weiss appreciated the psychodynamics of being a patient and stressed to trainees the importance of tuning into this aspect of patient care. As World War II loomed, he participated in the study of the efficacy and safety of the albumin-containing component of blood plasma as treatment for hemorrhage, and he chaired a national committee whose recommendation to the Surgeon General, based on this study, led to a revolution in the treatment of wounded soldiers with blood loss. Still reaching out to others, he voluntarily chaired monthly conferences at a local military base to keep otherwise isolated military physicians abreast of the latest developments in medicine. A friend noted: "Through these many channels . . . flowed his ever-increasing influence upon medicine of America."

Weiss stated succinctly his philosophy underlying his relation to and mentoring of faculty and trainees; the T.S. Eliot lecture quote he liked most was "What one must be judged by, scholar or no, is not particularized knowledge but one's total harvest of thinking, feeling, living and observing human beings."[84] Associates responded to him with reverence. Soma Weiss was "a man with a profound knowledge of medicine, a keen sense of humor, and the courage of his convictions, combined with a great kindness and consideration of others."[85] "His self-reliance, kindness, and sense of humor were felt by all who knew him and inspired their respect and devotion. He was a friend and a stimulating intellect to men of all ages." "Soma had the magic touch of making the day seem more meaningful. . . He was above all a mover of men, and there lies the secret of the legend."[86] Being at the Brigham was "like Camelot;"[87] we are "ever grateful for the inspiration he gave us," and for the "chance to be so intimate with him." Medical students described him as a "superstar" who exhibited "his loving attitude to patients and students."[88] Thus he is also remembered as a builder of people who continued his leadership in American medicine and often carried out the changes in education and medical care that Weiss envisioned.

Weiss died suddenly in January 1942, just four days after his forty-third birthday. His many friends and associates were devastated. Eulogies came from many corners, and many were expressed at the memorial service at Harvard Medical School in March. Graduating members of the Harvard Medical School Class of 1942 expressed their grief in their yearbook:

He has not gone from us! Not when these halls
Throb with his presence! When continually
We seem to breathe in from the very walls
The essence of his rich vitality!
Forever in our hearts he is the "Chief,"
The great physician, teacher, guide and friend,
A gay blithe spirit poised in bright relief
Against a world of pain. He could transcend
The narrow bounds of earth in daring flight
And give us wings for pathless space above,
Where we might soar in seeking for the light
Of greater knowledge through our greater love;
But, of all the gifts that crowned his healing art,
The rarest was his understanding heart.[89]

He was, indeed, the Osler of his day.

Table II

A Comparison Between the More Important Specific Therapeutic Remedies Available in 1913 and in 1943

1913	1943	
Salvarsan	Arsenicals	Placental hormones
Quinine	Liver extract	Vitamin A
Vermifuges	Heparin	Vitamin B, thiamin, niacin, riboflavin, etc.
Thyroid extract	Epinephrine	Vitamin C
Digitalis	Insulin	Vitamin D
Emetine	Thyroxin	Vitamin E
	Parathyroid extract	Vitamin K
	Adrenal cortex extract	Dihydrotachysterol
	Estrogenic hormones	Antitoxin
	Progesterone	Immune sera
	Androgenic hormones	Prostigmine
	Anterior pituitary	Thiouracil
	Pitressin	Sulfonamides
	Pitocin	Tyrothricin
		Penicillin

FIGURE 1-20 Therapeutic specifics, 1913 versus 1943. (From the 1943 PBBH Annual Report.)

among industry, academia, and hospitals that had produced insulin, penicillin, and heparin had only just begun—and the teaching hospital was the logical place from which to base the continued growth of clinical research and reap its rewards in transformed patient care.

Thorn likewise thought the teaching hospital was the crucial node in the expanding network of biomedical research taking shape in the postwar era. Much as the Manhattan project illustrated that the physical science of the postwar period was practiced on an entirely different scale from the elite foundation-based laboratories of the first few decades of the twentieth century, so too did biomedical research in the Thorn/Moore era progress from a small affair to "big science" in its own right. Between 1946 and 1956, the research budget of the PBBH increased by an order of magnitude,[90] and Thorn worked continuously to find research funds to support the growth of research, exemplified by his own work on the use of corticosteroids to treat Addison disease.[91] He had met the young aircraft magnate Howard Hughes in the 1940s, and by 1953 Hughes had funneled his considerable income to found the Howard Hughes Medical Institute (HHMI). Thorn became director of research of the HHMI shortly thereafter. The energetic endocrinologist also built relations with the Massachusetts Institute of Technology, leading to the creation of the Health Sciences and Technology track at HMS. Thorn's success at private funding and development efforts, however, would soon be dwarfed by the expanding public funding of biomedical research in the postwar decades. The National Institute of Health (NIH) became plural in 1948, the National Science Foundation was funded in 1950, and the NIH extramural research program expanded dramatically over the 1960s. Under Thorn's leadership, the PBBH received one of the first grants to build a Clinical Research Center, which opened with $2 million in NIH funds in 1960.

The transformation of therapeutics and research would come to redefine the role of the hospital in medical education as well. In the aftermath of the war, Thorn authored a set of essays on the "Hospital-Medical School Relationship" in which he projected the more general changing role of the hospital in medical education in the second half of the twentieth century. "Slowly," he noted, "but progressively, during the past decade, medical undergraduate teaching has shifted to the hospitals to permit closer correlation of instruction in fundamental science with the practical application in the care of patients and study of disease."[92] Where Flexner saw the teaching hospital as a place for students to encounter clinical material, Thorn saw the hospital as a grounded location for considering basic science in clinical context. In parallel, to attract basic scientists to academic hospitals, Thorn argued that "full-time" employees of an academic hospital should be considered members of the faculty of the medical school—even if they neither gave lectures nor received a specific salary from the school itself.

BIOGRAPHY

GEORGE WIDMER THORN, 1906-2004

Gordon H. Williams

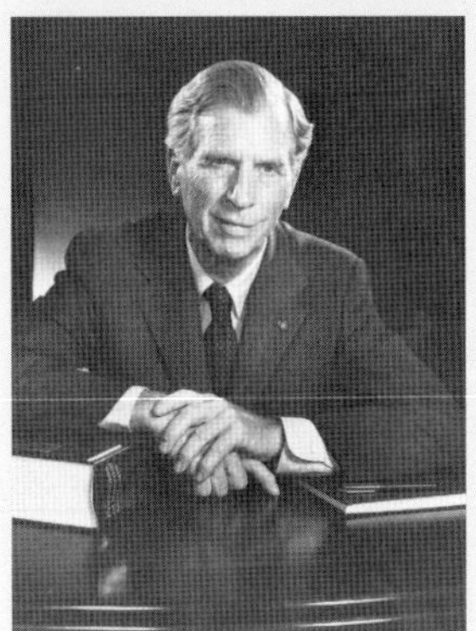

FIGURE 1-21 George Thorn.

George W. Thorn served as chair of the Department of Medicine at the Peter Bent Brigham Hospital (PBBH) from 1942 to 1972. He was born on January 15, 1906, in Buffalo, New York. He died on June 26, 2004, in Beverly, Massachusetts. Thorn attended Wooster College in Ohio and then entered the University of Buffalo School of Medicine in 1925. He became a protégée of Frank Hartman, an association that directed his research career toward the adrenal cortex. As a student, he documented that giving an adrenal extract to adrenalectomized rats allowed them to grow normally. As a research fellow with Hartman, he developed a method to prepare adrenal extracts, and was the first to demonstrate that giving the extract to an Addisonian patient markedly improved the individual's well-being. Hartman and Thorn received the Gold Medal of the American Medical Association for this translational research in 1932. Two years later he was awarded a prestigious Rockefeller Foundation fellowship for training at the Massachusetts General Hospital. There, his research was directed by Albright, Means, and Bauer, among others. In 1936, he went to the Johns Hopkins Medical School to conclude his fellowship and was appointed associate professor of medicine at Hopkins in 1938. The next few years brought great advances in the understanding of adrenal cortical physiology and pathophysiology, in which Thorn played a major role. Cushing syndrome's characteristics were clarified. Edward C. Kendall synthesized cortisone and cortisol and provided them to Thorn, who assessed their effects in a well-studied patient with Addison disease.

After the sudden death of Soma Weiss in early 1942, Thorn was appointed the third physician-in-chief at the PBBH and the ninth Hersey Professor of the Theory and Practice of Physic at Harvard Medical School (HMS). Beginning his second career as an academic administrator, while also continuing his research, he inherited a department consisting of six individuals: two residents and four senior physicians—James O'Hare, Charles Janeway, Sam Levine, and Lewis Dexter. During the next fifteen years, Thorn made substantial changes in the PBBH. It was the center of research on the adrenal cortex in animals and humans, including new approaches to measure the activity or insufficiency of the organ. The Reddy-Thorn method for measuring urinary 17-hydroxysteroids became the standard test of adrenal glucocorticoid function for nearly twenty-five years. His research efforts also assessed the adverse role adrenal steroid production played in other diseases, such as prostate cancer. After the discovery of aldosterone by Simpson and Tait in the mid-1950s, Thorn studied its role and regulation. His group defined both mineralocorticoid "escape"—the mechanism by which excess aldosterone production does not lead to edema and heart failure—and aldosterone's role in heart failure when escape does not occur because of hemodynamic impairment.

Administratively, Thorn made revolutionary changes in the delivery of medical care. He started the "General Medical Clinic," staffed by medical students, house officers, and faculty from all medical specialty groups. This "one-stop shopping" approach to patient care was the forerunner of the multispecialty clinical groups of the later twentieth and twenty-first centuries. Thorn expanded the Department of Medicine to capably address diverse medical problems, from cardiac to endocrine to renal. For example, he convinced John Merrill to become a nephrologist, not a cardiologist. Because of Merrill's career change, and his relationship with Joseph Murray, they and others performed the first successful kidney transplant.

In the late 1950s, Thorn began his third career as an academic fundraiser. He became concerned about the growing gap between laboratory research findings and their application to human disease. He believed this resulted both from the lack of laboratories performing research on humans and the inadequate training of physicians in the scientific method. Addressing the first issue, he created a clinical research unit with funds from industry. With other academic leaders, he lobbied the National Institutes of Health (NIH), which funded the first four general clinical research centers (GCRCs) for cutting-edge human research in 1961. One was awarded to HMS and was housed on E-Main at the PBBH. Over the next three decades, NIH-funded GCRCs were established in seventy-eight institutions, including each of the major Harvard academic teaching hospitals. Shortly thereafter, NIH addressed Thorn's second issue by establishing the Medical Scientist Training Program to provide funds to medical schools to support medical students in pursuit of a PhD. In a *New England Journal of Medicine* article, Thorn asserted that this program would train physicians in the scientific method, leading via rigorously designed studies to understand better human physiology and pathophysiology.

During this same period, Thorn became increasingly involved in identifying funding sources for junior investigators, particularly those with MDs or MD/PhDs, because of his concern that they might leave academia to enter private practice. Some of these funds came directly from his patients and some from foundations. He persuaded the Hartford Foundation to provide multiyear salary and research funding to junior physician-scientists, many of them at the PBBH. He contributed in profound ways to the function of the Howard Hughes Medical Institute (HHMI). This opportunity presented itself because of a tie from his Hopkins days with Verne Mason, the personal physician to Mr. Howard Hughes. During the mid-1950s, Mr. Hughes formed the HHMI, with funding from the Hughes Aircraft Company. The Medical Advisory Board, to which Thorn was appointed as a result of his friendship with Mason and other board members, determined that the HHMI would fund midcareer medical scientists at major medical centers, which initially included Harvard, Duke, Vanderbilt, Hopkins, Yale, and the University of Washington. After Hughes's death in 1976, Thorn, who was now emeritus at HMS and PBBH, became president of HHMI and one of three members of its Executive Committee. Over the next three decades, supported and directed by Thorn, HHMI support expanded to fund investigators at many additional academic health centers and medical schools and became the largest source of private funding for biomedical research in the United States. After he stepped down as president in 1984, he remained chair of its board until 1990. Continuing his efforts to increase the nongovernmental support of biomedical research, he became vice-president and chair of the Scientific Advisory Board of the Whitaker Heath Sciences Fund—a major funding source for medical research. He also was involved in expanding educational opportunities at HMS and elsewhere. He became one of the initial coeditors of *Harrison's Textbook of Medicine* and its editor-in-chief in the late 1980s.

During his more that half century as a physician-scientist, academic administrator, educator, and entrepreneur, Thorn received numerous honors. These included honorary degrees at Harvard and many other institutions, the Public Welfare Medal of the National Academy of Sciences, the George M. Kober Award of the Association of American Physicians, the John Phillips Memorial Award of the American College of Physicians, the Lifetime Achievement Award of the Massachusetts Medical Society, and, on two occasions, the Gold Medal of the American Medical Association. Yet, through all of his achievements, Thorn considered himself, above all, a physician. He began his medical career as a private practitioner. He delighted in making rounds daily on his patients with an entourage of students, fellows, and residents. Patients flocked to him from far and wide, including King Ibn Saud, Robert Frost, Judy Garland, and Spencer Tracy. In that setting, all who attended appreciated his personal warmth, his caring and gentle approach to patients, and his deep understanding of their needs. Indeed, George W. Thorn was uniquely able to "get into" other individuals' minds to ascertain how he could help them to help themselves, whether the individual was a patient, a medical student, a resident, a faculty member, or a wealthy businessperson. In many respects this was his most endearing quality, and it is the one by which those who knew him will always remember him.

Thorn's vision for the hospital would be complemented by that of Moore, who devoted his annual reports of the late 1940s to arguing for the essentiality of the teaching hospital to both undergraduate and graduate medical education in the mid-twentieth century.[93] In this new atomic age, Moore sketched out a vision of the teaching hospital itself as an atom structured around a nucleus of honesty, inquiry, and

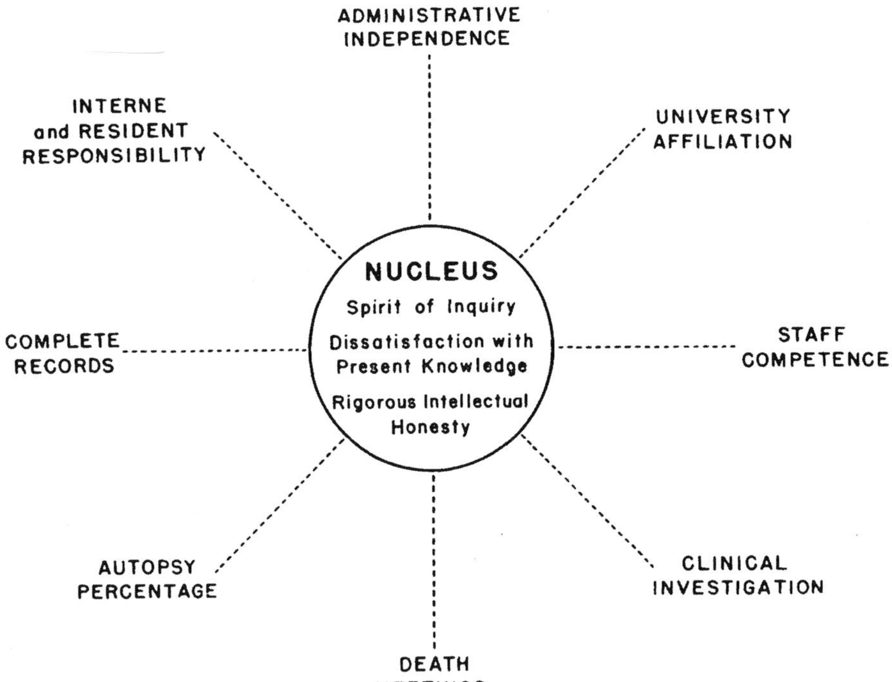

FIGURE 1-22 Francis Moore's hospital atom. (From the 1949 PBBH Annual report.)

the need to improve continuously the standard of care. This nucleus, unchanged since the days of Cushing and Christian, was surrounded by the expanding "outer electronic trappings of the hospital as an educational institution—well-kept records, high autopsy percentage, resident responsibility, clinical research, university affiliation, administrative independence."[94] Like Thorn, Moore described a role for the postwar academic hospital that extended well beyond the original Flexnerian conception, as the specialized spaces of the teaching hospital became ever more essential to both undergraduate and graduate medical education.

BIOGRAPHY

FRANCIS D. MOORE, 1913-2001

Nicholas E. O'Connor and Nicholas L. Tilney

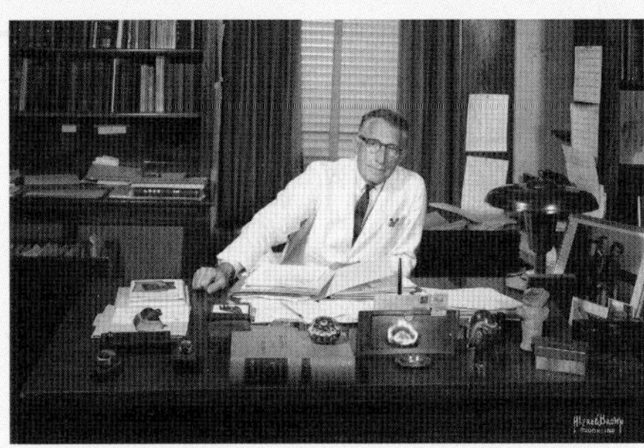

FIGURE 1-23 Francis Moore.

Francis Daniels Moore became the Mosely Professor of Surgery at Harvard Medical School and surgeon-in-chief of the Peter Bent Brigham Hospital in 1948. He was the youngest surgical chair in Harvard's history. For the next twenty-six years, he led his department through an unparalleled period of research and clinical innovation, bringing Harvard and the Brigham further international renown.

Moore began his own pioneering studies of the metabolic response to surgery and trauma, using isotope chemistry, while a surgical resident at the Massachusetts General Hospital. He continued this work at the Brigham in his laboratory and at the patients' bedsides, culminating in two classic books: *The Metabolic Response to Surgery* with M. Ball (1949) and *Metabolic Care of the Surgical Patient* (1959). These masterpieces changed the thinking of surgeons and their care of patients worldwide. Before Moore's work, their focus was primarily on operative methods to treat disease and trauma. After Moore's work, surgeons assumed total responsibility for the care of the patient, and this included altered physiologic states, electrolyte imbalances, endocrine responses, and nutritional requirements. From his research, attention to these changes became routine throughout the world. This achievement, which became the scientific basis for the metabolic care of surgical patients, was a major advance in surgery in the twentieth century. This recognition resulted in Moore's being on the cover of *Time* magazine in 1963.

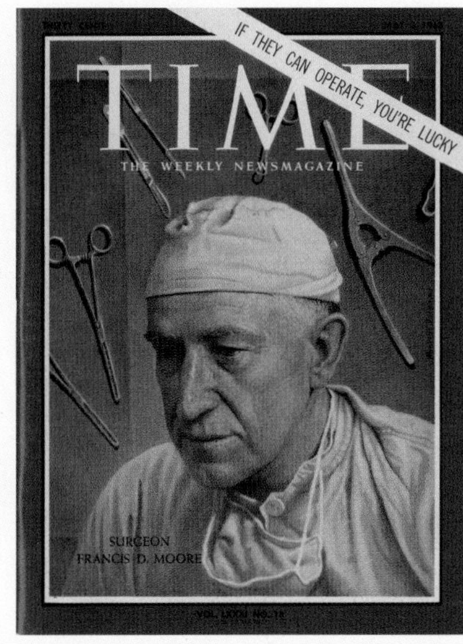

FIGURE 1-24 *Time Magazine*, May 3, 1963.

At the same time, other monumental advances were being nurtured by Moore in his department. David Hume, whom Moore termed "the restless genius," started experimenting with organ transplants, both in laboratory animals and, in collaboration with John Merrill, in patients with terminal renal failure (with limited results). After Hume was called back to the Navy in 1953, Moore persuaded Joseph Murray, who was working on skin transplants, to take over the program. Murray's success in human kidney transplantation in the 1950s and 1960s led to his receiving the Nobel Prize in Medicine or Physiology in 1990. In his acceptance speech, he credited Moore with providing the leadership, courage, and unselfishness that led to the success of transplantation.

In Moore's first year as chief, thoracic surgeon Dwight Harken developed the technique of closed mitral valvuloplasty. Ultimately, with the support of Moore and the cardiology service, Harken's procedure became standard therapy around the world. When Harken retired, Moore trainee John Collins returned to continue these innovations in cardiac surgery. Under Moore's directorship and encouragement, several new surgical facilities were established: the Bartlett intensive care unit (ICU) for the treatment of burns, trauma, and sepsis; the surgical bacteriology laboratory, directed by Carl Walter; and the bioengineering department under Philip Drinker, who played a signal role with Robert Bartlett in the development of the membrane oxygenator. In all of these endeavors, Moore provided leadership and support and was unfailingly generous in giving the credit to others. His standards in research and clinical care were exceedingly high, but his intellectual quest was always tremendously exciting.

Franny Moore brought all of his prodigious talents to bear in his teaching of Harvard medical students and in his training of his surgical residents. Saturday morning surgical clinics, for the first-year medical students, were meticulously planned and even rehearsed, bringing to the fore Moore's considerable dramatic talents honed in his undergraduate years as president of the Harvard Lampoon and the Hasty Pudding Club. Residents were continually prodded and quizzed by Moore as they presented the patient, who was then presented to talk about his/her experience. In one instance, the patient was Laure Bartlett Moore, his beloved wife, who later that same day underwent urgent surgery for acute cholecystitis! These clinics impressed on the students that surgical care of patients was a team effort demanding high attention to detail. That same challenge was evident in Moore's Monday afternoon chief's rounds with the house staff. At the beside of patients in the ICU, Moore probed the residents about the details of laboratory values, fluid orders, and medications, drilling in the responsibility to master all the aspects of patient care. Surgical Service meeting, held on Thursday evenings, included a review of deaths and complications of the whole department each week, with Moore and the chief resident officiating. As the focus was always on why and how to do better, these were the most interesting and intellectually challenging meetings of the week for the residents. Moore also regularly reviewed the research work of his residents and fellows. Here he was at his most expansive and engaging as he listened, exchanged, and encouraged. He was extremely helpful and generous with his time in honing the young investigators' talks as they prepared to present their work at national meetings.

To be a resident at the Brigham under FDM, as he was known, was both a challenge and a privilege: a challenge because of the level of talent and commitment of all residents and the surgical staff, and a privilege because of the close association with the awesomely talented chief. Francis Moore was the most accomplished surgeon-scientist of his generation, widely published, extensively funded, a famously magnetic speaker, and recognized and honored around the world. He and his wife, Laure, a childhood sweetheart, constantly hosted the residents at their home in Brookline or at their summer residence. He was an avid sailor, skippering his beautiful yawl *Angelique* in races to Bermuda and Halifax. He loved the arts, especially music, and had twin grand pianos in his homes, where he would play duets with his children or any of his visitors.

In 1992, with donations from friends and associates, Harvard Medical School created the Francis D. Moore Professorship in Surgery. Nicholas L. Tilney, a transplant surgeon-scientist and one of Moore's trainees, became the first incumbent. On Tilney's retirement in 2011, Michael Zinner, the current Mosely Professor of Surgery and surgeon-in-chief at the Brigham, appointed Francis D. Moore, Jr., to the professorship.

Francis Moore was a once-in-a-generation phenomenon. He used all of his wonderful gifts to the fullest for the benefit of his patients and students and for future generations of both.

At the same time, the "ecology of care" (to use a later metaphor of Moore's) delivered at the hospital—on view for students to behold—was becoming more complex every year.[95] Field medicine in World War II had mobilized surgical services on an unprecedented scale and mobilized networks for the development of surgical and pharmaceutical innovations, from plasma transfusion to penicillin. Techniques for managing combat injuries—aided by new means of producing, storing, and distributing plasma and other blood products newly fractionated from human blood—produced new possibilities for clinical care in the postwar hospital. At the Brigham, these developments derived from important research on blood fractionation conducted by E.J. Cohn and Charles Janeway (whose relationship was catalyzed by Soma Weiss) and took place in large part because of the lifework of Carl Waldemar Walter.[96] A resident at PBBH in the 1930s, Walter established the first blood bank for the Brigham in 1942; under his directorship, the blood bank blossomed at the PBBH and spun off additional innovations, such as the development of vacuum-collapsible bags and plastic tubing, which made blood all the more bankable.

The war had also led to remarkable changes in the management of trauma, including the emerging technology of artificial respiration and the creation of specialized spaces of care such as the intensive care unit. Dwight Harken had pioneered the use of postoperative intensive care for cardiac surgical patients, whereas the Bartlett Unit would accommodate the needs of a broader array of surgical patients. Such units involved the innovations of respiratory ventilation and close monitoring and soon spread to medical patients as well.[97] The physical plant of the PBBH changed more broadly to accommodate these new technological practices. Under the directorship of John Putnam Merrill, the PBBH opened one of the first "renal units" in 1949, installing two "artificial kidneys" to support patients with renal failure who otherwise clearly would have died.[98] A new Emergency Ward was opened in 1950.[99]

Other specialized units followed, including the 1963 opening of the Levine Cardiac Unit (LCU), a monitoring station that extended the principle of the Bartlett Unit to a population of patients hospitalized after life-threatening heart attacks. The LCU's creator and first director, Bernard Lown, could claim within two years of operation to have decreased mortality among post–myocardial infarction patients by more than 50%.[100] By 1971, coronary care units could

REPORT OF THE PHYSICIAN-IN-CHIEF

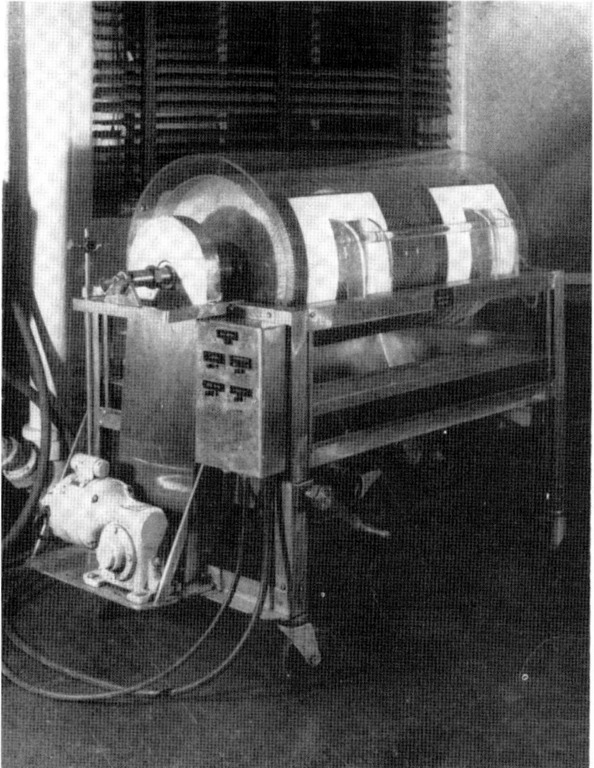

THE MECHANICAL KIDNEY

FIGURE 1-25 The PBBH's first artificial kidney.

be found in more than 5,000 hospitals in the United States, to be followed by the many other specialized units (the neonatal intensive care unit, the pediatric intensive care unit, etc.) now commonplace in the modern hospital.

Lown could only attribute part of the success of the new coronary care unit to specialized technologies of cardiovascular monitoring (limited at that time to the continuous electrocardiogram). Far more important was the attention of specialized nurses who had learned to monitor such equipment.[101] Labor conflicts among physicians, nurses, and management, however, would become more complex in the postwar environment after the minimum wage law went into effect in 1950 and the country was beset by a series of regional and national nursing shortages. In 1965, the hospital was forced to close a ward temporarily for shortage of nurses,[102] and in turn, the hospital director responded by conceding to nursing a greater voice in hospital management and stressing that the hospital needed to have nurses work to the fullest extent of their specialized training as allied healthcare professionals.

As the terrain of the hospital changed from undifferentiated medical and surgical wards into a collection of specialized spaces for clinical research and clinical care, Thorn and Moore expanded their departments of medicine and surgery, respectively, with an eye to the new differentiation of specialties and subspecialties by which the medical world was becoming ordered in the second half of the twentieth century. In the 1940s, Thorn changed the structure of the department of medicine from a general field into a set of divisions, the first three being cardiovascular (under Samuel A. Levine and Lewis Dexter), renal (under W. Putnam Merril), and endocrine/metabolic (under his own direction). This simple set would expand to thirty-two divisions and subdivisions by the time he retired. Likewise, Moore began to divide and expand his department of surgery to include a division of anesthesiology (under Leroy Vandam), plastic surgery (under Joseph Murray), cardiothoracic surgery (under Dwight Harken), and gynecology (under Somers Sturgis).

Yet, it was the clinical and research spaces created at the *intersection* of these specialities that enabled the Brigham to produce some of its most memorable therapeutic contributions in the postwar decades. This was exemplified by the collaboration among Vandam, Merrill, Murray, urologist J. Hartwell Harrison, and pathologist Gustave Dammin, that resulted in the first successful renal transplant in 1954, for which Murray would be awarded the Nobel Prize in Medicine or Physiology in 1990. The translation of research from bench to bedside would become an oft-repeated theme of Brigham medicine, including many items we now take for granted and epitomized by the concept of electrical cardioversion, devised by Bernard Lown in the late 1950s and early 1960s.

Woven through these narratives of progress and expansion, however, one finds darker refrains within the reports of Thorn and Moore. Some of these reflect complaints common to the expansile infrastructure of postwar American hospitals: there is not enough space, and the space that there is has become increasingly problematic.[103] Just over three decades after the

REPORT OF THE PHYSICIAN-IN-CHIEF

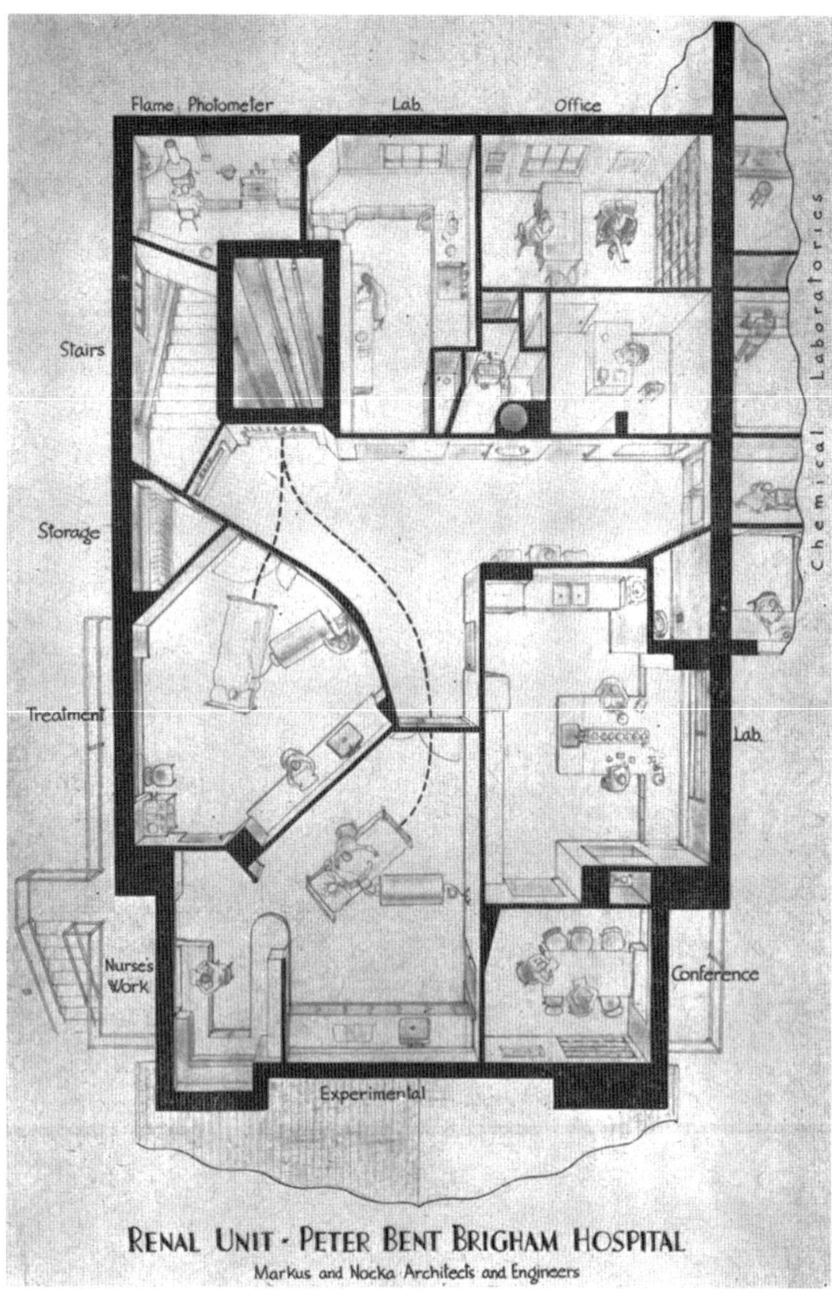

[26]

FIGURE 1-26 The PBBH's renal unit, 1951.

hospital's architecture had been praised as unsurpassed in the country, Francis Moore would recall in 1960 that the PBBH had been "physically obsolete the day it was opened," being more concerned with nineteenth century preoccupations with ventilation than with twentieth century concepts of infection control.[104] Apart from the old amphitheater, which Moore admired as a statement of the hospital's character as a teaching institution, he had choice words for every other aspect of its construction, and bitterly complained:

> *The architect had evidently spent most of his life on the Riviera and his previous forays into the hospital field had been subtropical. The sprawling nature*

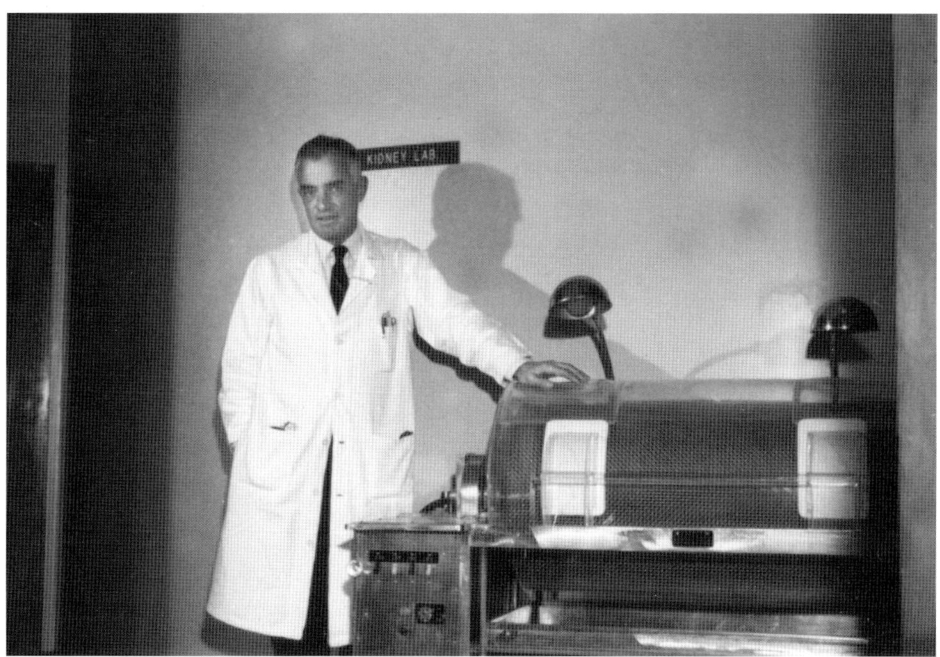

FIGURE 1-27 John Merrill with dialysis machine.

of the Brigham made it wasteful of heat; the long open corridors were useless in the New England winter, and one by one all have been covered. The pavilion system was completely abandoned by 1920. The hospital had no entrance and no exit. Hundreds of unidentified people came in and out every day, including grammar school students on their way to and from classes.[105]

The "small" hospital of the PBBH tried to make do with its limited pavilion model hospital by retrofitting old spaces in innovative ways. N.A. Wilhelm, the superintendant and director of the hospital for more than three decades, had apparently pondered the possibility of a "vertical hospital" early in the 1940s. However, as at so many other academic medical institutions, calls to build a new hospital that was better suited for the changing clinical care and research of the mid-twentieth century gave way to hopeful plans for gradual renovation.[106] With the idea of a vertical hospital shelved by 1943, Wilhelm instead focused his effort on "reconstructing and modernizing" the physical plant, starting with Wards E and F and their accompanying laboratories, operating rooms, and clinics.[107]

SPOTLIGHT

1948: "THE WORLD'S BEST MEDICINE IN THE WORLD'S WORST FACILITY"

James Dealy

Dissatisfaction with the Peter Bent Brigham Hospital's aging facility was a constant theme in the hospital's annual reports. In this excerpt from the 1948 report, James Dealy reflects on radiology facilities.

"In last year's Annual Report it was suggested that a review of how the last decade had altered the face of the X-ray Department might be a fitting theme for a subsequent report. There being no time like the present, herewith recorded are some observations—filled with miles of nostalgia—which may serve the purpose of illustrating both the dividends and the liabilities of increasing girth.

"When your writer arrived at the Brigham in 1948, the spirit was one of acquisition; the hospital had acquired a new Surgeon-in-Chief, the X-ray Department had acquired a new therapy machine (the newest one we have today) and Merrill Sosman had acquired *enfin* an office of his own. The area outside the office became the department's first viewing room, with only about one-quarter of the space sacrificed to contemporary film filing. This was not a serious compromise, for there was but one stereo, two-box illuminator and one dictaphone . . . with only two residents and two assistants to use them when the 'Professor' was not holding forth.

"All clerical work was transacted in the front office. Film filing was complicated by a multiplicity of numbering systems and lack of adequate storage space (the same basement storage space is somewhat more crowded today). To avoid the horrors of the subterranean, envelopes were stored at halfway points by clerks who found consistent reliance on their own ingenuity to find them. When they were sick, all was lost. Film control was even worse, for it was the practice to keep the films on the wards. The sheer mechanics of delivery and procurement and the dovetailing of these with film interpretation were a nightmare—brightened only by the cheery sight of ebullient little Nicky Chrysanthos as she made her hospital rounds with the precursor of the supermarket shopping basket.

"The heart of the technical side of the ground pike (manned by three technicians, one of them a full-time volunteer, and one student, as I recall), consisted of the "chest room" and the "bone room" (where the high voltage lines were cautiously placed behind a picket fence) flanking a single fluoroscopy room which contained an upright table that couldn't be turned down and a downright table that couldn't be tilted up. The patient had to be sent to another room for films (they still do, from this particular room). Fortunately, the darkroom was dark, for it did not pass well the exposure of illumination. Films in small lots were placed in open hoods to be blown dry in an hour . . . or so.

"This, then, was the essence of the physical plant wherein were conducted examinations on 17,132 patients, using 39,407 films in the process, and 2,230 x-ray treatments. No small part of the operation was the outright blood, sweat and tears of the resident staff. Endless hours at night were spent drying, clipping and filing films made after 3:30 P.M. Then came the logging, the filling of envelopes, the sorting of requisitions and, finally, the arrangement of films into an order of interpretation designed to second-guess which staff man would be the first to the department the next morning to inquire about his favorite patient."[108]

Renovation would become routinized in the life of the twentieth century teaching hospital, which continuously required more and newer spaces for physicians, patients, researchers, and evolving technologies of diagnosis and management.[109] What worked for Wards E and F in 1943 would work for C and D in 1946 and A and B in 1949. Even when the NIH provided the funding to build one of the nation's first independent Clinical Research Centers, the blueprint of Ward E-Main remained visible in the external plan of the cutting-edge clinical research unit.

Thorn hoped that renovations would render the hospital a new beacon of postwar modernism. "Indeed," he added in an early report on PBBH's renovation, "so extensive is the metamorphosis that 'before and after' photographs will be required to insure the recognition of many aspects of the institution by staff members now away."[110] However, many Brigham staff found the modernization more euphemistic than real and complained instead that the constant construction added more clatter and clamor to a largely unchanging cramped condition of care. As Merrill Sosman had already complained in 1945:

> *For 23 years the Radiologist has existed in one small corner of the general office, a veritable gold fish bowl, with no privacy and no office to call his own. Similarly we read our films and discuss our most intimate cases in a cubby hole off the main corridor of the department, open to curious patients, subject to the noises of their coughing or retching and the inevitable "Take a deep breath, Ho-l-l-l-d it" just across the corridor.*[111]

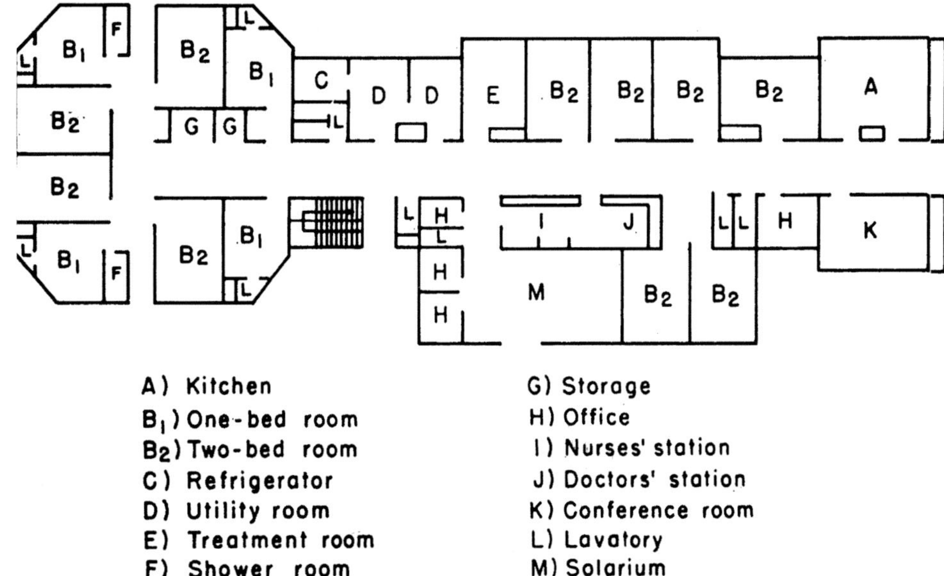

FIGURE 1-28 Floor plan of the Clinical Research Center, 1960.

This problem had only worsened by the 1950s, as the expansion of the hospital was hemmed in by two contradictory constraints. On the one hand, it had to fit more patients into the same amount of space; on the other hand, it had to respond to a patient base shifting from a largely "public" to a largely "private" model, in which paying patients came to expect their own rooms—and nice rooms at that. Pulling his hair for inspiration, Hospital Director Wilhelm initiated what would come to be known as the Brigham "minimal room" system, based on the ergonomics of train travel:

> *While occupying a roomette on a trip, great admiration suddenly developed for the designers of these Pullman car accommodations, who worked with square inches instead of square feet. Here was a very small room, which provided that precious ingredient everyone desires—privacy—and at a reasonable price. One would not care to be quartered too long in such a small area, but for a few days it was most acceptable. In addition to privacy, there were all the necessary facilities; wash basin with running water, drinking water, mirror and toilet—all skillfully arranged in a compact area of about 20 square feet! Why couldn't these same principles be applied to patients' rooms?*[112]

At the same time, increased funding was available for hospital construction through the 1946 Hill-Burton Act, by which Congress opened up federal funds for hospital expansion as the cornerstone of a hospital-based postwar public health system.[113] Although Moore, like many physicians of his day, was increasingly critical of the spectre of "socialized medicine," he found much to celebrate in the Hill-Burton Act's contribution to American teaching hospitals:

> *Support of the federal government in the building program of voluntary University Hospitals might be regarded by some as an inroad of socialized medicine. But in contrast to some other forms of federal support of medical care, it marks the return of public funds to the fountainhead from which has come the great advance in medicine and surgery in the last hundred years: the University Hospital.*[114]

PETER BENT BRIGHAM HOSPITAL

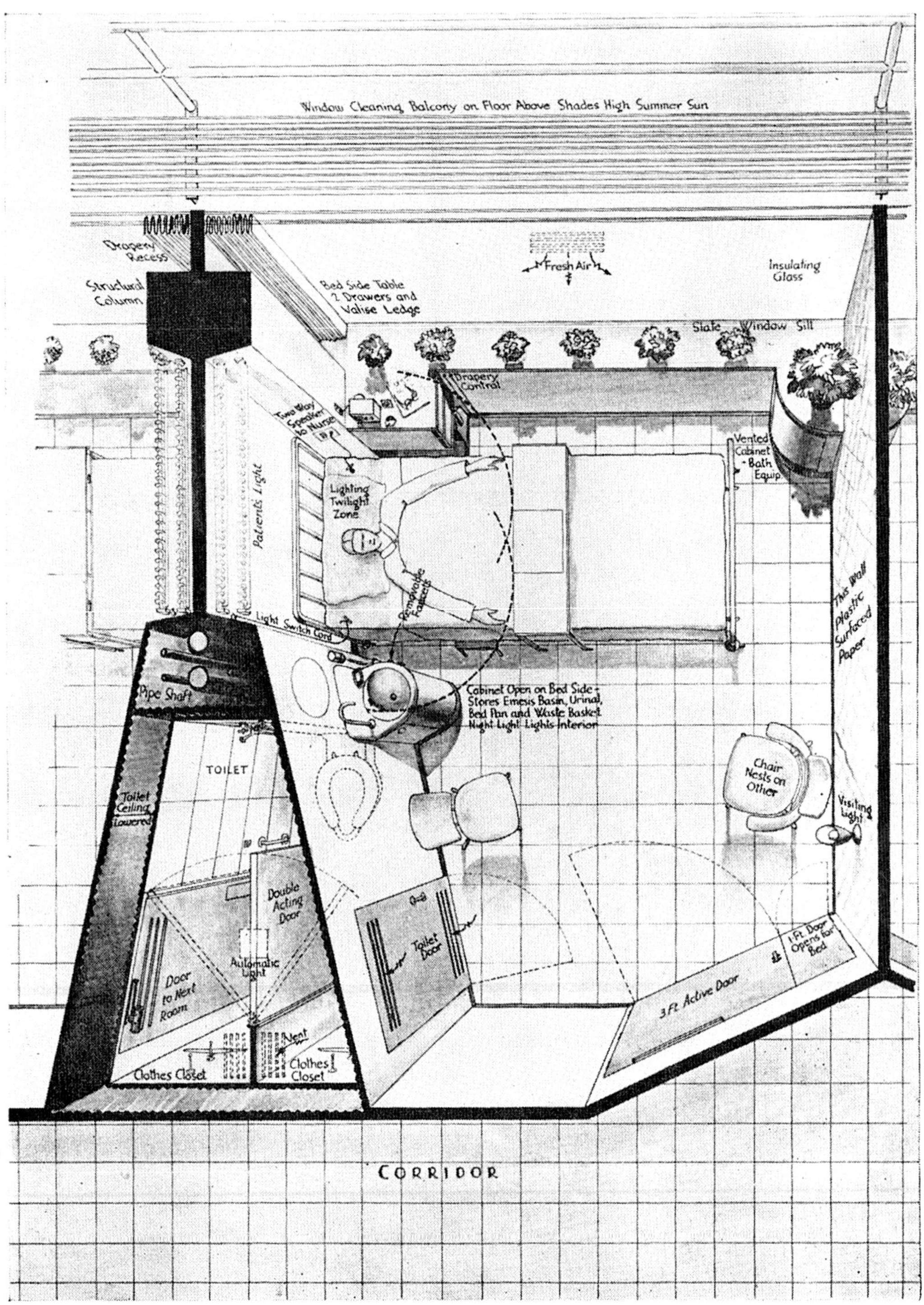

Designed by Markus & Nocka, Architects, Boston, Massachusetts

FIGURE 1-29 The "minimal room" design in 1950: Markus and Nocka, architects.

THE BRIGHAM AND ITS COMMUNITIES

The transformation and growth of the PBBH in the second half of the twentieth century reflected responses to changes in technologies as well as social conditions unimaginable by Flexner, Cushing, or Christian half a century prior. By the end of the 1950s, it was clear to all that the piecemeal revision of the PBBH was insufficient to manage the increasingly complex and voluminous work of clinical care, research, and teaching. Moore's critique of the obsolescence of the pavilion model in 1960 was paired with hopes that a radically redesigned, truly modern vertical hospital might rise from its ashes. By 1961, Moore's hopes had crystallized in the formation of a Hospital Planning Committee. As Charles Barnes, the Brigham's president, wrote,

> *[A] combination of the now separate facilities of the Boston Lying-in Hospital, the Free Hospital for Women, the Massachusetts Eye and Ear Infirmary, and the Peter Bent Brigham and Robert Breck Brigham Hospitals in close association with the Children's Hospital Medical Center will provide a potential in medical care, teaching, and research which will far exceed the total now provided by these institutions operating separately.*[115]

By 1962 this group was named the Affiliated Hospitals Center, Inc., and hinged on a real estate promise. As part of this deal, the PBBH agreed to sell land to Harvard between 1962 and 1975, beginning with the site that would become the Countway Medical Library on the site of the former PBBH nurse's residence. By 1967, the Free Hospital for Women and the Boston Lying-In Hospital had merged to form the Boston Hospital for Women and, along with the PBBH and Robert Breck Brigham Hospital, had authored a joint venture working agreement called *A Plan for a Medical Center*, having decided not to wait for the Massachusetts Eye and Ear Infirmary and Children's to agree.[116]

Further progress would be muddled by serial departures of leadership in the joint venture, as well as by economic and political setbacks. However, the chief blow to the new Brigham came in 1969 when, on the eve of breaking ground on the long-anticipated vertical tower for patient care, Harvard backed away from its prior promise to deliver parcels of land across Francis Street. As Moore would later note, as part of the 1969 occupation of University Hall by Students for a Democratic Society, students at Harvard College and HMS had demanded that the University cease its "exploitative" development activities in poorer neighborhoods such as Roxbury and Dorchester.[117] To Moore, the idea that the expansion of a teaching hospital, whose identity was formed in its orientation toward students, would be hobbled by the antipathy of students themselves was a grotesque perversion of logic:

> *This small group of students had become intensely interested in the Affiliated Hospitals, and, as is so often the case with student protest, the issue became a deeply emotional one with a firm conviction that there was something innately evil about the Affiliated Hospitals Center. This was an unreasoned hate, oriented towards a target rather than carrying a mission. It was intent on bringing down people and institutions without respect to any good that might result for the sick or the community itself, and without the presentation of any sensible alternative plan.*[118]

However, Moore came to realize that the anger that had motivated so many of the students was built around a nucleus of a reasonable critique of the Brigham and HMS. Like so many other urban academic medical centers, the PBBH had been built on the basis of accessibility to a poor urban "public ward" population that functioned as a substrate of medical education and medical research in ways that did not always prioritize the "care of sick persons in indigent circumstances" that Peter Bent Brigham had originally described. As Moore admitted:

> *[T]he events of last summer showed that amongst our students there was another group demonstrating remarkable ability and surprising devotion to the actual task at hand: betterment of the living conditions of the people in the Francis Street area. These students, less given to public protest, had actually*

gone to live in this area and had spent hot summer days trying to improve the lot of the residents of the area, and had brought to light a feature of University administration that was truly most unfortunate and contrary to any social aim of a public institution: namely, that having purchased these plots of land, the University gave the landlord function over to a real estate operator who had little regard for niceties, who let the dwellings deteriorate beyond repair, and who seemed to be motivated solely by a desire to make the dwellings so uninhabitable as to drive the residents away.

Many of us concerned with the Hospitals and the University felt a sense of responsibility: As members of the Staff of the Brigham Hospital we should have been aware of what was going on in these neighborhood dwellings and should have insisted on decent management of inhabited dwellings.[119]

The Brigham could, and should, do a better job of demonstrating its commitments to the communities it was supposed to serve. To move forward, its leaders perceived a need to build more community centers, talk more clearly with students about community outreach, and—in what would become a frequent refrain for Moore and Thorn over the 1960s and 1970s—do a better job of making its community commitments clear. And as K. Frank Austen writes elsewhere in this volume, such community commitments were, indeed, clarified (with Austen himself, along with Eugene Braunwald, HMS Dean Robert Ebert, and social scientist Stephen Miller playing key roles) before the merger would take place.

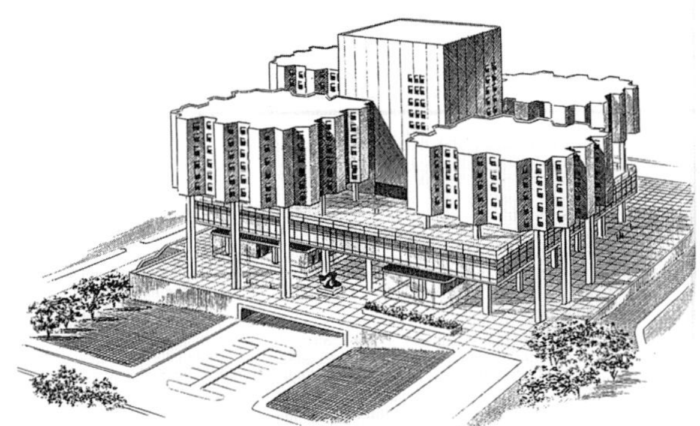

FIGURE 1-30 Affiliated Hospitals building design concept, 1969.

The Brigham had, in fact, invested in community health for several decades, if not always in the most visible ways. Thorn had seen the need for an expanded "Out-Door Department" in the aftermath of World War II, as the hospital took on "increased obligation for the medical care of the neighborhood surrounding our institution."[120] The Out-Door Department had been expanded into an Out-Patient Department in 1947;[121] and by 1961 the Brigham had taken on responsibility for emergency cases from Brookline, Roxbury, Jamaica Plain, and West Roxbury. This had led to the renaming of the Emergency Ward the "Emergency Service"—a joint project of surgery and medicine—and the opening of a refurbished Emergency Service building in 1966.[122]

By the early 1960s, though, reflecting national attention to the need for what would soon be termed "primary care," the hospital director became concerned that an academic institution like the Brigham might be seen as merely a collection of specialists with little interest in the general care of the community, and he worked to reorganize the general clinics to be more accessible to the daily needs of local populations:

Under the new arrangement, each patient is under the guidance of one physician, who is responsible for the patient's total care. Patients do not have to shuttle back and forth between various specialty clinics. In contrast to the former custom whereby a doctor was assigned to the clinic for a short period of time, the reorganization of the clinic provides for the continuous and long supervision of a patient by a single physician.[123]

Thorn would likewise worry openly that the PBBH's success in producing "physician-scientists" might paradoxically alienate it from the surrounding communities that it served; the hospital also needed to be successful in "improving patient care beyond the hospital walls."[124] In 1963 he suggested this trend might be stemmed by creating more physician *social* scientists (a proposition that placed him increasingly at odds with his surgical counterpart). As Thorn admitted:

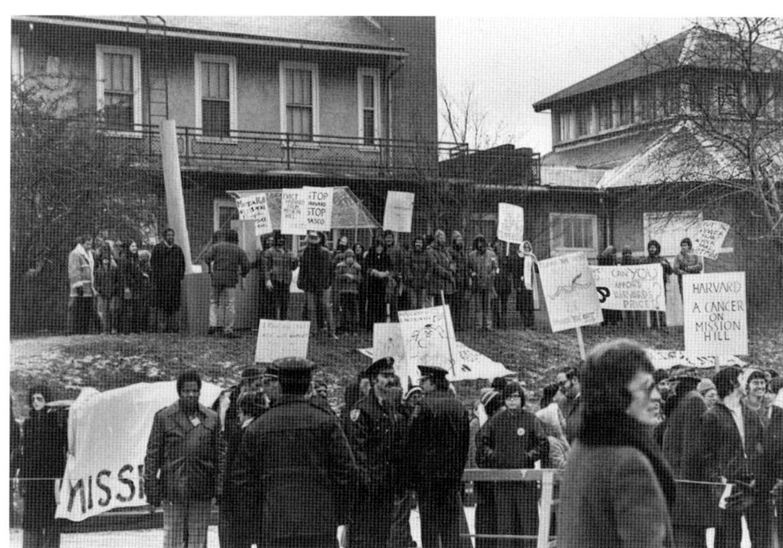

FIGURE 1-31 Harvard student protests, circa 1969.

"Some will argue the fact that the teaching hospital need not accept responsibility for medical care beyond its walls, stating that this is the province of departments of preventive medicine or schools of public health." However, he considered that preventive medicine and public health could only be realized through engagement with academic medicine:

> *In reviewing the methods by which a department of medicine can and perhaps should move in relation to these particular problems, it is pertinent to suggest that here is a key role for the social scientist... The university hospital with its problems of patient care, undergraduate and postgraduate physicians' training as well as the education of nurses, dietitians and technicians, its research program in clinical investigation as well as basic science, would appear to be an ideal laboratory for the social scientist.*[125]

This reflected changes in the province of academic medicine far beyond Flexner's original 1910 vision. As Washington University's William Danforth wrote in the *Journal of the American Medical Association* in 1969:

> *The obligations of medical schools to society differ from those of an earlier day in being more complex and frequently only partially defined... All of us in medicine must certainly feel a deep sense of responsibility, not only for patients under our care, but also for the future of biochemical and biophysical research and the social consequences of this work, for the relevancy of medical curricula, for the substandard health of the poor and the black, for the rising cost of medical care, for the quantitative as well as the qualitative aspects of the education of physicians and other health professionals, for population control, for the purity of air and water; and so the list could go on and on.*[126]

After its plans for a "vertical hospital" were blocked by student protests alleging the Brigham's perceived disinterest in the communities it served, the hospital began a public campaign of community center construction. At the same time, as Andrew Jessiman and Ann Conway write elsewhere in this volume (and catalyzed by the efforts of Jessiman, Richard Nesson, Joseph Dorsey, and economist Jerome Pollock), the new Harvard Community Health Plan began to develop prepaid health programs, including for those in the nearby Mission Hill Housing Project.[127] These years likewise saw the establishment of the Martha Eliot Health Center (catalyzed again by Jessiman's efforts), the Southern Jamaica Plain Health Center, and a hospital-based

Spanish-language clinic. Additionally, as part of this response, by 1971 the hospital's trustees had "elected representatives of minority and neighborhood groups to the governing board of the Hospital."[128] In 1970 the PBBH hired Harold May, an African-American surgeon and former Tuskegee Airman who had been director of a hospital in Haiti for 15 years, as the head of a new division of community health and medical care. These forms of institutional outreach to the communities would become common across academic hospitals in the 1970s, as largely urban institutions sought to shake off critiques that they functioned parasitically off of the racial and economic disparities of American cities. In his final reports, Thorn stressed that finding ways to serve better the surrounding communities of the Brigham would be more vital to the future of the institution than any physical expansion of the hospital plant itself.

FROM PBBH TO PARTNERS

The Thorn/Moore partnership would end in 1972 with Thorn's retirement. Moore would follow suit a few years later, and they would be followed by the dynamic cardiologist Eugene Braunwald and the enterprising vascular surgeon John Mannick. And yet, however larger-than-life one might paint a figure such as Eugene Braunwald (indeed, quite large, as he was able to serve as editor of *Harrison's Principles of Internal Medicine*, author of the definitive textbook on heart disease, and chair of medicine at both PBBH and the Beth Israel Hospital at the same time), unlike the Christian/Cushing, Weiss/Cutler, or even the Thorn/Moore eras, it was no longer possible to sketch out the character of the activities of the teaching hospital in terms of the visions of the physician- and surgeon-in-chiefs alone.

This was a product of two related changes. The first involved new relations with local partner institutions. The Robert Breck Brigham Hospital (RBBH), funded by Peter's younger brother, had opened its Mission Hill facility in 1914, soon serving as a pioneering teaching hospital devoted to arthritic and rheumatological conditions. The Boston Lying-In Hospital, founded in 1832, had been one of the nation's first maternity hospitals, while the Free Hospital for Women had been founded in 1875 "for poor women affected with diseases peculiar to their sex or in need of surgical aid." The Boston Lying-In Hospital and the Free Hospital for Women merged in 1966 to form the Boston Hospital for Women (BHW), and in 1975, the three institutions (PBBH, RBBH, and the BHW) formally merged. With the stroke of a pen, academic medicine and surgery no longer defined the hospital—they shared it with gynecology, obstetrics, neonatology, anesthesiology, neurology, psychiatry, orthopedics, radiation medicine, and a rapidly growing list of other departments—including nursing. Braunwald's role in editing *Harrison's*, for example, would be matched by Stanley Robbins and Ramzi Cotran's eponymous stewardship of the *Pathologic Basis of Disease*, or Radiologist-in-Chief Herbert Abrams' authorship of the first textbook in interventional radiology, the eponymous *Abrams' Angiography*. By 1975, the merged hospital had appointed a vice-president for nursing, Marion L. Metcalf, whose annual report was understood to be as essential to the institution as Braunwald's or Mannick's.

The second change was more internal to the departments, a byproduct of growth. The Department of Medicine Thorn handed to Braunwald in 1972 was the polar opposite of the depleted pool of physicians that had awaited Thorn when he began his tenure as physician-in-chief in 1942.[129] As Thorn himself had described, the Department had grown into an unrecognizable and in many ways impossible bureaucracy, like a small town that suddenly realizes it has turned into a sprawling metropolis. As he noted in his final annual report:

> *Consider the breadth of activities encompassed by our department of medicine. At one end of the spectrum we have a full scale Division of Medical Biology with its great strength in biophysics and biochemistry—stronger in talent than many of the basic science departments now functioning in medical schools. Supplementing this area of scientific investigation are mathematicians and laboratories of steroid biochemistry, bacteriology*

and physiology—the latter being primarily related to cardiovascular and pulmonary function. These laboratories are supplemented by the clinical divisions, numbering more than fifteen, responsible for the care of patients and advances in the application of new knowledge. The clinical divisions include renal, endocrine-metabolic, hematology, neurology, and psychiatry as well as units devoted to the care and study of alcoholics and other drug addictions, a psychology testing laboratory, a division of clinical pharmacology and one of communications medicine![130]

If Thorn and Moore had presided over a "golden age" of expansion for American biomedical research largely centered on the academic hospital, Braunwald and Mannick would inherit a series of challenges in its aftermath, in an age, after the passage of Medicare and Medicaid, of increasing national attention to the costs of medical care. They were, paradoxically, taking over at a time when an incredible array of new benefits of biomedicine and meaningful discoveries might yet further impact the morbidity and mortality of individuals and communities, yet at the same time inheriting an incredibly complex bureaucracy in an era of increasing financial self-examination. This is not to state this would be an era of contraction; indeed, just the opposite took place. Under Mannick, the funding for surgical research continued to expand, from $1.25 million to $12 million by end of his tenure, and the surgical staff grew from 23 to 68 full-time surgeons. Under Braunwald, the total full-time faculty in medicine grew from 180 to more than 500, and the research income in the Department of Medicine rose from less than $10 million per year as of 1981 to more than $80 million per year by the time of his retirement in 1996.[131] However, it did take place in an era mandating the justification for such measures and practice. If the Brigham of Thorn and Moore represented the growth spurt of American academic medicine, the Brigham of Braunwald and Mannick required tools for managing a sustainable trajectory of growth and development.

BIOGRAPHY

JOHN A. MANNICK

Anthony D. Whittemore

In 1976, John A. Mannick succeeded Francis D. Moore as the surgeon-in-chief of the Peter Bent Brigham Hospital and Moseley Professor of Surgery at the Harvard Medical School. A graduate of Harvard College and Harvard Medical School, his surgical training at the Massachusetts General Hospital set him on course for an outstanding surgical career. He was recruited to the faculty at the Medical College of Virginia under the leadership of former Brighamite David M. Hume, where his clinical interest in vascular surgery developed, and his research career in transplant biology and immunosuppression began to take shape. In 1973, he became surgeon-in-chief at the Boston University Medical Center, prior to his move across town to the Brigham.

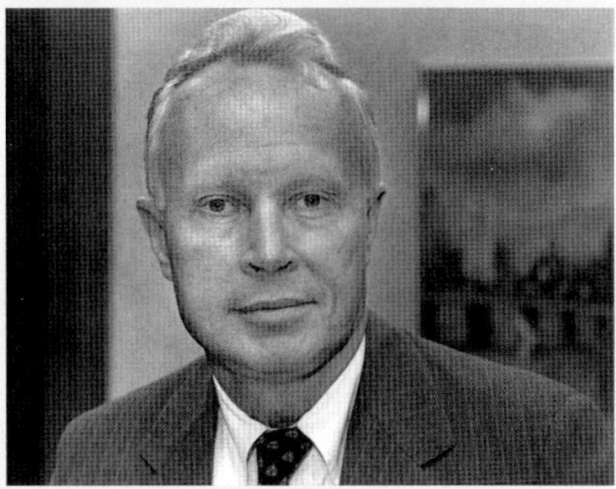

FIGURE 1-32 John Mannick.

During his eighteen years of leadership, from 1976 through 1994, in which the Brigham affiliated with the Robert Breck Brigham Hospital and the Boston Hospital for Women, Mannick expanded the Department of Surgery from 25 to 70 active surgeons, with an attendant increase in operative cases from 8,000 to 25,000 per year. He created the divisions of vascular, thoracic, and trauma surgery and nurtured substantial programs in the emerging fields of cardiac and pulmonary transplantation. He maintained a major focus on research, as department funding increased from $1 million to $12 million annually.

During this time, the surgical education program expanded to accommodate the demands created by the new divisions and the increased operative volume. In addition, the program made the challenging transition from the independent "super chief" general surgical service, run by a sixth-year resident/junior attending physician, to three services fully staffed around the clock by attending physicians. Moreover, the breadth of general surgery became more diversified, reflective of the development of more challenging and sophisticated subspecialty procedures. Subspecialty training became the norm after general surgical board eligibility. As an increasing number of fellows were added to the specialty training programs, constant vigilance by staff surgeons, to ensure adequate operative experience for the general surgical residents and specialty fellows, became essential. Of the graduates of the training program, 92% entered academic practice with full-time faculty appointments.

Mannick maintained an active research laboratory that was continuously funded throughout his career and well beyond his assumption of emeritus status. His primary interest and the bulk of his 250 original publications reflect his investigative efforts aimed at a better understanding of the immunosuppressive response to trauma and sepsis.

BIOGRAPHY

EUGENE BRAUNWALD

Thomas H. Lee, Jr.

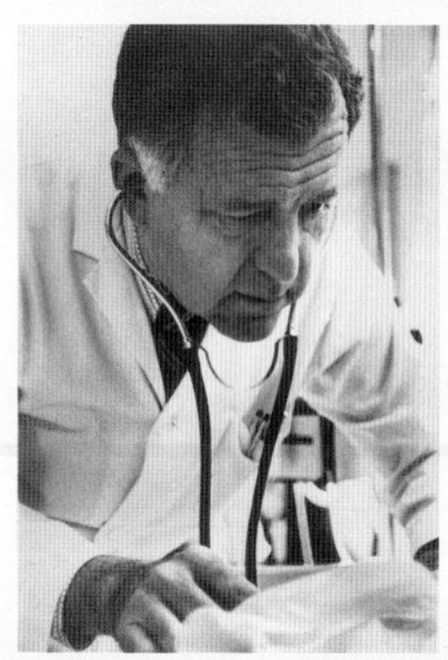

FIGURE 1-33 Eugene Braunwald.

Eugene Braunwald was chair of the department of medicine at the Brigham and Hersey Professor of the Theory and Practice of Physic at Harvard Medical School (HMS) from 1972 to 1996. During his tenure, the Brigham moved to front ranks of the world's great departments of medicine and a generation of leaders of academic medicine received their training on its wards and in its laboratories.

Braunwald's career reflects the rise of American academic medicine in the second half of the twentieth century. He was born in 1929 in Vienna and had an idyllic childhood until the *Anschluss*, the 1938 annexation of Austria by Nazi Germany, which led to widespread persecution of Jews. The family had a harrowing escape, first to England, and then to Brooklyn, where Braunwald completed his high school requirements at age sixteen. He attended New York University (NYU) for his undergraduate and medical education. He was the last applicant admitted to his class at the medical school, reflecting the Jewish quotas at the time, and he graduated first in his class. He married his classmate, Nina Starr, who later became the first female cardiac surgeon as well as the first surgeon, male or female, to perform a mitral valve replacement, just a day after the first aortic valve replacement by Dwight Harken in 1960.

In the spring of 1953, while an intern at the Mount Sinai Hospital, Braunwald learned that he would not be permitted to continue his residency because of his likelihood of being drafted. Thus he signed on for a research fellowship at Mount Sinai and then for a second one at NYU with Andre Cournand, a future Nobel laureate who developed cardiac catheterization. His fellowships were extraordinarily successful, and this helped him secure an appointment at the National Institutes of Health (NIH). The NIH years, 1955-1968, unparalleled in research productivity, established him as cardiology's leading investigator while he was only in his early thirties. Highlights of his many accomplishments include the following:

- Recognition that myocardial infarction is a dynamic process that plays out over hours and that interventions that reduce oxygen consumption can reduce the damage to the heart and improve prognosis.
- Discovery and characterization of hypertrophic cardiomyopathy, a common cause of sudden death.
- Development of diagnostic techniques, including measurement of left ventricular ejection fraction and trans-septal cardiac catheterization.
- Description of the natural history of aortic stenosis, recommending that surgery be performed when patients develop chest pain, heart failure, or syncope.

In 1968, Braunwald left the NIH to participate in creating a new medical school at the University of California, San Diego, his first experience as a leader of a department of medicine. Unfortunately, cutbacks to the University of California system were introduced by governor Ronald Reagan. Braunwald realized that his ambitious visions for the school would not come to pass in his lifetime. When the opportunity to succeed George Thorn at the Brigham arose, Braunwald took it, becoming the tenth Hersey Professor at the HMS and the fourth physician-in-chief at the Peter Bent Brigham Hospital.

When Braunwald arrived in Boston in July 1972, he learned that plans for a new hospital to house the old Peter Bent Brigham Hospital, the Robert Breck Brigham Hospital, and the Boston Hospital for Women were on hold because the required Certificate of Need had been rejected. Later, he learned that funding from HMS to support the revitalization of the Brigham's Department of Medicine would be minimal at best. His Boston tenure was off to a rocky start. For the next several years, Braunwald addressed the complex politics of the merger of the three hospitals and the opening of the new facility, while also creating innovations to advance his department from "good" to "great." He hired Marshall A. Wolf to direct the housestaff program. Together they developed several additional new residency tracks: primary care, one of the first in the country; research, the "hemi-doc" track; and global health. By the end of the 1970s, physician educators generally considered the Brigham's medical residency to be the best place to launch a career in academic medicine. He created a faculty practice plan for all clinical activities for full-time members of medicine. The funds that came to his division chiefs and to him were used to subsidize clinical activities that were inadequately compensated (e.g., infectious diseases), research, and teaching. He fostered a close relationship with the Harvard Community Health Plan (HCHP), an innovative new staff-model health maintenance organization. He appointed and mentored new division chiefs who embodied the "triple threat" model Braunwald had helped create at the NIH—physicians who excelled at teaching, research, and patient care. The result of these and other streams of work was the emergence of the Brigham's Department of Medicine as a world leader in patient care, teaching, and research. Braunwald is the first to say that he did not accomplish this progress on his own, noting that his close relationships with Marshall Wolf, Brigham president H. Richard Nesson, and HCHP medical director Joseph L. Dorsey were critical to the success of the triple threat culture.

Braunwald stepped down as chair of medicine in 1996, but did not retire. He had created the Thrombolysis in Myocardial Infarction research group in 1984 and led it until 2010. In 2012, he devoted most of his time to leading clinical trials that improve the treatment of myocardial infarction, heart failure, and other aspects of cardiovascular disease. Asked what other Brigham research experience was most satisfying, he cited the SAVE (Survival and Ventricular Enlargement) study, which demonstrated first in rats and then in humans that the angiotensin inhibitor drug captopril reduced damage (i.e., infarct size) from myocardial infarction. In the subsequent SAVE study, a large multinational randomized trial, captopril reduced deaths after myocardial infarction by 19%. Braunwald loved the SAVE experience because it began where he began—in a laboratory, exploring a physiological concept with animal models. Then it moved to human research, then to a large clinical trial, and, ultimately, by effecting a change in the practice of medicine, to a substantial innovation in care.

Eugene Braunwald was a member of the editorial board of *Harrison's Principles of Internal Medicine* from 1967, while the sixth edition was being planned, until 2009, with the publication of the seventeenth edition. The current, eighteenth edition of this major text is dedicated to him, "our colleague, teacher, mentor, and friend. . . His indelible impact on the institutions he has led, the practice of cardiology, medical education, this textbook, and the many individuals whom he has trained will continue to be felt in future generations."[132]

Medical financing and medical research had become increasingly complex in an era of managed care and competition from for-profit hospital chains and for-profit contract research organizations.[133] Patient care had also become equally complicated through the further burgeoning of specialties and technologies, despite the formal advent of primary care. The importance of managing this complexity was underscored by the 1977 appointment of H. Richard Nesson (for whom the backbone holding the hospital together, the Nesson Pike, would later be named) as Vice-President of Ambulatory and Community Care. Praising Nesson's appointment, Braunwald called for the continuing need for people who could manage complexity and who could buttress the hospital's new emphasis on primary care as well as specialty care; he hoped that Nesson's leadership might help clinical care at the Brigham "put the patient together again."[134] Nesson launched a primary care residency program in 1978; one of the first graduates of this program, Phyllis Jen, would redesign the series of primary care clinics through which the Brigham continues to train physicians while closely listening to and meeting the needs of its surrounding communities.

By January 1, 1975, as noted earlier, the legal merger of the PBBH, RBBH, and BHW finally had taken effect with the official formation of the Affiliated Hospitals Center (AHC). PBBH was now one division of a larger hospital spanning three campuses, which hoped soon to occupy a consolidated structure. For many years still, this would be an aspirational future that nonetheless colored and motivated organizational tasks. Ground was finally broken on the new hospital tower in December 1976; an artist's sketch of the new tower formed the cover of the AHC's annual report in 1977; the same cover in 1978 was graced with a photograph of the completed shell of the tower; and the move of laboratory faculty began in 1979 and of clinical services in earnest in 1980. In that year, the AHC became the Brigham and Women's Hospital.

The structure of the new hospital tower reflected a fundamentally different vision of the ordering of clinical, research, and teaching spaces from the "pavilion hospital" of the late nineteenth century. An edifice

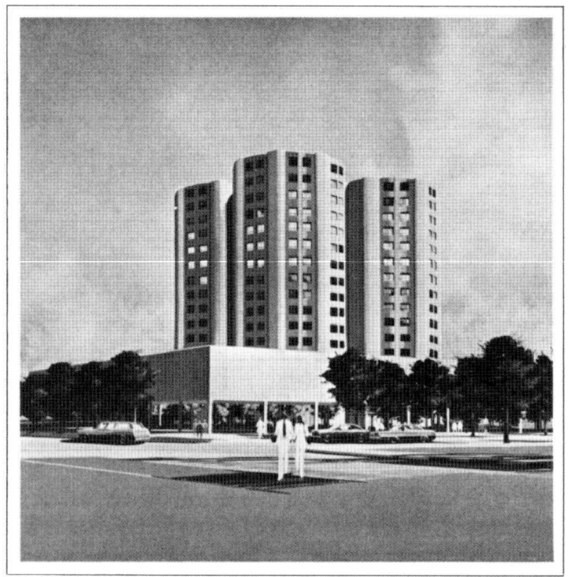

FIGURE 1-34 Artist's sketch of the new tower. *Annual Report* cover, 1977.

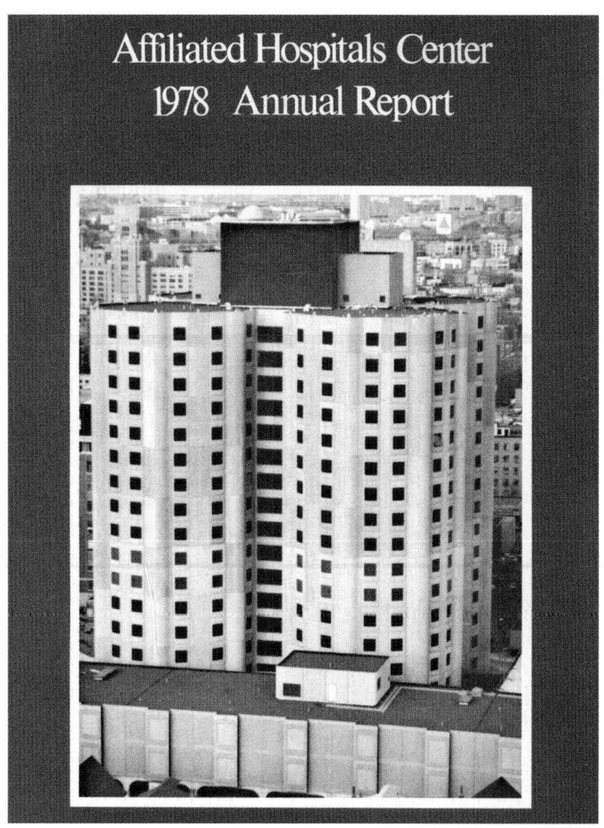

FIGURE 1-35 Photograph of the completed shell of the tower. *Annual Report* cover, 1978.

a monthly bulletin published for employees, medical staff,
corporation members, trustees, campaign workers and auxilians
AUGUST 1980
Inside
BRIGHAM and
WOMEN'S HOSPITAL

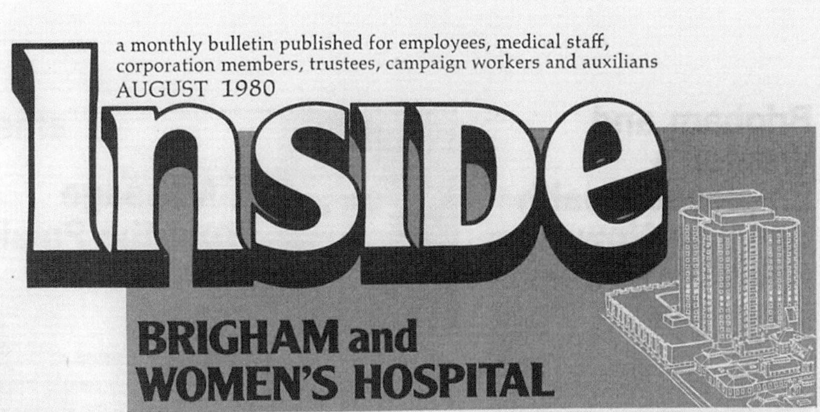

It's Goodbye, Divisions . . . Hello, Brigham and Women's !

TA-DAY IS
1980
JULY
9
191 WEDNESDAY 175
Everyone take Notice
Attn. Everyone! effective Immediately
Please claim any personal belongings or articles left in the nurses station and throughout the unit. We are presently cleaning and organizing everything in the unit for the move to the new hospital in July. We are discarding unclaimed articles.
Thank you Bill.
J. King

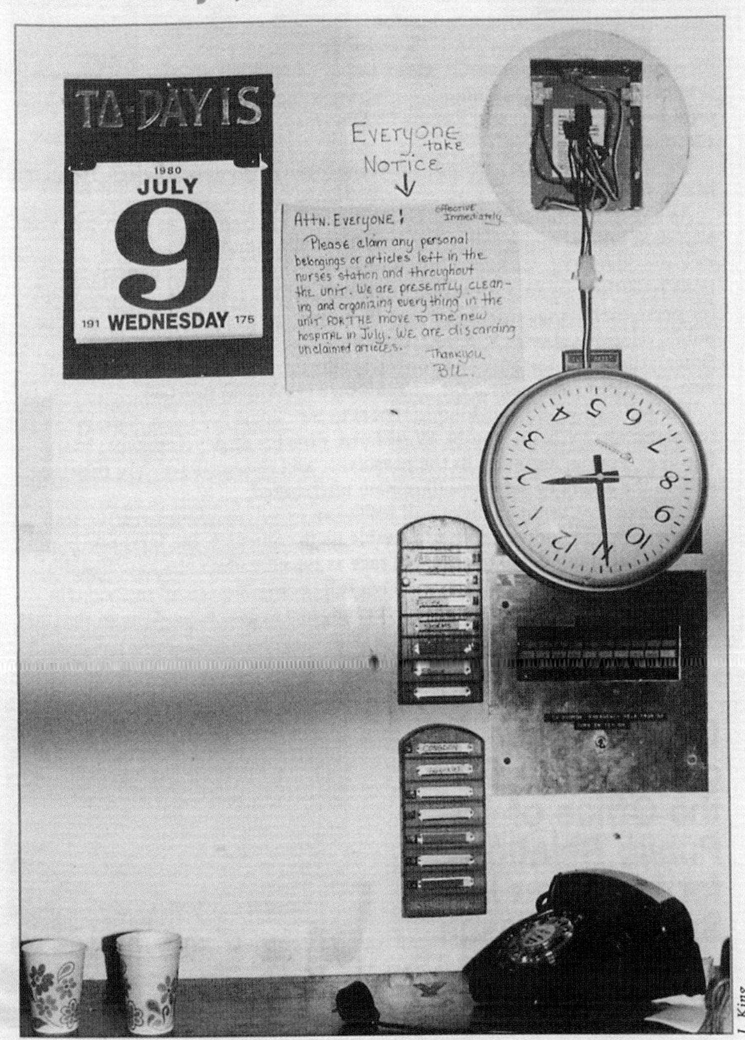

It was a task that could have boggled the mind of the most brilliant strategist. But the first phase of the Brigham and Women's Hospital's move to a new facility went well, on schedule and with a minimum of surprises, according to Brigham and Women's director of relocation Arthur Stomberg.

On Wednesday, July 9, nearly 250 patients were moved from units in the Peter Bent Brigham Hospital to new units on floors 7,8,9,10,11 and 12 of the new bed tower—an event accomplished in a remarkable nine hours. It took a full nursing staff (supplemented by nurses from nursing administration, staff education and the School of Nursing), as well as a temporary manpower pool of more than 100 volunteers from numerous departments, 20 administrators, 16 unit management coordinators, six special transport teams for critically ill patients, two special code teams for potential emergencies, 20 handymen/engineers and 40 movers and supervisors from an independent moving firm. It also took a lot of cooperation and hard work from everyone on the Brigham and Women's staff—from housekeeping and security to those in administrative departments who held down the fort while coworkers assisted in the patient moves.

For nursing staff, whose priority was assuring patient care, comfort and safety, move day was the cul-

Continued on pages 10–14

FIGURE 1-36 The move to Brigham and Women's Hospital. From *Inside Brigham and Women's Hospital*, August 1980.

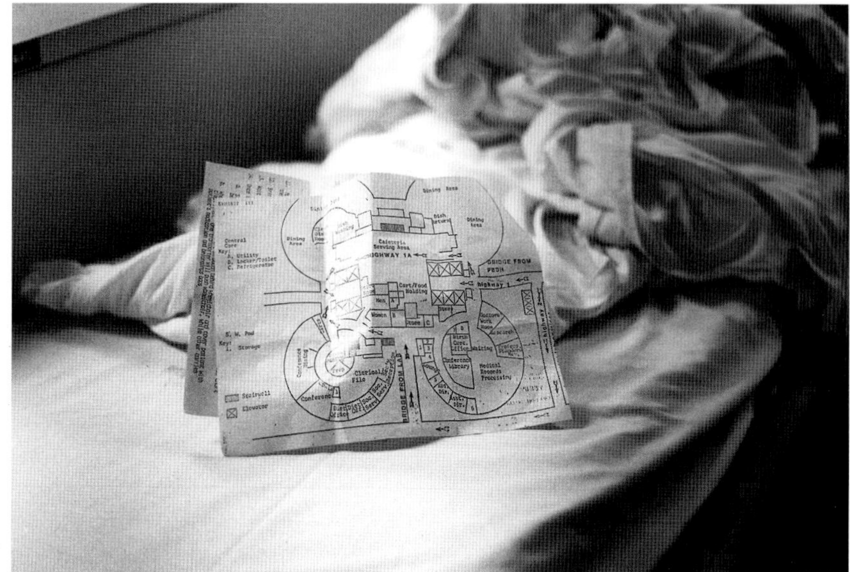

FIGURE 1-37 Blueprint of the tower on a hospital bed.

of patient care and medical education (the "tower") would rest on a "platform" of diagnostic and therapeutic services: the clinical laboratories, the operating rooms, and the radiology suites.[135] Eyeing the possibilities for further transformative spaces of patient care as the ground was first broken on the new building, the director of nursing expressed hope that the new building would allow for the more complex gradations of levels of care: unit, bed, stepdown, specialty ward.[136] The tower, once built, greatly expanded the capacity of the hospital, although the move from ward to tower would prove emotional for medical and nursing staff alike. The radial design of tower pods allowed for easier monitoring of patients from centrally located nursing stations, although physicians soon grumbled that the curving hallways gave them no safe place to gather for morning rounds. For those who could not wait for the congested elevators at peak times, the sixteen-floor stairwell offered a means of combining cardiovascular exercise with clinical care.

CONCLUSIONS

It is a central irony of the institution that only at the end of the twentieth century could the Brigham claim to have the physical plant of a twentieth-century hospital. Paradoxically, at the very moment that the Brigham could boast a "vertical hospital" that compared with its chief rival across Boston, new economic realities forced both hospitals to rethink that rivalry. In 1994, BWH and MGH announced the formation of what would become the state's largest healthcare provider, Partners HealthCare, with Richard Nesson as its first chief executive officer and Samuel Thier as its first president.

The Partners merger shook the healthcare field and helped to set off a scramble for other hospital mergers across most major metropolitan areas within the United States.[137] In Massachusetts, the Spaulding Rehabilitation Hospital and McLean Hospital immediately joined the partnership, which would continue to expand throughout the early twenty-first century. Braunwald stepped down as chair of the medicine department in 1996, to be replaced by Victor Dzau, who himself would be succeeded in 2005 by Joseph Loscalzo. Mannick likewise stepped down as chair of the surgery department in 1994, replaced by Michael Zinner. Later chapters in this work follow their roles in the further development of the Brigham, along with the careers of many other department chairs in a complex institution no longer defined by the fields of medicine and surgery alone.

BIOGRAPHY

VICTOR J. DZAU

Peter V. Tishler

Serving in several positions at the Brigham at different times, including chief resident, clinician/cardiologist, care provider, and chair of the Department of Medicine, Victor Dzau has a tremendous affection for and appreciation of the Brigham as an exemplary hospital, healthcare system, research enterprise, and educational resource.

Dzau returned to the Brigham after completing his cardiology fellowship at the Massachusetts General Hospital. He thrived in this then-relatively small hospital. His research on the pathobiology of the renin-angiotensin system paved the way for both elucidating the importance of this system in cardiovascular disease and creating therapeutic cardiovascular medications. He moved briefly (1990-1994) to Stanford University as chief of cardiology, then chief of medicine and director of research, but "ran" back to the Brigham to assume similar roles as Hersey Professor of the Theory and Practice of Physic (1996-2004). This caused him some early anxiety, because "so many greats had been at the Brigham prior to me." He innovated profusely. He passionately embraced the work of young physicians Paul E. Farmer and Jim Y. Kim in Partners in Health. Making Farmer and Kim and their missions available to others, he created the Division of Global Health in 2003. He led in the creation of new divisions, including Women's Health (with Paula A. Johnson), Pharmacoepidemiology and Pharmacoeconomics (with Jerome L. Avorn), and several not-so-conventional programs. As a devout researcher and director of research at the Brigham, he encouraged interdisciplinary investigations and worked with others, including physicians Michael A. Gimbrone, Jr. and Dennis L Kasper, to create the Biomedical Research Institute. And, of course, his fostering of major genetics/genomics research at the Brigham, which is exerting "an important impact on medicine," was the beginning of the current huge effort in these spheres of human investigation.

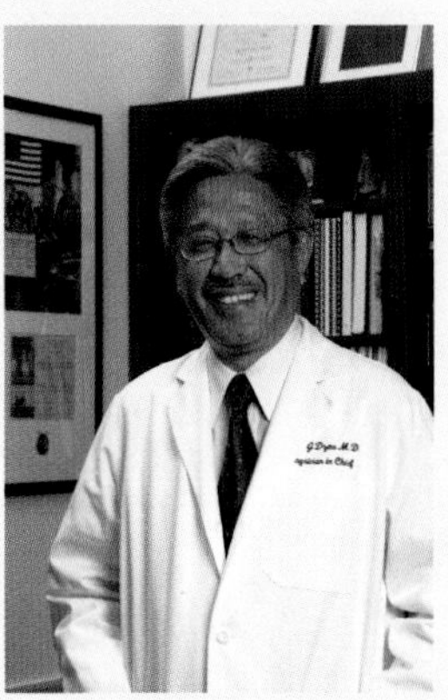

FIGURE 1-38 Victor Dzau.

In the manner of Francis Weld Peabody, Victor was dedicated to the care of patients with "wisdom and mercy" and to shaping the "right minds" of young physicians to practice this way. He was convinced that the pipeline of eminent trainees at the Brigham was unparalleled and that the Brigham was among the best in patient care and education. He clearly embraces all goals of contemporary medicine.

Victor left the Brigham in 2004 to join Duke University as the James C. Duke Professor of Medicine and chancellor and chief executive officer of its healthcare system. He returns to the Brigham every year to attend the annual lecture on global health that is named in his honor and to reconnect with his friends and former associates. At Duke, he is leading efforts similar to those that he led at the Brigham. Additionally, he is leading in the period of medical readjustment to meet the federal mandate of increased care for populations while decreasing the costs of medical care. He states: "Physician scientists, evidence-based medicine, specialty medicine, and community medicine will all come out with the right balance and the right way."[138]

BIOGRAPHY

MICHAEL J. ZINNER

Peter V. Tishler

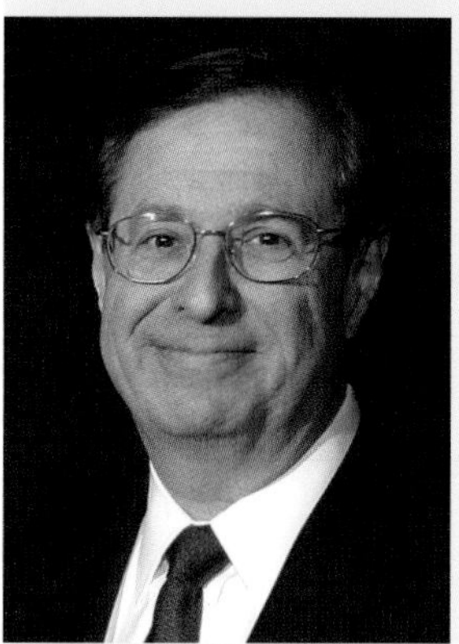

FIGURE 1-39 Michael Zinner.

Michael Zinner is currently surgeon-in-chief and chair of the department of surgery at Brigham and Women's Hospital; clinical director of the Dana Farber/Brigham and Women's Cancer Center; executive director of the Center for Surgery and Public Health, Brigham and Women's Hospital, Harvard Medical School, and Harvard School of Public Health; and Moseley Professor of Surgery at Harvard Medical School. He received his MD at the University of Florida School of Medicine in 1971 and completed his residency in surgery at the Johns Hopkins Hospital in 1979. He was chief of surgery at the UCLA School of Medicine for six years before assuming his post at the Brigham in 1994.

Zinner's role and activities at the Brigham reflect his enthusiasm and energy. He is totally committed to nurturing, successful care of patients and to the education, training, and mentoring of younger colleagues. Many of his protégés have assumed leadership roles at the Brigham and throughout the nation. Zinner encourages individual research by members of his staff. He is personally involved, as are others, in the Center for Surgery and Public Health, which he developed in 2005 in collaboration with Harvard Medical School and Harvard School of Public Health. Established to bridge the gap between public health and surgical quality, safety, and access, its mission is "to save lives and improve the value of surgical care at the population level."

The size of the Department of Surgery has increased significantly since Zinner arrived. This includes the number of surgical beds and patient visits to the surgical clinics and also the number of full-time surgical staff. A major attraction of surgeons to his department is his enthusiasm, directness, and love of colleagues. This love affair must be mutual.

BIOGRAPHY

JOSEPH LOSCALZO

Peter V. Tishler

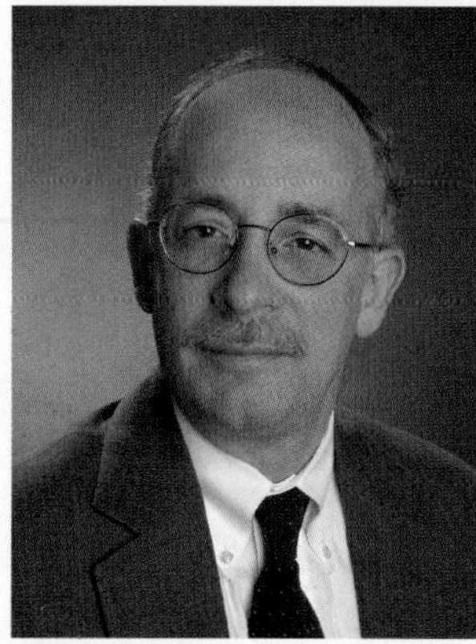

FIGURE 1-40 Joseph Loscalzo.

Joseph Loscalzo is the current chair of medicine and physician-in-chief at the Brigham and the Hersey Professor of the Theory and Practice of Physic at Harvard Medical School. He received his AB and PhD in biochemistry and MD from the University of Pennsylvania. He completed his residency in internal medicine and fellowship in cardiology at the Brigham and was medical chief resident in 1983-1984. He served on the staff of the Brigham and the Brockton-West Roxbury VA Medical Center until 1994, when he joined the faculty of Boston University School of Medicine. He rose rapidly to become the Wade Professor and Chair of Medicine, professor of biochemistry, and director of the Whitaker Cardiovascular Institute. He returned to the Brigham as Hersey Professor in 2005.

Loscalzo belongs to an illustrious group of physicians who have held this position since the opening of the Brigham: Henry A. Christian (1913-1939), Soma Weiss (1939-1942), George W. Thorn (1942-1972), Eugene Braunwald (1972-1996), and Victor J. Dzau

(1996-2004). All Hersey Professors have contributed in major ways to the growth and development of the Brigham. Loscalzo brings unique characteristics to this role. He is quiet and soft-spoken and wonderfully articulate and perceptive. And he has a quick sense of humor! He has had a passion during his entire professional life for science and research, progressing from relatively classical aspects of biochemistry through vascular biology to futuristic systems biology/network medicine as applied to the human condition. He is a cardiologist through and through, is actively involved in the progress and innovation in cardiology, and sees patients on the wards and in clinic. He is equally dedicated to the training of physicians and to fostering the intellectual development and research productivity of members of his staff. He cares for patients and is concerned, in the words of Francis D. Moore, that patients be treated "with wisdom and mercy." The extraordinary number of local and national awards to Joe Loscalzo, including honorary degrees and visiting professorships, is phenomenal for this relatively young man.

Joe is a man for all seasons.

Looking back on the major phases of the Brigham's evolution over the twentieth century—the foundational era of Cushing, Christian, Weiss, and Cutler, the growth years of Thorn and Moore, and the maturation of a complex institution in the Braunwald and Mannick era—raises a set of issues that will resonate throughout the rest of this volume. First, even before a spadeful of earth was turned to lay the foundations for the hospital on the corner of Francis Street and Huntington Avenue, the Brigham was understood by its founders and staff not just as a hospital, but as a physical manifestation of the abstract ideal values of American academic medicine. As an iconic American teaching hospital, the Brigham's internal and external spaces were designed to balance what Sir William Osler referred to as the three cardinal values of academic medicine: patient care, clinical research, and medical education. Second, however, we find that that design was neither perfect nor always prescient. As the pace and character of academic medicine changed over the twentieth century, new spaces were needed: novel research spaces, such as the Clinical Research Center; novel spaces for care, such as the Levine Cardiac Unit. However, in both of these cases, the new technological and structural capabilities of late-twentieth-century biomedicine needed to be superimposed on an architectural background based on nineteenth-century principles of pavilions and covered walkways. Tracing the piecemeal re-imagination of the spaces of the Brigham provides a palpable reminder of the contingent and path-dependent progress of modern medicine.

Third, as we review the development of Brigham and Women's Hospital at a century's remove from the founding of the PBBH, it is clear that Osler left out an important part of the Brigham's mission when he described the balance of clinical care, medical research, and pedagogy. This fourth task is the responsibility of the hospital to its *communities*: to the citizens of the neighborhoods around the Brigham, to its thousands of employees, and to populations halfway around the world who nonetheless can receive the Brigham's high standard of care through global outreach programs. Osler stated during his famed appearance at the PBBH in 1913: "There should be no difference, from a university standpoint, between a large clinical community and a chemical laboratory. I mean to say that they should be conducted on the same lines and that the directors of both should spend most of their time in their workshops."[139] At the time, Osler implied that the directors of the PBBH should remain physically within the hospital—their "workshops," where their clinical community resided under their watchful gaze. As the Brigham has extended and redefined its own mission over the ensuing century, its gaze has been extended and redefined in parallel.

The following chapters continue to use the Brigham as a historical vehicle to explore continuity and change in the ideals and practice of academic medicine in spheres that include biomedical research, clinical medicine, medical education, and the broader communities of care. They point to both triumphs and challenges, with the challenges often leading to adjustments and progress that often could have not been foreseen. As Osler concluded his 1913 address:

> *It is not a bad thing to have little frictions and difficulties, which really enable you to shake down more comfortably afterwards. And if you face them in the proper spirit they will work out and adjust themselves without any doubt. After all, it is a matter of give and take, of feeling that you are a part of a great organization, that you are taking a very important step in medical education, that this is a great thing for the city and for the country in the future development of medicine.*[140]

REFERENCES

1. David McCord, *The Fabrick of Man: Fifty Years of the Peter Bent Brigham.* (Boston: Published for the Hospital by the Fiftieth Anniversary Celebration Committee, 1963).
2. Oglesby Paul, "Leadership: A Short History of the Peter Bent Brigham Hospital," Unpublished Manuscript, 1999, Oglesby Paul Papers (H MS c291), Harvard Medical Library in the Francis A. Countway Library of Medicine, box 2, ff20.
3. Morris J. Vogel, *The Invention of the Modern Hospital, Boston, 1870-1930* (Chicago: University of Chicago Press, 1980); David Rosner, *A Once Charitable Enterprise: Hospitals and Health Care in Brooklyn and New York, 1885-1915* (New York: Cambridge University Press, 1982).
4. Kenneth M. Ludmerer, *Learning to Heal: The Development of American Medical Education* (New York: Basic Books, 1985), pp. 9-20.
5. Charles E. Rosenberg, *The Care of Strangers: The Rise of America's Hospital System* (New York: Basic Books, 1987).
6. Abraham Flexner, *Medical Education in the United States and Canada: A Report to the Carnegie Foundation for the Advancement of Teaching* (New York: Carnegie Foundation for the Advancement of Teaching, 1910).
7. Ludmerer, *Learning to Heal,* pp. 29-101; Thomas N. Bonner, *Iconoclast: Abraham Flexner and a Life in Learning* (Baltimore: Johns Hopkins University Press, 2002).
8. Ludmerer, *Learning to Heal,* p. 58.
9. Michael Bliss, *William Osler: A Life in Medicine* (New York: Oxford University Press, 1999), pp. 168-207.
10. Paul, "Leadership," p. 4; Vogel, *The Invention of the Modern Hospital,* pp. 82-3; Nicholas L. Tilney, *A Perfectly Striking Departure: Surgeons and Surgery at the Peter Bent Brigham Hospital, 1912-1980* (Sagamore Beach: Science History Publications, 2006), pp. 4-7.
11. Thomas Francis Harrington, *The Harvard Medical School: A History, Narrative, and Documentary, Volume III* (New York: Lewis Publishing Company, 1905), pp. 1173-4.
12. Ibid, p. 1183.
13. Ibid, p. 1182.
14. Ibid, pp. 1182-4.
15. F.B. Mallory, "The Present Needs of the Harvard Medical School," *Science* 24 (1906), p. 338.
16. "Opening of the New Harvard Medical School Buildings," *BMSJ* 155 (1906), pp. 352-3.
17. Flexner, *Medical Education in the United States and Canada,* p. 92.
18. Ibid, p. 109.
19. Paul, "Leadership," p. 6; Henry P. Walcott, Arthur J. Cabot, and Charles F. Adams 2nd to Alexander Cochrane, June 27, 1902, Peter Bent Brigham Hospital Ledger, p. 169, Box 6, ff 1, Peter Bent Brigham Hospital records, 1830-1987 (inclusive), 1913-1980 (bulk). BWH c3. Harvard Medical Library, Francis A. Countway Library of Medicine, Boston, Mass. (hereafter PBBH Archives).
20. Paul, "Leadership," p. 6; Ludmerer, *Learning to Heal,* p. 221. See also Alexander Cochrane and E.D. Codman to J.S. Billings, 12/2/05, Peter Bent Brigham Hospital Ledger, p. 65, Box 6, ff 1, PBBH Archives.
21. Edward F. Stevens, *The American Hospital of the Twentieth Century,* Third Edition (New York: F.W. Dodge Corporation, 1928), p. 24.
22. Vogel, *The Invention of the Modern Hospital,* pp. 85-6. On Christian and Cushing's early leadership, see Christian, "Report of the Physician-in-Chief," *Annual Report,* 1931, pp. 112-121.
23. *1912 Travels of the Medical Staff, Peter Bent Brigham Hospital,* Box 42, ff12, PBBH Archives. This volume has also been digitized and made available through Harvard's HOLLIS Library catalog.
24. Harvey Cushing, "Report of the Surgeon-in-Chief," *Sixth Annual Report of the Peter Bent Brigham Hospital for the Year 1919* (Cambridge: The University Press, 1920), pp. 55-7.
25. William Welch, "Address," in *Founders Day Program, Peter Bent Brigham Hospital, November 12, 1914,* Box 7, ff 2, PBBH Archives.
26. Letter from Henry A. Christian to James B. Conant, May 3, 1938. Henry A. Christian papers (H MS b68), Harvard Medical Library in the Francis A. Countway Library of Medicine.
27. Letter from Herrman L. Blumgart to Henry A. Christian, 1935. Henry A. Christian papers (H MS b68), Harvard Medical Library in the Francis A. Countway Library of Medicine.
28. Schnitker, M., Letter to Henry A. Christian, October 12, 1938. Henry A. Christian papers (H MS b68), Harvard Medical Library in the Francis A. Countway Library of Medicine.
29. H.L. Blumgart, Castle W.B., Means J.H., and Thorn G.W., Memorial Minute, *Harvard University Gazette,* January 19, 1952.
30. Harvey Cushing, "Report of the Surgeon-in-Chief," *Eighteenth Annual Report of the Peter Bent Brigham*

Hospital for the Year 1931 (Boston, 1932), p. 77; Nicholas L. Tilney, *Invasion of the Body: Revolutions in Surgery* (Cambridge: Harvard University Press, 2011), pp. 7-15.

31. Cushing, "Report of the Surgeon-in-Chief," *Eighteenth Annual Report,* p. 77.

32. Henry A. Christian, "Report of the Physician-in-Chief," *First Annual Report of the Peter Bent Brigham Hospital for the Years 1913 and 1914* (Cambridge: The University Press, 1915), pp. 121-133.

33. Harvey Cushing, "Report of the Surgeon-in-Chief," *First Annual Report of the Peter Bent Brigham Hospital for the Years 1913 and 1914* (Cambridge: The University Press, 1915), pp. 46-69.

34. Harvey Cushing, "Report of the Surgeon-in-Chief," *Ninth Annual Report of the Peter Bent Brigham Hospital for the Year 1922* (Cambridge: The University Press, 1923), p. 54.

35. Francis Weld Peabody, *The Care of the Patient* (Cambridge: Harvard University Press, 1927), p. 48; see also Oglesby Paul, *The Caring Physician: The Life of Dr. Francis W. Peabody* (Boston: Countway Library of Medicine, 1991).

36. Henry A. Christian, "Report of the Physician-in-Chief," *Seventeenth Annual Report of the Peter Bent Brigham Hospital for the year 1930* (Boston, 1931), p. 120.

37. Ibid.

38. Henry A. Christian, "Report of the Physician-in-Chief," *Ninth Annual Report of the Peter Bent Brigham Hospital for the Year 1922* (Cambridge: The University Press, 1923), p. 105.

39. Henry A. Christian, "Report of the Physician-in-Chief," *Twenty-Fifth Annual Report of the Peter Bent Brigham Hospital for the Year 1938* (Boston, 1939), pp. 101, 102-3. See also Samuel A. Levine, *Coronary Thrombosis: Its Various Clinical Features* (Baltimore: Williams and Wilkins, 1929).

40. Harvey Cushing, "Report of the Surgeon-in-Chief," *Eleventh Annual Report of the Peter Bent Brigham Hospital for the Year 1924* (Boston: Wright & Potter, 1925), p. 70.

41. Cushing, "Report of the Surgeon-in-Chief," *Eleventh Annual Report,* p. 73; Vogel, *The Invention of the Modern Hospital,* p. 87.

42. Cushing, "Report of the Surgeon-in-Chief," *Eighteenth Annual Report,* p. 76.

43. "25th Anniversary Play Program," Box 7, ff5, PBBH Archives.

44. John Shillito, "Cushing: The Clinical Surgeon," in *Harvey Cushing at the Brigham,* Peter McL. Black, Matthew R. Moore, and Eugene Rossitch, Jr., eds. (Park Ridge, IL: American Association of Neurological Surgeons, 1993), pp. 77-89.

45. Ibid.

46. Eugene Rossitch, Jr., Matthew R. Moore, and Peter McL. Black, "Cushing: The Surgical Innovator," in *Harvey Cushing at the Brigham,* op. cit., pp 107-18.

47. Michael Bliss, *Harvey Cushing. A Life in Surgery* (New York: Oxford University Press, 2005), pp. 476-8.

48. Henry A. Christian, "Report of the Physician-in-Chief," *Fifteenth Annual Report of the Peter Bent Brigham Hospital for the Year 1928* (Boston, 1929), pp. 151-4.

49. Harvey Cushing, "Report of the Surgeon-in-Chief," *Fourteenth Annual Report of the Peter Bent Brigham Hospital for the Year 1927* (Boston, 1928), p. 70.

50. Joseph F. Dinneen, "The Hospital Orderly They Call 'Doctor,'" *Collier's Weekly,* December 1, 1951, p. 57.

51. John F. Fulton, *Harvey Cushing: A Biography* (Springfield, IL, Charles C. Thomas: 1946), p. 706.

52. Ibid., p. 419.

53. Francis Moore, "Report of the Surgeon-in-Chief," *Forty-Third Annual Report of the Peter Bent Brigham Hospital for the Fiscal Year Ending September 30, 1956* (Boston: 1956), p. 112.

54. Dinneen, "The Hospital Orderly They Call 'Doctor,'" p. 58.

55. Ibid.

56. Francis D. Moore, "Memorial Established for Adolph." *Brigham Bulletin,* Vol. IV, No. 10, February and March, 1957, p. 4.

57. Harvey Cushing, "Report of the Surgeon-in-Chief," *Eighteenth Annual Report,* p. 110.

58. Dinneen, "The Hospital Orderly They Call 'Doctor,'" p. 58.

59. Moore, *Forty-Third Annual Report,* p. 113.

60. Charles Hatcher, *All in the Timing: From Operating Room to Board Room,* (Bloomington, IN: Authorhouse, 2011), p. 79.

61. Dinneen, "The Hospital Orderly They Call 'Doctor,'" p. 60.

62. Moore, *Forty-Third Annual Report,* p. 113.

63. Hatcher, *All in the Timing,* p. 79.

64. George Thorn, "Report of the Physician-in-Chief," *Forty-Third Annual Report of the Peter Bent Brigham Hospital for the Fiscal Year Ending September 30, 1956* (Boston: 1956), p. 74.

65. Moore, *Forty-Third Annual Report,* p. 114.

66. Ibid., pp. 70-1.

67. Henry A. Christian, "Report of the Physician-in-Chief," *Twenty-Fourth Annual Report of the Peter Bent Brigham Hospital for the Year 1937* (Boston, 1938), pp. 101-8.

68. See also Marilyn King, *The Peter Bent Brigham Hospital School of Nursing: A History, 1912-1985* (Boston: Brigham and Women's Hospital).

69. Tilney, *A Perfectly Striking Departure,* pp. 93-4.

70. William Hollingsworth, *Taking Care: The Legacy of Soma Weiss, Eugene Stead, and Paul Beeson* (San Diego: Medical Education and Research Foundation, 1994).

71. George W. Thorn, "Report of the Physician-in-Chief," *Thirtieth Annual Report of the Peter Bent Brigham Hospital for the Year 1943* (Boston, 1944), p. 24.

72. "Art as Applied to Medicine." http://www.hopkinsmedicine.org/about/history/history7.html, accessed August 8, 2012.

73. Ranice W. Crosby and John *Max Brödel: The Man Who Put Art into Medicine* (Berlin: Springer-Verlag, 1991), p. 249.
74. Matthew R. Moore, John Shillito Jr., and Eugene Rossitch Jr., "Mildred Codding: An Interview with Cushing's Medical Artist," *Surgical Neurology* (1991), p. 341.
75. Ibid, p. 341.
76. Ibid, p. 342.
77. Merrill Sosman, "Report of the Roentgenologist," *Thirtieth Annual Report of the Peter Bent Brigham Hospital for the Year 1943* (Boston, 1944), p. 56.
78. Soma Weiss, "Self-Observations and Psychologic Reactions of Medical Student A.S.R. to the Onset and Symptoms of Subacute Bacterial Endocarditis," *Journal of the Mount Sinai Hospital New York* 8 (1942), p. 1079-94.
79. Hollingsworth, *Taking Care,* pp. 236-7.
80. Ibid., p. 56.
81. Ludmerer, *Learning to Heal,* p. 28.
82. John Laszlo and Francis A. Neelon, *The Doctors' Doctor: A Biography of Eugene A. Stead, Jr., MD* (Durham, NC: Carolina Academic Press, 2006), pp. 155-6.
83. Hollingsworth, *Taking Care,* p. 54.
84. Soma Weiss, Letter to Dr. C. Sidney Burwell, March 29, 1940. Soma Weiss papers, Harvard Medical Library in the Francis A. Countway Library of Medicine.
85. C.S. Keefer, Soma Weiss, 1899-1942, *New England Journal of Medicine* 226 (1942), pp. 505-6.
86. Eugene A. Stead, Jr., "Eugene A. Stead, Jr.: 1937-1939," in *The Harvard Medical Unit at Boston City Hospital, eds.* Maxwell Finland and William B. Castle (Volume II, Part I, Boston: Francis A. Countway Library of Medicine, 1983), pp. 334-5.
87. Robert J. Glaser, "Soma Weiss, M.D., posthumously Hersey Professor of the Theory and Practice of Medicine," (Palo Alto: Alpha Omega Alpha, Video, 1994), video interview with Drs. Paul B. Beeson, Richard V. Ebert, Jack D. Myers and Eugene A. Stead. http://www.alphaomegaalpha.org/leaders.html.
88. Personal letter to author by Dr. Frank J. Lepreau, Jr., July 14, 2008.
89. "To the Memory of Soma Weiss," *The Aesculapied,* (Boston: Harvard Medical School, 1942), p. 5.
90. George W. Thorn, "Report of the Physician-in-Chief," *Forty-Fifth Annual Report of the Peter Bent Brigham Hospital for the Fiscal Year Ended September 30, 1958* (Boston, 1958), p. 23.
91. Paul, "Leadership," pp. 28-9.
92. George W. Thorn, "Report of the Physician-in-Chief," *Thirty-Fifth Annual Report of the Peter Bent Brigham Hospital for the Year 1948* (Boston, 1949), p. 32.
93. Francis D. Moore, "Report of the Surgeon-in-Chief," *Thirty-Sixth Annual Report of the Peter Bent Brigham Hospital for the Year 1949* (Boston, 1950), p. 39.
94. Ibid, p. 41.
95. Francis D. Moore, "Report of the Surgeon-in-Chief," *Fifty-Second Annual Report Peter Bent Brigham Hospital 1964-1965* (Boston, 1965), p. 25.
96. On Cohn, see Angela Creager, " 'What Blood Told Dr. Cohn': World War II, Plasma Fractionation, and the Growth of Human Blood Research," *Studies in History and Philosophy of Biological and Biomedical Sciences* 30 (1999), p. 377-405.
97. Tilney, *A Perfectly Striking Departure,* pp. 207-9; Moore, "Report of the Surgeon-in-Chief," *Forty-Third Annual Report,* p. 77; Moore, "Report of the Surgeon-in-Chief," *Forty-Fourth Annual Report of the Peter Bent Brigham Hospital for the Fiscal Year Ended September 30, 1957* (Boston, 1957), p. 126.
98. George W. Thorn, "Report of the Physician-in-Chief," *Thirty-Sixth Annual Report of the Peter Bent Brigham Hospital for the Year 1949* (Boston, 1950), p. 25; Thorn, "Report of the Physician-in-Chief," *Thirty-Eighth Annual Report of the Peter Bent Brigham Hospital for the Year 1951* (Boston, 1952), p. 27.
99. George W. Thorn, "Report of the Physician-in-Chief," *Thirty-Seventh Annual Report of the Peter Bent Brigham Hospital for the Year 1950* (Boston, 1951), p. 19.
100. Charles B. Barnes and Alan Steinert, "Report of the Chairman of the Board and the President," *Fifty-Second Annual Report Peter Bent Brigham Hospital 1964-1965* (Boston, 1965), pp. 7-8.
101. George W. Thorn, "Report of the Physician-in-Chief," *Fifty-Second Annual Report Peter Bent Brigham Hospital 1964-1965* (Boston, 1965), p. 25.
102. F. Lloyd Mussells, "Report of the Director," *Fifty-Second Annual Report Peter Bent Brigham Hospital 1964-1965* (Boston, 1965), p. 13.
103. Rosemary Stevens, *In Sickness and in Wealth: American Hospitals in the Twentieth Century* (Baltimore: Johns Hopkins University Press, 1999).
104. Francis D. Moore, "Report of the Surgeon-in-Chief," *Forty-Seventh Annual Report of the Peter Bent Brigham Hospital for the Fiscal Year Ended September 30, 1960,* p. 52
105. Ibid.
106. For similar complaints regarding hospital renovation in this period, see Annemarie Adams, *Medicine by Design: The Architect and the Modern Hospital,* 1893-1943 (Minneapolis: University of Minnesota Press, 2008).
107. N.A. Wilhelm, "Report of the Superintendent," *Annual Report,*1943, pp. 19-20.
108. James Dealy, Forty-Seventh PBBH *Thirtieth Annual Report of the Peter Bent Brigham Hospital for the Year 1943* (Boston, 1944), pp. 123-4.
109. Stephen Verdeber and David J. Fine, *Healthcare Architecture in an Era of Radical Transformation* (New Haven: Yale University Press, 2000).

110. George W. Thorn, "Report of the Physician-in-Chief," *Thirty-First Annual Report of the Peter Bent Brigham Hospital for the Year 1944* (Boston, 1945), p. 21
111. Merrill Sosman, "Report of the Radiologist," *Thirty-Second Annual Report of the Peter Bent Brigham Hospital for the Year 1945* (Boston, 1946), pp. 85-6.
112. N.A. Wilhelm, "Report of the Director," *Thirty-Seventh Annual Report of the Peter Bent Brigham Hospital for the Year 1950* (Boston, 1951), pp. 10, 13.
113. Stevens, *In Sickness and in Wealth*, pp. 216-26.
114. Moore, "Report of the Surgeon-in-Chief," *Thirty-Eighth Annual Report*, p. 58.
115. Charles B. Barnes, "Report of the President," *Forty-Eighth Annual Report of the Peter Bent Brigham Hospital for the Fiscal Year Ended September 30, 1961* (Boston, 1961), p. 6.
116. Charles B. Barnes and Alan Steinert, "Report of the Chairman of the Board and of the President," *Fifty-Fourth Annual Report Peter Bent Brigham Hospital 1966-1967* (Boston, 1967), p. 7.
117. Sims McGrath, "Report of the President," *Fifty-Sixth Annual Report Peter Bent Brigham Hospital 1968-1969* (Boston, 1969), p. 7
118. Francis D. Moore, "Report of the Surgeon-in-Chief," *Fifty-Sixth Annual Report Peter Bent Brigham Hospital 1968-1969* (Boston, 1969), p. 40.
119. Ibid, pp. 40-1.
120. Thorn, "Report of the Physician-in-Chief," *Thirty-First Annual Report*, p. 21.
121. Charles S. Pierce, "President's Report," *Thirty-Fourth Annual Report of the Peter Bent Brigham Hospital for the Year 1947* (Boston, 1948), p. 3.
122. F. Lloyd Mussells, "Report of the Director," *Annual Report*, 1961, p. 10; "Report of Dr. Mussells," *Fifty-Sixth Annual Report Peter Bent Brigham Hospital 1968-1969* (Boston, 1969), p. xiii.
123. F. Lloyd Mussells, "Report of the Director," *Forty-Eighth Annual Report of the Peter Bent Brigham Hospital for the Fiscal Year Ended September 30, 1961* (Boston, 1961), pp. 10-11.
124. George W. Thorn, "Report of the Physician-in-Chief," Peter Bent Brigham *Hospital Fiftieth Annual Report 1962-1963* (Boston, 1963), p. 21.
125. Ibid.
126. William H. Danforth, "A New Flexner Report?" *JAMA* 209 (1969), p. 930.
127. William E. Hassan, Jr., "Report of the Director," *Fifty-Fifth Annual Report Peter Bent Brigham Hospital 1967-1968* (Boston, 1968), pp. 12-13.
128. George W. Thorn, "Report of the Physician-in-Chief," *Fifty-Eighth Annual Report Peter Bent Brigham Hospital 1970-1971* (Boston, 1971), p. 41.
129. George W. Thorn, "Report of the Physician-in-Chief," *Fifty-Fourth Annual Report Peter Bent Brigham Hospital 1966-1967* (Boston, 1967), p. 3.
130. George W. Thorn, "Report of the Physician-in-Chief," *Fifty-Ninth Annual Report Peter Bent Brigham Hospital 1971-1972* (Boston, 1972), p. 47.
131. Paul, "Leadership," pp. 35, 38.
132. Dan L. Longo, Dennis L. Kasper, J. Larry Jameson, Anthony S. Fauci, Stephen L. Hauser, Joseph Loscalzo, "Dedication: Eugene Braunwald," in *Harrison's Principles of Internal Medicine* 18th edition (New York: McGraw Hill, 2012).
133. Kenneth Ludmerer, *Time to Heal: American Medical Education From the Turn of the Century to the Era of Managed Care* (New York: Oxford University Press, 1999); Jill A. Fisher, *Medical Research for Hire: The Political Economy of Pharmaceutical Clinical Trials* (New Brunswick: Rutgers University Press, 2009); Adriana Petryna, *When Experiments Travel: Clinical Trials and the Global Search for Human Subjects* (Princeton: Princeton University Press, 2009).
134. Eugene Braunwald, "Report of the Physician-in-Chief," *Sixty-Third Annual Report Peter Bent Brigham Hospital 1975-1976* (Boston, 1976), p. 42.
135. Peter Keating and Alberto Cambrosio, *Biomedical Platforms: Realigning the Normal and the Pathological in Late Twentieth-Century Medicine* (Cambridge: MIT Press, 2003).
136. Marion L. Metcalf, "Annual Report, Department of Nursing," *Sixty-Third Annual Report Peter Bent Brigham Hospital 1975-1976* (Boston, 1976), p. 12.
137. John A. Kastor, *Mergers of Teaching Hospitals: in Boston, New York, and Northern California* (Ann Arbor: University of Michigan Press, 2001).
138. Interview with Dr. Dzau by Peter Tishler in November 2011, http://videocenter.brighamandwomens.org/videos/victor-dzau-md (last updated June 18, 2013).
139. William Osler, cited in Cushing, "Report of the Surgeon-in-Chief," *Sixth Annual Report*, pp. 56-7.
140. Ibid, p. 57.

CHAPTER 2

EDUCATIONAL LANDMARKS AND LUMINARIES

EDUCATIONAL LANDMARKS AND LUMINARIES

Joel T. Katz, Ann C. Conway, and Nicholas L. Tilney

Through the unlikely convergence of Peter Bent Brigham's altruism and Harvard Medical School's (HMS's) opportunism, a carefully designed medical education experiment connected the disjointed medical and scientific training movements emerging in the late nineteenth century. In doing so, it produced a new teaching model and resultant generation of academic leaders well out of proportion to the Peter Bent Brigham Hospital's (PBBH's) quite modest footprint. In addition, the wave of innovation introduced at the new institution in the early twentieth century extended, by design, the revolution in medical education initiated at Johns Hopkins two decades before. The educational enterprise that arose on Boston's Francis Street was carefully constructed to create an ideal training environment, many aspects of which were not possible in Baltimore or at existing Harvard hospitals. The PBBH's unique blend of science, charity, and full-time staff became the blueprint for the modern teaching hospital. The story of educational innovation at the Brigham and its antecedent and affiliated institutions provides insight into the indelible mark left on the restructuring of U.S. medical education in the twentieth century.

BUILDING EDUCATION AT THE BRIGHAM

When Brigham wrote his last will and testament in the 1870s, medicine as practiced in the United States was far different than that practiced today. There were few effective therapies, save for opium (pain relief), quinine (malaria), and digitalis (temporary relief of dropsy, now known as congestive heart failure). Furthermore, the few beneficial interventions were outnumbered by countless ineffective treatments, many of which, in retrospect, were clearly harmful (e.g., mercury used for many disorders). Early in the nineteenth century, hospitals were often unsanitary institutions, reserved for the poor, untreatable, and dying. Although the post–Civil War emergence of both professionalized nursing, with its emphasis on cleanliness and ventilation, and the emerging understanding of the germ theory would begin to change this grim picture, anyone who could afford care at home avoided hospitals completely.

The state of medical education remained equally dismal and completely unregulated in the second half of the nineteenth century. There were no standards for medical training; at the turn of the twentieth

century, the majority of practicing doctors had not completed medical school.[1] Medical schools were for-profit, unregulated businesses, run, at best, by self-declared teachers and, much more likely, by fiscal opportunists and charlatans. A one- to two-year undifferentiated internship-like experience existed, under the term "Pupil" or "House Pupil,"[2] but it offered no scientific rigor, balance of clinical experience, or appropriate supervision. Physician training in the cities was largely limited to apprenticeships at private doctors' offices caring for wealthy patients and in rural areas as apprenticeships to generally untrained practitioners.[3]

However, some reason for hope was brewing. As Brigham finalized his last will in 1877, medical breakthroughs began to challenge existing theories of humors and miasmas. Biochemical advances began to elucidate metabolic pathways and the roles of hormones in human health and disease. Pasteur and Koch visualized bacteria and proposed causality (1870s).[4,5] Advances in vaccination demonstrated promise in combating some of the most devastating and feared scourges of the time, such as anthrax (1881) and rabies (1885). Early "antisepsis" measures improved operative mortality; anesthesia made surgery more merciful. In 1895, the discovery of roentgenography opened a new field of diagnostic possibilities. These advances, which largely occurred in Europe, attracted relatively little attention from U.S. physicians and medical educators.

Brigham's bequest was not intended to address educational needs or to strengthen the emerging scientific foundations of medical practice. He was a merchant abolitionist, not an academic. Hospital endowments at the time typically "were based on particular ideologies of dependence and class" and focused on providing options for populations at risk and without economic means or social status to provide for themselves;[6] the purpose of such settings was often terminal institutionalization. Brigham's endowment was no exception. In fact, his nephew, Robert Breck Brigham, specifically designated his will to provide for the "treatment of incurables." At that time, there was admittedly little that could be done for those who suffered from rheumatic diseases who formed the preponderance of early patients at the soon-to-be-named Robert Breck Brigham Hospital.

During the twenty-five years stipulated by Peter Bent Brigham for the strengthening of his trust, major social and political forces intervened to change the face of medicine.[7] The Industrial Revolution transferred the national focus from rural to urban, from agrarian family units to individuals. At the same time, the scientific revolution promoted a novel perspective that paved the way to redefine medicine as academic, democratic, and corporate. Scientific advances validated the field and the claims of physician legitimacy.

In this rich and turbulent milieu, a major breakthrough in U.S. medical education came at the Johns Hopkins Hospital, established with great fanfare in 1889, which became the inspiration for the Harvard-Brigham experiment.[8] The new Hopkins medical curriculum stressed the emerging link between science and health, including an original, longitudinal, cohesive, and scientifically grounded curriculum from medical school to postgraduate training. In addition, the supporting philanthropists insisted that women be admitted as students.[9,10] At the graduate level, the Hopkins founders designed the modern residency system after the German tradition of a structured apprenticeship as a prerequisite to independent academic practice.[11] Changing professional attitudes set the expectation for deferred personal fulfillment in favor of constant availability, thorough due diligence, and increasing independent responsibility.

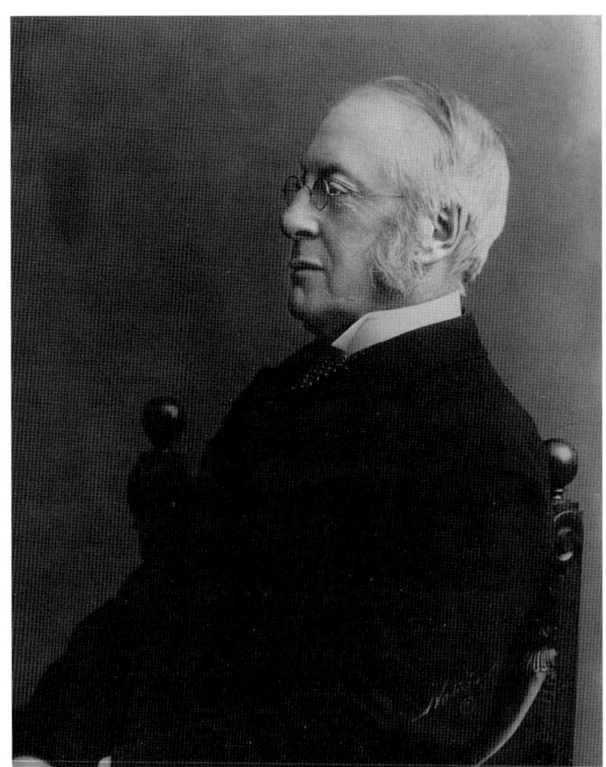

FIGURE 2-1 Charles Eliot.

In parallel with the activity ongoing in Baltimore, Harvard College President Charles W. Eliot established a personal and university goal to transform Harvard's medical school from what he felt was a "diploma mill"[12] and a weak trade school, at best, where he knew "nothing about the quality of the Harvard Medical students—more than half of them can barely write"[13]—to a refined center for scientific medicine.[14] Flexner's 1910 study of existing U.S. medical schools, including Harvard, concluded that "a large majority" were "highly unsatisfactory," operating without standards, meaningful admissions requirements, coherent curriculum, or assessment of either students or faculty.[15]

At that time, admissions criteria for Harvard College greatly exceeded those for its medical school, which, like most other medical schools, did not require a college degree; neither entry nor promotional examinations were required.[16] To accomplish this ambitious reinvention, President Eliot needed to create a new hospital that was not subordinated to the hopelessly entrenched fiefdoms of the private, largely Brahmin Boston physicians. With an eye on resources, Peter Bent Brigham's will, which had increased to more than $5,000,000 value by the turn of the twentieth century, provided an opportunity too enticing to ignore. If anchored to Harvard's mission, this endowment would become a large proportion—almost a quarter—of the entire medical school endowment, enough to sway the Harvard trustees to consider a new site for the medical school. Thus plans for the school's buildings were relocated from Allston to Roxbury's former Ebenezer Francis estate to meet the stipulation in Brigham's will that the new hospital provide care for the indigent of Suffolk County.[17] "The Harvard authorities no doubt always had a weather eye for securing an owned or closely allied hospital. When land was purchased on Longwood Avenue ... a large excess area was preserved for that purpose."[18] Lawsuits between the family heirs and the hospital trustees delayed the opening of what was to become the showpiece for Harvard Medical School.

According to David McCord, "Medically-imaginative Boston was tormented by the dazzling success of the Johns Hopkins Medical School. The Hopkins not only introduced to American medicine many European discoveries and techniques, but the medical faculty controlled its teaching hospital appointments simply by owning and operating the hospital in which they were made."[19] President Eliot and the trustees drew on this and many aspects of the groundbreaking Hopkins model in crafting the Brigham. By creating a new hospital at a new location, Harvard and PBBH trustees could recruit from a national rather than a local talent pool and thereby avoid the pitfalls of established hierarchy and entrenched referral patterns that ruled local institutions such as Massachusetts General Hospital (MGH), in favor of innovation, accomplishment, and scientific productivity. Medical historian Kenneth M. Ludmerer wrote of the period: "For the modern medical school to do its work, it needed to control strong teaching hospitals deeply rooted in university medicine."[20] President Eliot wrote:

> *I feel as if the Medical School were embarking on a happier future. Ever since I have been a member of the Medical Faculty I have seen clearly what a handicap on the school it was that the University had no hold on the hospital appointments. Hereafter, the school will be able to reach all around the country for the very best men to fill vacancies.*[21]

As was the case at Johns Hopkins Hospital, whose excellence was based on its academic leaders Osler (physician-in-chief), Halsted (surgeon-in-chief), and Welch (chair of pathology and first dean of the medical school), Harvard chose three gifted proponents of scientific medicine to design this new hospital in Boston and to craft its carefully considered, innovative educational methods. Perhaps not coincidentally, Henry Christian (physician-in-chief), Harvey Cushing (surgeon-in-chief), and William Councilman (pathologist-in-chief), known as the "Three Cs," all shared academic pedigrees split between Harvard and Hopkins. Christian and Cushing were considered to be among the superstars of their era despite their surprising youth—ages 37 and 41, respectively. Osler strongly advised Cushing to come to Boston. President Eliot recruited Christian as Dean of the Medical School (1908-1912), which gave him the ideal vantage from which to construct and expand on Eliot's vision of a center for scientific medicine. In addition, the Brigham endowment required that Christian create something new: scientific charity, an essential partnership between Harvard's teaching mission and Brigham's stipulation for the provision of indigent care.[22]

In time, these missions—charitable care and science—grew so seamlessly intertwined that the initial schism was largely lost, and the relationship emerged as a central and necessary ingredient of well-functioning academic medical centers. At the twenty-fifth year PBBH celebration, Reginald Fitz, one of the very first Brigham interns and by then a distinguished internist and future HMS assistant dean,[23] imagined the hospital's founder observing what his bequest had created:

> *Peter Bent Brigham, if he could see his hospital now, situated at the very heart of one of America's great medical centers, was fully realizing how fruitful had been its first twenty-five years. He was looking ahead happily, knowing that the next twenty-five years of the hospital will continue to make life more hopeful and to make cure more possible for sick persons in indigent circumstances in the county of Suffolk and for sick people the world over.*[24]

Although it may have been unintentional, the first great and lasting educational achievement of the new Brigham was to redefine what is now widely known as the "academic medical center" as a site simultaneously serving the missions of charity, training, and discovery, and where the "neighborhood" was inclusive of human health needs throughout the world.

BIOGRAPHY

WILLIAM T. COUNCILMAN (1854-1933), Legendary Teacher

Joel T. Katz

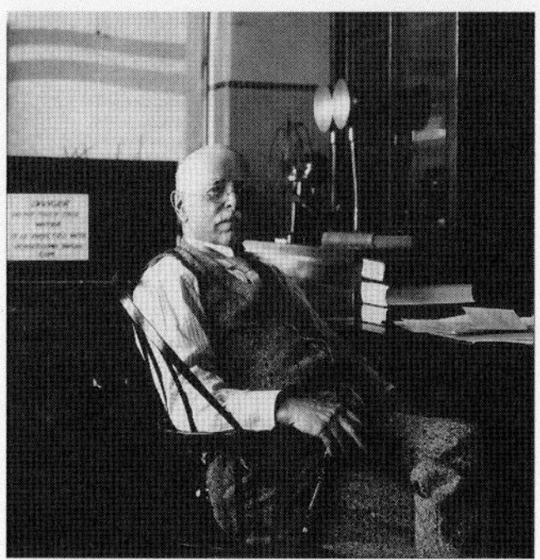

FIGURE 2-2 William Councilman.

From the early days led by the distinguished William Thomas Councilman, "education and teaching have been both a core value and an historic tradition of the Department of Pathology" at Brigham and Women's Hospital, says Frederick Schoen.[25] Generous and informal, a shrewd and independent thinker, Councilman's broad scope and affable style made him an "inspiring teacher for the young."[26] His pedigree included study under Welch at Hopkins and collaborations with the premiere European (e.g., von Recklinghausen, Cohnheim, Weigert, Chiari) and American (e.g., Abbott, Tyzzer, Mallory, Wright) pathologists of the day. Councilman joined Harvard Medical School (HMS) faculty two decades ahead of the other two of the "Three C's" (Christian and Cushing) in 1892, where he compiled and delivered the full curriculum of pathology lectures to adoring second-year HMS students.[27]

With his appointment as the first PBBH pathologist-in-chief in 1913, time for his outside interest in horticulture was greatly curtailed, and he took it on himself to design and maintain the hospital planters—characteristic of the tenderness toward living things that he extended to his students. "It is an important thing that people should be happy in their work," Councilman stated, "and if work does not bring happiness there is something wrong; and both at the University and at the Hospital there was that wonderful happiness in work."[28] Relative to the training mission, he famously stated, "It seems to me that the most important thing for the teacher is to awaken interest and enthusiasm in his students and to provide them with opportunities of following the interest which is aroused, for in this way we progress."[29]

A NEW SYSTEM FOR MEDICAL EDUCATION

Christian and Cushing, under the authority of the founders of the new hospital, designed teaching methods with great care and forethought over a number of preparatory years. Both had trained in Europe and participated in the building design and systems development of the Brigham, as did the soon-to-be superintendent of nursing, Carrie Hall. In this, the planners capitalized on a bold and progressive spirit to design a hospital suited to conquer previously untreatable disorders. Many of the innovations began as refinements of the traditions of the great teaching hospitals of Britain and Germany and addressed the buoyant promise of new scientific horizons and the simultaneous need for increased educational rigor, resident supervision, and personal responsibility. Christian and Cushing gave these tenets form, resulting in "an entirely new hospital system" for education.[30]

The prioritization of education was apparent even in the structural design of the building. The chiefs "considered intimate personal contact in their daily teaching with their junior staff of cardinal importance in perpetuating the high standards envisioned for the institution."[31] The Brigham educational system they created was novel in many ways and was "especially valuable at this period in medicine and in medical education, when there is need of breaking away from the traditions and professional custom and lay inertia which now do so much to restrict the usefulness of both medical schools and hospital."[32] In an ironic mishap, the initial hospital included no amphitheatre for teaching purposes, foreshadowing the 1980 Brigham and Women's Hospital (BWH) tower construction that included no student or resident call-rooms.

The Brigham and HMS alliance established the first full-time teaching model—appointment to the staff and admitting privileges required an HMS appointment.

Previously, admitting and teaching physicians had private practices that occupied their principal attention and determined their prioritization. But at the new institution, attending physicians were (initially) forbidden from having a private practice, and Christian gave up his practice on Marlboro Street when the hospital opened. The PBBH "established a system by which the staff members tacitly agreed to bring all their patients, both free and private, to the Hospital so that all of their work might be done within its walls—an arrangement rather widely known as the 'Boston System.'"[33] (Cushing resisted and ultimately reversed this mandate, and some rare exceptions were made.[34]) In return, the staff were "paid 'liberal' salaries"[35] to discourage seeking remunerative activities outside the medical school. Research was expected and rewarded for faculty who ultimately depended on the medical school for their appointment. Stringent admissions criteria and a coordinated four-year curriculum assured that the medical students were of uniformly high quality and intent. The medical school–hospital alignment fostered a rich learning environment and for the first time offered the school leverage to determine curriculum and secure some control over the quality of the teachers.

BIOGRAPHY

HARVEY WILLIAM CUSHING (1869-1939), Legendary Teacher

Joel T. Katz

"It is the poor teacher whose student does not surpass him."[36] Thus the mercurial pioneering brain surgeon and inaugural PBBH surgeon-in-chief, Harvey Cushing, set the high benchmark for success and path to future scientific discovery, and inspired a profound loyalty. Although Cushing—a fourth-generation physician—had only recently been a surgery resident at Hopkins, by the time he returned to Boston he was considered the leading neurosurgical specialist in the world. When he left PBBH two decades later, he had trained the next generation of neurosurgeons to carry the field forward. Cushing was unusually multitalented, having attained professional-level expertise as an athlete, artist, and biographer.

Cushing had an energetic, exacting, and inspirational teaching style, and, as a workaholic, he led by example. "The battle of the Marne was nothing compared to the stress and strain of being Cushing's assistant," commented a PBBH trainee.[37] Despite his demanding approach, he showed a softer side as he and his wife frequently invited the surgical house staff to their home for Christmas. In his 1963 PBBH history, poet David McCord wrote that "the names of Cushing and PBBH are solidly joined" in the same way that "Henry J. Bigelow and MGH are names the medical world will couple for all time."[38]

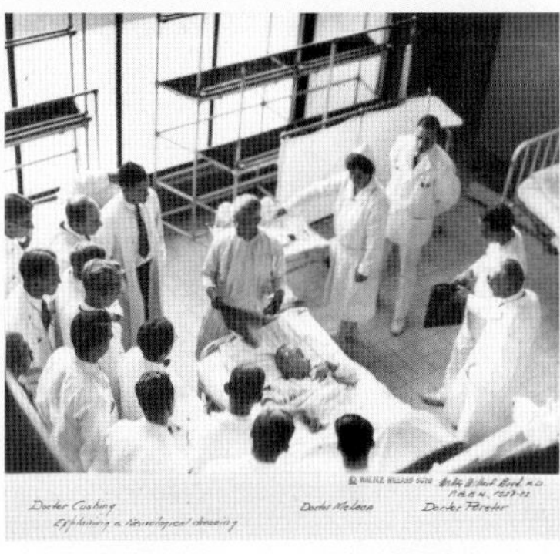

FIGURE 2-3 Harvey Cushing teaching.

FOUNDATIONS OF THE MODERN RESIDENCY

The new residency system drew on and expanded the most advantageous aspects of the Hopkins and European models, with significant alterations to meet the needs of prioritizing both science and charity. Although it was at Hopkins that the term "residency" was first coined, the Brigham was the next to adopt this ambitious model and, in doing so, refined and codified the structure as the template for the U.S. post-graduate training system, establishing ties between training and scientific investigation that required an organized hierarchy of ascending independence and a system of close association between faculty and trainees.[39]

The first house officers (i.e., "interns") had to be medical school graduates, a requirement initially pioneered at Hopkins. They served 16-month terms, were appointed quarterly, and worked in exchange for room, board, and clean white uniforms. Housing for trainees, including the chief resident, was in quarters above the Brigham rotunda. Four 4-month rotations were designed by Christian and Cushing, sequentially focusing on routine laboratory work, taking patient histories, head of the ward (intermediate care), and outpatient department.

This gradual escalation in responsibilities was designed by the chairs to optimize the attainment of clinically useful skills and minimize the danger to patients by deferring full independence until practical skills had been attained. Newspaper accounts at the time cited the safety advantage of house officers having at least eight months of experience in the hospital before stepping into largely independent care roles. Within a few years of the hospital opening, house officers were asked to differentiate themselves along medical or surgical tracks, the first such intern-level specialization in the United States.

House officers were now to be supervised by "assistant residents," a newly defined group of physicians at an intermediate training level who had declared their allegiance to surgery or medicine. These physicians were accepted into this rigorous course of training as a pathway into the newly emerging careers that encompassed expertise in clinical care, research, and teaching. A pyramidal selection and promotion process required the demonstration of excellence before promotion to the next level, with some trainees unable to move on at the institution.[40] According to the *Boston Evening Transcript*, "The PBBH appears to be the only one in America having a paid, resident staff above the grade of house officer. The system is in partial effect at the Johns Hopkins Hospital, but not consistently and liberally carried out."[41] Assistant residents served one-year renewable terms—generally a total of four to six years—after which they often moved into leadership roles in academic medicine (e.g., as department chairs). Three assistant residents were appointed in 1912, two in surgery and one in medicine. In addition to supervising clinical care, they were welcomed into the work of research that was conducted by the staff physicians and the medical school faculty. The names of trainees were increasingly included as authors on papers, heralding a period of intellectual honesty and increased discovery.

One resident physician (a role that would subsequently be known as "chief resident") was appointed for a two-year term to oversee the other trainees and hospital operations. In this role, he served as "assistants to the department chairmen" and was largely assured of a faculty appointment when one became available.[42] Often this experience was followed by a year-long tour of European medical centers as the entry point into the fraternity of academic leaders. Each of the first seven Brigham chief residents in internal medicine received academic appointments, compared with only three of twenty former assistant residents who were not selected chief resident.[43]

Francis Weld Peabody, the first Brigham resident to hold the position, was, unlike his chairs, a product of the Boston Brahmin elite; he was also the nephew of President Eliot. Peabody was appointed resident physician in 1913 six years after graduating from HMS, having completed his internship at MGH, residencies in medicine and pathology at Johns Hopkins, and postdoctoral study periods at The Rockefeller Institute in New York and in the Berlin chemistry laboratory of Nobel laureate H. Emil Fischer. He already had published widely read papers on typhoid fever, heart disease, and poliomyelitis. As an indication of the momentum possible from this position, within five years of completing his assignment as resident physician, Peabody was a full professor at HMS and director of the Thorndike Memorial Laboratory, training ground for the next generation of great clinical scientists, such as Henry Christian's successor, Soma Weiss.[44]

Although ambulatory settings had largely been ignored in clinical training, Christian and Cushing felt that this experience was required to produce outstanding doctors. In contrast to the sporadic and inflexible ambulatory schedules in vogue at the time, the novel Out-Door Department was designed to provide "easy patient access" and to be "open all day so that any one desiring treatment can come at any time

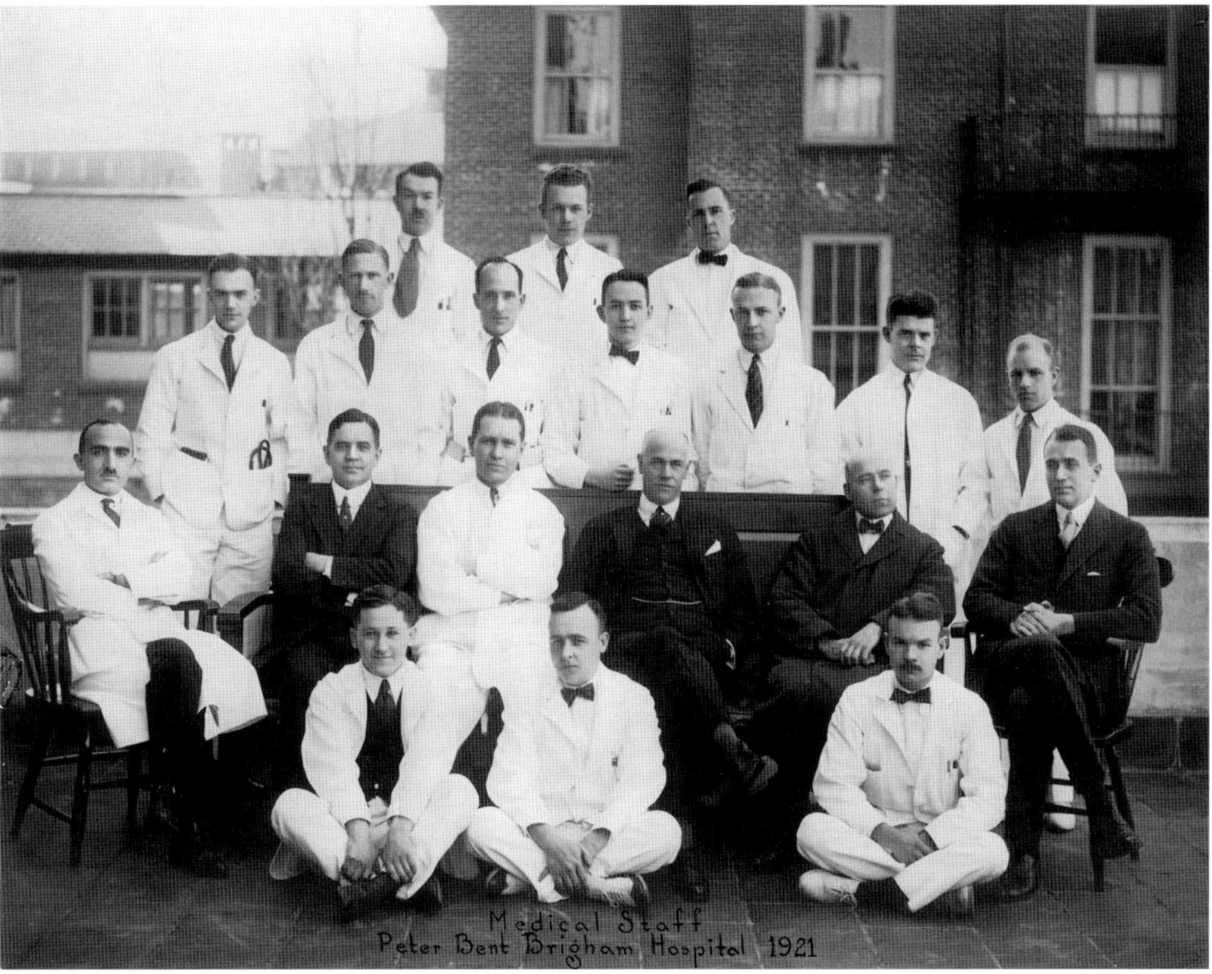

FIGURE 2-4 Peter Bent Brigham Hospital staff, 1921.

that is convenient or possible for him."[45] House officers were allotted thirty minutes to see a new patient, and fourth-year medical students an hour and a half, thus matching the patient needs to what was safe and educationally sound. "The result was greater satisfaction among patients, who lost less time on clinic days and received more thorough evaluations" by the trainees.[46] The value of this new model was apparent, and the practice spread quickly to other teaching hospitals throughout the country. As David McCord put it, "The Christian clinic proliferated into clinics elsewhere, often involving the service of some teacher-doctor once (and perhaps always at heart) a Brigham man."[47]

Under the watchful eyes and high expectations of the chairs, the trainees were granted an unprecedented level of responsibility, well beyond the Hopkins blueprint. This approach fit both the rigorous training plans and the accepted norms for indigent care. As *The Boston Evening Transcript* reported:

> *The visiting physician and surgeon are in control of the two sides (medical and surgical) of the hospital work; their assistants are not as in America young men who rotate in their functions, and remain at most only two years in the hospital, but assistants who live in the hospital for terms of perhaps six or eight years at a time. The only practice of these hospital assistants is the work of the hospital itself, and they will be instantly available in any patient's crisis.*[48]

Assuredly, Brigham trainees were hardworking—some may say abused—by their long hours. And indeed they were long, although the interns realized that their lot was better than those at Hopkins. There, the house staff entered the hospital on July 1 each academic year and did not leave the building until the following year. Testimonials from the period suggest, however, that at the best academic centers the prevailing opinion was that the reward was a rich and exhilarating learning environment. Lewis Thomas fondly recalled that "No job I've ever held since graduating from medical school was as rewarding as my internship," which he completed at the nearby Boston City Hospital.[49] A distinguishing feature of this new model—born at Hopkins and refined at the Brigham—was that work and learning were seamlessly integrated; science was not just memorizing facts, but was a way of thinking. Individual responsibility included establishing an evidence basis for therapy. Christian established teaching's paramount importance through the tradition of visiting physicians and surgeons *pro tempore*. Today, the hospital continues to host distinguished national or international scholars to teach for an extended period.[50] A related tradition—for the house officers to regale and occasionally mock that physician by writing and performing humorous theatrics—did not survive.

Residents were expected to explore disease in great depth, including the expectation that trainees conduct clinically relevant research—what Osler once called "the highest function of a hospital." Patient care was expected to move from a vocation to a way of thinking, as a means to an end to advance the profession. Evidence of this new focus on investigation was the great emphasis of early Brigham leaders on the importance of pathology; Cushing in the first annual report noted the high rate of autopsies (81 of 118 fatal cases), although permissions from some racial and ethnic groups could be difficult to obtain.[51] Furthermore, the unique design of the hospital with pavilions extending out from a 220-yard central brick pathway (the "Pike") augmented the rich learning environment by fostering collegiality and the high degree of camaraderie characteristic of the Brigham. The horizontal Pike design "forces community engagement; everyone runs into everyone else making the hospital like a true family."[52] House officers and residents lived in rooms within the upper floors of the hospital. They were uniformly single, overwhelmingly male.

BIOGRAPHY

SAMUEL A. LEVINE, 1891-1966, Legendary Teacher

Peter V. Tishler and Joel T. Katz

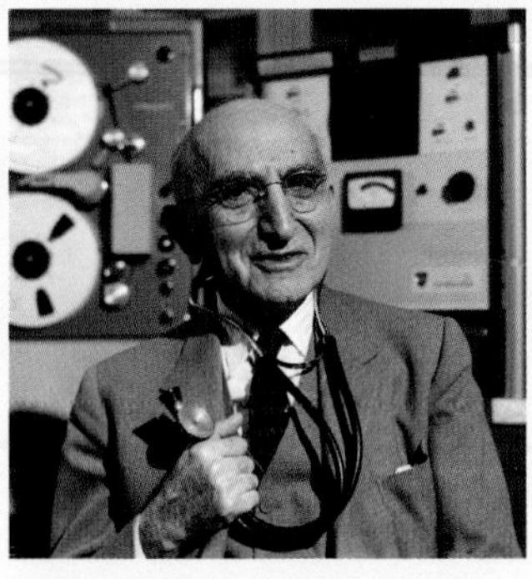

FIGURE 2-5 Samuel Levine.

Samuel Levine's lifetime influence on local, national, and international medicine spanned the Brigham's first fifty-plus years, commencing with his being the first student clinical clerk and then a house officer at the new Brigham in 1913 under Henry A. Christian. Following a brief period on the Beth Israel (BI) faculty, he returned to the Brigham after a dispute over authorship order led to his "fortuitously" being relieved of his faculty position at the BI.[53] With the exception of time out for service in World War I, "SAL" remained an innovative and influential Brigham staff member until his death in 1966. He spent much of his service time in Great Britain, interacting with British cardiologic luminaries James Mackenzie and Thomas Lewis as well as William Osler and Clifford Allbutt. This was the start and the only "formal" part of his cardiologic education.

He and Paul Dudley White at the Massachusetts General Hospital were responsible for the development in Boston of clinical cardiology, a discipline that began after the invention of the electrocardiograph machine at the turn of the twentieth century. Early on, he described the first antemortem diagnosis of coronary thrombosis (1918), and in 1923 he collaborated with surgeon Elliott Cutler to create the Cutler-Levine cardiotomy and valvotomy for mitral stenosis. He was a close associate of other cardiologic pioneers, including William Dock and Brigham-trained Tinsley R. Harrison.

Levine was most widely known as a beloved teacher of a generation of cardiologists. He had a brilliant mind and boundless energy and personally delivered the entire content of the Harvard Medical School (HMS) cardiac pathophysiology and cardiology continuing medical education (CME) courses. He taught cardiovascular medicine to countless individuals, both at the bedside and in a postgraduate course he gave each summer from 1921 to 1956. He nurtured a younger generation who also became leaders in clinical and research cardiology, such as his fellows W. Proctor Harvey and Bernard Lown. Even his first Brigham teacher and mentor, Henry A. Christian, dedicated a book "to Samuel A. Levine, a devoted pupil who has taught me much of cardiology."

H. Richard Tyler recalls:

> *Sam Levine, of course, was everybody's role model as a pleasant, outgoing, eminent cardiologist who impressed you at the bedside. The first day I came to the Brigham ... Sam Levine came on the ward and said, "Let's go see this patient." He took a history, he did an examination and I said, "Do you want to see the X-rays?" Levine said, "No, let's talk about him," and made the diagnosis from his bedside. He said, "Now we'll look at the X-ray," and of course it confirmed just what he said. I was terribly impressed that here was a man [who] was clearly a doctor ... and a role model that you would try to emulate.*[54]

As a prolific writer, he taught physicians in a wider sphere, with more than 180 journal publications, including "Coronary Thrombosis: Its Various Clinical Features," printed in the journal *Medicine* in 1929, and books, including *Clinical Auscultation of the Heart* with W. Proctor Harvey in 1949 and 1959 and his landmark textbook *Clinical Heart Disease*, first published in 1936, in which he gratefully acknowledged Soma Weiss. He also gave lectures worldwide.

He contributed practically to improving the care of patients with heart disease, supporting Bernard Lown financially and politically in creating the Brigham's Levine Coronary Care Unit in 1964, developing a chair for convalescence of patients with myocardial infarction, and advocating their early graduation from bed to chair convalescence. Marshall A. Wolf has said: "Dr. Levine saved the Brigham by attracting a robust clinical practice to the Brigham at a time when there were many empty beds."

His recognition and reputation burgeoned during his lifetime, and he became a full professor of medicine at HMS in 1948. In 1954, a patient endowed a professorship in his name at HMS and the Brigham, occupied by J. Sidney Burwell from 1955-1959, George W. Thorn from 1967-1972, Barry M. Brenner from 1976-2009, and Joseph V. Bonventre since 2010.

At the time of his death, Tinsley R. Harrison wrote: "I have not known a keener bedside clinician, a more inspiring teacher, a kindlier physician, a more loyal friend, a nobler gentleman nor a sweeter human spirit. Without Sam Levine the world will never again be quite the same."[55] Paul Dudley White wrote tributes in several medical journals, paying homage to SAL as a "colleague and close friend ...for fifty years," and "an inspiration to us all."[56] W. Proctor Harvey, evaluating his fellowship with SAL in 1997, exclaimed: "What a wonderful experience and a wonderful man!...I admired him and respected him for everything that he was as a teacher, a father, and a great clinician."[57] Bernard Lown, in his 1996 book *The Lost Art of Healing*, devotes many pages to Samuel Levine the clinician, teacher, and human being. His tribute to Levine is touching. Theirs was a *bona fide* personal and professional relationship that grew over many decades, beginning with Lown's "youthful arrogance" and culminating in his acknowledgment that Levine "remains a lifelong role model."[58] Theirs was not a one-way relationship; they both loved and learned from each other. SAL continued to instruct Lown during his final illness.

Samuel A. Levine "brought a buoyant spirit and incorrigible optimism to the bedside."[59] What a wonderful legacy he has left to medicine and humanity!

SURGICAL TRAINING IN THE NEW HOSPITAL

Cushing's Hopkins mentor, William S. Halsted, was responsible for much of the evolution of modern surgery and the education of young aspirants.[60] He developed a program of postgraduate training in surgery that has continued without significant alteration to the present: a graded series of responsibilities, with a final year of independence. After considerable time on the hospital wards as medical students, Halsted's chosen disciples dedicated years of focused commitment to developing their surgical skills that emulated Halsted's insistence on precise and gentle dissection with minimal blood loss and strict adherence to the principles of antisepsis. From this novel surgical culture came the recognition that standards of surgical treatment and care should be established. Although nearly anyone could operate on patients regardless of training and experience until well into the twentieth century, surgical leaders gradually formed professional societies such as the American College of Surgeons and an expanding series of credentialing and specialty boards. These mandated appropriate years of training, set the numbers and range of supervised operations, and assessed clinicians with formal examinations.

Having learned the Hopkins system well, Cushing was a stern taskmaster during his tenure at the Brigham.[61] Once in Boston, Cushing organized a dog course in aseptic technique for the Harvard Medical students based on the one he had orchestrated at Hopkins. This course remained popular well into the 1980s and stimulated generations of students to enter surgery. Despite limiting his practice to neurosurgical cases, Cushing stressed to his faculty and residents that they must be expert in all aspects of surgery. He taught his detailed surgical techniques to large numbers of young acolytes who gained positions of prominence in the United States and abroad, and in time, trained many other academic surgeons. The two general surgeons on Cushing's staff—John Homans, ebullient, voluble, and iconoclastic, and David Cheever, correct, precise, and serious—were dedicated to both patient care and teaching the house staff. The third departmental faculty member, Walter Boothby, was one of the few individuals in the United States to dedicate himself to the field of anesthesia.

With his protean interests and enthusiasm, Eliot C. Cutler, Cushing's successor, carried on this tradition from 1932 to 1947, believing firmly in a structured residency program of increasing and faculty-supervised responsibility and exhorting the building of a strong foundation of surgical education based on Halsted's principles. Cutler was always teaching—at the bedside, in the operating room, and at numerous sessions for the house staff. His 1939 *Atlas of Surgical Operations*, coauthored with colleague Robert M. Zollinger, became immensely popular among trainees throughout the country, went through many editions, was treasured by generations of surgeons and their trainees, and was a prototype for the many specialty atlases that have since emerged.

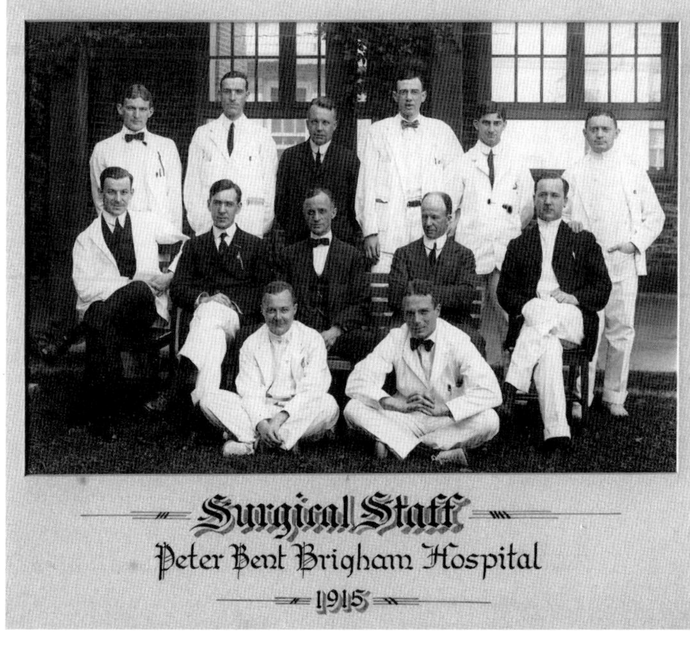

FIGURE 2-6 Peter Bent Brigham surgical staff, 1915.

Other Training Programs

The Nursing School was another important educational responsibility of the new institution. In 1912, the hospital reported:

> *It is expected that the hospital, while primarily for the relief and care of the sick of Suffolk County, will be rich in the clinical material for the education of both medical students and nurses. The active dispensary service which will be maintained will furnish ample opportunity for the study and solving many of the social and economic problems confronting the nurses of today.*[62]

With this bold statement, the hospital expressed an impressive commitment to extend the educational experiment to nurses (discussed more fully later in this chapter by Marilyn King). Superintendent Carrie M. Hall, a proponent of the progressive model of nursing emerging at the turn of the century, was tasked with implementing this lofty challenge. The PBBH School of Nursing (1912-1985) and the Nursing Service charted an ambitious and innovative course toward leadership in the field. The three-year curriculum was to incorporate scientific education with the "nursing arts"—the latter often encompassing the many housekeeping tasks for which nurses were traditionally responsible. Designed by Hall, the curriculum was considered very progressive for its time, with newly established admissions requirements, a preliminary period of scientific didactics (e.g., chemistry, bacteriology, hygiene, dietetics), and clinical rotations at affiliated hospitals, as well as public-health oriented courses such as one on "social problems."

However, the reality of nursing's weak status at the time presented many challenges, as captured in the advice Christian gave graduating nursing students:

> *Be cautious of the spoken word; it is far wiser to remain silent rather than to chatter... Never criticize the methods of treatment or the ability of the physician in charge of your patient... In nursing his patient you become partner in his work and must help in every way to further his plan of treatment.*[63]

As was seen in other teaching hospitals of the time, Hall's broad vision for a scientific curriculum was considerably circumscribed by the hospital's need for inexpensive student labor.[64]

BIOGRAPHY

CARRIE MAE HALL, 1873-1963, Legendary Teacher

Jackie Somerville and Mary Lou Etheredge

Carrie Mae Hall, the first principal of the Peter Bent Brigham Hospital School of Nursing and superintendent of nursing, dedicated her life to caring for patients and elevating educational standards for nurses. "The most important work of the nurse is bedside nursing," Hall declared, an art "resting solidly on education and science." During her twenty-five-year tenure Hall helped transform the hospital into one of Boston's leading healthcare institutions. By creating a highly regarded school of nursing and nursing service, Hall not only assured excellent care for the hospital's patients, but also established her own reputation as a national nursing leader.

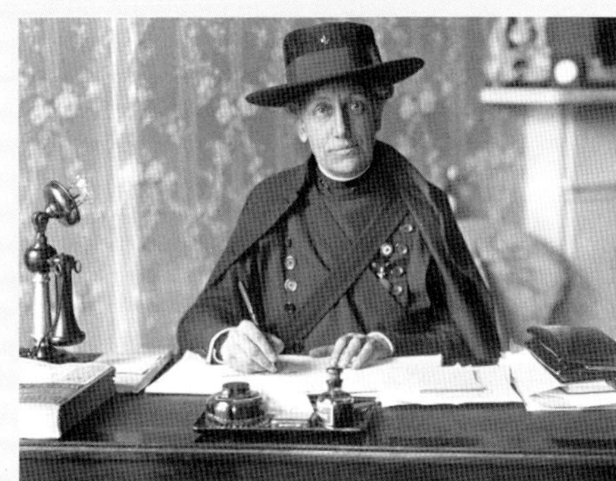

FIGURE 2-7 Carrie Hall.

Born in 1873, Mary (as she was called by her family) was her parents' oldest child and only daughter. She started caring for others early, taking charge of the family home and the care of her father and two younger brothers when her mother died in 1893. This experience reinforced her loyalty and commitment to caring and no doubt influenced her decision to study nursing.

Carrie Hall entered professional nursing during its formative years, enrolling in the Massachusetts General Hospital Training School for Nurses in 1901. The training school was one of a trio of important nursing schools that had opened in 1873 (the others were in Connecticut and at Bellevue Hospital in New York City) and were based on the Nightingale model, which combined practical experience with formal classroom instruction.[65] Hall's leadership abilities were recognized early, and she was appointed the head nurse of a unit while still a student nurse. She stayed on at Massachusetts General Hospital as a head nurse after completing her training, eventually leaving to become assistant matron at Quincy Hospital and then superintendent of the Margaret Pillsbury General Hospital in Concord, New Hampshire. Hall's natural inclination toward leadership and her thirst for learning soon led her to enroll in an eight-month course in hospital economics for nurses at Columbia University's Teachers College, which was the first program for nurses to be based at a university.

In 1912, Hall became principal of the School of Nursing and superintendent of nurses at the Peter Bent Brigham Hospital. She brought with her innovative ideas about nursing education promoted by national nursing leaders. These ideas ranged from establishing more robust entry requirements for schools of nursing to forming affiliations with colleges and other hospitals for the purposes of providing well-rounded learning experiences for students.

From the start, Hall ensured that patients admitted to the Peter Bent Brigham Hospital were cared for by a disciplined cadre of nurses and that students attending the School of Nursing acquired the scientific knowledge and practical experience they needed to provide excellent care. The student population grew quickly, from five students in 1912 to eighty-six in 1916. To her students, Carrie Hall represented strength, authoritative wisdom, and strict discipline—traits that she consistently demonstrated in combination with respect and fairness. At the same time, she was admired as a dedicated nurse and teacher, someone who put the interests of patients first and who was a "stickler for doing the right thing." Privately, she was known as a gentle and warm woman with a wonderful smile and a good sense of humor, who was caring and steadfast and had "a great love for and tolerance of young people." She also loved her summer home at Sagamore Beach and was an expert at darning and crocheting, although this side was a part of herself that she largely reserved for family and friends.

Hall's students may have sometimes chafed under her firm adherence to rules and discipline, but they knew that the rigid structure she imposed was designed for their benefit and that of patients. Her high standards would serve as the foundation for the profession of nursing. In later years, alumna Mary Gilmore would recount how students appreciated "Miss Hall's" efforts, remarking that her "example of integrity, courage, and kindness will continue to be a[n] inspiration to the graduates of her school as long as that school and Brigham traditions exist."[66]

During World War I, Hall interrupted her tenure at the Peter Bent Brigham to become the chief nurse of the Peter Bent Brigham-Harvard Unit, which the Red Cross organized in 1917 in France. Gertrude Gerrard, a graduate of the Peter Bent Brigham Hospital School of Nursing who was with Hall in France, recalled, "It was almost wholly a tent hospital and practically a swamp after the frequent rains...How Miss Hall ever spread our five hundred-bed personnel over that 1,000 bed hospital, I have never understood. But she did it, along with a great many other difficult things."[67] After a year, Hall was appointed head nurse of the American Red Cross in Great Britain and later chief nurse of the American Red Cross in France. Serving until 1919, she was highly decorated for her leadership and received many medals and citations, including the Royal Red Cross Medal and the Florence Nightingale Medal from the International Red Cross.

Although Hall considered her war years as "the smallest part" of her career, they reinforced her view of patient care as the central mission of nursing. On returning to the Brigham in 1919, she re-immersed herself in the work of educating nursing students. She also became active in nursing education nationally, serving on the Board of the National League of Nursing Education from 1922-1932 and as its president from 1925-1927. These were pivotal times, marked by change and reform, for nursing and nursing education. Hall played a central role throughout, chairing and participating in numerous committees at the state and national level working to elevate educational standards, working conditions, and economic security for nurses. Two key reports—*Nursing and Nursing Education in the United States*, also known as the Goldmark Report, published in 1923, and *Nurses, Patients, and Pocketbooks*, a report by the Committee on the Grading of Nursing

Schools, published in 1928—guided much of the discourse at the national level. Carrie Hall remained an active voice shaping this discourse until her retirement in 1937.

Hall's lifelong commitment to nursing did not end with her retirement, as she remained active in the American Red Cross and the American Nurses' Association, and served as a member of the state Public Safety Committee. Through these activities she continued to direct her intelligence and organizational and leadership abilities toward advancing the care of patients and the profession of nursing. In 1963, at the fiftieth anniversary of the Peter Bent Brigham Hospital, General Robert Cutler, honorary chair of the Board of Trustees of the School of Nursing, remembered Hall as being "dedicated throughout her life to two basic principles: quality in education and quality in service," and as "a leader and pioneer in American nursing, in time of war and in time of peace. Generations of skilled nurses grew up under her wise, strong compassionate teaching, a teaching that [is] viewed today in the light of tomorrow."[68]

As a corollary to their teaching commitment, Christian and Cushing introduced a new and comprehensive method of record keeping that fostered patient care, education, and the opportunities for clinical research. Recall that Cushing himself earlier began a tracking system for vital signs in the operating theater that led to many important advances, including discovery of the "Cushing reflex." "Henry A. Christian, chief of medicine of the Peter Bent Brigham Hospital, considered the creation of a set of complete, typed hospital records of all patients at the hospital to be the institution's 'greatest single achievement.'"[69] As Chapter 6 notes, standardization of forms and records was also a Brigham management emphasis, as were early efforts in quality improvement, such as Christian's study of patient flow through the Out-Door Department. In addition to improving communication and enforcing discipline, the patient records in their pasteboard covers were also a gold mine for residents doing clinical research; they were able to tabulate extensive follow-up of many disease states or the results of surgical intervention. Many academic careers opened with publications of those studies.

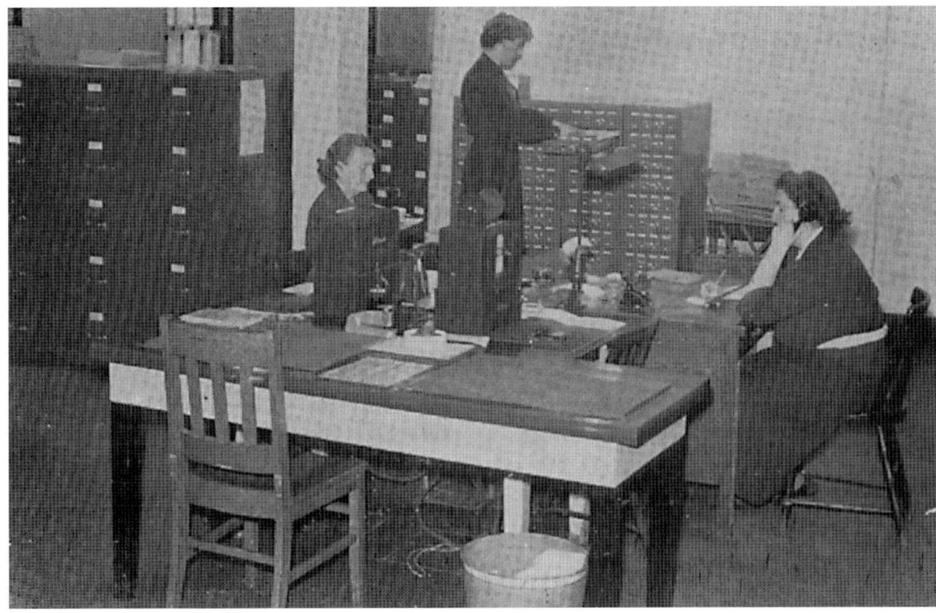

FIGURE 2-8 Peter Bent Brigham Hospital records room, 1951.

On April 30, 1913, amid "scaffolding and plaster,"[70] Sir William Osler paid a visit to officially inaugurate the new hospital.[71] The carefully considered and executed Brigham educational structure embedded the idea of medicine as calling, and Osler's presence sanctioned a symbolic new beginning. After touring the facilities, Osler reflected on what this meant for medical education. "I have no doubt...that you can develop here a scheme for the instruction of the student that will be better than any that has yet been devised."[72] Famously, in his speech that day Osler described the hospital and its teaching programs as "a new and perfectly striking departure" and concluded his remarks by stating: "You are taking a very important step in medical organization and...for the country in the future development of medicine."[73]

The opening of the Brigham was soon followed by the opening or relocation of neighbor institutions in what was to become known as the Longwood Medical Area circling the marble HMS edifice: Children's Hospital (relocated 1914), Forsyth Dental Infirmary for Children (1914), The Infants Hospital (1914), The Robert Bent Brigham Hospital for Incurables (1914), the Harvard School of Public Health (1922), Boston Lying-In Hospital (relocated 1923), and Beth Israel Hospital (1928).[74] Several of these institutions were to merge into the BWH complex many decades later.

REFLECTIONS ON EDUCATION: THE BOSTON HOSPITAL FOR WOMEN

The Boston Hospital for Women (BHW), created in 1966 with the cooperation of HMS, was the merger of two institutions with storied histories, both distinguished for their medical achievements as well as in the education of generations of physicians and surgeons: the Boston Lying-In Hospital (BLI) and the Free Hospital for Women (FHW). The BLI, founded in 1832, presents a history of not only the evolution of the hospital but also of the field of obstetrics itself. The number of great teachers associated with the BLI is impressive, starting with its founders, Walter Channing and Enoch Hale. Channing was an extraordinary figure who became Boston's most prominent obstetrician and the first professor of midwifery at HMS (1818); he was remembered as a "vivid and entertaining" teacher.[75]

William Richardson, the chief of staff for many years, served effectively as a mentor and in July 1894 encouraged George Haven to perform the first cesarean section at the hospital. As a lecturer in the medical school, Richardson was remembered as "forceful and dramatic."[76]

Alfred Worcester was house officer in 1883, at a time when yet another puerperal fever epidemic raged in the hospital. After hearing of the innovative use of antiseptics by August Breisky of Prague, Worcester began the use of antiseptic technique.[77]After initial doubts, Richardson also encouraged the use of antiseptic technique. This and the initial use of rubber gloves by Franklin Newell helped put an end to this pestilence associated with maternity hospitals. Remembered as an exemplary teacher, Newell later cofounded one of the first obstetrical clinics in the country.[78]

In 1930, S. Burt Wolbach at the BLI established the first pathology department in a maternity hospital, one of many "firsts" that led the way for obstetrics teaching innovation and impact. In his 1942 book, *Safe Deliverance,* former Lying-In Obstetrician-in-Chief Frederick Irving described the Lying-In's educational achievements, which included the establishment of the first free outpatient prenatal clinic, the first well-baby clinic, and the first teaching obstetrical clinic.[79] By 1942, 550 house officers, 8,000 medical students, and 6,500 nurses had been trained at the BLI.[80]

The FHW was founded in 1875 by William Henry Baker, who had studied with Marion Sims, founder of the New York Hospital for Women. One of the hospital's educational innovations was evidenced early on, when Baker demonstrated that gynecology could be taught to students in a public clinic in spite of the opposition of the older members of the profession who held that it was immodest and that the public would never permit such instruction.[81]

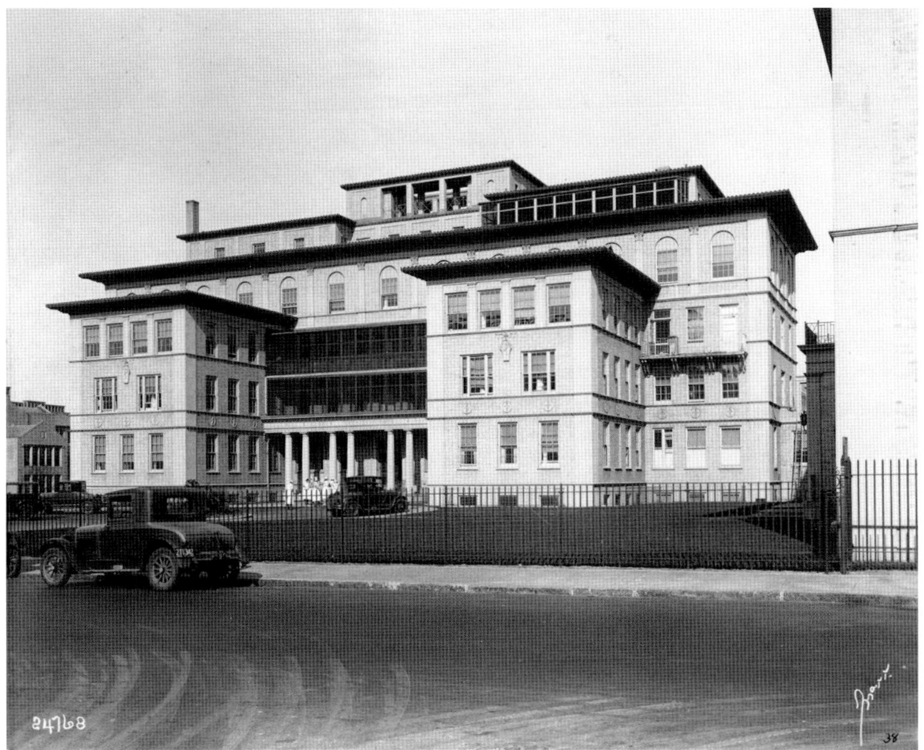

FIGURE 2-9 Boston Lying-In Hospital, 1927.

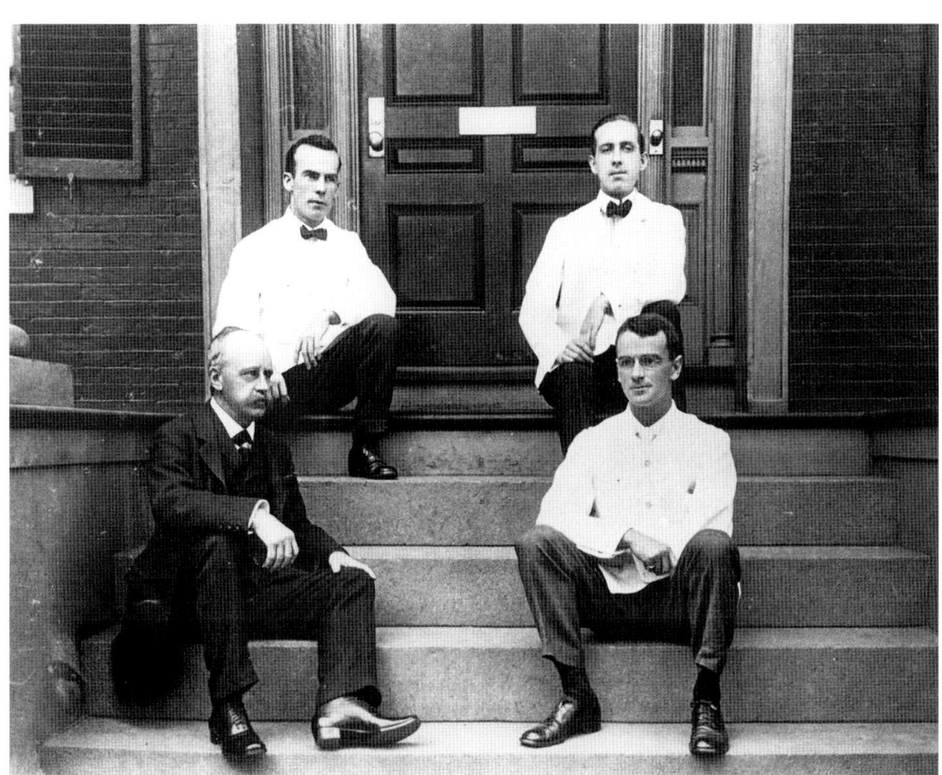

FIGURE 2-10 Boston Lying-In Hospital staff, circa 1900. William Richardson is at lower left.

There were extraordinary opportunities for teaching at the FHW, particularly in the Outpatient Department, which grew each year. In one example, almost 3,000 patients were seen in 1879, at a time when the clinic was closed during the summer.[82] The number grew even more after the FHW moved to Brookline in 1895. Another teacher at the FHW was William Graves, who had studied in Vienna and started out in pathology at the hospital.[83] Graves enhanced the FHW's reputation for excellence even more; by the first decade of the new century, HMS stated that it "was expecting more from the FHW than from any other hospital in respect to the development of the science of surgery in gynecology, but also in the laboratory investigations of causes and processes of women's diseases."[84] Graves worked in close tandem with Superintendent Hannah Ewin, who had started a nursing school at the FHW in 1895.[85]

The educational relationship between the Brigham, the BLI, and the FHW was longstanding. In the 1920s, Harvey Cushing proposed a fused house officer service between the three institutions, with HMS paying salaries. Each resident was expected to devote time to research.[86] The BLI formalized a teaching relationship with the FHW in 1951, when the obstetrical and gynecology training programs, which had been informally associated since 1922, were combined. The BLI and FHW integrated residencies to provide the three years of the combined training needed for certification by the American Board of Obstetrics and Gynecology. Finally, the 1966 merger between the FHW and the BLI, in cooperation with HMS, to form the Boston Hospital for Women, was one of the foundations for the 1975 overall merger of the PBBH, Robert Breck Brigham Hospital, and Boston Hospital for Women that created BWH.[87]

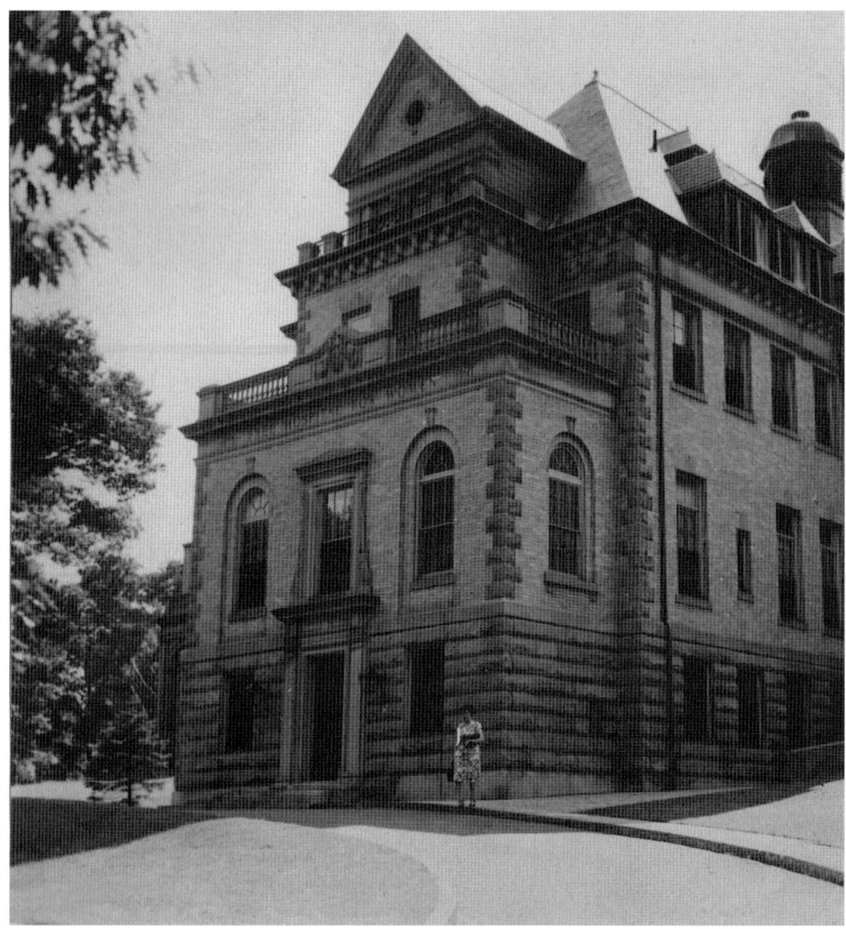

FIGURE 2-11 Free Hospital for Women, 1970s.

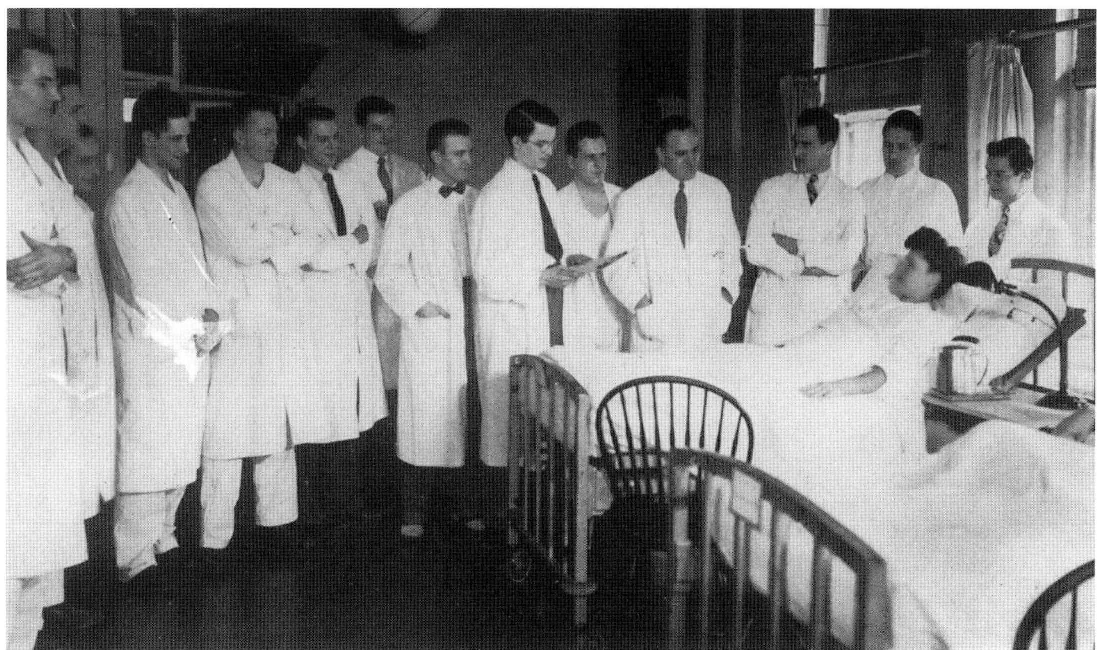

FIGURE 2-12 Duncan Reid leading rounds at Boston Lying-In Hospital, 1947.

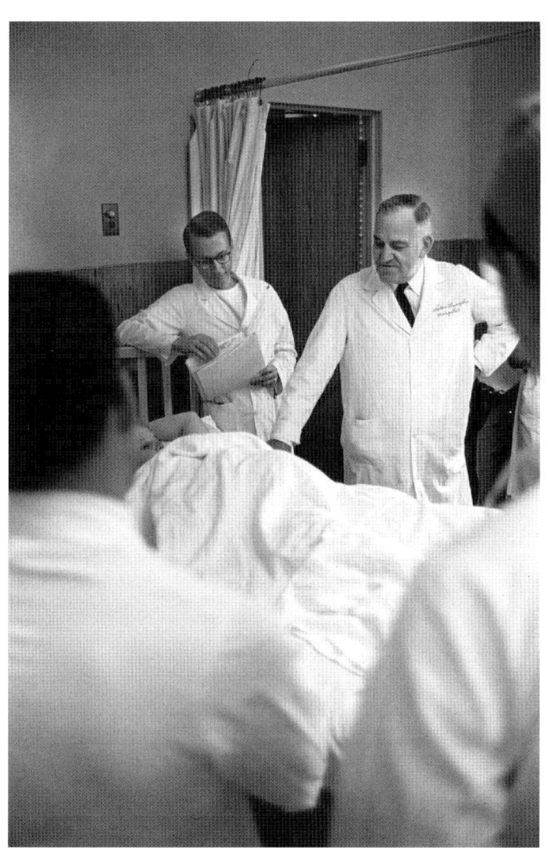

FIGURE 2-13 Duncan Reid leading rounds at Boston Hospital for Women, 1968.

These legacies of hospital, educational and research development would thrive after the 1975 merger and subsequent move to the BWH tower in the early 1980s. The educational mission of the Boston Hospital for Women lives on in the work of the Center for Women and Newborns, the Mary Horrigan Connors Center for Women's Health, and the multidepartmental Division of Women's Health and Gender Biology.

REFLECTIONS ON EDUCATION: THE ROBERT B. BRIGHAM HOSPITAL

The Robert Breck Brigham Hospital (RBBH) opened in 1914 through a bequest of Robert Breck Brigham, Peter's nephew. It would become the first American teaching hospital devoted exclusively to the care of arthritis and rheumatic disease. There were many notable educators in its history, including Joel Goldthwaite, the progressive orthopedic surgeon and planner of orthopedic surgery hospitals during World War I. Goldthwaite also established the underlying philosophy of treatment at

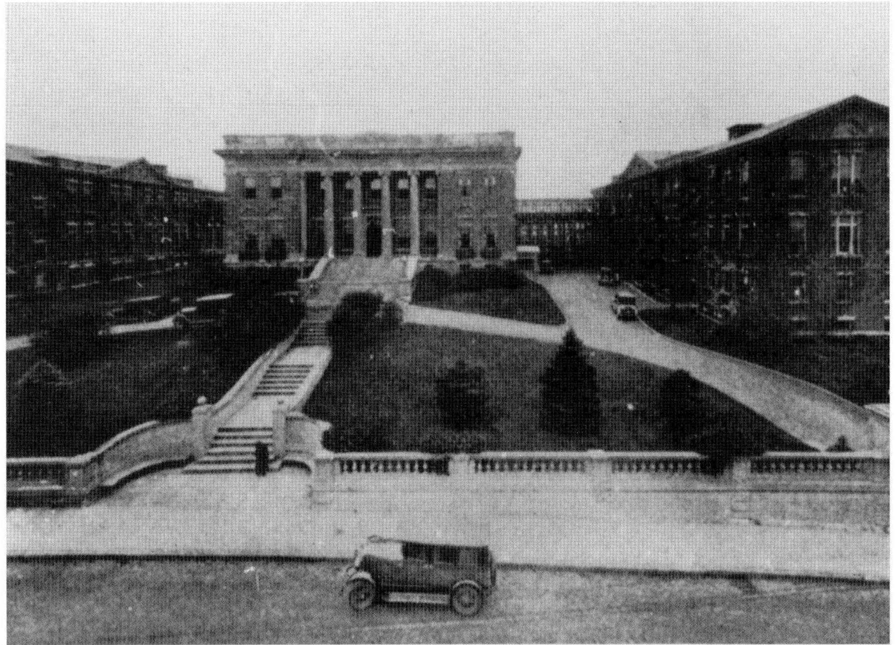

FIGURE 2-14 Robert Breck Brigham Hospital, circa 1928.

RBBH, which was based on a holistic sense of the patient, incorporating their family and social context. He also established the first hospital occupational therapy department, encouraged associated training programs, and formed an orthopedic nursing school at the hospital. Another early teacher was Loring Swain, who emphasized an integrative approach to care, including the importance of spiritual concerns.

The RBBH had an educational mission that existed in tandem with a progressive approach, emphasizing the community as well as medical education. Both Tufts and HMS students attended ward rounds in the 1930s, although it would not be until 1966 that the RBBH would officially become a Harvard teaching hospital.

In part because of financial obstacles during the early years of the RBBH, care was provided by referring physicians. In 1933, the first full-time physician, E. Douglas Taylor, was appointed.[88] Taylor held a weekly clinic to educate students and community physicians; his teaching was oriented toward promoting awareness of rheumatic disease, particularly approaches designed to emphasize a positive, rehabilitative approach.

The relationship between the RBBH and PBBH was cemented after World War II, with encouragement from George Thorn, chief of medicine at the PBBH. Residents from his department began to rotate through the "Robert Breck" and clinical research fellows were appointed.

Arthur Hall and Peter Barry were early RBBH clinician-educators who influenced many subsequent rheumatologists, including the legendary teacher Ronald J. Anderson, who became the initial RBBH director of clinical training programs in 1971 when the first rheumatology and immunology fellowship was established. Clement B. Sledge, chief of orthopedic surgery, was a pioneer in joint replacement surgery, succeeding gifted teacher Sydney Stillman. Physician-in-Chief K. Frank Austen elevated the RBBH immunology research program to worldwide renown and played a central role in the merger that created what is known today as the BWH.[89,90]

BIOGRAPHY

JEAN MARLENE JACKSON, 1942-2008, Legendary Teacher

Ronald J. Anderson

Jean Marlene Jackson, a rheumatologist and internist at the Brigham and Women's Hospital for nearly 30 years, was the embodiment of excellence as a clinician and teacher. Her skills and commitment to the care of patients and the education of developing physicians defined her career.

To understand the challenges Jackson faced and the areas in which she was a pioneer, one should first appreciate the era in which she trained as a physician. Jackson applied to medical school in the mid-1960s, when fewer than 10% of the students were women. Harvard Medical School had accepted its first woman student only two decades previously, and only a handful of women had been residents in the Department of Medicine at the Peter Bent Brigham Hospital. During the application process, female applicants were frequently asked to justify why they should "take the place of a male" in the entering class. This was asked of Jackson several times.

After graduating from the University of Rhode Island, she entered the University of Maryland Medical School. During her third year she rotated as an extern at the Good Samaritan Hospital, a Johns Hopkins institution focusing on the area of rheumatology, orthopedics, and rehabilitation, in many respects similar to the Robert Breck Brigham Hospital. The "Good Sam's" clinical director was the legendary Mary Betty Stevens, a gifted and devoted clinician and teacher who served as a role model for Jackson as well as for numerous medical students and residents.

Jackson came to the Robert Breck Brigham Hospital in 1970 as a research fellow and worked on humoral immunity in the laboratory of Peter Schur. Her clinical interest in juvenile rheumatoid arthritis was sparked by James Sydney Stillman, the former physician-in-chief who had created investigational and therapeutic programs for children afflicted with arthritis at a time when treatment modalities for these conditions were minimal. Although she had no formal training in pediatrics, Jackson participated actively in programs related to juvenile rheumatoid arthritis in her fellowship and subsequently throughout her career. By the 1980s she was appointed to the staff of Boston's Children's Hospital Medical Center, where her clinical skills and teaching had a major impact on a generation of pediatricians and pediatric rheumatologists.

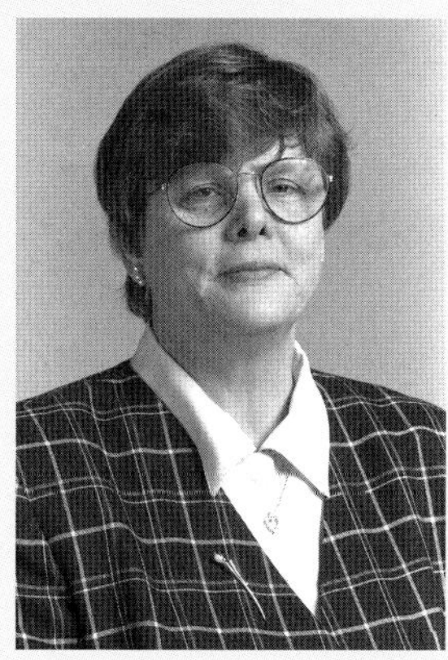

FIGURE 2-15 Jean Jackson.

After completing her fellowship in 1972, Jackson returned to the University of Maryland to serve as chief medical resident and then joined the faculty as clinical director of rheumatology. In 1975 she returned to the Robert Brigham as a full-time clinician-teacher, with an appointment at Harvard Medical School. Although this mode of practice is currently standard, only a handful of physicians on the Harvard faculty in the 1970s functioned in this role. She served as an attending physician at the Robert Breck Brigham and also as the first female attending physician on the General Medical Service at the Peter Bent Brigham Hospital.

For the next thirty years, before and after the merger of these two hospitals, she was a revered and highly effective teacher, role model, and mentor to the house staff and medical students. Jackson had an imposing presence, related in part to her almost encyclopedic knowledge of medicine and her height of close to six feet, which could initially be intimidating to house staff and medical students. On meeting a patient, however, her innate warmth and compassion would radiate and a relationship of trust would develop. She was a master of the art of bedside teaching. Her ability to perform and teach the physical examination was extraordinary and done in a manner that was sensitive to the patient and the audience.

Jackson believed strongly that the essence of being an effective physician was a persistent effort to understand the patient, the illness affecting that patient, and the effect of the illness on the patient's life. She incorporated these concepts into the care of her patients and stressed them in her interactions with physicians at all levels. She held her students to the highest of standards, but acknowledged their efforts with sincerity and gratitude. Despite her forceful personality and unbounded enthusiasm for her work, she never involved her personal ego, doing only what was best for the patient. Her fellow physicians, the nursing staff, allied health personnel, and others dedicated to patient care appreciated her compassion, skills, and dedication to excellence and profited from the experience.

In the final four years of her life, Jackson was limited by complications related to metastatic breast cancer and was unable to continue practicing medicine. Still in good spirits, she remained an exemplary teacher on a different level, teaching her colleagues how to care for individuals with a terminal illness. She stressed that patients always need hope and concern, irrespective of their prognosis, and if a physician no longer performs a physical examination during a visit, it is an indication that hope no longer exists. In recognition of her skills and commitment, a Special Award for Teaching was presented to her by the Department of Medicine in 2007. After her death, in 2008, the Jean M. Jackson Award for Excellence in Bedside Teaching was established and is awarded annually.

Jean Jackson was truly a pioneer in both establishing the role of women in clinical medicine at the Harvard teaching hospitals and defining the role of the full time clinician-teacher. Her aim was to be the best physician possible and to instill this goal and desire in others. Buoyant and enthusiastic, she was a nurturing individual who was always available for advice and support. I had the joy and honor to be associated with Jean for over thirty years. Her warmth, character, skills, commitment to excellence, and compassion for others were transmitted to those she trained, her coworkers at all levels, and to the many patients fortunate enough to have been under her care.

POSTWAR GROWTH AND THE EDUCATIONAL EXPERIENCE AT THE BRIGHAM

Medical school education underwent significant changes after World War II. Some schools experimented with new approaches to presenting the material taught in the first two years. Rather than teaching the sciences in individual, discipline-specific courses, they taught relevant material drawn from each of the sciences in units organized around individual body organs or organ systems. This approach was adopted as a means of integrating, as much as possible, content across the sciences as well as basic science and clinical disciplines. In virtually all schools, clinical clerkships were moved from the fourth year (the Osler model) to the third, with the fourth year more frequently devoted to rotations in hospital clinics and to inpatient services in clinical disciplines not represented by the routine clerkships.[91]

In the 1940s and 1950s, ever more effective therapies began to allow recovery from relatively commonly encountered medical conditions, such as rheumatic fever, pernicious anemia, syphilis, and tuberculosis. Expertise in certain surgical and medical areas attracted patients to the Brigham with uncommon conditions, especially in the fields of kidney disease, endocrinology, hematology, and heart diseases. With advances in available therapies and the advent of Blue Cross and later Medicare and Medicaid to pay for them, the volume and complexity of patient care increased. One result was that their burgeoning clinical responsibilities placed increasingly heavy demands on young physicians. Residents took call every other night and every other weekend.[92] Despite their onerous schedule, the Brigham was characterized by a heady atmosphere in which to train. The emphasis was on quality, excellence, and camaraderie.

Research also became more and more a priority in physician training. Reflecting on the role of research in medical education in the thirty-fifth Peter Bent Brigham Annual Report for the year 1948, George Thorn noted its ever-expanding role:

> *Slowly, but progressively, during the past decade, medical undergraduate teaching has shifted to the hospitals to permit closer correlation of instruction*

in fundamental science with the practical application in the care of patients and study of disease. Such a shift has been made possible by the presence on the hospital staff of men with fundamental training in the medical sciences...The University has signified its willingness to cooperate with the hospitals in making joint appointments available for medical scientists working in the clinical hospital units.[93]

The breadth of surgery and surgical education also expanded substantially after World War II. Not only had the returning surgeons increased their own expertise and innovations in the care of the wounded, but new technologies were enhancing the scientific basis of the field. The new surgeon-in-chief at the Brigham in 1948, Francis D. Moore, a surgeon-scientist of renown, enthusiastically exploited these advances for patient care and resident education and was himself a most dynamic and charismatic "father" of many surgical graduates. The virtual revolution in surgery and its applied sciences also encouraged the growth of specialties that included gynecology, heart and vascular surgery, organ transplantation, and others.

Physicians' personal lives were affected by the intensity of the experience. Although in other parts of the United States, more and more residents were married and lived outside of hospital confines, the tide turned slowly at the Brigham and residents continued to live at the hospital.[94] "At that time, the Brigham had a rule that you couldn't change your marital status after you came as a house officer, so I got married 4 days before we came so I didn't have to get someone's permission," recalled one 1951 house officer.[95]

Grand Rounds were patient-oriented and attended by the full faculty. The hospital's first salaried neurology consultant, H. Richard Tyler, recalls:

In the front row would be George Thorn, Franny Moore, and the Head of Radiology. They interacted with each other; you would learn tremendously as each one baited the other. For example, the radiologist would remark, "George, go up and read the X-ray," as he taught Thorn how to read an X-ray. But of course, in teaching George Thorn, he taught everybody in the audience.[96]

Pathology played a critical role in the clinical and research missions: "Everybody had post-mortems in those days and there would be no question that as an intern you would always feel terrible if you didn't get a post-mortem. [The autopsy rates ran] between 70-95%."[97] The procedure was laborious, including preparation of 2 × 2 inch lantern slides for later presentation and a serious commitment of time for all involved.

Desperately needed funding was required to support the increase in research activities of trainees at the Brigham after World War II. Fortunately, this process was expedited by newly established government grants as well as private philanthropy. No philanthropy went further than that given by a patient of Thorn, the reclusive aircraft industry tycoon Howard Hughes, who launched The Howard Hughes Medical Institute (HHMI), the landmark biomedical research charity. Beginning in 1954, Thorn, who became HHMI's director of research in 1956,[98] was asked to play key roles in the organization and used its monies to steady the financial course at the hospital and to launch important research and educational programs. When cash was low, Thorn also opened the emergency room to ambulances that had previously been directed to other charity institutions, further enriching the educational experience.

Tyler recalls that when he joined the Brigham faculty in 1956, his entire yearly salary, $7,500, was paid by HHMI, noting that "at that time the Brigham was a small hospital, 250 beds or so, and was known as the research hospital: a very small staff, but highly endowed with research." By this time, most physicians pursued extra years of specialized training. Thorn was a great proponent of this departure, often assigning students areas of specializations whether or not they desired them. Thomas O'Brien recalls that Thorn called him to his office and announced that he should become an infectious diseases specialist, at a time when the fledgling Brigham microbiology lab needed leadership; O'Brien dutifully complied, and in 2013, forty-five years later, he was still leading the now greatly expanded, state-of-the-art laboratory facilities.

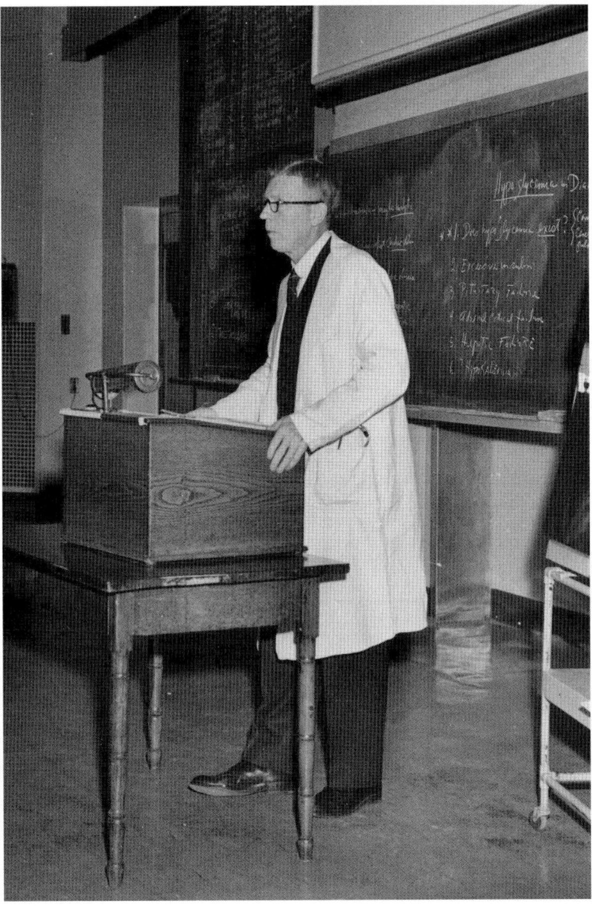

FIGURE 2-16 George Thorn.

A DEMOCRATIC APPROACH TO EDUCATION

Over the years, "The Pike"—the original open pathway and later closed corridor connecting the series of low buildings that comprised the PBBH—became a symbol of affection and a central focus for educational activities, much as did "The Yard" at Harvard College. Impromptu gatherings along the Pike served as forums for consultation and starting points for grand research collaborations. As funding improved, Moore and Thorn exploited the opportunities provided by new faculty and new areas of research; the expectations for trainees to participate in and get credit for their research contributions also increased. At the Brigham, "senior faculty would look out for junior faculty where the chief of internal medicine went to great lengths to ensure that the younger instructors received proper credit of authorship for their investigative work."[99] In this vein, the legendary Brigham teacher, Richard Gorlin, often removed his name from publications so that his trainees would receive the credit and not be overshadowed by his well-established fame.[100]

The "Doctor's Dining Room" was the hub of the hospital, a site where the lowliest and loftiest physicians met at mealtime, providing an opportunity for clinical and scientific discourse that was decidedly unusual in academia. Through the early 1960s, service was with silver and cloth napkins.[101] Although the cuisine was not glamorous,[102] staff at all levels dined together, creating a collegial and relaxed air and time of great teaching that Marshall A. Wolf described as "lunch with the stars."[103] Tyler also reflects on this unusually high level of access that contributed to the *esprit de corps*. "If you wanted a consultation, you always knew who ate at 12:30, who ate at 12:45 and you'd go and you'd have dinner with them and sit at their table."[104] An evening meal occurred about 10 or 11 o'clock every night, "and staff would frequently come back and eat with the residents and interns."[105] Former resident Phillip J. Snodgrass recalls: "I learned more good medical stories at midnight snacks than I ever heard in daily rounds."[106] This positive atmosphere facilitated innovative cross-disciplinary teaching and investigations, such as were possible in areas of mutual strength and interest: metabolism, pernicious anemia, kidney injury and transplant, heart failure and valvular surgery, and endocrine physiology and gland resection.

Friday night open bar was a regular fixture into the 1970s, occasionally with heavy consumption; even in the 1990s the residual Friday "Liver Rounds" persisted as an opportunity for residents and staff to relax with friends on the hospital grounds.[107] An important result of this institutional philosophy was the warm relationship that existed between trainees in each of the departments, apparently in contrast to other major regional and national medical centers. The mutual respect and affection was the consequence of the intimate size, architectural elements such as the horizontal Pike design, and shared purpose. This mutuality was echoed loudly at the very top, particularly by Surgical Chiefs Moore and Mannick and Medical Chief Thorn. The leadership demonstrated genuine respect for both clinicians and investigators and offered the possibility for everyone to do both, based on their own abilities.

A number of prominent leaders chose to see patients and teach exclusively, which was supported at the highest levels.[108] Eugene Eppinger, for example, who started at the Brigham as an intern in 1931, recognizing that a research-intensive environment needed master clinicians, gave up his fledgling investigative career to become the hospital's only full-time clinician.[109] With that, he took charge of the medicine training as program director and demanded excellence and dedication at every level while cementing the HMS relationship where he was assistant dean.

Kenneth H. Falchuk recalls that after an exhausting night on call in 1966, he showed up unshaven to rounds conducted by Eppinger. Eppinger disapprovingly requested that he go shave and change his attire; Falchuk then inquired, "Where should I meet the team?"

Eppinger sternly replied, "The team will wait right here until you look presentable."[110]

Marshall A. Wolf, who was an intern in 1963 and became medicine training director in 1972, also remembers: "You did not want to be called to Dr. Eppinger's office."[111]

Eppinger's stringent standards led to more than just housestaff foreboding. He was considered the "doctor's doctor" of the time and as such attracted complicated and vexing referral cases that helped keep the wards full of interesting patients. He also had an eye toward quality and turned to the house officers for solutions, sometimes spontaneously. Wolf recalls that on one occasion as an intern he was called to Eppinger's office, and although he came directly, it was not quickly enough for Eppinger's taste. Eppinger asked him, "What took you so long to get here?"

Wolf replied that there were sections of the hospital where overhead pages could not be heard and bravely added: "In some hospitals they apparently have 'bell-boys' to solve this problem." At the end of the day, Wolf was again summoned overhead to come to Eppinger's office. This time, Eppinger's secretary handed him and all the house officers brand new bell-boys (the predecessor of pagers), purchased that day.[112]

BIOGRAPHY

BERNARD LOWN (1921-), Legendary Teacher

Joel T. Katz and Peter V. Tishler

Bernard Lown, a Lithuanian Jew who escaped the impending Holocaust at age fifteen, is a boundary-defying cardiologist well known as a scientist, humanist, critic, and inspiring teacher. Lown developed the human cardiac defibrillator in 1962 based on Paul Zoll's demonstration that a heart could be restarted after open heart surgery with delivery of a 110-volt alternating current shock. He founded Physicians for Social Responsibility in 1961 and later co-cofounded International Physicians for the Prevention of Nuclear War, for which he received the Nobel Peace Prize in 1985.[113] (His mother always thought he would win a Nobel Prize.) Marshall A. Wolf, one of his trainees, describes Lown as "a brilliant clinician who was also interested in the patient as a human being."

Before arriving at the Brigham, Lown proved that the causation of arrhythmias and fatalities from digitalis was often the result of diuretic-induced hypokalemia. This challenged and disproved the hypothesis of Samuel A. Levine and led to Levine inviting Lown to be his cardiology fellow at the Brigham in 1950. Lown studied the pharmacology of the digitalis preparations, advocated the routine use of digoxin because of its superior properties and lesser risk, and published a book on the use of the digitalis preparations with Levine. He pioneered in the creation of a

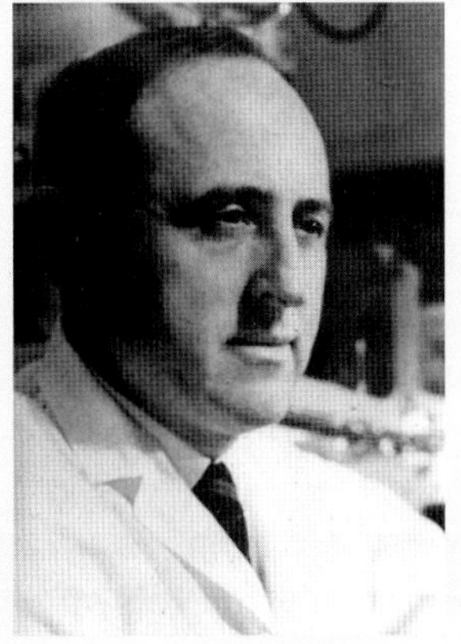

FIGURE 2-17 Bernard Lown.

coronary care unit at the Brigham in 1965—the Levine Coronary Unit (LCU), which was among the first in the country. His treatment of patients with an acute myocardial infarction included not only close observation in the LCU, but also lidocaine prophylaxis to prevent arrhythmias (his finding, in 1968), defibrillating if necessary, and rapidly mobilizing patients from bed (his therapy, with Levine) to reduce the likelihood of thrombotic events.

Lown had the ability to connect deeply with his patients regardless of their social or medical situation. Exemplifying his unique style, a trainee recalls a physical examination rounds session in the early 1990s during which Lown was asked to demonstrate cardiac auscultation for assembled students and medicine residents. Lown entered the room, introduced himself to the elderly woman patient, and held her hand while asking probing and sympathetic questions about her life, past and present, eliciting details previously unknown to the team. Near the end of the discussion, he gently percussed her chest wall and left the room with the team. When asked about auscultation of the heart, Lown explained that hearing the patient's story and feeling her pulse revealed all that he needed to know—establishing a diagnosis of mitral stenosis as a consequence of rheumatic fever, which had now progressed to heart failure.[114]

Lown was a magnetic teacher and worked hard to demonstrate that technology is no substitute for high-quality interpersonal interactions with patients. His establishment of the Lown Cardiovascular Research Foundation in 1973 is his monument to these important basics of medical practice and medical care. By his example, the physicians in the group, while minimizing the use of invasive procedures, achieve therapeutic success rates that are as good as if not superior to those of other cardiologic practices. In 1987, he founded Satellife, an organization that distributes health information to practitioners in nations without access to basic medical information that ensures quality care, and in 1997, he founded ProCor, a global network that promotes access to cost-effective preventive strategies and noninvasive medical management of cardiac disease.

Lown's lesson that technology cannot surpass the human touch became the focus of his 1996 memoir, *The Lost Art of Healing*. In reference to this work he stated:

> *Now the doctor, by virtue of accepting science so totally, creates a total imbalance, forgetting the art of healing, forgetting the art of engagement, forgetting the art of listening, forgetting the art of caring and ceasing to invest time with the patient. So I believe medicine has lost its human face.*[115]

In recognition of Lown's unique and lasting contributions, in 2010 the Brigham established its first hospital-wide faculty teaching award—the Bernard Lown, M.D. Award for Excellence in Teaching.

ADDITIONAL EDUCATIONAL PROGRAMS

The powerful chiefs of surgery and medicine cautiously and sometimes begrudgingly opened up opportunities for specialists outside the core departments to assume care and teaching responsibilities for their patients. Neurology is an example. In 1956, Tyler became the first full-time neurological consultant and was soon followed by David M. Dawson; they were eventually allowed to devote ten beds to the care of such patients. Medicine interns were assigned to rotate with them, joined by a neurology resident from Boston City Hospital, when available. Once the medicine program director was satisfied with the quality of the experience, the first Brigham neurology training slot, shared with the adjacent Children's Hospital, was opened in 1962. The neurology training program expanded from one to three years' duration, and eventually, in 1988, Tyler's successor, Martin A. Samuels—one of the first faculty at the research-intensive HMS to be appointed full professor as a clinician-educator—gained the endorsement of chairs Eugene Braunwald and John A. Mannick and the trustees to elevate neurology to full departmental status.

The pathology residency, established in 1958 and now the longest continually funded such program in the country (National Heart, Lung, and Blood Institute and National Research Service Award), also steadily grew in scope and influence. With a strong research focus, 50% of residents trained since 1974 held both MD and PhD degrees, a figure that increases to approximately 70% for residents selected after 1990. As a consequence of the mentoring and academic focus, "over 25 [current] chairs of Pathology departments throughout the country trained at BWH."[116]

Moore's successor as surgeon-in-chief in 1976, John A. Mannick, and his director of education, Anthony D. Whittemore, expanded surgical training to accommodate the new surgical divisions and increased operative volume. Increasingly sophisticated imaging methods and the advent of minimally invasive techniques contributed significantly. The breadth of general surgery itself increased, reflective of new, more challenging, and more sophisticated subspecialty procedures. Fellowships in subspecialty training following board eligibility in general surgery were now available for individuals intending to specialize.

LEVELING THE PLAYING FIELD AND REACHING OUTWARD

By the 1960s and 1970s, the strict, pyramidal method of promotion had created a competitive training environment that was widely prevalent in academic hospitals of the time. "Being a resident in the early 1970s was like being in the Marine Corps," recalls Eugene Braunwald. "There was a sink-or-swim mentality."[117] The hostile tone was set early, during the harrowing intern selection process. Through the early 1970s, aspiring medical students were invited to interview for the medicine training program in two large groups—half HMS students and half the top students from the remaining U.S. medical schools. Students were paraded through seven rooms where faculty grilled them on minute areas of their own expertise, often biochemistry or obscure philosophical challenges, "until the applicants broke."[118] Surgery used similar methods.

As an example, Tyler recalls being asked, "Do foxes eat grasshoppers?" at his Brigham internship interview, which he somehow felt preferable to the purely factual oral examination he was hammered with at his MGH interview.

> *The question I was asked at the Brigham, I thought, was probably the most intelligent way of finding out what I did because they knew I didn't know [all the answers], so [the Brigham approach] first, picked out the bluffers and second, the next part of the question was, You don't know, how would you figure it out? I think that question more than anything else persuaded me that the Brigham was more interested in me as a person, rather than just someone who could spit back facts.*[119]

The faculty could then go on to pit one applicant against another, asking one to critique the other applicant's answers.[120] When Wolf became the medicine residency director in 1972, he was assigned the task to "recruit the future faculty"[121] and recognized that this selection process, combined with the pyramidal, competitive promotions, led to attracting and promoting exactly the wrong personal qualities one hopes for in the most effective physicians. He and Braunwald did away with both the pyramidal and competitive aspects of house officer selection and began a focus "to look at the human qualities of the people we recruit,"[122] apparently a first for academic programs in the United States.

Braunwald and Wolf next set out to alter the toxic aspects of the culture of the medicine training program and rectify the woeful lack of diversity by making extra efforts to identify and attract more women and minority physicians, creating flexible schedules that allowed for parenting, engaging trainees in intern selection and program governance (via weekly "Mouse Club meetings"), scheduling sessions for reflection (the Humanistic Curriculum cofounded with William T. Branch, Jr.), and reducing overnight call frequency from every-other-day to every-third-day—all trend-setting moves.[123] When the affiliated hospitals united to form the BWH in 1980, the distinction between "private" and "ward" patients was also eliminated, bringing to fruition a long-overdue sense of equity consistent with the more progressive ethos of the time. In his biography of Eugene Brauwald, Thomas H. Lee, Jr. wrote: "These changes helped set a new tone, and the Brigham Department of Medicine became known as a serious but happy place."[124] In doing so, Wolf "humanized the training programs, relieving some of the work-related stress and encouraging staff and teachers to be compassionate and helpful to the trainees."[125] Wolf credited the changes as exemplifying "the hopeful spirit that permeates the Brigham."[126]

Braunwald and Wolf set out to reconcile the increased clinical demands with their desire to encourage scientific investigation by establishing the first hybrid physician-scientist training options in the country. As science expanded in the postwar period, there was increasing need for more methodological training than had been expected in the early Brigham days. Braunwald was committed to providing his trainees what he felt were the essential ingredients for a successful academic career: in-depth engagement in patient care, inspiring mentors, strong team building, encouragement to ask original and important questions, and feeling the "thrill of the chase."[127] Braunwald and Wolf created scheduling flexibility to allow for carefully selected residents to alternate time on the wards and in the laboratory sufficient to maintain academic momentum—what they called a "Research residency"—and also implemented the forerunner of the current "Short-Track" training model, whereby scientifically bent trainees can move through clinical training at an accelerated pace.[128]

Proving the value of such reforms, from the very first, many Research Residency trainees went on to distinguished academic careers, among them Edward Benz (president and chief executive officer, Dana-Farber Cancer Center), Jeffrey Drazen (editor, *New England Journal of Medicine)*, Peter Libby (chief, BWH Cardiology Division), Thomas Musliner (executive director, Merck Pharmaceuticals), Paul Farmer (Kolokotrones University Professor, Harvard College, and chair, HMS Global Health and Social Medicine Department), and Jim Kim (director, World Bank).

Partly as a result of house staff and student advocacy, as well as the availability of federal funds, more educational opportunities were offered in community settings, including experiences in neighborhood health centers and other ambulatory settings. Primary care became a priority. In 1975, Braunwald noted:

> *After a period in which most progress in medicine was made by examining, in great depth, individual organs and organ systems, it is time to "put the patient together again" and to build up a strong cadre of general internists capable of seeing the patient as a whole and serving as models for students and residents.*[129]

This approach would be championed by Braunwald along with H. Richard Nesson and Wolf,[130] who established two of the pioneering programs to train primary care physicians embedded within an academic medical center—one based at the Brigham and the other at the newly established Harvard Community Health Plan, which was an independent, staff-model health maintenance organization with some shared staff and patients. The value of this trend was reinforced as care shifted from inpatient to outpatient settings and primary care providers emerged as gatekeepers in the new healthcare systems of the 1990s.

The 1970s merger of PBBH with the Boston Hospital for Women and the Robert Breck Brigham Hospital, and the eventual 1980 move into the new Tower as Brigham and Women's Hospital, meant that professional cultures, including those of medical education, had now to be brought together. Although based on justified pride in the accomplishments of the program in the separate institutions and their various departments, the "parochialism" which Associated Hospitals Center President F. Stanton Deland had referred to in one annual report would have to be overcome in approaches to medical education as well. The 1996 Partners Healthcare merger between BWH and MGH, which resulted in the consolidation of a number of residency and fellowship training programs, including orthopedics, neurology, dermatology, plastic surgery, and oncology, has required valuable, but in some cases contentious, redefinition of the educational mission. Currently, there are sixteen Partners Healthcare-wide Accreditation Council for Graduate Medical Education (ACGME)–accredited residencies and fellowships rotating at the Brigham, compared with thirty-seven that have remained independent.[131]

BIOGRAPHY

MARSHALL ALAN WOLF (1937-), Legendary Teacher

Joel T. Katz

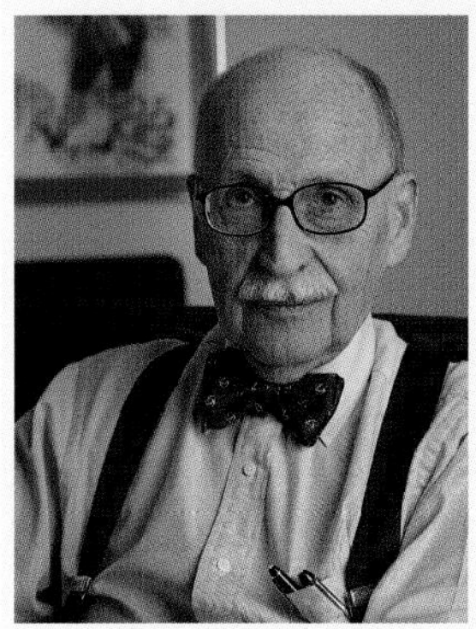

FIGURE 2-18 Marshall Wolf.

As the *Brigham and Women's Magazine* reported in 2011:

> *Marshall Wolf, emeritus vice chair for Medical Education at the Brigham and Women's Hospital (BWH), is known as a straight-talking, no-nonsense physician with extremely high standards—a combination that can be intimidating. He is also described as one of the most generous, nurturing, and effective mentors in medicine. Wolf, who is legendary for launching the careers of some of medicine's great leaders, has trained thousands of doctors in a way that brings out the best they have to offer. "He has one of the most effective mentoring styles I've ever seen," marvels Jim Kim, currently head of the World Bank and a former BWH and Wolf trainee.*[132]

Wolf arrived at the PBBH in 1963 as a Harvard Medical School clerk and stood out for his brilliance and attitude. After training in medicine and cardiology, Wolf was hired by the fourth chair of medicine, Eugene Braunwald, to direct the residency program (1972-2000). This would become a legendary partnership: Braunwald the prodigious scholar and Wolf the kind-hearted teacher, both exacting and visionary.

Wolf's first realization as program director was that the intern selection process in place at all academic hospitals of the time—including a grueling series of oral examinations—fostered a competitive and often hostile environment among the interns who survived, not the type of traits he was looking to perpetuate. He reorganized the selection process to identify previously undervalued characteristics, such as kindness, collegiality, and creativity. "Medicine," he told applicants, "is not a competitive sport." Next, he eliminated the pyramidal promotions structure that had been present for half a century at the Brigham and at other teaching hospitals, so that all qualified interns could have the option to return as assistant and senior residents.

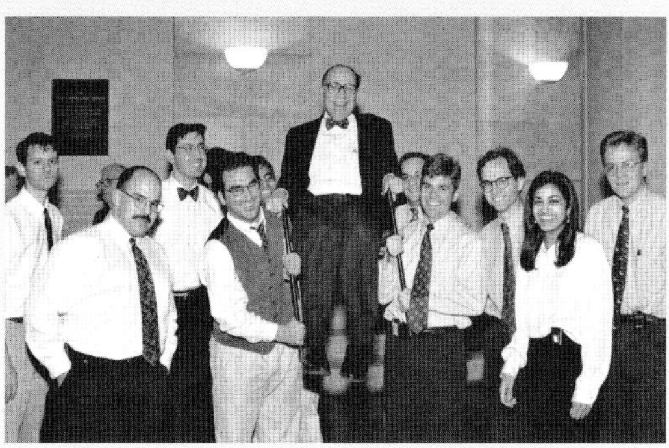

FIGURE 2-19 "Medical residents and students hoist Wolf in an affectionate salute to his untiring commitment to mentoring young doctors-in-training, at a ceremony at Harvard Medical School in 1997." Originally published in the *Brigham Bulletin*.

These innovations gradually opened the doors to a new group of medical students who had been steered away from academic medicine at Harvard, particularly woman physicians.

With Braunwald's support, Wolf developed one of the foremost academic primary care residency programs in the country, and a number of other innovative models for preparing future leaders. Former pupil Jeffrey Drazen, editor-in-chief of the *New England Journal of Medicine* and a senior physician at Brigham and Women's Hospital (BWH), said, "He makes medicine fun...Marshall is a terrific teacher, and he keeps people motivated in medicine. He understands what excites people intellectually and is able to stoke that fire."[133] Wolf was also "instrumental" in the success of Partners In Health (PIH), founded by Kim and Paul Farmer before their residency. He "tailored a research residency program that allowed Kim and Farmer to share a residency and to become internists while splitting their time between Haiti, the focal point for PIH, and the BWH."[134]

In 1996, Wolf received the second annual Harvard Medical School Excellence in Mentoring Award after being nominated collectively by hundreds of his former trainees. In recognition of his championing the careers of aspiring woman and minority physicians, Wolf was the recipient of the Harvard Medical School Harold Amos Distinguished Faculty Diversity Award in 2007.[135] His many lasting educational innovations over decades of sustained leadership led the Association of Program Directors in Internal Medicine to recognize Wolf with their inaugural Distinguished Medical Educator Award in 2008.

"We have the most generous and nurturing mentors at the Brigham and the best and brightest residents. The young people who pass through these doors continue to inspire me," says Wolf.[136]

THE RESIDENCY DUTY HOURS CONTROVERSY

Although many enduring aspects of the educational ethos remained, during the 1980s and 1990s, the BWH residency experience strained under rapid changes in the healthcare environment. In 1984, the death of Libby Zion at New York Hospital led to the implementation of duty hour regulations that created extraordinary pressure on existing training and supervision models without additional resources.[137] The complexity of care needed by sicker patients with short hospital stays meant that residents were asked to do more in fewer hours, without additional supervision, and less time to reflect. Payment reform pushed the resident experience toward clinical care, with fewer means for hospitals to pay trainees to participate in research. At BWH, residents were also increasingly called on to provide care at affiliated hospitals such as the Parker Hill Hospital, Veterans Administration Hospitals in Brockton and West Roxbury, Sydney Farber Cancer Center (now the Dana-Farber Cancer Institute), Faulkner Hospital, and South Shore Hospital; these sites assuredly enriched the patient mix and introduced great new teachers, but also added responsibilities to already overextended trainees.

Some observers, such as BWH Sleep Medicine Division Chief Charles A. Czeisler, posited that the system created unnecessary hazards. In 2006, The Institute of Medicine's *To Err is Human* (coauthored by BWH's David W. Bates) highlighted that even the most modern hospital is a potentially dangerous place, spurring a patient safety emphasis in clinical care and education.[138,139]

The BWH Divisions of Sleep Medicine and General Internal Medicine examined the issue through pioneering studies of the relationship between trainee fatigue and patient safety, wherein medicine and surgery residents conducted their patient care activities while connected to electrodes to monitor brain waves and followed by trained observers; saliva was analyzed to measure hormone levels, such as melatonin. Surgical resident schedule changes implemented in 2006 by Surgeon-in-Chief Michael Zinner and Surgery Program Director Stanley Ashley were based on these findings. These included implementation of night float teams and shift lengths limited to twelve hours and represented the most dramatic surgical training frameshift since the time of surgical education pioneers Halsted at Hopkins and Cushing at the Brigham.[140] These studies were also cited as critical justifications for the ACGME reforms. Although debate remains about the efficacy of ACGME reforms—a 2009 Medicare study by Brigham medicine residency graduate Kevin Volpp found they had little impact on clinical outcomes[141]—the subject continues to be examined.

On the medical side, recent educational redesign efforts at BWH have piloted models that address the phenomenon of "work compression"—where residents have more and more to accomplish in fewer hours—leaving them with less time for reflective decision-making. BWH has developed an inpatient "Integrated Teaching Unit" pilot for the inpatient internal medical residency, which includes reduced clinical load, less frequent time on call, and a dual-attending model using faculty known for their teaching expertise.[142] The model inspired medical historian Ludmerer to remark:

> *The current study clearly demonstrates the educational benefits of developing a rich learning environment. It reminds us that what matters most in residency training are not simply the hours of work but what residents do during those hours. Today we should be focusing less on the time residents spend at work and more on the educational character of that work.*[143]

Technology increasingly offers trainees intriguing new ways to improve technical and clinical decision-making skills as well as new ways to communicate. In 2004, BWH established the STRATUS Patient Simulation Center, a high-fidelity simulation center used for the training of all Brigham residents, which provides important training in both procedural (e.g., central line placement, surgical techniques) and cognitive (e.g., teamwork training, clinical reasoning) elements of care improvement.

EDUCATION AND THE COMMUNITY

New conceptions of physicians' responsibilities to the wider local and world community have grown in ways that the Brigham founders could not have imagined. The BWH and HMS currently partner with the Indian Health Service and support bidirectional educational exchange programs with the Navajo Nation and other tribes; these programs have accelerated the entry of Native Americans into medical professions.[144] Through a number of channels, including the Brigham's collaboration with Partners in Health, a nongovernmental organization founded by Farmer and Kim,[145] numerous international medicine training experiences are now available to students, residents, and faculty. Two of these are the Howard and Doris Hiatt Global Health Equity Residency Program and a related program in global surgery, which teach unique skills of advocacy, program development, economics, and human rights.[146] The Department of Surgery has also created important new training opportunities in health services research through their Center for Surgery and Public Health. The Harvard School of Public Health's Program in Clinical Effectiveness was designed by Brigham faculty and is considered the premiere training program of its kind in the country.

Unique niche fellowship programs have been developed in emerging multidisciplinary fields such as informatics, medical management, patient safety, refugee medicine, and gender-based health. The Brigham's training programs extend into allied health professions as well, and the hospital offers a residency in clinical nutrition (one of the oldest such programs in the country) as well as a highly regarded hospital chaplaincy training program.

In recent years, BWH and HMS have responded to monetary challenges to develop new collaborative funding models, which have helped to sustain opportunities for innovation and joint educational aims. Brigham educators played a key role in creating "Harvard Catalyst," the integrated "human research laboratory" Clinical Translational Science Center at HMS, led by Principal Investigator Lee Nadler, dean for clinical and translational research and professor of medicine at the Brigham. Joseph Loscalzo and Thomas Michel played central roles in establishing the Leder Human Biology and Translational Medicine Program at HMS. BWH has long been a leading participant in curricular reform and the HMS Academy, working closely with HMS to examine pedagogy's relation to the changing healthcare landscape—just as it did in the years of the formation of the original institution.

CONCLUSION

At its inception and inauguration in 1913, the Brigham educational model was unique. Capitalizing on the newly emerging scientific foundations of medicine and expanding on the Johns Hopkins template with a coordinated curriculum and a new breed of teaching hospital, the Brigham grew in ways not possible in Baltimore and became the first full embodiment of the university-owned model—based on the European template, drawing its initial faculty from Hopkins, and designed with medical education at the heart of the mission. Changes in the methods and attitudes of training marked a critical inflection point in what has become state-of-the-art. The Brigham's operational design incorporated a new educational and teaching model, one built on forming a cadre of physician-leaders through a rigorous, shared educational experience. This experience would lead to many of the hallmarks of medical education at the Brigham: an emphasis on overarching commitment to excellence, research and scientific rigor as core components of resident responsibility, a hierarchical system designed to promote the "best and the brightest," innovations in ambulatory training, and full-time, conjoined teaching relationships with HMS. These foundational values

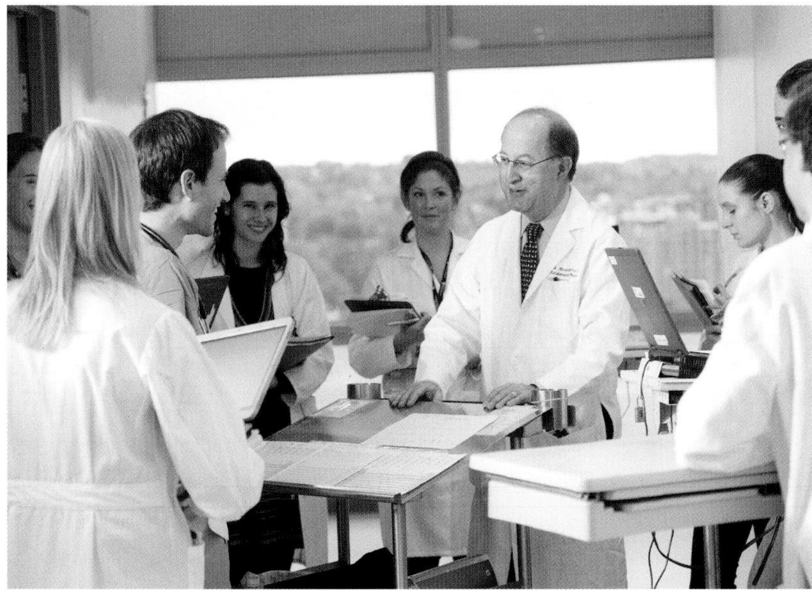

FIGURE 2-20 James Kirshenbaum teaching.

would mark the Brigham medical education for the coming century.

Educational programs at the PBBH, the RBBH, the Lying-In, the Free Hospital for Women, the Boston Hospital for Women, and finally Brigham and Women's Hospital, through their unique commitment to what are now considered cornerstones of professionalism—selfless dedication, altruism, social justice, and discovery—helped raise medicine from a trade to a calling. Groundbreaking innovation was fostered in the rarified but also egalitarian and collegial Brigham atmosphere. The story of education at Brigham and Women's Hospital is one of steady innovation paralleled by medical milestones that were, indeed, "striking departure(s)" that set the stage for the successful and groundbreaking modern academic teaching hospital Osler famously predicted at its opening ceremony.

A LEGACY OF EXCELLENCE: THE PETER BENT BRIGHAM HOSPITAL SCHOOL OF NURSING, 1912-1985

Marilyn Givens King

"Nurses are essentially doers. The skilled hand, however, must be directed by the intelligent mind."[147]

—Carrie Hall, fifteenth Peter Bent Brigham Hospital Annual Report, 1929

When the Peter Bent Brigham School of Nursing opened the doors to the first group of students in 1912, nursing education, like medical education, was in flux. As Isabel Hampton pointed out in 1893, nursing education could mean anything, everything, or next to nothing.[148] There were no clear standards to promote quality in the young profession. Nearly every hospital had a nursing school, the primary purpose of which was to provide students to be low-cost nursing staff. Education in many instances was a secondary consideration. Carrie Hall, a Massachusetts General Hospital nursing school graduate who had just completed a year of postgraduate study at Teachers College at Columbia University, aimed to set a different standard at the Peter Bent Brigham nursing school.[149]

To implement her vision for nursing education at the Brigham, Hall designed the program based on the most current ideas about professional reform in nursing education, what she later called her "radical" ideas.[150] To understand the history of this exemplary school, it is important to first understand the professional reform movement in nursing education as it existed in the early 1900s, and the ideas Hall used from this movement in developing the Brigham nursing program.

A New School of Nursing Opens

On November 7, 1912, the first group of students arrived at the new Peter Bent Brigham Hospital to begin their education in nursing. They found a hospital in the final stages of construction, no patients, and an unfinished nurses' residence hall. Still, the excitement of this grand experiment in nursing education and practice was palpable. Susie Watson, the science instructor, provided the following vivid description of the setting on her arrival. "There was no iron fence; piles of mason's supplies and boards, with roadways leading between the buildings; and, in the middle of the street. . . mud, mud on every side."[151] The only building ready for occupancy was hospital superintendent Howard's house, where the pupil nurses and faculty lived until the nurses' residence and classroom building was completed.

Arrival of the first group of students was the culmination of months of planning by Hall and Howard, which included not only the building design for the nurses' residence, but choosing faculty and nursing staff, designing the curriculum, and selecting candidates for the first class of pupil nurses.

Faculty and students went to work immediately, holding classes in Howard's living room. Science courses and laboratory work were taught in one of Christian's laboratories at the Harvard Medical School.[152] Students also learned practical nursing techniques and hospital housekeeping. And on January 25, 1913, the five probationers "took brooms and dustpans and went with Miss Johnson to A-Main, where they labored to make it clean and shining. The next day our first patient was admitted."[153]

Educational Reform at the Brigham

It is rare that an opportunity arises to develop a new program in a new institution where there are no established traditions creating barriers to reform. For Carrie Hall, the Brigham provided her with a clean slate on which she could build a program that was to become a showcase for the professional reform movement in nursing education. Professionalizing strategies Hall implemented at the Brigham included the following:

1. A three-year program based on a college semester, with a six-month probationary term
2. A four-month preliminary course that included the sciences and nursing arts
3. Assignment of credit hours to create college equivalence for the nursing courses
4. An eight-hour duty shift when on day duty, with twelve-hour shifts for evenings and nights until 1921
5. A requirement that applicants have a high school education or its equivalent
6. A requirement that students be age twenty-one or older for admission[154]

Although these ideas may seem quite ordinary by contemporary standards, they were quite extraordinary in 1912. This was an era when most nursing programs were one to two years in length with little in the way of content. Courses consisted of a series of lectures primarily provided by busy physicians. Pupil nurses typically worked twelve-hour days with one half day off per week, and students entered nursing programs with diverse educational backgrounds. There were no standards regarding educational preparation for admission to nursing education programs. At a time when only 9% of seventeen-year-olds in the nation graduated from high school, Carrie Hall successfully recruited and admitted such students.[155] Students began their nursing education with a six-month probationary term, the first four months of which was a preliminary course that included the

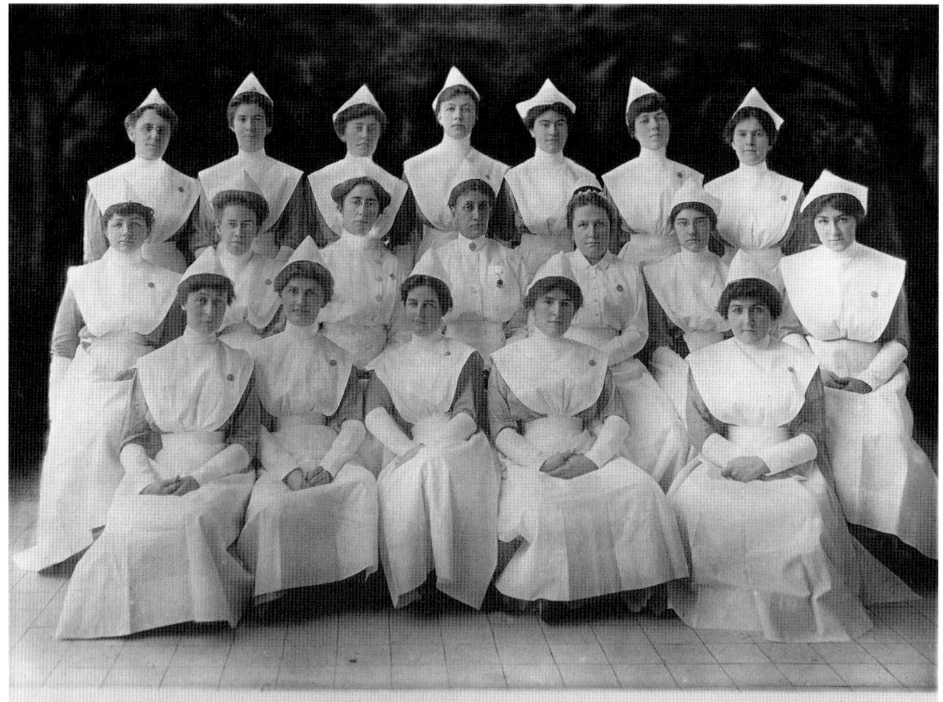

FIGURE 2-21 Peter Bent Brigham School of Nursing Class of 1915.

science and nursing arts courses, in which students were introduced to hospital housekeeping as well as nursing procedures and techniques they would use in daily patient care.[156]

Because hospital "housekeeping" is much more than simply preparing tidy-looking rooms, students also learned the scientific principles behind such work in their science courses and applied hospital housekeeping techniques in the care of the nurses' residence.[157] According to Carrie Hall, this taught students the importance of cleanliness and order in preventing the spread of communicable diseases. It also taught pupil nurses two important facts: "namely, that the 'head often saves the heels,' and the value of cooperation."[158] Bernice Sinclair, class of 1924, graphically described this experience. "I was most unpopular when I routed my companions from their beds so I could strip the bed, turn the mattress, and remake it exactly as I had been taught. Five beds before the eight o'clock class was no small assignment."[159]

In addition to hospital housekeeping, the nursing arts course included content on the skills and procedures pupils would use once they began ward work. Students learned how to take vital signs and how to perform patient hygiene, slush baths, bandaging, and hypodermic injections (including care of the syringe and needles). The classroom also provided greater freedom and opportunity for questions and discussions.[160]

Following successful completion of the preliminary course and the probationary term, students were capped and began full-time ward work. During the second half of the first year, students studied materia medica and urine analysis. In the second year, students continued to work full-time on the wards along with studying clinical courses in medical and surgical diseases. Obstetrics and pediatrics were in the third year, offered through affiliations with other hospitals. Elective affiliations in public health nursing, mental nursing, and infant nursing were also available. Students also sat for lectures on special disease nursing and on modern social problems in relation to nursing and caring for the ill.[161]

Although the rigor of the program Carrie Hall developed for the Peter Bent Brigham Hospital School of Nursing set it apart from the norm in nursing education in the early twentieth century, like other hospital schools, the students were also there to provide a nursing staff for the hospital. These dual demands placed a heavy burden on students. The hours were long, the work demanding, and the discipline strict. Records of the school, however, are replete with examples of students finding joy and camaraderie in the difficult and emotionally demanding experiences they encountered during the three years they were in the program and in the lifelong friendships that developed during their school years.

Life of the Pupil Nurse

Students at the Brigham, as with other nursing programs in Boston and beyond, were in many ways cloistered. They lived on the premises of the hospital, worked long hours, and in the early years had only one half day off on Sundays. Discipline in the school and on the wards was strict. Nursing Arts Instructor Johnson developed a document she titled "Points for Probationers" that spelled out the rules. The probationers were instructed to obey orders only from the head nurse and senior nurse, to know what was expected of them rather than guess, to be observant and keep the ward in order, to stay busy and never go from the ward to service rooms empty-handed (as there were always pitchers, bouquets, glasses, and so forth that needed attention), to learn the names of doctors, and not to talk to patients or one another, as this was unacceptable behavior. Students were also admonished not to "nurse hard things" but to learn from their offenses. Added to the list of forbidden activities were gossiping and telling funny stories.[162]

Students, however, being youthful and exuberant, took these rules in stride, and injected a touch of humor. For instance, they developed what they referred to as "The Nurses' Ten Commandments." Commandment number four advised students to:

> *Remember the Sabbath Day to make it useful. Six days shalt thy hurry and lose thy head, but on the seventh is the day of rest. In it thou shalt do thy dish count, sign up thy breakage, fine comb thy heads, and weigh all thy patients within thy gates. For in six days we have bathed our patients, cleaned our Diet Kitchen, scoured our Utility Room, and scrubbed the bedside tables. Wherefore there is no dust on the seventh day, so we bless this day and make it useful.*[163]

Another commandment stipulated that students should "not kill either time or patients, nor thine own conscience; but pediculi, mice, and water-bugs, them only shalt thou kill with all diligence."[164]

Although the Ten Commandments were written to poke fun at the strict discipline and rules, the nature of nursing work and the high expectations of students in carrying out this work are clearly evident. Nursing work in the early 1900s was quite different and very labor-intensive compared with contemporary nursing in the twenty-first century. Antibiotics did not yet exist, anesthesia was still quite rudimentary, and treatment procedures and methods were limited. Hospital stays were two weeks at a minimum, with patients kept on bed rest for much of the time, particularly after surgery. Most patients were admitted to large open wards, with the only privacy being obtained through placement of heavy screens the nurses were required to move into place. Much of the meal preparation took place in the ward diet kitchen, with students carrying heavy trays to each patient on the ward.

In her 1924 annual report for the School of Nursing, Carrie Hall provided a detailed and rich description of a typical day on the ward.[165] For instance, a probationer or first-year student would be assigned to "begin preparations for serving the breakfasts... This includes serving the trays, giving each patient the kind of diet which is prescribed for him, and giving careful attention to the special diets which have been prepared."[166] Another probationer would be assigned to check the utility room to "see that it was in proper order for the day."[167] This student would also be responsible for taking care of patients' flowers, dusting, and making sure the bathrooms were in order.

Following breakfast, nurses were assigned patients for whom they provided bedside care, which included:

> *bathing the patient, attention to hair, nails, and teeth, making the bed with the patient in it, and*

sometimes transferring the patient to another bed. It includes all the care of the bed, keeping it clean and dry, the sheets tight, without wrinkles, free from crumbs or other material in order that the patient's skin may be kept in good condition, no pressure sores allowed to appear, and involves attention to every phase of the physical well-being of that individual.[168]

Each student was assigned between two and nine patients. This routine was to be completed by 10 am in preparation for the physicians to make their rounds.

Throughout the day, the junior and senior nurses were busy with admissions and discharges, preparing patients for surgery and postoperative care, or assisting with a number of tests and treatments. These included "gastric lavages, gastric analyses, phthalein tests, two-hour renal tests, glucose tolerance tests, Meltzer-Lyon tests, infusions, transfusions, paracenteses, lumbar punctures," as well as "the Sippy regime, the administration of insulin, and other special treatments."[169] Poultices were another common treatment. Nurses also escorted patients to the X-ray rooms, operating rooms, eye laboratory, photographic room, clinics, metabolism laboratory, cystoscopy room, and so on.[170] By the time a student graduated from the program, she was a competent nurse and prepared to take on a variety of roles outside the hospital, which typically included private duty home nursing or public health nursing. These "graduate" nurses were usually only hired by the hospital to fill in when there was a shortage, such as during epidemics. The opportunity for excellent clinical training was perhaps the primary strength of the hospital-based nursing education programs. However, this model, based on students serving as unpaid workers putting in long and intense hours on the hospital wards, was, over time, also its greatest weakness.

National Studies of Nursing Education: The "Worn Out Apprenticeship Plan"

Students from the Brigham School of Nursing staffed the hospital wards until the 1950s. This was not unusual for a hospital training school, and nursing leaders have a long history of speaking out against the abuses of this diploma school system of nursing education. Leaders Isabel Hampton Robb and M. Adelaide Nutting began to advocate for change in the education of nurses as far back as the 1890s.[171] Between 1920 and 1950, there were three major studies of nursing education in the United States. The first, the Goldmark Report, funded by the Rockefeller Foundation, was released in 1921. One of the significant recommendations of this study was the creation of central, or university, schools to pool resources and improve the quality of nursing education. Hall believed that the Harvard Medical Center had superior facilities for the establishment of such a school. She stated:

We believe that no other center in the country offers greater advantage for a well-rounded preparation in nursing...[but] Until co-operation both financial and educational is secured, the schools of nursing in the hospitals comprising this medical center must continue to carry on under the worn out apprenticeship plan with such fusion of courses and exchange affiliations as may seem practicable, while continuing to give as good instruction as is possible to provide outside of university class rooms and laboratories.[172]

The Goldmark Report also recommended (1) a cost analysis to determine the true cost of the school to the hospital, (2) the need for a permanent paid nursing staff to reduce hospital reliance on students to staff the wards, (3) a twenty-eight-month curriculum that would reduce unnecessary clinical practice by pupil nurses, and (4) an eight-hour duty shift for the three shifts. Hall was successful in implementing the eight-hour duty shift recommendations in the early 1920s. She was not successful with the other recommendations, although she continued to advocate for changes until her retirement in 1937.

The next significant study was by the National League of Nursing Education (NLNE). The first full report was released in 1931 and noted an important trend in nursing and nursing education. As early as 1928, graduate nurses were already experiencing high under- or unemployment. There was now documentation of an oversupply of nurses in the United States. Recommendations were "to reduce and improve the supply of graduates in some hospitals entirely, in others in part; to help hospitals meet the costs of graduate service; and to get public support for education."[173] This committee also pointed out that a hospital's need for a cheap labor source was not a legitimate reason to maintain a nursing education program.

Hall again pointed out that accomplishment of these recommendations "means the uprooting of the present well-entrenched apprenticeship system and the securing of separate endowments for schools of nursing."[174] However, the boards of trustees still had not yet seen "their way clear to providing a stable graduate nursing service in the hospital."[175]

The third study with significant implications for nursing education was published in 1948 under the title *Nursing for the Future* and became known as the "Brown Report." This study, conducted by Esther Lucille Brown and funded by the Russell Sage Foundation, recommended that the nursing profession take steps to close poorer quality diploma schools as well as schools run by specialty hospitals. The report also recommended improving the quality of education in the better schools and ultimately moving nursing education into academic settings. In her research, Brown once again confirmed that the conflict that existed between education and service could not be resolved as long as nursing education was housed in and run by hospitals.[176]

PBBHSON Responds

Carrie Hall's successors after her retirement in 1937 continued to advocate for change. Lucy Beal, Hall's immediate successor, was successful in implementing curriculum changes as well as increasing graduate nurse staffing in the hospital. She also successfully moved the school through the first accreditation process in the late 1930s.[177] In 1939 the Brigham School of Nursing underwent an accreditation review by the NLNE in connection with its newly initiated program of accreditation for schools of nursing throughout the country. On this first visit, the Brigham was granted accreditation.[178]

Elsa Storm, Beal's successor as the director of the School of Nursing, shepherded the school through the remainder of World War II and into the postwar years, which were marked by an ongoing nursing shortage. This shortage meant ongoing long hours of work for student nurses. With an upcoming accreditation visit, Storm was concerned with this state of affairs, and with good cause. Following the 1950 visit, the NLNE visitors recommended withholding accreditation because of the ongoing issues with both heavy class and clinical workloads for students and faculty. Some nursing faculty lacked adequate educational credentials for their positions. Miss Storm resigned her position shortly after the loss of accreditation.[179]

Dorothy Vernstrom, the first non-Brigham graduate to hold the director's position since Carrie Hall, succeeded Elsa Storm. She immediately went to work to address the issues raised in the accreditation report, which entailed changes in the curriculum, clinical practice expectations, and the hiring of additional nursing staff to reduce the practice burden on students. In 1961, the school was notified by the National League for Nursing (NLN) that it had received reaccreditation, albeit with the stipulation that:

> *This approval will not extend beyond December 31, 1963 unless steps are taken to solve problems and to improve the program...The board expressed concern about problems in the areas of faculty organization, curriculum development—especially the relationship of instruction and clinical experience, and the evaluation of the program. It was also noted that a number of faculty members need to improve their preparation for their present position.*[180]

Verstrom eventually resigned, and Margarita Farrington, who took over as director of the school after Vernstom's resignation, at last regained full accreditation for the PBBHSON. For the remaining years of the school's existence, accreditation was no longer an issue.[181]

With these changes, however, the cost balance for the hospital began to shift. The cost of maintaining the school was becoming a significant drain on the hospital budget. Throughout the remaining

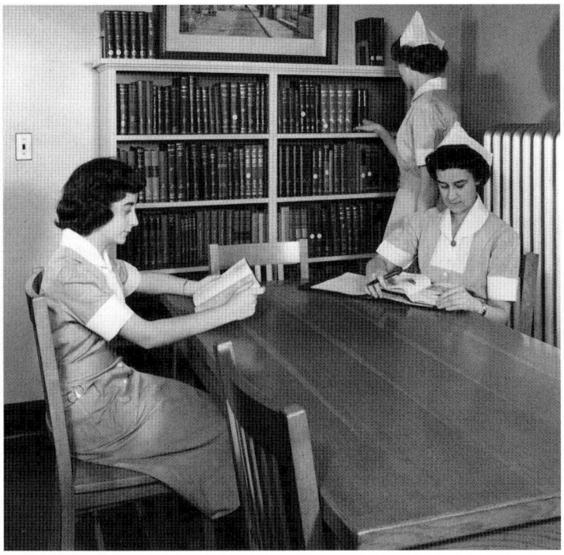

FIGURE 2-22 Peter Bent Brigham School of Nursing students in library, 1959.

history of the School of Nursing, efforts were made to identify financial resources to support the school. In the 1970s and 1980s, monies became available from the federal government through the Federal Nurse Training Act. Brigham leadership took advantage of these opportunities to obtain resources to support students in their education. Ultimately, however, the cost of maintaining the school was too much for the hospital. In a 1976 letter to Shirley Egan, then associate director of the School of Nursing, Alan Steinert, president of the Peter Bent Brigham Hospital, stated, "It is essential that the school become as self-sustaining as possible."[182] Despite best efforts by the Advisory Committee, the school was unable to raise the needed endowment to provide ongoing support to the school. The final recommendation of a task force established in January 1983 to evaluate options for continuing the school was to close the school following the graduation of the Class of 1985.[183]

Conclusions

Founded on the principals and standards of nursing education that were being promoted at the turn of the twentieth century, the Peter Bent Brigham Nursing School quickly established a national reputation as one of the top training schools in the country. Maintaining this status was not always an easy task, as the school had to contend with societal demands resulting from national involvement in two world wars, the Great Depression, the changing roles and status of women in society, and changes in hospital economics. Professional standards also continued to evolve. Nursing leadership worked for greater control of education through the development of admissions criteria, a standard curriculum, and nurse registration. All of these issues had an impact on the Brigham.

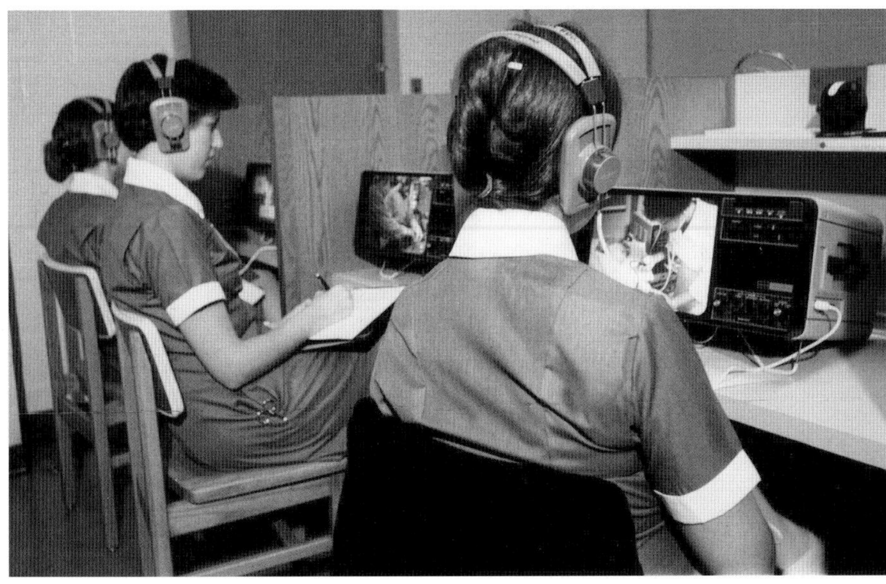

FIGURE 2-23 Peter Bent Brigham School of Nursing video lessons, 1970s.

Perhaps Carrie Hall's greatest legacy was her success in instilling a sense of professionalism in nursing school graduates. Many of these women went on to make unique contributions to the school, to nursing, and to society.[184]

Friendship, loyalty, practicality, and optimism—words that aptly characterized the student experience at the Brigham from 1912 when those first five students arrived until 1985 with the graduation of the final class. What binds these generations of graduates together is commitment to high-quality patient care and a vision for the future of care, the legacy of Carrie Hall and her staff from that November day in 1912.[185]

HARVARD MEDICAL SCHOOL AND BRIGHAM AND WOMEN'S HOSPITAL

Jeffrey S. Flier, Dean, Harvard Medical School (2007-present)

From its birth in 1913 to the present moment, the Peter Bent Brigham Hospital, incorporated into what is now Brigham and Women's Hospital, has been an essential partner in the life of the complex entity that is Harvard Medical School (HMS). Between the founding of the school in 1782 and the opening of the Brigham in 1913, medical education underwent dramatic changes in the United States that are outlined elsewhere in this volume. The introduction of scientific training into the preclinical curriculum and the increasing importance of in-hospital experiences for medical students exemplify the kinds of changes that occurred during this period. Like most other schools at that time, HMS did not own any hospitals, so education requiring hospital experience involved arrangements between the school and independent hospitals. Massachusetts General Hospital (MGH), Boston City Hospital, Boston Lying-In Hospital, McLean Hospital, and Children's Hospital were the main sites for clinical training of HMS students at the time of the Brigham's founding, although no formal affiliation agreement existed until 1949. The move of HMS to the Longwood Medical Area in 1906 was influenced by the site chosen for building the Brigham. Beyond the geographic proximity, Brigham leadership sought from the outset to develop the closest possible scientific, clinical, and educational relationship to the medical school next door, which began by allowing HMS to nominate its initial chief of surgery, Harvey Cushing, and chief of medicine, Henry Christian. This set the stage for increasing HMS involvement in faculty appointments at all of its affiliated hospitals.

Before examining the high points of the Brigham-HMS relationship, it would be useful to describe the elements of what we now often call the "Harvard Medical community," or as it is more commonly known, Harvard Medicine. Harvard Medical School is one of the eleven schools of Harvard University. It is the oldest of Harvard's graduate schools and the farthest removed physically from the main campus in Cambridge. HMS admits 165 MD students per year into a four-year medical curriculum and about 120 PhD students. We have formal affiliation agreements with sixteen clinical and research affiliates, including four major teaching affiliates—the Brigham, MGH, Beth Israel Deaconess Medical Center, and Boston Children's Hospital—where our students receive clinical education in their third year and throughout much of their fourth year as well. By these agreements, the hospital affiliates, which are independent fiscal entities, have agreed to uniquely align themselves and their faculties to HMS. As a consequence, these entities are universally referred to as "Harvard teaching hospitals," to the benefit of Harvard and the hospitals.

Harvard Medical School directly hires and houses approximately 200 faculty in the "Quadrangle" in its

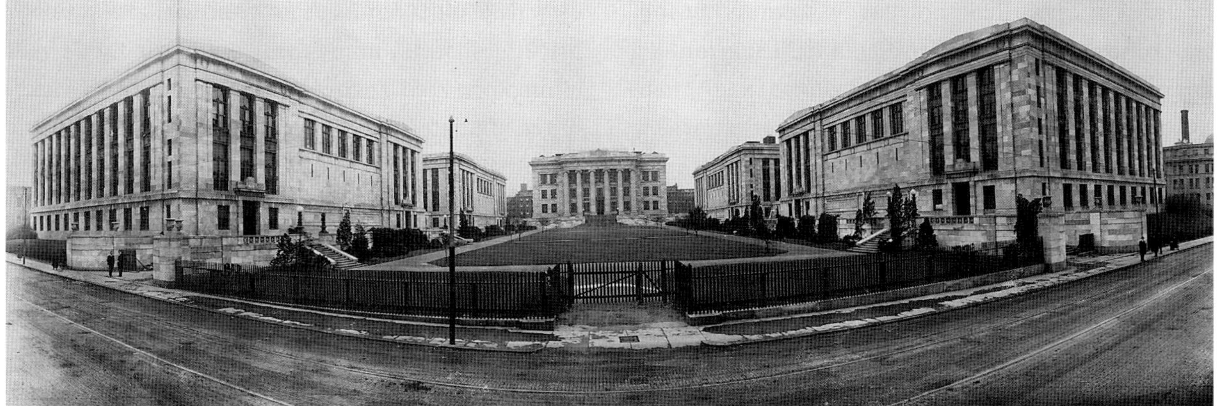

FIGURE 2-24 Harvard Medical School, 1930s.

basic and social science departments. An additional 8,000 full-time and another 4,000 part-time faculty are employed by the affiliates, all of whom must hold HMS faculty appointments granted by the school and Harvard University. This relationship is considered by all parties to be critical to the success of the school, the affiliated institutions, and the faculty members themselves.

The Brigham and HMS are interrelated across a broad array of activities. As noted, all Brigham faculty are granted a rank ranging from instructor, an annual appointment currently with little review, to professor, which represents the highest level of achievement and recognition. Currently, the Brigham has 956 HMS instructors, 515 assistant professors, 296 associate professors, and 220 professors. Among the professors, a small number hold endowed professorships through HMS, which provides both honor and financial resources to the incumbent. These Brigham faculty members reside academically in one of fourteen clinical departments overseen by HMS (e.g., medicine, surgery, and radiology), and a minority—currently about twenty faculty—also hold appointments in a Quad basic science department. Many Brigham faculty members play important roles in the education of medical students, both during the two preclinical years as masters of the student societies, course directors, or tutors, and during the clinical clerkships, now called the Principal Clinical Experience (PCE). About one third of HMS students participate in the PCE at the Brigham.

HMS students are a vital component of the life of the Brigham, its faculty, and its programs. Brigham faculty members are also integral to life at HMS, where many participate in and lead preclinical courses. Many students pursue the now-required scholarly projects with Brigham faculty, in areas from basic science to clinical studies and social science. The Brigham is a highly sought-after hospital among our graduating students who are seeking residency and fellowship training. As a result, many of our outstanding students—HMS is the most selective medical school in the country—eventually become faculty there. One fifth of our students are in the Health Science and Technology Program, which is a joint venture between HMS and the Massachusetts Institute of Technology. A Brigham faculty member has been the HMS leader of this program for many years, first Joseph Bonventre, and currently David Cohen, both of whom are professors of medicine.

According to the model by which HMS operates, each affiliate conducts research programs in its own research facilities. However, a significant component of Brigham research is conducted in space within the New Research Building, leased from HMS. One major element of this arrangement is a Brigham genetics program, located strategically near the HMS Department of Genetics, where faculty members, including Steve Elledge, Raju Kucherlapati, Mitzi Kuroda, Richard Maas, and Christine Seidman, have joint roles. Another area of strategic alliance is in neurology. Dennis Selkoe, professor of neurology at the Brigham, played a key role in founding and co-led the Harvard NeuroDiscovery Center, originally the Harvard Center of Neurodegeneration and Repair. Funded by a large anonymous gift to HMS, this program leverages neuroscience expertise across all of Harvard, through pilot grants, cores, and other community-building efforts, with the dean of HMS serving as the chair of its advisory board. A major segment of the animal facilities utilized by Brigham faculty are managed by HMS.

Over time, many clinical and research programs at the Brigham have become tightly linked to those at HMS. I will highlight just a few of these. HMS and the Brigham have deeply interrelated and synergistic programs in the area of global health. This alliance in global health arose out of the passion and accomplishments of two individuals, Paul Farmer and Jim Kim. These two physicians graduated from HMS one year apart, and both received doctoral degrees in medical anthropology from Harvard. They both did internal medicine residencies at the Brigham, where Farmer also completed subspecialty training in infectious diseases. While students, they cofounded the organization Partners In Health (PIH) and became national leaders in the field of global health with faculty appointments in medicine at the Brigham and in the Department of Social Medicine at HMS. This department has been renamed Global Health and Social Medicine (GHSM) and is chaired by Farmer. While pursuing their efforts at HMS and PIH, in collaboration with residency director Joel Katz, Farmer and Kim also pioneered a highly competitive global-health equity track in the Brigham Internal Medicine residency program, a program that may well become a national model. A Division of Global Health Equity at the Brigham houses the faculty for this program, and many of these faculty members also hold appointments at HMS in GHSM. Together, GHSM, the Division of Global Health Equity, and PIH function as a highly effective and mutually beneficial superorganism. Although at times the borders between these entities can blur, creating administrative ambiguity and financial complexity, I believe these issues are greatly overshadowed by the innovative and transformative work of this group.

A second example of the HMS and Brigham collaborative relationship is in the realm of clinical research. Since 1961, the Brigham had an outstanding National Institutes of Health (NIH)–funded General Clinical Research Center (GCRC) in which complex human experiments were conducted. Three other HMS affiliates also had similar programs. When NIH announced in 2006 that the GCRC program would be replaced by Clinical Translational Science Centers (CTSC) and that Harvard institutions could have a total of only one center, there was much uncertainty and some consternation at the thought that these fully autonomous programs would likely be ending. In the end, after extensive discussion, it was agreed that HMS would submit the grant, with HMS Dean for Clinical and Translational Research Lee Nadler, professor of medicine at the Brigham, as principal investigator. This decision was made with the full cooperation of and involvement of all preexisting holders of GCRCs, including the Brigham. There was also agreement about institutional support in the form of financial contributions, totaling $15 million per year for five years, from Harvard University, HMS, and each of the affiliated hospitals. A complex multi-institutional governance structure was established, demonstrating both the effect of external pressure and the capacity of HMS leaders to rise to the occasion. The grant was funded on the first attempt, and the federal support of $24 million per year is the largest among CTSCs nationwide. A far more integrated "human research laboratory" is the new identity of the previously independent and uncoordinated GCRCs. Brigham faculty play a key role in the leadership of this program, today named Harvard Catalyst. Its leadership team includes, among others, Elliott Antman, who leads the educational effort, and Barbara Bierer, who leads the regulatory program. Harvard Catalyst, including its Brigham components, is a national model for CTSCs.

HMS is heavily involved in graduate education in biomedical science, with nearly 700 students enrolled in PhD programs of the Division of Medical Sciences, which is part of the Graduate School of Arts and Sciences at Harvard, and home to many of the most highly rated graduate programs in the world. David Golan, professor of medicine (hematology) at the Brigham and professor of biochemistry and molecular pharmacology at HMS, is dean for graduate education at HMS. He jointly oversees the MD-PhD program with Dean for Medical Education Jules Dienstag, and the program director, Loren Walensky, Harvard Medical School associate professor of pediatrics. Our MD-PhD students often choose Brigham labs for their research, and the Brigham is a preferred site for their residencies and often their subsequent faculty careers. Brigham leadership, including Joseph Loscalzo and

Thomas Michel, played a critical role in creating a new and exciting track in our graduate program, the Leder Human Biology and Translational Medicine Program. This program creates new opportunities for hospital-based faculty to train graduate students in medical science related to faculty research.

It should be evident by now that HMS and the Brigham are very tightly and importantly aligned in a way that immeasurably strengthens both institutions with respect to both function and reputation. It should not be forgotten, however, that there are constant challenges to this close relationship, resulting in part from the fact that each institution maintains independent governance and finances. Furthermore, a rarity among American medical schools is the fact that HMS had no history of receiving funds, sometimes referred to as a dean's tax, from the clinical affiliates. During prosperous times, when all institutions were experiencing financial success, this situation could afford to be ignored. During periods of financial difficulty with flat or falling NIH budgets, poor endowment returns, and problems with the national economy, this model will likely not be sustainable. Two responses to this period of financial challenges have been particularly notable. First, the partner institutions and HMS developed a plan to provide new funds from all organizations to compensate their clinical educators. In a second important effort, there was agreement for a three-year period to provide modest financial support to HMS from the affiliates, support that is proportional to the size of their HMS faculty. An extension of this support will be an important indicator of the strength of the bonds that tie us together.

Indeed, we must all acknowledge the dramatic changes that will likely shape our institutions, both jointly and individually, over the coming decades. In the realm of clinical medicine, it is clear that the share of economic resources flowing into the U.S. health-care sector is unsustainably large. By one means or another, forces will emerge to profoundly alter this flow of resources over the coming years, hopefully while improving, rather than reducing, the quality and safety of the care that we deliver. The Affordable Care Act—whatever your views on its benefits and/or failures—will not by itself correct this unsustainable course. Whatever changes take hold through further regulation or market forces, it will almost certainly involve an enhanced need for primary care, care coordination, and interprofessional teams, as well as more appropriate, and perhaps limited, utilization of some specialty services. How institutions like BWH respond to this challenge will have material impact on the future of the hospital, HMS, and our critical, essential relationship. Although extremely deep in specialty and tertiary care, BWH also is a leader in primary care and is dedicated to planning for systems redesign, so I am especially hopeful about how BWH may contribute in the future. Many factors will also push HMS to institute important changes to our educational curriculum. Among these will be a need to have greater ambulatory—as opposed to inpatient—experience, new models of team training, and greater recognition of the new pedagogical models that suit students steeped in the digital age. In all of these areas, HMS will work closely with Brigham faculty, who are key players in the design and conduct of our medical education program. Finally, the future of biomedical research is evolving in response to fiscal realities and the need to increase the success with which we translate basic research into safe and effective therapies. I am convinced that HMS and the Brigham, as well as our other affiliates, will need to work together more effectively if we are to succeed and remain the leaders that we are today.

A model through which strategic planning and cooperation leverage our individual strengths and resources will far outpace the model of the past century, where, with a few important exceptions, our institutions pursued largely separate, individual agendas in independent, albeit successful, pursuit of scientific excellence. The success or failure of this more collaborative approach will occupy the future leadership of HMS and the Brigham for decades to come. I am committed to substantially dedicating the remaining period of my deanship to realizing this vision.

FORMER RESIDENTS REFLECT ON THEIR TRAINING YEARS

While historical events and milestones establish the architecture of the Brigham's contributions to academic medicine, this is only part of the story. Adding the personal reflections and stories of trainees, who inhabited those walls while building careers and lifelong friendships over long hours of mutual toil, provides vivid color and rich texture to complete the picture. The essays below by former Brigham and affiliate hospital trainees over the past seven decades infuse substance, humor, and important life lessons learned.

—Joel T. Katz

NOSTALGIA FOR OBSOLETE DISEASES AND THE LESSONS THEY TAUGHT

Thomas Francis O'Brien

Thomas O'Brien was a PBBH intern and resident in medicine in 1954-1956 and 1961-1962. Between his junior and senior residency years, he was an active duty captain in the U.S. Army Medical Corps and completed postdoctoral research at Harvard. He is currently a senior physician in the BWH Division of Infectious Diseases, medical director of the BWH Microbiology Laboratory, and co-director of The World Health Organization Collaborating Centre for Surveillance of Antimicrobial Resistance.

Medicine aspires to make all diseases obsolete, either prevented or else cured whenever diagnosed. So nostalgia about obsolete diseases seems misplaced...but it happens.

When I was an intern back in the first half of the Peter Bent Brigham century (1954-1955), there was a senior staff member at PBBH who had spent his entire career caring for patients with syphilis and learning everything about it. A decade earlier, however, he and his disease, and all of the intricate manifestations and feeble treatments of it that he could nuance so lovingly, had been blindsided by penicillin. He was still recovering from his loss and trying to convey all that knowledge to us. But we weren't interested. We had enough other diseases and were pleased to jettison one.

At a later Grand Rounds, a hematologist was diagramming the action of vitamin B_{12} when our eminent cardiologist, Sam Levine, launched into an unscheduled lecture on the clinical syndromes of terminal pernicious anemia, an interest of his before Minot and PBBH's William Murphy had found its cure. He stood with his thumbs hooked in the vest pockets of his London-tailored tweed suit—as in his portrait now in the Bornstein Amphitheater—lost in reverie about patients lingering through lemon-colored edematous skin, dyspnea, palpitations, abdominal pain, diarrhea, fevers, numbness, spasticity, depression, stupor, coma, and death. We saw pernicious anemia as blood smears and diagrams of B_{12}, but had no idea of its once-doomed patients.

Severe, protracted uremia seems obsolete here now but was our worst problem as interns then. PBBH had just fabricated the first artificial kidney in the United States and became a magnet for patients with acute kidney failure seeking to survive the three to four weeks it took their kidneys to recover. Uremia made them hard to like—sick, demented, raving, biting, cursing, combative, needing restraints, and thirst-crazed when requiring fluid restriction. When a bouquet was given to one, he threw the flowers on the floor, tilted back his head, and chug-a-lugged down all the water in the vase.

For each hemodialysis, a surgeon ligated and threaded catheters into the major artery and vein of a wrist (or reluctantly, thigh). Because none could be reused, the hemodialyses had to be a week or more apart to get through the duration of acute kidney failure. Hemodialysis could lower potassium, but patients remained sick and demented, their mortality remained high, and its benefits controversial. Hemodialyzed patients were then thought to be kept sick by accumulating toxins that couldn't be dialyzed. Whatever! What we knew as house staff was that they remained very difficult to care for.

So when this PBBH experience prompted the Army a few years later to assign me to its hemodialysis unit, it didn't seem like a great thing. But it gave me the opportunity to help make uremia obsolete. I was able there to design and fabricate the first indwelling vascular access devices that allowed repeated hemodialyses through the same site, to then use them to dialyze patients more often than before, and to find and report that this strategy minimized uremic symptoms. Patients had remained ill not because of undialyzable toxins, but because the prior technology had not let them be dialyzed enough. Belding Scribner then used, improved, and adapted this method and this finding to treat patients with chronic renal failure and extend their lives by decades.

Looking back now, the nostalgia probably wasn't for the obsolete diseases themselves as much as for the times and difficult work they shaped, the remarkable colleagues and suffering patients, and for the slowly acquired specialized savvy and skills that went obsolete with the diseases. War stories from forgotten wars. This was much of the Brigham for the first third of its century, and being there to hear those memories before they faded was a privilege.

Some of those diseases may also have made especially clear lessons about patient care that may be applicable but less apparent for other patients. Halfway through my intern year, a difficult uremic patient taught me one of those lessons. He was in the one single room of Ward F, about or below where the Duncan Reid Conference room is in BWH now. I was not his primary intern, but the one who covered that service on alternate nights, and a big part of my sleep deprivation on those nights was his typical raving, combative uremic behavior. A part of me knew that it was not his fault, but a big part also had trouble not disliking him.

He was Richard Herrick, who soon got from his identical twin brother, Ronald, the first successfully transplanted kidney. His surgeon would be Joe Murray, who became a Nobel Prize winner for this procedure. Because of his special circumstances, Herrick was around the hospital longer than the patients surviving acute renal failure, who were usually discharged before full recovery. So I had a chance to talk with him after he was fully convalescent from his uremia, and he was a very nice guy: articulate, thoughtful, and pleasant.

The lesson for me as an intern was: don't judge patients while they are sick. Impressions, if made at all, have to be deferred until patients are fully recovered. If they are still unpleasant then, that's different.

SAFE DELIVERANCE

Donald Peter Goldstein

Goldstein, professor of obstetrics, gynecology, and reproductive biology at HMS, graduated from Williams College in 1953 and Cornell University Medical College in 1957. He completed his fellowship and residency in obstetrics and gynecology at the Boston Lying-In and Free Hospital for Women in 1963, followed by two years at the National Cancer Institute in Bethesda. He served as gynecologist-in-chief (1974-1987) at the Division of Pediatric and Adolescent Gynecology at Boston Children's Hospital. He co-directs the New England Trophoblastic Disease Center with Ross Berkowitz.

I started my combined Ob/Gyn residency at the Boston Lying-In/Free Hospital for Women on July 1, 1960. You might say, though, that I started the program three years earlier when, after graduating from Cornell Medical School, I spent two years as a surgical house officer at Boston City Hospital and one year as a Josiah Macy Fellow in Reproductive Endocrinology in the Gyn-Endocrine Laboratory at the PBBH run by Somers Sturgis, chief of gynecology. The two years of surgery was a prerequisite for the Ob/Gyn residency program because at that time gynecology was considered a surgical specialty, and many general surgical operations were performed at the Free Hospital. My fellowship year was spent studying the endocrine function of heterologous ovarian transplants in Millipore filter chambers and ovarian follicle atresia using the anterior chamber of the rat's eye, an immunologically privileged site.

I became interested in the specialty of obstetrics and gynecology during my third year in medical school largely because of Cornell's superb teaching program at that time. The specialty appealed to me because the practice of Ob/Gyn required knowledge and skills in the fields of internal medicine, surgery, neonatology, pediatrics (in conjunction with obstetrics), geriatrics, and pathology. The interview process for acceptance into the residency was quite different than it is today. Interviews were conducted in the record room of the Free Hospital. The interview committee consisted of ten to twelve members of the combined department including chiefs from the Free Hospital (George Smith), Boston Lying-In (Duncan Reid), Peter Bent Brigham (Somers Sturgis), and Massachusetts General (Howard Ulfelder). You were expected to return the next year for a final interview before acceptance. At the interview I was questioned about plans for my career and particularly about my interests in research and teaching, reflecting the philosophy of training leaders in women's health care.

Until 1951, obstetrical and gynecologic training at Harvard were separate, similar to the Hopkins model. Then in 1951 the program was combined so that residents received training at both the Lying-In and the Free Hospital. The residency program consisted of three very intensive years divided into quarter rotations. Patients were either private or clinic-based. The first three months were spent on labor and delivery and in the obstetrical clinics. The Lying-In pioneered the development of specialty clinics to provide specialized care for high-risk problems. The Varicose Vein Clinic was run by Joseph Mullane, a vascular surgeon from St. Elizabeth Hospital. Injections of Sotradecol, a sclerosing agent, was used to treat symptomatic varicosities with excellent results. The Cardiac Clinic, originally established by Paul Dudley White of the MGH, and run by his successor George Sturgis, was populated largely with patients whose pregnancies and lives were threatened by valvular disease from rheumatic fever. The Diabetic Clinic was managed by Priscilla White of the Joslin Clinic, a pioneer in the management of pregnant diabetics. The obstetrical care of these complicated patients was conducted by Luke Gillespie and John Driscoll. At that time virtually all primiparous diabetic patients were induced at thirty-seven weeks because of the risk of intrauterine fetal demise. Their cesarean section rate, needless to say, was about 50%. Because Rh incompatibility was still a significant problem, the Rh Clinic was overseen by Louis Diamond and Stewart Clifford, the pediatric hematologists from Boston Children's Hospital who helped develop Rhogam (anti Rh(D) immune globulin), and Charles Easterday, who managed these patients obstetrically. The risk of intrauterine fetal death with all its medical and emotional aspects was also significant with these patients and required both expert and empathetic care. Early induction followed by exchange transfusions immediately after birth were the primary therapeutic modality.

Reid's Special Clinic (actually family planning) was established despite prohibitive federal and state regulations. Birth control pills were dispensed without charge (courtesy of a wealthy Boston woman), and tubal sterilization procedures and pregnancy termination were facilitated. Multiparous patients with cardiac problems, most commonly due to mitral stenosis, were the most likely candidates for tubal ligation. The main indication for pregnancy termination was suicidal ideation, which required a psychiatric consultation and an overnight stay in the hospital in a room with bars on the window!

Managing obstetrical patients in the early 1960s was quite different than the technology-driven practice of today. Ultrasound had not been introduced. Fetal monitoring was primitive and unreliable. Fetal scalp sampling for determining acidosis was also just being developed. There was no prenatal genetic testing. Placenta previa was diagnosed with placentograms and digital examination of the cervix using an operating room double setup, in case an emergency cesarean delivery was necessary. X-ray pelvimetry was frequently performed during obstructed labors to determine whether cesarean section would be required. The section rate for primiparas (nondiabetic) was about 6-7%, in marked contrast to the current rate of about 35%. Spinal anesthesia was used for cesarean section and deliveries. Epidural anesthesia was just being introduced.

Labor was routinely conducted under scopolamine-induced twilight sleep, and deliveries were almost always performed with the use of Irving forceps. Frederick Irving, Reid's predecessor as chief of staff, had developed an axis-traction forceps that could be used for rotations, deep transverse arrests, outlet forceps, posterior presentations, and even after-coming head of breeches. His philosophy and that of his successor was that a properly applied and executed forceps delivery over a generous episiotomy was preferable to a cesarean section. They therefore required residents to utilize forceps for most deliveries, and the low section rate in those years was due largely to the wisdom of that teaching. In my opinion, the decline in the use of forceps and the increase in cesarean section rates was due in large part to concern about malpractice litigation. It is lamentable that most residents today have little or no training in their use.

On admission all patients were bathed, received an enema, and were thoroughly shaved. Fathers were not allowed in either labor or delivery rooms and usually did not see their wives until the day after delivery when she was fully awake and back in her room. A far cry from today, when fathers routinely share with their wives the joy and miracle of childbirth.

The residency program was highly structured. There was a Blue Book that outlined the procedures to be followed for each obstetrical procedure or emergency. Although in retrospect this seems rather rigid, it instilled confidence in dealing with critical situations. One of my most memorable events was the management of a cardiac arrest that occurred in the middle of the night immediately after delivery of a ten-pound baby after a long and difficult labor. In the 1960s, open cardiac massage was the treatment of choice for cardiac arrest, and many residents carried a scalpel in anticipation of just an event. After the patient was successfully resuscitated she could not understand why she had two episiotomies, one on her bottom and the other on her chest. For the first three months we were only allowed to deliver multiparous patients with outlet forceps who did not require advanced operative obstetrics. During the second three months, we began to do more advanced forceps deliveries. The second six-month period was spent in the specialty clinics, assisting at and doing cesarean sections and supervising the junior residents in labor and delivery.

After the first year, three months were spent in the pathology laboratory with John Craig and Shirley Driscoll signing out biopsies, placentas, curretings, and surgical specimens. Then off to the Free Hospital for another three months of pathology with Robert Ehrmann and staff. After six months of pathology we spent three months in the gynecology clinics. In addition to the general gynecology clinics there were three specialty clinics—urology with Hathorn Brown, cervical dysplasia clinic with Paul Young, and infertility clinic with William Mulligan. The specialty clinics were overseen by the attendings, but the gynecology clinics were largely supervised by remarkably competent and knowledgeable nurses (they were the nurse practitioners of today) who lived in a residence across the street known affectionately as "menopause manor." The bulk of the resident's surgical cases were referred from these clinics. After three months in the clinics, we scrubbed with the private gynecologists for three months, followed by three months as assistant chief, and finally three months as chief, during which you were in the operating room all day, five days a week, doing a wide variety of gynecologic procedures.

The Saturday morning pathology conference was the highlight of the week because the attending had to justify his management if the pathology and the surgery didn't quite match. It was, in a sense, an open tissue committee, which sometimes led to a spirited discussion. Patients were admitted for surgery the day before and were seen and examined by the attending who would be assisting at the operation. The chief resident had to explain what procedure was planned and why. These were excellent teaching sessions where the principles and practices of gynecology as seen through the eyes of the attending were revealed. Although the Free Hospital was housed in an outmoded building, the staff and operating rooms were first rate, and the patients received excellent and loving care. Because there were no subspecialties or fellows in the 1960s, we were trained to do the full panoply of gynecologic operations including infertility surgery (no in vitro fertilization), radical pelvic surgery for cancer, and urogynecologic procedures. Laparoscopy wasn't introduced until the late 1960s, so all surgery was either vaginal or abdominal, and the volume on both the private and clinic service was heavy.

After completing rotations at the Free, we returned to the Lying-In for the last six months of the program. The assistant chief and chief had complete responsibility for all clinic patients. Reid and staff were always available for consults and were active mentors. There was genuine camaraderie and a close working relationship between the residents and attendings. Fuller pavilion housed the complicated patients, including those preeclampsia, third-trimester bleeding, and pelvic infections. Reid or his surrogate made rounds with the chief daily and came in at night for emergencies, if warranted. During the last three months the chief resident had to be present 24/7, but was allowed to go home every other night until midnight.

Training in the 1960s when there were no subspecialties and none of the technical advances we take for granted today provided me with a much broader surgical and obstetrical experience. This shaped my career by providing me with the skills needed to pursue my interests in oncology, reproductive medicine, high-risk obstetrics, urogynecology, and adolescent gynecology, which most trainees today do not enjoy. In retrospect, the lack of technology compelled us to rely more on our clinical judgment, which improved the quality of the care we provide.

HOME AWAY FROM HOME

Robert M. Quinlan

Quinlan is currently the director of The Comprehensive Breast Center at UMass Memorial Medical Center and professor of surgery at the University of Massachusetts Medical School. He began his internship at PBBH in July 1970 and finished as the Cabot Fellow in December 1975. He spent two years at Philadelphia Naval Hospital before joining the staff at Johns Hopkins working at their new oncology center until returning to Memorial Hospital to become their first full-time chief of surgery, an affiliation he has continued for thirty-two years. He served as president of the New England Surgical Society, the MA Chapter of the ACS, and the New England Cancer Society, and continues active practice in breast and thyroid surgery.

Forty-two years ago, the Peter Bent Brigham became my home away from home. Travel to and from Belmont, Massachusetts, happened in the dark, and daylight was seen on days off. Our call schedule was Monday, Wednesday, Saturday, and Sunday followed by Tuesday, Thursday, and Friday. This resulted in a 140-hour work week, unless a colleague was sick, and then you lived there.

We eight interns met Francis Moore on arrival June 23, 1970, and were not handed a syllabus on how to become a good intern. He did advise, however, to learn a hobby—"a surgical hobby." Finding our way to the laundry, OR, patient floors, and our chief resident was our responsibility. We managed.

Seven of the eight interns were on call together and would gather in the closed cafeteria at 10:00 pm to eat toast with peanut butter and drink coffee. It was a mutual leaning on each other. Although I've switched to tea, peanut butter has been a daily staple at play or at work. My daily routine is still to be up before 5:00 am and usually in bed reading by 10:00 pm whether working or sailing.

My fondest memories include calls to 311 (Moore's extension); Richard Wilson, a hero to the residents; and Richard Burleson (Burley), my first super chief on ward service. Sadly, both Wilson and Burleson left us too soon.

We were taught to touch the blood that was set up for a case knowing it would be there in the morning and be personally responsible for X-rays needed. You were in the OR before the attending, "always" according to Botsford. Patient data was carried in your head or on small index cards. This changed in the ensuing six years, but it seemed that the important data was easily remembered.

My first OR assignment was to help Wilson with a kidney transplant in Room 2. The procedure was being filmed. The chief resident was out with hepatitis. Despite never having seen a transplant and struggling to tie my first knots in a very public situation, Wilson was patient and instructive. Memories from the Children's year were the sick kids and the quiet expert care given to them by Robert Gross. On a visit to his office to discuss patients, I was given a copy of his new atlas of children's surgery and some advice on a nonoperative day: "It is OK to have a light day." (I regret at this time not listening to this suggestion.) Doing small people surgery was certainly good for technique. Judah Folkman came in the second half of the year after Gross's retirement. Folkman was the first scientist-surgeon I had met almost on a daily basis. Folkman's mind was never still, always questioning *why* and *what if*? His humor and kindness only complimented his genius.

Technical advice given with clarity and patience by Dick Wilson, Lou Plzak, Alan Baker, John Lamberti, John Sanders, Bud Sandberg, and Mort Kahan lives forever in my subconscious. Appreciation of tissue planes, stay in the middle, known to unknown, tension and counter tension, sew toward and tie away, and many other basic surgical principles are often lost amidst all the other information texted, tweeted, and emailed into the modern-day OR.

Moore's genius and his questioning from a very basic level to highly advanced information gathering was an art that permeated his daily life in understanding a complex clinical problem—go to simple questions to begin and then escalate in a logical progression to the answer that he left in the air for you to look up and report back. Murray's expertise, kindness, loyalty, and *equanimitas* will always be a personal goal. He never forgot a name and always thanked everyone for helping. You also felt that Nate Couch, John Brooks, Fred Morgan, Nick Tilney, and Alan Birtch knew what it was like to be a resident and had a word of encouragement at just the right time.

All the attendings knew their patients and took care of them one at a time, giving until the problem was solved. They took responsibility for the problem with backup. Moore would call from the office on Sunday afternoon, if he had been away, to catch up on patients. He would troop around to see patients, and his suggestions would grow exponentially. I usually needed to report later that night or he would call me with another question regarding Mrs. So-and-So. There would be a request to flush a cecostomy tube one more time before I turned in—which was not frequent, the turning in that is!

A "FOREIGN MEDICAL GRADUATE" AT THE PBBH

Murray F. Brennan

Born in Auckland, New Zealand, Brennan obtained his medical degree at the University of Otago in 1964 and completed surgical residencies at University of Otago and at PBBH. He specializes in the treatment of soft tissue sarcomas, endocrine tumors, and pancreatic and stomach cancers. He was chair of the Department of Surgery from 1985 until June 2006 and is currently vice-president for International Programs. He is the Benno C. Schmidt Chair in Clinical Oncology at Memorial Sloan-Kettering Cancer Center.

Coming to the Brigham forty years ago as a foreign medical graduate (FMG), now more politically correctly described as International Medical Graduate, was a real challenge. There were plenty of FMGs at the Brigham at this time, but they seemed to be very transient: "here today, gone tomorrow." The residency in general surgery, with five categorical interns destined to finish, was quadrangular, with many external residents added at the junior levels, making it diamond-shaped. Francis Moore, the chief of surgery, was a challenging taskmaster and an intellectual inspiration, although he was not always kind to FMGs, who were actually considered "try-outs" for the complete residency. It was very difficult to avoid feeling bad for a young FMG who began on the unusual starting date of December 31. As his wife was arriving on January 1, he had to disappear to collect her at the airport. Disappear he did—from the program!

For someone who was single, as I was, the every second night sleeping in the hospital did not seem too onerous. Every other Saturday afternoon was reserved for sleep! The on-call rooms above what was the main lobby of the old Brigham were clustered to say the least. The first woman, Robin Goodfellow, entered the general surgery residency in 1972, followed by Susan Chambers and Jeanne Petrek in subsequent years. Even so, there was little concern about the "coeducational" on-call room environment. Certainly, no one was awake long enough to even think about who was sleeping where. Of note also, the first African American resident was probably Howard Smith in 1972, followed by Frank Smith (no relation) in the following year.

I have no doubt that this was one of the finest residencies in the nation at that time. It was an amazing opportunity to develop lifelong friends from the cadre of residents. We certainly thought that we were "special," if only because we had to educate ourselves. The Ward Service allowed for almost complete independence. It was a courageous senior professional staff member who would even consider visiting a patient on the ward service without a formal invitation from the chief resident. Gynecology was done by the general surgery residents. In retrospect, the commonest operations done by the senior residents at that time were hysterectomy for pelvic inflammatory disease and bilateral adrenalectomy for metastatic breast disease. Nothing was more complex than a hysterectomy in a young woman with extensive inflammatory fibrosis. Adrenalectomy by a bilateral posterior approach was a much easier operation, and it became common. The response, although transient, was surely dramatic. The image of a woman entering the hospital with a walker or in a wheelchair and leaving just a few days later essentially pain-free remains an indelible example of the power of endocrine ablation for metastatic breast cancer.

All of the tubal ligations and therapeutic terminations were done on the ward service. There was concern by some residents with a religious background regarding the moral and ethical correctness of sterilizing young, invariably poor women, unable or unwilling to consider birth control, other than by termination. The tubal ligations were done with somewhat primitive peritoneoscopes, with poor optics.

No frozen section was allowed. Imagine the consternation when the pathology of the fallopian tube returned a week later as "portion of round ligament."

Conferences were wide and varied and, when led by Moore, had everyone's attention. However, the Friday afternoon conference in the pathology lab was a lost cause. The moment the lights went out, everyone in the room except the person speaking was fast asleep.

The hospital pager was an overhead speaker system. One always dreaded the "call 311," the office of the chief. Every time we heard that, we feared that someone was about to have a "corrective interview" or even be fired, although this rarely happened. Challenging other memories include the first presentation by a distinguished California urologist of a transsexual operation that rendered Moore speechless, a rare event. Joe Murray, future Nobel laureate, the kindest and most generous attending who was solicitous of the resident's welfare, often included a resident in his mid-craniofacial procedures, lasting twelve-plus hours. The hospital ward A-third, designed for the famous and the affluent, was supported by a very senior nursing and ward staff that at most institutions would long be retired. For the resident, this was frustrating. The common "joke" was that at least it was close to a good hospital. A-third was, indeed, quite close to a very good hospital!

There was limited if any noncardiac thoracic, but there was plenty of cardiac surgery. The Veterans Administration Hospital was completely run by the residents. Certainly some of our endeavors there would be questioned by a modern institutional review board.

Forty years later, would I do it again? You bet! The best of it all was the lifelong friendships that I developed: Nick Tilney, Gordon Vineyard, Steve Rosenberg, Bob Bartlett, Arnie Coran, Alan Baker, Paul Sugarbaker, Alden Harken, Bob Osteen, Mort Cahan , Ned Cabot, Bob Quinlan, and *many* more.

THE GIFT THAT KEEPS ON GIVING

Nick P. Perencevich

Perencevich is a graduate of Harvard Medical School, having done his first two years of medical school at Dartmouth. His internship, residency, and fellowship were all at PBBH (1972-1978). He practiced general surgery in Concord, New Hampshire, for twenty-three years. He is an instructor and adjunct associate professor of surgery at Dartmouth's Geisel School of Medicine. He is actively engaged with the Clinton Health Access Initiative and the Human Resources for Health Program training surgeons in Rwanda, Africa.

My internship group in 1972-1973 was Tom Aiken, Chuck VanBuren, John Pelligrini, Susan Chambers, Jim Fredrickson, Frank Smith, Ned Cabot, and myself. We had John Lamberti and John Sanders as our chief residents. Francis D. Moore, Sr., was our chief of surgery. John Brooks and Nick O'Connor administered the program.

I was blessed to have folks like Murray Brennan, Steve Rosenberg, Paul Sugarbaker, Gordon Vineyard, and Roger Christian ahead of me as senior residents and young attending physicians. They all had an interest in cancer, and that got me going in the same direction. Gordy and Paul had me doing colonoscopies a full decade before gastroenterologists dreamed about doing them. We all loved working with Dick Wilson even though he often deflated our egos after we felt we had done most of a big case with him, like saying that he "could teach a chimpanzee to do the case." The Oreo cookies in his mask when he returned to the table after looking at the microscopic pathology were a common feature. It was a real hit to the program when Steve Rosenberg took Brennan, Sugarbaker, and John Baker to the National Institutes of Health in the summer of 1974. Some of us, including some wonderful new residents who left their laboratories, got fast-tracked to fill the slots. That same summer I got married, and several fellow residents made it to our wedding in West Virginia. I'm still lucky to be married to the same wonderful woman.

Burbank Hospital in Fitchburg, Massachusetts, was also a junior and senior residency rotation while I was in training. My exposure to smaller community practice, surgeons like Fred Ross and George Walker, and the nature of the work was a large factor in my deciding to eventually do community practice. My wife and I both felt what it would be like living and working in a place like Fitchburg.

After my second senior year (pgy-4, now) I was able to do an extra clinical year in Glasgow, Scotland, an exchange that was arranged by Moore and Sir Andrew Kay. I had hoped to become a gastric surgery expert, but cimetidine had just come out in the United Kingdom, and damn it, it worked. Nonetheless, I learned to do upper endoscopy, watch ulcers heal, and operate on my own. I had a great year and have stayed in touch and visited recently with Scottish surgeons Stewart MacPherson and Dudley Booth, both part of the exchange. I, like many of us who went to Glasgow, loved working with Douglas Clark.

I returned from Scotland in June 1977, to my chief residency, which was an intense six months. I loved the whole experience, because nothing was like it before or since. Moore had retired, and Mannick had been chief since 1976. We didn't know each other, but Mannick was very kind to me. Two attending physicians oversaw the ward (then being called for the first time the Cushing service): Francis Moore, the former chief, who was still operating, and a young Glenn Steele, who had just joined the staff to work with Dick Wilson. I had the advantage of having these two superstars, at different ends of their clinical careers, at my bidding. I valued their expertise and got to know them well in and out of the operating room. I also had second-year residents I didn't know. Two of them, Chip Moore and David Brooks, came from good surgical bloodlines. It was easy to pick the cases for them—I would just clear it with their fathers. Even then, Chip and David could operate circles around me.

I left the Brigham in January 1978, did two years in the Air Force (the old Berry Plan), and joined a private practice in Andover, Massachusetts, which allowed me to teach fourth-year medical students at the Brigham. I subsequently practiced in Concord, New Hampshire, for many years, retiring in 2010, and recently began work in Rwanda, Africa, in a program that has Brigham roots. My boss was Robert Riviello, a Global Health surgeon from the Brigham. In preparation, Chip Moore let me into the Brigham OR on two occasions to observe and retool.

My Brigham training was a blessing and a curse. The training taught us a clear way to manage our patients and to be open to change as science progressed. Even the Scotland experience and the rotation in Fitchburg gave us insights on other ways to do things. However, being mostly out of academic practice during my career, I realized that much of the care around me was not based on the principles I was used to, hence the curse. I experienced much frustration and personal tongue biting at times while in community practice. In retrospect, at the Brigham we were indeed taught what accountable care organizations now call "evidence-based care management protocols." We called that "do what's right," reflecting our being drilled to know what was right and how that could change. The 1970s Brigham Department of Surgery in retrospect was a true accountable care organization. This curse for me is now disappearing with the good changes I see in nonacademic medicine and medicine as a whole.

There is still a part of me at the Brigham. My daughter Molly L. Perencevich is a Brigham-trained internist, now a gastroenterologist there. Her husband Jeremy is a Brigham orthopedist, and their daughter was born at the Brigham. The Brigham seems to be a gift that keeps on giving.

THREE YEARS FLASHED BY

Daniel W. Cramer

Cramer graduated from the Colorado University School of Medicine and served for two years in the Public Health Service at the National Cancer Institute before completing his residency in obstetrics and gynecology at the Boston Hospital for Women (1973-1976). Cramer's research focuses on the epidemiology of gynecologic cancers with a particular focus on ovarian cancer. He shares joint appointments at BWH and Dana-Farber Harvard Cancer Center, where he is professor of obstetrics, gynecology and reproductive biology at HMS and professor of epidemiology at Harvard School of Public Health.

October 1, 1973, was my first day of work at the Boston "Lying-In" Hospital at 221 Longwood. At that time there was not a combined internship/residency program. Successful applicants would complete an internship elsewhere and join the Obstetrics and Gynecology (Ob/Gyn) residency on a quarterly basis. The departure of the graduating resident and arrival of the new would occasion a "change party" every three months—some of these with legendary excesses that were recounted by more senior residents.

Built in 1927, the Lying-In was a rectangular structure set back from Longwood by a uterine-shaped driveway. Two smaller attached square buildings flanked the hospital's columned entryway connected by two rows of screened porches above it. To the right was a separate building that fronted Longwood. All of the original buildings were clad in tan brick with a distinctive, double row of green soffits supported by corbels and tiled on the top. After almost half a century, the hospital was now a patchwork of renovations. On the left a curved addition called the Richardson House was added in 1932, which mirrored the architecture of Vanderbilt Hall on the other side of Louis Pasteur Ave—nicely done but noticeably unsymmetrical with the building on the right. The soffits had been removed from the two square buildings flanking the entryway, and two metal boxes of plopped on top to expand the operating room space. The porches were closed in by the same ugly commercial metal. At the back of the hospital, other changes included a fourth-floor addition to the Labor and Delivery Area that perched precariously on fourteen three-story-high concrete stilts.

It was not Indian summer, the day I began work, but chilly, damp, and colorless gray. My first thought was "I'm going to have to spend the next three years of my life here" as I reconstructed the matrix of circumstances and decisions that brought me there. I enjoyed my Ob/Gyn clerkship during medical school and remember being allowed to do a forceps delivery. I had completed a student project analyzing data related to levels of human placental lactogen during pregnancy that resulted in a paper published in the "Gray" journal. Still, I had opted for an internal medicine internship, thinking that this was the best path to an academic career, and I matched with the program in Ann Arbor. During an internship elective, I met a superb representative of academic Ob/Gyn, Robert Jaffe, then also at Ann Arbor. Later, he would suggest I consider the Boston Hospital for Women program that Kenneth Ryan had just been selected to lead.

Global events also played a role. In 1970, the Vietnam War still smoldered, and doctors were subject to the draft. In autumn that year, I received my "Greetings" telegram, ordering me to report for an induction physical at a Detroit armory. Fortunately, during medical school, I had applied to the Public Health

Service as an alternative and received the news in November that I had been accepted. I would serve my "war" years at the Biometry Branch of the National Cancer Institute in Bethesda (we were known as the "yellow berets"). During that time, I worked on cancer statistics, learned a little about NIH bureaucracy, and met Brian MacMahon, an epidemiologist, at the Harvard School of Public Health. So here was the convergence: Boston, neat! Ob/Gyn and Public Health at Harvard, wow!

I would spend many, many hours on the Labor and Delivery (L & D) floor at the Lying-In. This had a great view of Fenway Park, and on a summer evening call of night between deliveries, I would look out at the lights and imagine being there with a hot dog and a beer. I recollect now that a large proportion of deliveries involved elective outlet forceps under spinal anesthesia. If you were lucky, Lucy Lee was on call with you. Literally, in a minute, she could get a spinal in. Although the days of inhalation anesthesia for vaginal delivery had passed, a few of the private obstetricians still ordered twilight sleep (scopolamine and morphine) for their laboring patients. In the next room, there might be a patient in premature labor on an intravenous-alcohol drip to stop contractions. Talk about dazed and confused! Today's Ob residents might be uncomfortable here, but one of the constants they would recognize is the joy of shepherding mothers and their families through childbirth and receiving their gratitude. Then, as now, the vast majority of the deliveries were safe and uneventful.

During residency, time was split between the Lying-In and the Parkway, or "Free Hospital" for Women. This was a handsome building subjected to fewer drastic renovations than the Lying-In. Here, one found wonderful relics of the Parkway's beginnings—a bronze bust of Graves, a portrait of one of the Boston doyennes who founded the hospital, and beautiful nineteenth-century grandfather clocks. A door on the top floor led to a gigantic attic space filled with other treasures, including two huge Chinese floor vases that I imagined were donated by a patron and judged either too valuable (or ostentatious) for public view. At that time, many well-known gynecologists practiced at the Parkway including Robert Brown, Tom Griffiths, Robert Kistner, Thomas Leavitt, and Robert Knapp, the newly appointed head of the Parkway. Then, as now, hysterectomy was the most common procedure, and the outcomes were good and the patients grateful. But what stayed with me was the sadness and suffering that usually came with diagnosis and treatment of advanced cervical, endometrial, or ovarian cancer. There must be something that could be done to prevent these in the first place, I thought.

Ryan would move the residency toward the one recognized today. Internship and residency were combined. Fellowships in maternal-fetal medicine, gynecological oncology, and reproductive endocrinology and infertility were introduced or strengthened. The year 1973 saw the Roe v. Wade ruling and the formation of a committed Family Planning Service at the Lying-In. The three years I thought I would dread flashed by. I got my degree in epidemiology from the Harvard School of Public Health, with my thesis focusing on ovarian cancer. I remained on the Faculty splitting my time as a generalist and doing epidemiologic research. The three years became ten, then twenty, then thirty and now going on forty. The Boston Hospital for Women merged with the Peter Bent and Robert B. Brigham Hospital to become Brigham and Women's, the Parkway was sold to become condominiums, and the Lying-In was renamed the Richardson-Fuller Building part of BWH (I still have my office space there). Subsequent to the merger, the L & D and Gyn areas have moved several times, but long ago, I came to realize it is not the building that matters. Strong hospitals and departments are built on traditions of care and service established by our predecessors, carried on by dedicated faculty and staff, and reinvigorated by our new trainees. I have never regretted my decision go into Ob/Gyn and come to Boston.

SCHOLARSHIP IN WOLF'S CLOTHING

Don Ganem

A graduate of Harvard College and HMS, Ganem completed medical training at PBBH 1977 to 1979; he was chief medical resident 1982-1983. He was an infectious diseases fellow and ultimately rose to professor of microbiology/immunology and medicine at the University of California, San Francisco. Currently, he is global head of infectious disease research and vice-president of the Novartis Institutes for Biomedical Research. His research explores the molecular biology of human viral pathogens and the diseases that they cause, including identifying KSHV as the causative agent of Kaposi's sarcoma. Ganem is a member of the National Academy of Sciences, the Institute of Medicine, and the American Academy of Arts and Sciences.

The only time I ever heard Eugene Braunwald tell us something that wasn't true happened on the very first day of my internship, in late June of 1977. All the new interns had been summoned to his office that morning, shortly after we had been issued our whites and beepers. "Ladies and gentlemen," he began, calling us to attention. "The internship is not a year of scholarship."

He went on to explain that this year was a year in which our emphasis should be on mastering the details of patient care. The needs of the patients—for diagnostic testing, for pain relief, for emotional support, for continuity of care—were to take precedence over all other aspects of our lives, including attending lectures and conferences. By the end of this year of total immersion, we would be expected to have developed the clinical reflexes that are the *sine qua non* of the practicing physician. The book learning, the journal clubs, the displays of clinical erudition—all of that could come later.

We all took this message to heart and applied ourselves first and foremost to the bedside. It wasn't until much later that I realized that despite the deliberate oversimplification of Braunwald's memorable opening line, the internship had nonetheless been a year of intense scholarship—of *clinical* scholarship. For example, we did a lot of lab work ourselves—urinalysis, urine and sputum Gram staining, crystal exams on joint fluid, even the plating of cerebrospinal fluid specimens after midnight. We were taught that the examination of these fluids was not "lab testing," but was properly part of the clinical examination of the patient. So we learned to master both the performance and the interpretation of these procedures. During that process, a huge amount of information was transferred over the microscope in the house officer lab—both from our peers and from experienced fellows and chief residents.

Unlike today's attending rounds, which are heavily focused on management and discharge planning, we spent a lot of time on attending rounds discussing differential diagnosis, pathophysiology, and the scientific basis of therapeutics. But these discussions were not dry didactic exercises. They were all presented in the context of the management of the patient in question—so much so that we were unconscious of where the science ended and the caregiving began. The culture of the Brigham was so steeped in intellectual rigor and clinical scholarship that we could no more have avoided assimilating it than we could have avoided breathing atmospheric oxygen. So the internship was in fact a year of scholarship—one in which, as in all other scholarly endeavors, standards were set, learning was transmitted, and tests (here, all unwritten) were passed.

This Brigham tradition of clinical scholarship goes back many generations, but there's no question that its formulation and transmission to the house staff in the modern era was shaped first and foremost by our training director, Marshall Wolf. At his morning report, every doubtful or controversial assertion was challenged with a "Show me the data" from either Marshall himself—or from all of us eager to become his acolytes. (Needless to say, Marshall's requests of this type were always more courtly than our own). But for all its rigor, Marshall's pedagogy, like his doctoring itself, was always characterized by compassion, empathy, and warmth. He knew we were already putting a great deal of pressure on ourselves to excel, and he mastered the art of holding us to a high standard without adding any further to our self-imposed burdens. I know of no other single clinician whose example was more influential in my career and count myself lucky to have traveled, however briefly, in his orbit.

F-MAIN LIVES

Thomas H. Lee, Jr.

After graduating from Cornell University Medical College, Lee trained in medicine (1979-1982) and cardiology (1982-1985) at the Brigham. He married his co-intern, Soheyla Gharib, and their three daughters were born at Brigham and Women's Hospital. Lee is chief medical officer of Press Ganey, Inc., associate editor of the New England Journal of Medicine, and professor of medicine at HMS. He continues to see patients in the Phyllis Jen Center for Primary Care at the Brigham, on the sacred burial grounds of F-Main.

Like most people who worked at the Brigham before July 1980, I divide the world into two types of people—those who remember F-Main, and those who do not. I am, of course, in the first group. I was an intern and resident in internal medicine from 1979 to 1982, and I spent most of my first summer taking care of "ward" patients (those without private doctors or private insurance) on that unit at the end of the Pike of the old Peter Bent Brigham, about where the Jen Center is today. The patients were sick and poor. Attending physicians ventured onto the unit once a day, and then only briefly. We had no air conditioning, and I remember sweat dripping off my chin onto the progress note paper, smearing the ink from my handwritten notes. You had to call the laboratories to get test results, and the tip of my index finger was so tender from dialing the rotary phones that I would use my pen to dial.

But the care was great. The house staff and the nurses ran the show, and, for them, F-Main defined the cultural heart and soul of the Brigham—forever.

For the record, let me say that we live in a better world today—where patients are triaged to floors without consideration of their insurance status, and where patients who might benefit from close monitoring can virtually always be admitted to one of the Brigham's many intensive care unit (ICU) beds. But in the old hospital, there were only four medical ICU beds, and patients had to be desperately ill to warrant admission to them. That meant very sick poor patients were triaged to what we called "The Small Ward" of F-Main—a collection of stalls with one bed each across from the nurses' station.

In that era, we learned how to take care of septic shock without any built-in monitoring equipment. There were no arterial lines or pulmonary artery catheters on F-Main, but you could do a pretty good job with a Foley catheter, a blood pressure cuff, and looking at the neck veins (or placing a central venous pressure line). We used bedside monitors to detect cardiac arrhythmias—when we could find them.

Residents a little older than me still swear by a story about an incident one night in the late 1970s, when a resident mentioned to the family of a patient with chest pain that we had run out of cardiac monitors. They disappeared, and an hour later they reappeared with a cardiac monitor that said "Beth Israel Hospital" on the side. The monitor was plugged in and immediately put to use.

The patients in the Small Ward needed 1:2 nursing (one nurse for every two patients). Male patients who were more stable could be transferred to the Large Ward, in the back of F-Main. I am personally bitter that I arrived at the Brigham in 1979, a little too late to participate in the era when the Large Ward was in fact one big room, with the beds arranged in a circle. That open ward was called The Big Top—a large circle of poor sick men, many with severe psychosocial problems that would contribute to wild scenes at times. But a lovely social support system characterized the Big Top (which had time to develop because lengths of stay could be weeks or months). There was a saying that "No one ever dies under the Big Top" because, when patients would start to deteriorate, one of the other patients would see it and shuffle over to the nurses' station to let them know. The deteriorating patient would then be transferred and might die in the Small Ward—but not under the Big Top, not in front of his friends.

In that era and in that setting, we did everything for our patients. We did the electrocardiograms, cutting and taping the single-channel tracings onto progress note paper. We did the urinalyses in the small laboratory, where we also boiled urine to try to detect Bence Jones proteins so we could diagnose multiple myeloma without calling hematology consults. To my knowledge, none of us ever got a positive result. Nor did anyone ever diagnose tuberculosis by doing morning gastric aspirates and staining them for acid-fast bacteria.

But the discipline and the urge to try to do *everything* one could *by oneself* to take care of one's patients—that was a big part of F-Main culture. I remember being criticized by my senior resident for calling a gastrointestinal disease consultation for help with a diagnostic dilemma without checking with him. He said, "We call consultations for procedures that we cannot do. We don't call them to think for us—not until we have really read and tried on our own." I don't think it would be wise to try to do that today—there has been so much progress in the years since, you need specialist and subspecialists and sub-subspecialists right away to give state-of-the-art care.

But in that era, it was good for us in many ways. It made us read and think and stop experts in the Pike to run cases by them. It made the 10 o'clock meal and other trips to the cafeteria important components of patient care. It made you think about your patients all day long. In that precomputer era, I stamped a 3 × 5 card for every patient and wrote down their problems, medications, and key laboratory results. When they went home or died, I would throw the card in a wooden box. That box still sits on my bookshelf in my office, and every now and then, I flip through those cards. I am always struck by how few medications they were on. And I am struck by how many of the patients I still remember in detail.

If the house staff were at their very best when they were on F-Main, the nurses were exceptional as well. They were young, smart, strong, ready for responsibility and adventures. The atmosphere on F-Main crackled. Tempers were lost. Practical jokes were played. Romances began (and ended). And great care was delivered.

When the new hospital opened in 1980, we moved patients down the hall into the Tower, and soon the scene of so much chaos was eerily quiet. F-Main had probably always been kind of dirty, but suddenly the dust balls seemed so much more prominent. It was sad.

A few of us asked and were stunned to be given permission to use the empty F-Main for a farewell party. Today, I cannot believe that hospital administrators gave us that permission—loud music, a tremendous amount of alcohol (the nurses station was the bar), and close dancing until 2 am on a hot, sweaty night. Of course, those hospital administrators were all there. They were sad, too. I look often at the pictures from that party, of George Schreiner giving a very funny speech, with a sign behind him saying "F-Main: Best Care Anywhere."

As the years go by, and there are fewer and fewer of us who came of age on F-Main around, we feel like those aging veterans at the VA who would talk about having fought in "The Big One" (World War II). Eventually, we'll all be gone, too. But I like to think that the discipline and pride and dedication that we learned on that unit will always characterize the Brigham—and in that way, F-Main lives.

THE MEANING OF "HOUSE OFFICER"

Theodore N. Pappas

Pappas is a graduate of the Ohio State University College of Medicine. He completed his surgical residency at Brigham and Women's Hospital (1981-1988). His research has focused on upper gut and colonic motility, surgical innovation, and surgical history, leading to more than 200 peer-reviewed publications. He is the interim chair of surgery, distinguished professor of surgical innovation, and vice dean for medical affairs at Duke University School of Medicine.

It was 1981 and I was a brand new intern at the Brigham hospital. I had attended medical school at Ohio State, a very busy clinical experience, but was not quite ready for every-other-night call and 120-hour work weeks. My first rotation was on neurosurgery and I cross-covered one of my fellow interns, Wally Koltun, who was on the urology service. At that time, to get a weekend off you had to cover two nights in a row, Thursday/Friday, and then you could leave the hospital on Saturday. We would get to the hospital Thursday morning at about 4 am and leave at noon on Saturday, continuous call for fifty-six hours. Needless to say, this was well before anyone thought of an 80-hour work week. During my first month of this schedule, after I had already taken call on a Thursday night, I somehow forgot that I was also on call on Friday night and I went home. At the time that Koltun expected me to take sign-out he could not find me. I was startled when he called me at home to let me know I was supposed to be at the hospital taking call. I quickly came back to the hospital to a relieved Koltun who was worried that I had quit and gone back to Ohio. It was quite an adjustment to figure out how to live my life and still spend over 100 hours per week in the hospital. I remember I was so struck by the reaction I had to this on-call experience that I wrote a letter to the editor of the *Journal of the American Medical Association*.[186] I am probably the only intern in the rich history of the Brigham who managed to parlay a near-missed call night into a publication.

By the time I got to the end of the month, it was time to cross-cover again for Koltun, because he was due his intern-year vacation (one week). As he handed me his pager, I asked him who was covering the alternate nights while he was out of town for the week. He reminded me that it was I covering myself, and therefore I was going to do nine nights in a row in the hospital. This was an epiphany, as I realized that I needed to bring nine pairs of underwear and socks and a few clean shirts to the hospital, as I would have to live in my 6 × 6 foot call room during that 232-hour on-call stretch. The meaning of the words "house officer" became indelibly printed in my mind.

My next harrowing experience occurred on the following rotation, which was on the Cutler service. I first learned about the Demartel-Wolfson clamp while I was rounding one day on Glenn Steele's patients. The Demartel was a metal clamp that was used to seal the end of a colostomy and was applied at the skin level, instead of maturing the colostomy in the operating room (OR). It was eventually removed at the bedside whenever the patient started to have crampy abdominal pain and was ready to pass gas. After a signal from the chief resident, the Demartel would be removed and the stoma matured at the bedside, and this would occur at about five or six days postoperatively, when the stoma was "stuck" and would not fall back in the abdomen. Unfortunately, I had no knowledge of what a Demartel clamp was, so I simply took it off on postoperative day one when I discovered it on the patient. Then I proudly presented this fact on rounds and was amazed when the entire team rushed into the room to see if the stoma had fallen back into the abdomen. Russ Nauta, the chief resident, was trying to figure out how he was going to get me to call Steele to tell him that we were going back to the OR to fish out this lost stoma. Fortunately a stoma-miracle occurred that day: it somehow stayed at the skin level and did not fall into the abdomen. I am certain that I am a professor of surgery at Duke today *only* because that stoma managed to say at the skin level. I am equally certain that if I had called Steele to tell him we were going back to the OR because of my ignorance, I would have been looking for an anesthesia residency.

When I started my training in 1981, the hospital was newly named the Brigham and Women's Hospital. We were a group of residents who managed the transition from the old Peter Bent Brigham Hospital to the new Brigham and Women's tower. During my internship we were still using the old emergency ward that opened onto Brigham Circle from the basement of the old Peter Bent Brigham building. Most residents and faculty still called the hospital the Peter Bent, because we spent much of our time in the original hospital buildings. Still, my recollection was that we thought we were special because we had helped to move into the new hospital and launch the new era of Brigham surgery. We somehow felt we were a link back to this rich history that included Cushing, Cutler, Dunphy, Zollinger, Murray, and Franny Moore. But we were also part of this new organization, the Brigham and Women's Hospital, and therefore very much part of a bright and important future.

CONJUGAL VISITS

Michael G. Muto

Muto is a graduate of the University of Massachusetts Medical School. He completed his residency in obstetrics and gynecology in 1987 and his fellowship in gynecological oncology in 1990 at BWH. Muto is director, Gynecologic Oncology Fellowship Program, BWH/DFCI, and associate professor of obstetrics, gynecology and reproductive biology at HMS.

The rumor was that the architect who designed the new Brigham tower had never built a hospital before: only hotels, motels and strip malls. Unfortunately it showed on every floor and in every corner of the building. After moving in, the old Lying-In nurses would remark sarcastically, "Don't worry, it will be better when we get to the *new* hospital." But, of course, they were in the new hospital, and nothing seemed to be right.

Nowhere was the design more deficient than on Labor and Delivery. Birth: the miracle of life, an experience characterized by overwhelming joy, happiness, and love. So where do we put the new labor floor, a floor on which patients will experience those first magic moments as parents? A floor on which the finest, most sophisticated obstetrical care in the world would be provided? Why not the basement? Why not design small, cold, windowless rooms with no connection to the outside world? No television, no music, just the constant sound of fetal monitors and the dulcet tones of labor nurses crying "push, *push*." At least the patients were only down in that infernal dungeon for twenty-four hours 2.4 times in their life. The medical staff was there forever, peering upward toward the domed skylights that sat atop the twenty-foot silos jutting into the plaza above. There was nothing to see in those skylights: the heavily frosted glass effectively blocked both sky and light. Evidently the architect determined that allowing unfiltered sunlight would ruin the dark, dank ambiance of this basement department.

The patients were just visiting. The labor nurses went home after eight or twelve hours. The resident staff, however, never left. Call schedules in 1983 were not supposed to exceed one in three nights, but frequently, as a result of sickness, vacations or, god forbid, pregnancy, residents were often called on to work extended shifts. Sleep was at a premium.

Of course, the architect had no idea that on-call residents slept. He had assumed that on-call meant working a shift. The new Brigham tower had been initially designed without overnight call rooms. Medical residents slept two to a room on the as yet unopened upper floors of the tower. They were lucky to enjoy a beautiful view of the city, with big windows and excellent ventilation. Down on L & D, we slept in the subbasement below the labor floor. Our second home was a long corridor with a dozen doors leading to tiny rooms and a handful of bathrooms. There was no air circulation, just a series of sleep cells. The fact that it was nestled next to the nuclear pharmacy only added to the charm of the place. Nothing is more reassuring than a "Caution: Radioactive Materials" sign next to your bedroom. There were at least fourteen heavy doors on that narrow hall, which, because of the spring closures, would slam with a jarring metallic crack that reverberated through the narrow corridor. An obstetrical or anesthesia resident returning to his or her call room entered the corridor through a heavy main door. Slam. The sound echoed, amplified, and resonated, penetrating into your exhausted sleep-deprived brain, pulling you from restless coma to a startled state of full alertness. Sounds are always exaggerated just as you are trying to get to sleep; even the slightest noise can startle you. It's this very reason we stay carefully quiet in the OR while patients are put to sleep or awakened. Hearing is the last thing to go and the first thing to return, and nowhere is that more evident than in those tiny call rooms when the metal doors slammed.

Bang. The main door of the corridor slams and the resident now moves down the row of doors jiggling the door handles to find an open room. Opens the door and slam. Drops off the beeper, grabs a towel and goes back into the hallway to the bathroom. Slam goes the call room door. Slam goes the bathroom door. Slam goes the call room door. One resident to bed, half a dozen slams. Everyone is now awake. Repeat, repeat, and repeat. The door-slamming cycle stops just long enough to catch the sharp trill of the beeper piercing the echoing chambers.

Brigham beepers were a technical marvel. Unlike MGH beepers, which lacked any display screen, forcing you to call the page operator to retrieve every message, the technologically advanced BWH pagers would display four-digit extensions on blinking red light-emitting diode screens. The problem was the numbers were both largely illegible and displayed individually. The beeper would beep, you pushed the button, and then, one by one the red numbers would flash. It was torture. 5... long pause... 4... long pause... 3... 5... Labor floor. The second most hated extension in the hospital. The first, the infamous 5... 6... 3... 6 was the emergency department. The beepers went off continuously; residents would fall asleep while the numbers slowly displayed. They would be paged again. Then, the phone call, the crash of the receiver, a curse, followed by the groan of a very tired physician climbing out of a very uncomfortable bed in an asphyxiating room nestled next to stockpiles of radioisotopes. Slam, slam, slam went the doors.

Now sometimes sounds in the call rooms were more interesting. Heated telephone conversations with floor nurses, or calls home to loved ones, spouses... children. "I promise mommy will be home tomorrow night." Sometimes there were offensive bathroom sounds, often accompanied by offensive bathroom smells. Two-hundred-pound anesthesia residents mixed with Brigham cafeteria chili is a heady mix indeed. Sometimes the sounds were provocative. A whisper, a giggle, a conversation, or a muffled cry of joy and passion. The rhythmic creaking of a call room bed was hard not to notice. These sounds would build to a quiet crescendo and then... slam, slam, beeper, beeper, curse, groan. It was intrusive and it was unfair, but compared with the other sounds and smells of the corridor, this behavior was amusing and, in many ways, life-affirming.

Then someone complained. Some joyless person walked into the chair's office and complained. Kenneth Ryan was a brilliant, compassionate, and effective leader, but could be strangely awkward in social situations. He was not humorless, but he was not exactly a laugh-a-minute either. It was left to Ryan to address the issue of sex in the call rooms. How would he do it? There was no email system, and a staff note seemed a bit too public. Ryan chose an interesting forum.

Every Wednesday an obstetrical service meeting known as Meconium Rounds was held in a crowded conference room off L & D. The room was always packed with residents, medical students, and senior faculty. Ryan would sit at the head of the table and review the complicated cases of the week. It was usually a tense affair because residents needed to be prepared to defend how they had managed complicated obstetrical cases. In this tension-filled room, Ryan decided to make his move. "I would like to remind the resident staff that the call rooms are to be used for sleep only." The room fell entirely quiet. Then one senior resident, known for his lack of tact, said: "What do you mean?" Ryan's lip quivered in that certain way it did only when he was stressed or angry. "There shall be no conjugal visits in the call rooms." Again a long, pregnant pause. "Even with my wife? We are trying to have a baby and I'm never home at the right time!" Another painful silence. Ryan repeated: "There shall be no conjugal visits with anyone at any time."

For about a week or so after that meeting, the sounds in the corridor were much less interesting. Then, the natural order of the world was restored.

JUST AFTER THE DAYS OF GIANTS

Rebecca M. Baron

A native of Skokie, Illinois, Baron is a graduate of Stanford University undergraduate and Harvard Medical School. She did her internal medicine residency (1994-1997) at BWH and pulmonary and critical care medicine fellowship (1997-1999, 2000-2002) at the Harvard Combined Pulmonary and Critical Medicine Fellowship program; she served as chief medical resident in 1999-2000 at BWH. Baron currently is an investigator in sepsis and lung injury, attends in the medical intensive care unit, and is director of the BWH Pulmonary and Critical Care Medicine Fellowship Program.

Although I can't claim that I "spun my own crits" or donated my own blood for transfusion as in the "good ole days," it is sobering still to realize that much has changed and evolved since I and my classmates were internal medicine residents in the mid-1990s. Nonetheless, I endorse the prevailing timeless view that residency at the Brigham and Women's Hospital represented "best of times and the worst of times"—sometimes the worst of times at the time, and only the best of times in retrospect.

My memories as a house officer from 1994-1997 are dominated by perpetual motion, with the need to keep moving to keep ahead of the always-impending onslaught of admissions. The 1990s represented a time of change and expansion at BWH and in medicine in general, before the structural aspects of resident staffing had adapted to meet this need. There were no "work hours" or "caps" as there currently are, and therefore, as interns and residents, we admitted every patient that came to us over a given time period, regardless of how many patients that was. Thus produced the prevailing mantra, "You can hurt me, but you can't stop the clock." Just as our "light" schedules were poked fun at by more senior "giants" who trained before us, it is incredulous to current generations that I could admit ten to twelve patients per night as an intern (and twenty to twenty-four patients as a resident) every third-fourth night and not sleep for twenty-four to thirty-six hours on some rotations. Furthermore, in contrast to the current status that includes both physician's assistant and other "uncovered" services and limitations on house staff work hours, producing the need for a lot of "card-flipping" rather than bedside daily rounds, every medicine patient was cared for and rounded on daily by house staff teams. Our program director, Marshall Wolf, would admonish us if every patient wasn't seen every day by our team on morning rounds. I recall him saying once, "Patients in the hospital expect to be intruded upon by large groups of doctors every morning."

Conversely, the experiences of carrying out all of this work, at all hours of the day and night, with relatively limited supervision by attending physicians (as compared with my current intense workload as an attending) produced a unique and special environment of camaraderie amongst the house staff. We were all in this together, and the impulse and generally accepted norm was to do as much as possible to limit the amount of work your colleagues would have to take over for you when you left (thus further extending the numbers of hours you spent in the hospital). Marshall Wolf was and is revered by all medical trainees, not only as a brilliant physician and teacher, but also as the man who did anything possible to support and help the house staff, and this beneficence still permeates the corridors at BWH. One of Marshall's many wisdoms was the need for food at all conferences. I have many memories of competing for the last row of seats in the conference hall so that we could eat, then put our heads back against the wall and nap for a brief period until our pager went off yet again. Our knowledge base expanded exponentially, such that we gained a level of comfort with extremely sick patients fairly quickly and of necessity. In the mid-1990s, we were only partially computerized and thus had to spend much of our day in the bowels of the hospital tracking down medical records and X-ray films. With all of these obligations, multitasking and efficiency were critical for our survival.

I am incredibly proud to have trained at BWH, and I still use on a daily basis the experiences and lessons I learned from that important time. Moreover, the relationships and friendships that grew out of that special period are indelible, producing a cohort of colleagues who are forever bonded by these shared experiences. I have learned firsthand that regardless of the rules and regulations that are decreed regarding residency training, the BWH Internal Medicine Residency legacy will adapt and excel, keeping true to its principles and legacy.

REFERENCES

1. Clinton Sandvick, "Enforcing Medical Licensing in Illinois: 1877-1890," Yale Journal of Biology and Medicine (2009), pp. 67-74.
2. Kenneth Ludmerer, *A Time to Heal: American Medical Education from the Turn of the Century to the Era of Managed Care* (New York, NY: Oxford University Press, 1999), p. 81.
3. William Hollingsworth, *Taking Care: The Legacy of Soma Weiss, Eugene Stead, and Paul Beeson* (Chapel Hill, NC: Professional Press, 1994), p. 24.
4. John Tyndall, Louis Pasteur, *Les Microbes Organisés, leur Rôle dans la Fermentation, la Putréfaction et la Contagion* (Gauthier-Villars Press, 1878).
5. Robert Koch, "UntersuchungenüberBakterien: V. Die Ätiologie der Milzbrand-Krankheit, begründetauf die Entwicklungsgeschichte des Bacillus anthracis [Investigations into bacteria: V. The etiology of anthrax, based on the ontogenesis of Bacillus anthracis]," *CohnsBeitragezur Biologie der Pflanzen* 2 (1876), pp. 277-310.
6. Ann Conway, "Organizational Symbolism in the Peter Bent Brigham Hospital 1913-1938: A Cultural History," (PhD diss, BrandeisUniversity, 1993), p. 65.
7. Paul Starr, *The Social Transformation of American Medicine* (New York, NY: Basic Books, 1984), p. 79.
8. Ludmerer, p. 25.
9. "Women—or The Female Factor, "in "About Johns Hopkins Medicine," Johns Hopkins University School of Medicine. http://www.hopkinsmedicine.org/about/history/history6.html, accessed September 2012.

10. In contrast, Harvard Medical School did not admit women until 1945.
11. Ludmerer, p. 25.
12. Henry K. Beecher, Mark D. Altschule, *Mediciene at Harvard: The First 300 Years* (Hanover, NH: University Press of New England, 1977), p. 87.
13. Edward H. Cotton, *The Life of Charles W. Eliot* (Boston: Small, Maynard and Company, 1926).
14. Ludmerer, p. 14.
15. Flexner, Carnegie Report, 1910, p. 1.
16. Ludmerer, p. 4.
17. David McCord, *The Fabrick of Man* (Boston: Published for the Hospital by the Fiftieth Anniversary Celebration Committee, 1963), pp. 14, 22.
18. David Cheever, "Peter Bent Brigham Hospital 40th Anniversary: Teaching," *Brigham Bulletin* 3 (1953), p. 3.
19. McCord, p. 21.
20. Ludmerer, p. 18.
21. Cheever, p. 32.
22. Rosemary Stevens' *In Sickness and in Wealth: American Hospitals in the Twentieth Century* (Baltimore: Johns Hopkins University Press, 1999) extensively discusses the development of a scientific charity orientation—part of an overall reformist movement to encourage effective resource use and recipient self-help—in twentieth century teaching hospitals.
23. "Reginald Fitz," Office of the University Marshall, Harvard University. http://www.marshal.harvard.edu/fitz.html, accessed September 2012.
24. Reginald Fitz, *At the Heart of a Great Medical Center: A Record of Past and a Promise for the Future 1913-1938* (Boston: PBBH, 1938), p. 27.
25. Frederick Schoen, "Education and Training in the BWH Department of Pathology," PBBH History Essay, 2012.
26. Harvey Cushing, "W. T. Councilman: 1854-1933," *Science* 77 (1933), pp. 613-6.
27. Ibid., p. 616.
28. Ibid., p. 615.
29. Ibid.
30. Benjamin Baker, "The Finished Brigham Hospital," *Boston Evening Transcript*, October 9, 1912, p. 21.
31. George W. Thorn, "Report of the Physician-in-Chief," *Forty-Fifth Annual Report of the Peter Bent Brigham Hospital for the Fiscal Year Ended September 30, 1958* (Boston, 1958), p. 23.
32. Baker, p. 21.
33. David Cheever. "Peter Bent Brigham Hospital 40th Anniversary: Teaching," *Brigham Bulletin* 3 (1953), p. 3.
34. McCord, p. 40.
35. Baker, p. 21.
36. McCord, p. 37.
37. J.E. Fulton, *Harvey Cushing, A Biography* (Springfield, Illinois, Charles C. Thomas, 1946), p. 539.
38. McCord, 41.
39. Starr, p. 115.
40. The hierarchical PBBH system of limiting advancement to a relatively small percentage of physicians fostered the training of leaders (although the definition evolved over time) and ultimately, specialists. Some observers would say that this was also a foundation of elitist attitudes that have dogged the profession.
41. Baker, p. 21.
42. Ludmerer, p. 86.
43. Ibid.
44. Oglesby Paul, *The Caring Physician: The Life of Dr. Francis W. Peabody* (Cambridge, MA: Harvard University Press, 2011).
45. Baker, p. 21.
46. Ludmerer, p. 111.
47. McCord, p. 36.
48. Baker, p. 21.
49. Lewis Thomas, *The Youngest Science* (Toronto: Bantam Books, 1983), p. 36.
50. The first "*Pro Tem*" was Professor William S. Thayer from Johns Hopkins Hospital.
51. Harvey Cushing, "Report of the Surgeon-in-Chief," *First Annual Report of the Peter Bent Brigham Hospital for the Years 1913 and 1914* (Cambridge: The University Press, 1915).
52. Michael Zinner, video interview by Peter Tishler, 2012, "BWH History Videos: The Brightest and the Best," http://brw.sites.vm2.broadcastmed.net/videos/michael-zinner-md.
53. Marshall A. Wolf, personal communication with Joel Katz.
54. H. Richard Tyler, interview by Peter Tishler, 2012, "BWH History Videos: The Brightest and the Best," http://videocenter.brighamandwomens.org/videos/h-richard-tyler-md.
55. Tinsley R. Harrison, "Tribute to Dr. Levine," *New England Journal of Medicine* 275 (1966), pp. 222-3.
56. Paul Dudley White, "Samuel Albert Levine," *American Heart Journal* 291 (1966), pp. 291-2.
57. Charles F. Wooley, "Proc, Dr. Sam, Uncle Henry, and The 'Little Green Book,'" *American Heart Hospital Journal* 3 (2005), pp. 8-13.
58. Bernard Lown, *The Lost Art of Healing* (Boston: Houghton Mifflin, 1996), pp. 3, 79.
59. Ibid. pp. 79-80.
60. Excerpted from Nicholas Tilney, Anthony Whittemore, Michael Zinner and Stanley Ashley, "Evolution of Surgical Education," PBBH History Essay, 2012.
61. J.E. Fulton, *Harvey Cushing, A Biography* (Springfield, IL: Charles C. Thomas, 1946), p. 539.
62. Prospectus, School of Nursing, Peter Bent Brigham Hospital (Boston, MA: The Hospital, 1912).
63. Henry A. Christian, "Graduation Address," *The Alumnae Journal*, Peter Bent Brigham Hospital School of Nursing 17 (1937), p. 8.

64. See essay by Marilyn King in this chapter.
65. M.P. Donahue, *Nursing: The Finest Art* (3rd ed.) (Maryland Heights, MO: Mosby, 2011).
66. Marilyn King, *The Peter Bent Brigham School of Nursing: A History, 1912-1985* (Boston, MA: Brigham and Women's Hospital, 1987), p. 84.
67. Ibid., p. 23.
68. We thank members of The Peter Bent Brigham School of Nursing Alumni Association for their thoughts and contributions.
69. Ludmerer, p. 36.
70. Harvey Cushing, "Report of the Surgeon-in-Chief," *Sixth Annual Report of the Peter Bent Brigham Hospital for the Year 1919* (Cambridge: The University Press, 1920), p. 54.
71. The hospital was apparently unable to pay for Osler's visit, so the ceremony was timed to coincide with his planned travel through Boston for other reasons. *Seventh PBBH Annual Report* (1920), p. 55.
72. Cushing, *Sixth Annual Report,* p. 56.
73. Cushing, *Sixth Annual Report,* p. 54.
74. McCord, pp. 18-19.
75. Ibid.
76. Frederick Irving, "Highlights in the History of The Boston Lying-In Hospital," Canadian Medical Association Journal 54 (1946), p. 176.
77. Ibid., p. 177.
78. Ibid., pp. 177-8.
79. Frederick Irving, *Safe Deliverance* (Boston: Houghton-Mifflin, 1942).
80. Irving, p. 178. In addition to *Safe Deliverance*, John Jewett's *The Boston Lying-In Hospital: A Sesquicentenium*, gives a full accounting of the Lying-In's history.
81. Elmer Cappers, *A History of the Free Hospital for Women* (Boston: Boston Hospital for Women, 1975), p. 19.
82. Ibid., p. 21.
83. Ibid., p. 42.
84. Ibid., p. 44.
85. This closed during World War I.
86. Cappers, p. 64.
87. "Historical Notes," Robert B. Brigham Hospital 1889-1984. Records, Bulk 1915-1980: Finding Aid. Countway Library, Harvard University. http://oasis.lib.harvard.edu/oasis/deliver/~med00058, accessed July 2012.
88. Ann Conway, *A History of the Robert Breck Brigham Hospital,* draft manuscript (1993), p. 40.
89. Jeffrey M. Drazen, "Presentation of the 2004 Kober Medal to K. Frank Austen," *Journal of Clinical Investigation* 114 (2004), pp. 1174-1176.
90. "Historical Notes," Robert B. Brigham Hospital 1889-1984.
91. Michael E. Whitcomb, "Responsive Curriculum Reform: Continuing Challenges," *Ten Stories of Curriculum Change* (American Association of Medical Colleges/Milbank Memorial Fund: 2000). http://www.milbank.org/reports/americanmedicalcolleges/0010medicalcolleges.html, accessed August 2012.
92. By 1953 the system had evolved into what was called "every other night and weekend," including a Saturday through Monday on-call (60-hour shift) resulting in a weekly average of 132 hours, *if* one could meet all the schedule goals, which was uncommon. Phillip J. Snodgrass, *A Life in Academic Medicine* (New York: iUniverse, 2007), p. 29.
93. George W. Thorn, "Report of the Physician-in-Chief," *Thirty-Fifth Annual Report of the Peter Bent Brigham Hospital for the Year 1948* (Boston, 1949), pp. 32, 35.
94. Ludmerer, p. 191.
95. Tyler interview.
96. Ibid.
97. Ibid.
98. "Development, 1954-1983," Howard Hughes Medical Foundation. http://www.hhmi.org/about/development.html, accessed September 11, 2012.
99. Ludmerer, p. 43.
100. Marshall Wolf, personal communication.
101. The cloth napkins— which each physician stored carefully in a box by the entrance—were replaced with paper in 1963 (personal communication, Marshall Wolf).
102. Ibid. Resident staff joked that on vacation they ran the risk of developing "acute peanut butter withdrawal."
103. Ibid.
104. Tyler interview.
105. Ibid.
106. Snodgrass, p. 32.
107. Marshall Wolf, personal communication.
108. Ibid.
109. George W. Thorn, "Report of the Physician-in-Chief," Fifty-Fifth Annual Report Peter Bent Brigham Hospital 1967-1968 (Boston, 1968), p. 30.
110. Kenneth H. Falchuk, personal communication.
111. Marshall A. Wolf, personal communication.
112. Ibid.
113. In a strange and beautiful twist of irony, Lown and fellow Nobel recipient Eugene Chazov leapt from their dais seats at an Oslo press conference to resuscitate Soviet photojournalist Lev Novikov, who had gone into cardiac arrest.
114. Joel T. Katz, personal communication.
115. Bernard Lown, http://www.humanmedia.org/catalog/program.php?products_id=54, accessed November 12, 2012.
116. Schoen, "Education and Training."
117. Kristen DeJohn, "Tapping Potential: Marshall A. Wolf, M.D," *BWH Magazine*, Spring 2011.
118. Tyler interview.
119. Ibid.
120. Marshall Wolf, personal communication.
121. Marshall A. Wolf, video interview by Peter Tishler, 2012, "BWH History Videos: The Brightest and the Best,"

http://brw.sites.vm2.broadcastmed.net/videos/marshall-wolf-md.
122. Ibid.
123. In 2012, the minority racial/ethnic breakdown is: *residents* (American Indian/Alaska Native (.029%); Asian 21.3%), Black/African American (5.65%), Hispanic/Latino (5.07%), Multi (.58%). For *physicians*: American Indian/Alaska Native (.026%); Asian (15.29 %%), Black/African American (2.65%), Hispanic/Latino (6.75%), Multi (.26%) and *fellows*: Asian 32.16%), Black/African American (2.19%), Hispanic/Latino (4.37%), Multi (.69%). The overall gender breakdown is: *residents*: (47.10% female/52.90% male), *physicians* (40.26 % female/59.74% male) and *fellows* (41.38% female/58.62% male) Source: BWH Human Resources, August 2012.
124. Thomas H. Lee, Jr., Eugene Braunwald and the Rise of Modern Medicine (Cambridge, MA: Harvard University Press), 2013, p. 241.
125. Kristin DeJohn, "Marshall A. Wolf, M.D," *Brigham and Women's* (2011), pp. 18-25.
126. Wolf interview.
127. Zinner interview.
128. The PBBH "short-track" model was adopted by the American Board of Internal Medicine to what was called the "Subspecialty Investigatory Pathway" (1983) and now the "Research Pathway" (2008), whereby selected trainees can enter specialty fellowship one year early.
129. Eugene Braunwald, "Report of the Physician-in-Chief," *Sixty-Third Annual Report, Peter Bent Brigham Hospital, 1975-1976* (Boston: 1976), p. 42.
130. Wolf reports that his own desire to train better primary care doctors was based on discovering his own inadequacies on finishing PBBH residency, when he could resuscitate a complex cardiac arrest but could not comment on a simple rash in a patient or family member. Marshall A. Wolf, personal communication.
131. Debra Weinstein, "Partners Graduate Medical Education Annual Report," 2010.
132. Kristen DeJohn, "Tapping Potential," BWH Profiles in Medicine, *Brigham and Women's Magazine,* Spring 2011, 18.
133. Ibid., p. 20.
134. Ibid., p. 18.
135. Underrepresented minority physicians trained by Wolf currently hold the positions of president and CEO of the Robert Woods Johnson Foundation; director of the National Heart, Lung and Blood Institute of the NIH; and director of the Indian Health Service, to name a few.
136. DeJohn, p. 25.
137. Zion, the 18-year-old daughter of *The Daily News* columnist Sidney Zion, died after admission to the hospital's emergency room. She was treated by an intern who had graduated from medical school only eight months before and had been on duty for twenty-four hours. Subsequently, Zion sued the hospital and local and national publicity led to New York State policy changes. In 2003, the Accreditation Council for Graduate Medical Education imposed an eighty-hour limit on training programs, prohibited trainees from direct patient care, and mandated at least one day off weekly. DarshakSanghavi, "The Phantom Menace of Sleep-Deprived Doctors," *The New York Times Magazine,* August 5, 2011. http://www.nytimes.com/2011/08/07/magazine/the-phantom-menace-of-sleep-deprived-doctors.html?pagewanted=all&_r=0, accessed July 2012.
138. Institute of Medicine, *To Err Is Human: Building a Safer Health System* (Washington, DC: National Academies Press, 1999).
139. H.T. Stelfox et al,. "The 'To Err Is Human' report and the patient safety literature," *Quality and Safety in Health Care* 15 (2006), pp. 174-8.
140. Zinner interview.
141. Kevin G. Volpp, Amy K. Rosen, Paul R. Rosenbaum, Patrick S. Romano, Orit Even-Shoshan, Yanli Wang, Lisa Bellini, Tiffany Behringer, Jeffrey H. Silber, "Mortality among hospitalized medicare beneficiaries in the first 2 years following ACGME resident duty hour reform," *JAMA* 298 (2007), pp. 975-983.
142. Graham T. McMahon, Joel T. Katz, Mary E. Thorndike, Bruce D. Levy, and Joseph Loscalzo. "Evaluation of a Redesign Initiative in an Internal Medicine Residency," *The New England Journal of Medicine* 362 (2010), pp. 1304-1311.
143. Kenneth M. Ludmerer, "Redesigning Residency Work Hours: Moving Beyond Work Hours," *The New England Journal of Medicine* 362 (2010), pp. 1337-1338.
144. Thomas D. Sequist, "Health Careers for Native American Students: Challenges and Opportunities for Enrichment Program Design," *Journal of Interprofessional Care* (2007), pp. 20-30.
145. Tracey Kidder, *Mountains Beyond Mountains* (New York: Random House, 2003).
146. Jennifer Joan Furin, Paul Farmer, Marshall Wolf, Bruce Levy, Amy Judd, Margaret Paternek, Rocio Hurtado, and Joel Katz, "A Novel Training Model to Address Health Problems in Poor and Underserved Populations," *Journal of Health Care for the Poor and Underserved* 17 (2006), pp. 17-24.
147. Carrie M. Hall, 15th Annual Report, 1929, Peter Bent Brigham Hospital School of Nursing Papers, Nursing Archives, Mugar Memorial Library, Boston University, Boston, MA (hereafter referred to as PBBHSON Papers).
148. Isabel Hampton Robb, "Educational Standards for Nurses," In Isabel Hampton Robb, *Educational Standards for Nurses with Other Addresses* (Cleveland: E. C. Koeckert, 1907), p. 5.
149. "Carrie M. Hall" biographical sketch, typed manuscript in the PBBHSON Papers; Carrie M. Hall, "Memoirs of the School of Nursing," *40th Anniversary of the Peter Bent Brigham Hospital,* PBBHSON Papers, 1954.

150. Ibid.
151. Susie A. Watson, "Reminiscences of Early Days," *The Alumnae Journal* 1 (1910), p. 6.
152. Ibid., p. 7.
153. Ibid., p. 7.
154. Marilyn G. King, "Conflicting Interests: Professionalization and Apprenticeship in Nursing Education: A Case Study of the Peter Bent Brigham Hospital School of Nursing During the Carrie M. Hall Years, 1912-1937." Doctoral dissertation, Boston University, 1987.
155. Nancy Woloch, *Women and the American Experience* (New York: Alfred A. Knopf, 1984), p. 54; Carrie M. Hall, "Report of the School of Nursing," *Eighth Annual Report of Peter Bent Brigham Hospital for the Year 1921* (Cambridge, MA: The University Press, 1922), p. 31; and *Ninth Annual Report of Peter Bent Brigham Hospital for the Year 1922* (Cambridge, MA: The University Press, 1923), p. 32, (hereafter referred to as Annual Report), PBBHSON Papers; Commonwealth of Massachusetts, *The Law Governing the Registration of Nurses and the Minimum Curriculum required by the Board of Registration of Nursing.* Document in the PHHHSON Papers; PBBHSON Student Records for Classes of 1915-1919, Brigham and Women's Hospital, Boston, MA.
156. Sally Johnson, "The Arrangement of Subjects Taught in the School of Nursing of the Peter Bent Brigham Hospital," in *Proceedings of the 20th Annual Convention of the National League of Nursing Education* (New York: National League of Nursing Education, 1914), p. 209.
157. Carrie M. Hall, "The Teaching of Hospital Housekeeping to Pupil Nurses," *Proceedings of the 21st Annual Convention of the National League of Nursing Education,* 1915, p. 134. Cleanliness and order in the patient's environment was stressed from the time of Florence Nightingale and was critically important to the control of communicable diseases prior to the discovery of antibiotics. See Florence Nightingale, *Notes on Nursing: What It Is and What It Is Not* (Dover Publications, 1860/1969), for her ideas about the patient environment.
158. Johnson, "The Arrangement of Subjects," p. 209.
159. Bernice J. Sinclair, "Graduation Address," *The Alumnae Journal* 25 (1945), p. 6.
160. Johnson, pp. 211-13.
161. Ibid., p. 210.
162. Sally M. Johnson, "Points for Probationers," [n.d.] typed manuscript in the PBBHSON Papers.
163. "The Nurses' Ten Commandments," *The Alumnae Journal* 1 (1920), p. 15.
164. Ibid.
165. Marilyn King, *The Peter Bent Brigham Hospital School of Nursing: A History,* (Boston: Brigham and Women's Hospital, 1987), p. 51.
166. Carrie M. Hall, "Report of the School of Nursing," Eleventh Annual Report of the Peter Bent Brigham Hospital for the Year 1924 (Boston: Wright & Potter, 1925), pp. 44-9.
167. Ibid.
168. Ibid.
169. Ibid.
170. Ibid.
171. Isabel Hampton Robb, *Educational Standards for Nurses with Other Addresses,* 1907; M. Adelaide Nutting, *A Sound Economic Basis for Schools of Nursing and Other Addresses* (New York: Garland Publishing, Inc., 1926/1984).
172. Carrie M. Hall, "Report of the School of Nursing," *Ninth Annual Report of the Peter Bent Brigham Hospital for the Year 1922* (Cambridge: The University Press, 1923), pp. 30-1.
173. May Ayres Burgess, *Nurses, Patients, and Pocketbooks* (New York: National League of Nursing Education, Committee on the Grading of Nursing Schools, 1928); Committee on the Grading of Nursing Schools, "Nurses' Production, Education, Distribution, and Pay," published by NLNE, May 1, 1930, pp. 35-36.
174. Carrie M. Hall, "Another Graduation," *The Alumnae Journal* 8 (1928), pp. 6-7.
175. Ibid., p. 7.
176. Esther Lucille Brown, *Nursing for the Future* (New York: Russell Sage Foundation, 1948), pp. 116-98.
177. Lucy H. Beal, "Report of the School of Nursing," *Twenty-Fourth Annual Report of the Peter Bent Brigham Hospital for the Year 1937* (Boston: 1938), pp. 35-7; *The Alumnae Journal* 17 (1937): 13.
178. Lucy H. Beal, "Report of the School of Nursing," Twenty-Seventh Annual Report of the Peter Bent Brigham Hospital for the Year 1940 (Boston: 1941), pp. 49-50.
179. Interview with Shirley Egan, July 1, 1985.
180. Letter to Dorothy Vernstrom from Frances K. Peterson, NLN, January 4, 1961, PBBHSON Papers.
181. Margarita M. Farrington, "School of Nursing," Peter Bent Brigham Hospital Annual Report 1962-1963 (Boston: 1963), p. 372.
182. Letter to Shirley Egan from Alan Steinert, October 29, 1976, PBBHSON Papers.
183. Executive Summary and Recommendation, Nursing School Task Force, Brigham and Women's Hospital, [no date, but in 1983], PBBHSON Papers.
184. King, *The Peter Bent Brigham Hospital School of Nursing,* p. 145.
185. Ibid., p. 148.
186. T.N. Pappas, "Adjustment reactions and the surgical intern," *JAMA* 248 (1982), pp. 31-32.

CHAPTER 3

AN ENGINE OF BIOMEDICAL RESEARCH AND CLINICAL CARE

PART 1: EVOLUTION OF BIOMEDICAL RESEARCH

I. INTRODUCTION

AN ENGINE OF BIOMEDICAL RESEARCH

Peter V. Tishler

The Brigham and Women's Hospital ranks among the top institutions nationwide in research innovation and productivity, both of which continue to grow. One crude measure of this ranking is the amount of funding for research available over time. In fiscal year 1996, for example, the Brigham spent approximately $141 million on research (direct and indirect costs), whereas in fiscal year 2010, this figure was approximately $555 million (second highest nationally). How did all this come about?

When the Peter Bent Brigham Hospital (PBBH) was conceived, resulting in large part from the bequest of Peter Bent Brigham for establishing a hospital "for the care of sick persons in indigent circumstances residing in Suffolk County," medical research in the United States was rudimentary. At the end of the nineteenth century, it was primarily descriptive, with investigators defining and categorizing disease entities. Seeds of more mechanistic research had been laid in several areas, as represented by the germ theory of disease etiology (e.g., Pasteur and Koch's discoveries in the 1870s and 1880s) and the detailed descriptive pathology of the human body by Virchow and others in the late nineteenth century. As these examples suggest, most medical research was carried out in institutions in Europe and particularly in Germany. It was common practice in this era for graduates of American medical schools with

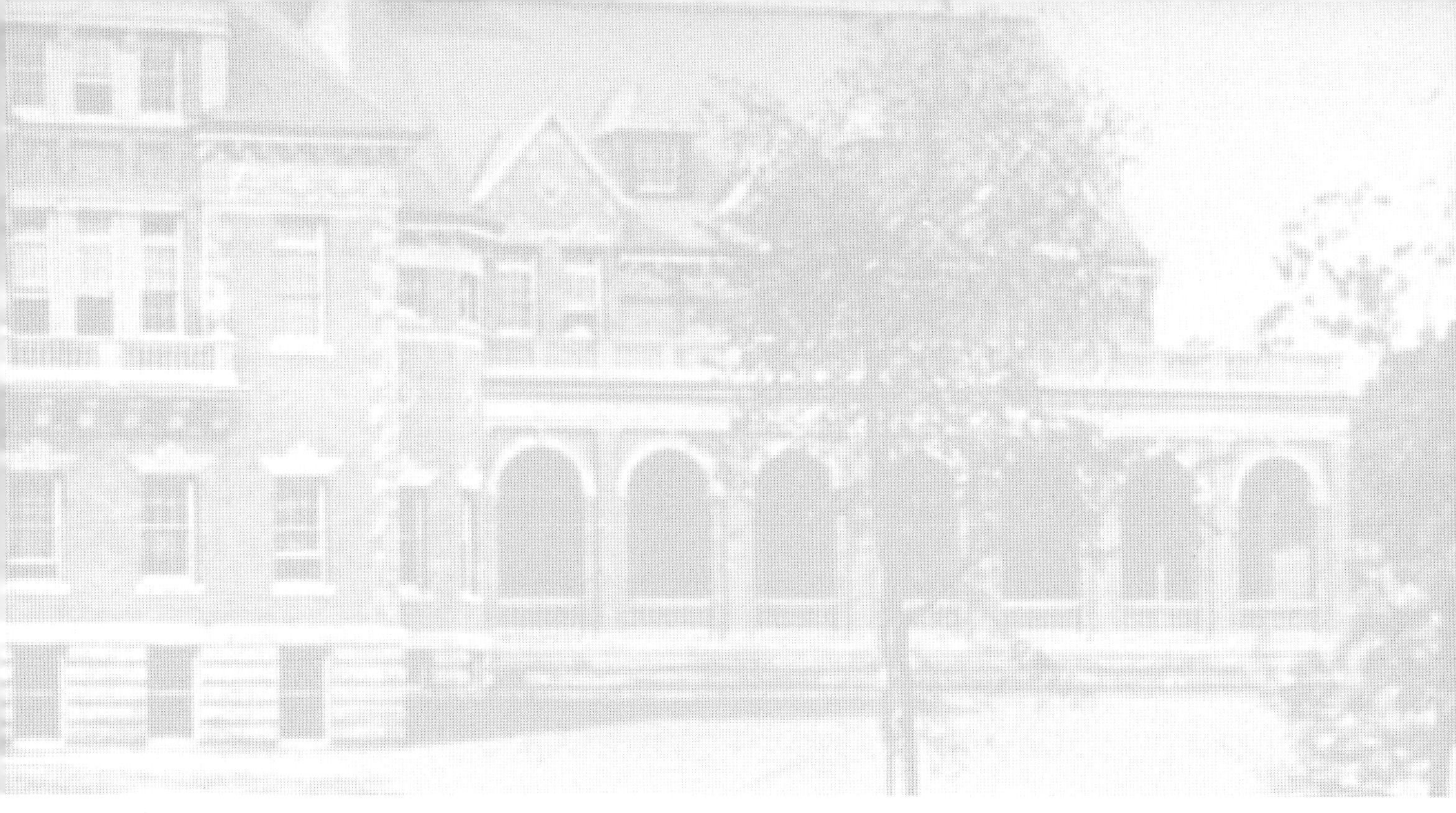

an interest in contemporary research to spend time in a laboratory of a well-known European investigator. This European influence on American medicine before World War I was pervasive, but limited to a small proportion of physicians with intellectual curiosity or great ambition. Those few individuals who returned from Europe to medical positions of prominence brought with them training in addressing mechanisms of disease that was ultimately passed on to younger trainees. Unfortunately, many individuals who journeyed to Europe for further education were not able to find institutions in the United States that would hire and support their research.

Things began to change in the early twentieth century, especially in its second decade. Most of the events underlying change generated circumstances in which the observation of patients with illness was markedly increased, resulting in markedly increased questions concerning the etiology and pathogenesis of disease. In 1910, Harvard Medical School (HMS) began its teaching affiliation with the nascent PBBH, its preferred teaching hospital owing to its proximity and academic purpose (HMS had moved to its current location in 1906). This was led by HMS Dean Henry A. Christian, who had trained in medicine at the pioneering Johns Hopkins School of Medicine (1895-1900) and was profoundly influenced by the educational importance of the uniquely affiliated Johns Hopkins Hospital.[1] Christian worked with the PBBH trustees to ensure that the Brigham would be composed of full-time clinical faculty, selected for research capabilities and interest as well as clinical expertise. He also negotiated an agreement that the HMS student curriculum would include mandatory clinical clerkships at the PBBH at its opening in 1913, modeled after his student clerkships at the Johns Hopkins Medical School and Hospital. Nationally, similar affiliations of hospitals and medical schools were occurring simultaneously or shortly thereafter. The enthusiastically received Flexner Report of 1910, with Flexner's insistence that medical schools establish a close and functional relationship with hospitals that can provide students a meaningful clinical apprenticeship, was an important stimulus to these affiliations. In virtually each case, the hospital administration and trustees granted medical schools the right to appoint the medical staff and use of the hospital for medical instruction as well as research. The overwhelming national acceptance of the Flexner Report led, by the early 1920s, to the establishment of clinical clerkships in virtually all teaching hospitals. The populations in teaching hospitals nationwide of intelligent, curious students and of physicians dedicated to patient care and teaching medical students burgeoned. As historian Kenneth Ludmerer has stated, "With so many observers, patients [whose length of stay in hospital was usually long] were studied carefully and thoroughly."[2] More questions about the nature and cause of the disease were asked. With more questions came the need for more patient-centered research, under the aegis of the teaching hospitals and the medical schools.[3] Now these institutions hired physicians to carry out research on their premises, providing them with facilities and equipment. By the late 1920s, in the words of Kenneth Ludmerer, the teaching hospital "represented the culmination of the process by which medicine became scientific."[4]

A simultaneous change in public perception of the efficacy of medical care and the role of the hospital in caring for the sick was occurring. Surgery became a hospital-based process in the early twentieth century, utilizing significantly more beds at the time than other medical specialties. The resultant major leap in surgical success rates contributed greatly to public confidence in hospital care.[5] The popularization of the Flexner report certainly added to this changing perception. Revolutionary and impressive theories and treatments, such as the germ theory in the late nineteenth century and the treatment of diabetes mellitus in the early 1920s, were well known. The emergence of new and diagnostically important technologies, usually hospital-based (e.g., X-ray, early clinical laboratory tests), became available. These events led to greater public expectations that medical research would lead to the further understanding and effective treatment of disease and that hospitals were essential in enabling this evolution.

An equally seminal event that contributed extensively to the evolution of clinical research was the establishment of the Rockefeller Institute for Medical Research and its hospital in the early 1900s. Conceived after its founders observed and funded medical research for several years nationwide, the Rockefeller was devoted from its inception to studying not only the causation of disease but the mechanism by which disease was caused. This mission was advanced in particular by Christian A. Herter, a physician at the Rockefeller who, in the words of A. McGehee Harvey, "recognized the need for research in physiological chemistry early in his career."[6] The new Rockefeller was a unique American institution, modeled after similar institutions in Europe, especially Germany.

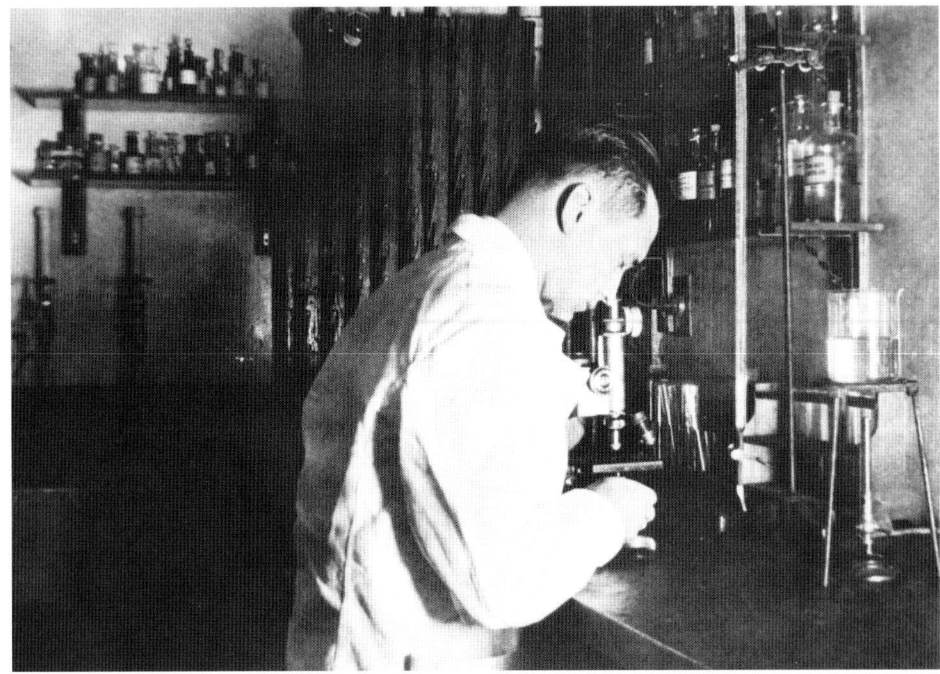

FIGURE 3-1 Early Peter Bent Brigham Hospital researcher.

Early graduates of the Rockefeller's training programs populated numerous medical schools and hospitals, spreading the gospel of physiological research. One such individual was Francis Weld Peabody.[7] A graduate of HMS in 1907, Peabody spent the better part of 1910 studying chemistry in Germany, followed by a fellowship at the Rockefeller Institute from 1911 to 1912. At the Brigham from its opening in 1913 to 1922, with time out for service in the world war, he was an early proponent and teacher of physiological research. At the Boston City Hospital (1922-1927), where he was the first chief of the Harvard Medical Unit and director of the Thorndike Memorial Laboratory, he trained a cadre of physicians (including Herrman Blumgart, William B. Castle, Cecil K. Drinker, Joseph T. Wearn, and Soma Weiss, physician-in-chief at the Brigham from 1939-1942) who further emphasized and expanded this type of clinical investigation in the later twentieth century. David Edsall, Jackson Professor of Medicine at the Massachusetts General Hospital (1912-1918) and dean at HMS (1918-1934), also had the research goal of studying the physiology of disease. Although he developed this approach before the Rockefeller Institute opened, studying in Europe in the late nineteenth century, he did send associates to the Rockefeller for training.

World War I exerted major influence on medical research. Many physicians joined the effort to care for the wounded, and many dealt with medical issues or wounds with which they had little experience. This led to questions of rather basic issues, such as acid-base balance and fluid physiology. Many of these issues were brought home after the armistice and investigated, beginning in the early 1920s, in hospitals.

Thus numerous factors contributed to the ascendency in the early twentieth century of medical research, particularly physiological research and clinical investigation, nationwide and specifically at the Brigham. World War II was an even greater major stimulus owing to major government funding, the tasks imposed on researchers as necessary for the war effort (e.g., the development of penicillin and streptomycin and of purified albumin solution for the treatment of soldiers with combat injuries) and the increase in numbers of medical students. Postwar,

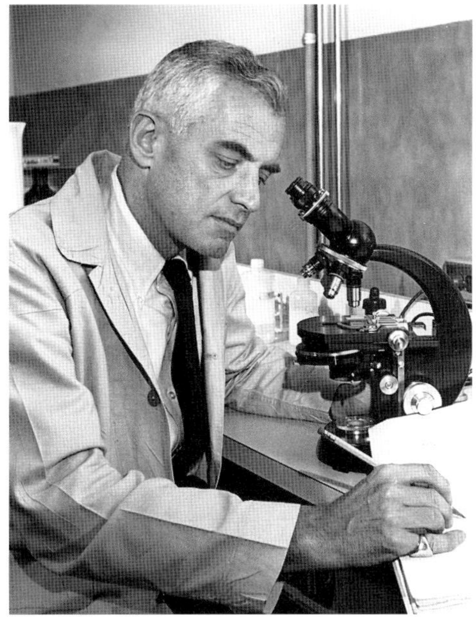

FIGURE 3-2 John Merrill with microscope.

innovations in biomedical statistics and clinical trial methodology (especially the randomized clinical trial) and continued major increases in federal spending on and training in medical research (i.e., the National Institutes of Health [NIH]), were critical. Eugene Braunwald, Arthur T. Hertig, Francis D. Moore, Joseph E. Murray, John C. Rock, George W. Thorn, and many others led the Brigham as this inquisitive research output burgeoned. Research that focused on the etiology, pathogenesis, and treatment of disease became the norm in the second half of the twentieth century, and the mechanisms by which these aims were studied evolved with amazing rapidity.

Perhaps the key initial discovery was Watson and Crick's formulation of the structure of DNA in the early 1950s. Their landmark description led rapidly to the introduction of molecular biology, emphasizing studies of the role of nucleic acids, the synthesis of proteins, and the function of the microscopic architecture of the cell. One major focus of the information accruing from molecular biology was in human genetics and genetic disease.[8] This effort began with the elucidation of the protein defect and the resultant pathophysiology of diseases caused by single gene mutations. It led sequentially to the identification and isolation of individual genes responsible for common genetic disease (e.g., sickle cell anemia, Huntington's chorea), then to the mapping of genes on chromosomes, construction of the human genome map, and, now, studies of the entire genome (genomics). Again, Brigham researchers Eugene Braunwald, Eva Neer, Elliott Kieff, Joseph Loscalzo, Christine Seidman, Nancy Berliner, their trainees, and many others led the way.

The first section in this chapter is devoted to research carried out by members of the Brigham staff since the founding of the hospital. We begin with a table that summarizes major accomplishments of many departments and divisions and follow with essays describing notable research in detail. Many of these essays include a consideration of both patient care and education, because these three major goals of hospital care are interrelated. These listings do not represent the only outstanding research at the Brigham. We shall also comment on the people who were seminal leaders and achievers in Brigham research, as well as in the other major professional disciplines of patient care and physician education. This includes essays on selected individuals and a listing of the awards and honors to the members of the medical staff.

In the twenty-first century, investigators focus on mechanisms of disease and mechanisms of control of disease at both the individual and population (public health) level. Given the amazing slope of research innovation and discovery in the last century, what can we expect in the near future?

NOTABLE CLINICAL AND RESEARCH ACCOMPLISHMENTS

Anesthesiology	
A new, pleasant 'vital capacity' induction, using Sevoflurane	Beverly K. Philip, Edward R. Road, James H. Philip
Development of continuous carbon dioxide monitor	James H. Philip, Daniel B. Raemer
First constant pressure fluid infusion system	James H. Philip, Beverly K. Philip
Cardiovascular Medicine	
Development of cardiac defibrillator	Bernard Lown
Demonstration of efficacy of angiotensin converting enzyme inhibitor in congestive heart failure and myocardial infarction	Eugene Braunwald, Marc Pfeffer
Elucidation of key role of inflammation in cardiovascular disease	Peter Libby, Paul M. Ridker
Design and conduct of large-scale, international clinical trials	Eugene Braunwald, Elliott Antman, etc.
Lipid-lowering therapy in patients with acute coronary syndromes	Christopher P. Cannon, Eugene Braunwald
Role of biomarkers CRP, BNP in risk stratification, treatment of acute coronary syndromes	Paul M. Ridker
Identification of novel fibrinolytic mechanisms in vascular disease	Douglas E. Vaughan, Daniel I. Simon, Joseph Loscalzo
Development of novel nitric oxide donor compounds for the treatment of cardiovascular disease	Jonathan S. Stamler, Joseph Loscalzo
Identification of a new disease class, the oxidative enzymopathies	Jane A. Leopold, Diane E. Handy, Joseph Loscalzo
Identification of genetic and acquired mechanisms of pulmonary hypertension	Ying Yi. Zhang, Stephen Y. Chan, Joseph Loscalzo

Dana-Farber Cancer Institute	
Creation of bone marrow models of multiple myeloma; identification of novel targets, therapies (proteasome inhibitor bortezomib; immunomodula-tory drug lenalidomide), increasing survival	Kenneth C. Anderson, Paul G. Richardson
The lung cancer EGFR gene mutation exists only in gefitinib-responsive lung adenocarcinoma. Patients are now EGFR-tested for the optimal therapy	Bruce E. Johnson, Pasi A. Janne, Neil L. Lindeman
Levels of tyrosine phosphoproteins are elevated in cells from patients with chronic myelogenous leukemia (CML); kinases could be therapy targets	Brian J. Drucker, Thomas M. Roberts
Development of 2nd-generation tyrosine kinase inhibitors for CML therapy	James D. Griffin
Targeted therapy for CML (imatinib) is therapeutic for GIST sarcoma, which has a similar molecular target	George D. Demetri, Jonathan A. Fletcher, Christopher D. Fletcher
Demonstration of the relation of telomeres and telomerase to cancer	Ronald A. DePinho, Lynda Chin
Leadership of successful trial of prostate cancer vaccine	Philip W. Kantoff
Application of genomics and gene array analysis to cancer characterization	Todd R. Golub, Margaret A. Shipp, Matthew L. Myerson
The normal VHL gene inhibits hypoxia-inducible factor and its downstream targets such as VEGF; oxygen regulates this response to hypoxia	William G. Kaelin, Jr.
The altered VHL gene in von Hippel-Lindau disease and kidney cancers permits development of vascular kidney cancers. VEGF inhibitors may be therapeutic	Jerome P. Richie, William G. Kaelin, Jr.
Monoclonal antibodies defined functional subsets of blood cells and characterized leukemias, lymphomas, myeloma	Stuart F. Schlossman, Ellis L. Reinherz, Lee M. Nadler
Immune manipulation of stem cell products reduces graft vs. host disease and promotes anti-leukemia activity in allogeneic transplantation	Jerome Ritz, Joseph H. Antin, Robert J. Soiffer, Edwin P. Alyea
International Prognostic Index classification of large-cell lymphomas developed, with distinct genetic signatures to predict treatment outcome	Margaret A. Shipp
Dermatology	
Description of cutaneous lymphocyte antigen; regulates T cell trafficking to the skin	Robert C. Fuhlbrigge
Glycosylated protein CD44 is the homing receptor for hematopoietic stem cells to bone marrow	Robert Sackstein, Charles J. Dimitroff, Robert C. Fuhlbrigge
Characterization of resident memory T cells, important in understanding immunologic memory	Lisa Z. Liu, Rachael A. Clark, Thomas S. Kupper
Identification of the tumor stem cell leading to melanoma	Robert C. Fuhlbrigge, Thomas S. Kupper
Development of a smallpox vaccine, safe for patients with immune dysfunction	Thomas S. Kupper, Robert C. Fuhlbrigge
Endocrinology	
First report of monogenic cause of hypertension (glucocorticoid-remediable aldosteronism)	Robert G. Dluhy, Richard P. Lifton
Identification of the extracellular calcium sensing receptor and its association with disease	Edward M. Brown

Discovery of mechanism of converting thyroxine to bioactive 3,5,3'-triiodothyronine	P. Reed Larsen
Design of sensitive methods and programs to screen for neonatal hypothyroidism	P. Reed Larsen
Identification of 'consumptive' hypothyroidism, usually found in infants	P. Reed Larsen
Gastroenterology	
Recombinant monomeric Fc fusion proteins generate long-acting Factors VIII & IX *in vivo*, that establish successful prophylaxis of hemophilias A, B	Richard S. Blumberg
General Surgery	
Inflammation promotes and amplifies injuries, e.g., acid aspiration	Herbert B. Hechtman
IgM antibody binds to membrane, activates complement and induces injury	Herbert B. Hechtman, Francis D. Moore, Jr.
Checklist minimizes mistakes and ensures proper patient care in OR	Atul Gawande
Genetics	
OurGenes, OurHealth, OurCommunity—Patient DNA stored for research	Elizabeth W. Karlson, Christine E. Seidman
Delineation of the inherited cardiomyopathies	Christine E. & Jonathan G. Seidman
Gene for tuberous sclerosis identified; its normal action defined	David J. Kwiatkowski
Hematology	
Defects in amount and function of globin mRNA occur in thalassemia, a first demonstration of the molecular genetic basis of a human disease	Edward J. Benz, Jr., Bernard G. Forget
Description of hemoglobin A1C and its relevance to diabetes mellitus	H. Franklin Bunn
Characterization of erythropoietin regulation by H1F1α	H. Franklin Bunn
Clonality of myeloproliferative disease	D. Gary Gilliland
TEL-AML1 translocation and modeling of leukemogenesis	D. Gary Gilliland
FIP1 translocation in eosinophilia and response to Imatinib	D. Gary Gilliland
Identification of rps14 as causative gene of 5q-syndrome	Benjamin L. Ebert
Nephrology	
Founding of nephrology as a subspecialty	John P. Merrill
Low birth weight is associated with reduction in nephron number, glomerular hypertrophy, greater renal disease progression, hypertension	Barry M. Brenner
Angiotensin-converting enzyme inhibitors and angiotensin receptor blockers reduce glomerular pressure, slowing renal disease progression	Barry M. Brenner
Glomerular hypertension leads to the final common path of progressive renal diseases	Barry M. Brenner
Discovery, isolation, and description of kidney ion transporters	Stephen C. Hebert
Genetic cause of focal segmental glomerulosclerosis identified	Martin R. Pollak
Discovery, characterization of KIM-1 molecule, a sensitive and specific marker for kidney injury	Joseph V. Bonventre

Neurology	
Pathogenesis of Alzheimer disease includes amyloid β-protein and the enzyme presenilin. The "Aβ or amyloid hypothesis" has led to worldwide research. Tau is found in neurofibrillary tangles	Dennis J. Selkoe
Role of α-synuclein established normally and in genesis of Parkinson disease, Lewy body dementia, other disorders	Dennis J. Selkoe
Neurosurgery	
Description of anatomy, pathology, surgery, secondary effects, and prognosis of intracranial tumors	Harvey W. Cushing
Obstetrics and Gynecology	
Discovery, characterization, site of synthesis, and biological effects of human placental lactogen	John B. Josimovich
Description of the syndrome of hypofibrinogenemia and clotting in pregnancy, its natural history, and identity with disseminated intravascular coagulation	Duncan E. Reid
Discovery and characterization of antigen CA-125, a widely used tumor marker	Robert C. Bast, Robert C. Knapp
Culture of human embryos, created from ova fertilized in vitro	Arthur T. Hertig, John C. Rock
Orthopedics	
Skin fibroblasts become chondrocytes in 3-dimensional culture. Genes regulated by chondrocyte-demineralized bone interaction identified	Julianne Glowacki
Vitamin D deficiency exists in patients with osteoporotic fractures	Julianne Glowacki
Bone marrow cells synthesize activated vitamin D; it transforms marrow cells to bone-forming osteoblasts. Vitamin D metabolism may be essential for bone homeostasis	Julianne Glowacki
Orthopedists designed and participated in evaluation of many artificial total knee replacements	Richard D. Scott, Clement B. Sledge, Thomas S.Thornhill, etc.
Autologous chondrocyte implantation	Thomas Minas
Establishment of Cartilage Repair Center for treatment of damaged arthritic cartilage	Andreas H. Gomoll, Thomas Minas, Timothy Bryant
Primary Care	
Studies focusing on patient safety, including adverse drug events: Up to 28% are preventable; most occur at medication ordering, most often in medical ICUs	David W. Bates, Laura A. Petersen
Computerized order entry reduces nonintercepted medication errors 50%	David W. Bates, Lucian L. Leape
25% of outpatients had an adverse drug event; 20% were preventable	Tejal K. Gandi, David W. Bates
Bar code technology and electronic medication administration reduce adverse drug events by 51%	Eric G. Poon, William W. Churchill, David W. Bates, Anthony D. Whittemore
Pulmonary and Critical Care Medicine	
Albuterol is an effective therapy of asthma	Elliot Israel, Michael E. Wechsler
Proteases contribute to the pathogenesis of obstructive lung disease	Scott T. Weiss, Edwin K. Silverman, Dawn L. Demeo
Lung mesenchymal stem cells repair emphysematous tissue injury	Shivraj S. Tyagi, Edward P. Ingenito

Stem cells demonstrated in human lung tissue	Piero Anversa, Mark A.Perrella, Joseph Loscalzo
Carbon monoxide protects against experimental sepsis and inhibits TLR4-driven inflammation	Rebecca M. Baron, Augustine M. K. Choi, Stefan W. Ryter
Radiation Oncology	
First linear accelerator-based radiosurgery	Ken W. Winston, Jay S. Loeffler
First dedicated total body irradiation machine	Peter M. Mauch
Image-guided brachytherapy for prostate, gynecological cancers	Akila N. Viswanathan
Radiation therapy of Hodgkin lymphoma optimized to maximize cure, minimize toxicity	Andrea K. Ng, Peter M. Mauch
Breast-conserving therapy	Jay R. Harris
Delineation of clinical risk groups on which prostate cancer management is based	Anthony V. D'Amico
Sleep Medicine	
The anterior hypothalamus is responsible for timing of sleep	John F. Fulton, Percival S. Bailey
Description of Pickwickian Syndrome, which popularized sleep apnea	C. Sidney Burwell
Human circadian pacemaker has an intrinsic period of ~24 hrs, and can be reset by light	Charles A. Czeisler, Richard E. Kronauer, Joseph M. Ronda
Urology	
A rat model of human rectal carcinoma after inserting ureters into the rectum identified nitrosamines from fecal bacteria as the causative agent	Ruben F. Gittes, Glenn D. Steele, Jr.
Genes causing benign prostate hypertrophy identified in a transgenic mouse model	Jerome P. Richie, Philip Leder

THE BIOMEDICAL RESEARCH INSTITUTE: A BLUEPRINT FOR THE FUTURE OF RESEARCH

Jacqueline Slavik and Barbara E. Bierer

The Brigham and Women's Hospital has a long history of unique and prolific research contributions, all largely attributable to the entrepreneurial energies of individual investigators. To Gary Gottlieb, the former president of the Brigham, the changing nature of research, coupled with increasing demands for infrastructure, resources, and space, all necessitated a new approach to its organization, governance, and support. In 2002, Gottlieb assembled a group of senior Brigham physicians, scientists, and hospital leaders to define the future of the hospital's research enterprise. This strategic planning committee, after considering both novel opportunities for basic, translational, clinical, and interdisciplinary research and the challenges confronting the research enterprise, recommended the formation of an integrated research institute. In 2005, the Brigham and Women's Hospital Biomedical Research Institute (BRI) was formalized. Its mission is to accelerate the pace of scientific discovery by fostering groundbreaking, interdepartmental, and interdisciplinary research within its research community and to provide a clear voice both within and outside the hospital for all Brigham researchers.

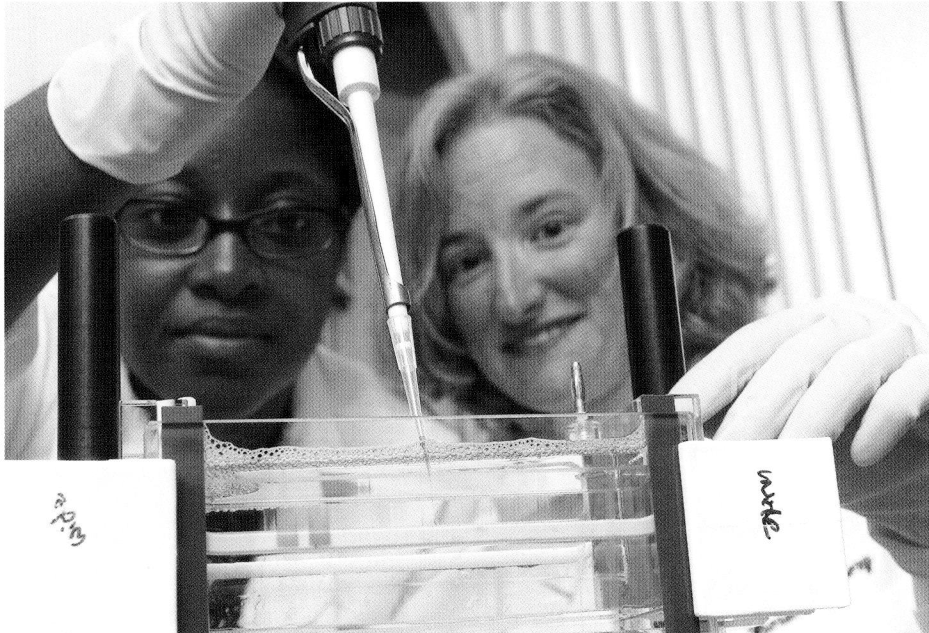

FIGURE 3-3 Yolonda Colson, Director of the Women's Lung Cancer Program (right) watches postdoc Kendra Taylor (left) loading cell lysates onto a gel prior to electrophoresis in order to identify unique cell proteins involved in the modulation of the immune system and stem cell behavior.

The BRI initially established eight research centers to foster collaborative research initiatives. A ninth center, the Patient-Centered Comparative Effectiveness Research Center, was added recently. Five research centers relate directly to the Brigham's five centers of clinical excellence (cancer, cardiovascular, neurosciences, orthopedic and arthritis, women's health).

The research centers couple the hospital's clinical focus and research strengths to both create a more expansive, inclusive research climate and strengthen the conduct of translational research. By developing successful models for collaboration, the centers also foster the BRI's local and national identity, facilitate peer-reviewed program and center grant funding, define areas of excellence for philanthropic

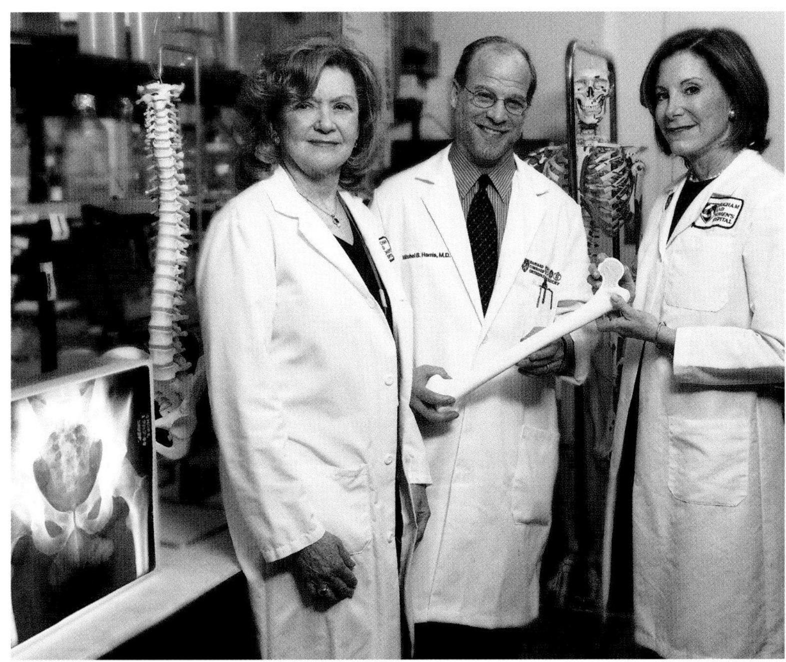

FIGURE 3-4 Left to right: Julie Glowacki, Director of the Skeletal Biology Program in the Department of Orthopedic Surgery; Mitchell Harris, Chief, Orthopedic Trauma Service; and Merle LeBoff, Director of the Skeletal Health and Osteoporosis Center and Bone Density Unit.

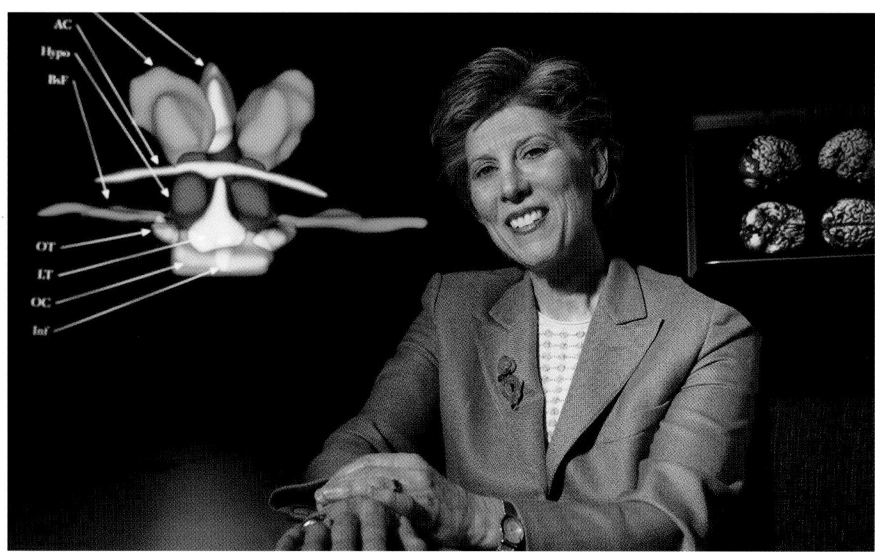

FIGURE 3-5 Jill Goldstein, Director of Research at the Connors Center for Women's Health and Gender Biology and Director of Research on Gender Neurobiology and Women's Mental Health in the Department of Psychiatry.

fundraising, and describe organized opportunities for industry collaborations. In addition, five resource- and technology-based programs provide tools for centers. Collectively, this infrastructure allows diverse clinicians and scientists to communicate more effectively, collaborate more easily, and respond nimbly to opportunities and challenges as they arise.

The BRI is governed by an executive and a Research Oversight Committee ("the ROC"), which foster transparency and accountability in decision making and planning new strategic initiatives. The Executive Committee includes an appointed director, co-director, and past-director, each serving two-year terms, plus the executive director and senior vice-president for research. The ROC, which is composed of the Executive Committee and many other appointees, has formulated five strategic operational themes: shared mechanisms of disease, personalized medicine, targeted therapeutics (including regenerative medicine and stem cells), comparative effectiveness, and health disparities. These strategic themes guide the BRI's activities, including interdisciplinary workshops, funding opportunities, and communication/educational offerings.

The BRI has undertaken exceptional funding initiatives. The Fund to Sustain Research Excellence (supported by the BRI, hospital leadership, and the Department of Medicine), which has provided $50,000 grants to more than sixty investigators while they await grant support from the National Institutes of Health, has had a great impact, both in terms of return on investment (awardees have brought in more than $58 million in funding) and in engendering a sense of support in the research community. Research Excellence Awards have been given to innovative investigators (junior researchers) since 2008 at the bi-annual research poster session and, since 2012, at the annual Research Day, at which research across the hospital is celebrated in a highly visible fashion. A "microgrant" program, initiated in 2012, provides $750-2,000 rapidly for acute needs for short-term funding. The BRI also funds or grants awards annually for junior faculty career development ($30,000/year), travel ($500) for junior faculty and trainees, collaborative projects (generally $50,000-100,000), and novel research (generally $50,000). The *OurGenes, OurHealth, OurCommunity* study, discussed elsewhere in this volume, was initiated and funded by the BRI. The first BRIght Futures Fund Prize ($100,000), awarded at Research Day in November 2012, was established by philanthropy to support novel research.

The BRI has sponsored many interdisciplinary research workshops to enable investigators across the Research Centers to learn about one another's research, connect with potential collaborators, and discover scientific resources. Topics have included diverse problems such as aging, space research, obesity, vitamin D, cancer immunology, novel imaging techniques, inflammation, and technology and innovation. The BRI sponsors other events to enrich the research community, including leadership retreats and scientific poster sessions. The biggest event is the annual Research Day, to celebrate Brigham research and encourage conversations on dissemination of research progress, education, stakeholder engagement, collaboration, and funding. The BRI and the Brigham Office for Research Careers in the Center for Faculty Development and Diversity also co-host a monthly career development series.

The BRI also serves as a voice, often via online communication, for the research community with respect to hospital and legislative policies and other issues. It has developed several online communication initiatives for this purpose. The Research Connection Email and LIVE Lunch Series provides researchers with weekly event and announcement information from the Research Administration, the Center for Clinical Investigation, and the Center for Faculty Development and Diversity's Office for Research Careers. The Brigham's "Find a Researcher" online directory of faculty research profiles helps scientists to both locate like-minded individuals and make Brigham science more accessible to the public, including other scientists. The BRI Web Development Service assists researchers who want a presence on the Brigham public web site. The BRIght Ideas campaign encourages investigators to share their research, awards, honors, and grants with the Communications office. Researchers use the Eureka! Innovation Intake Form to disclose novel inventions and other phenomena.

In summary, nearly 1,000 investigators drive the research mission at the Brigham, and 3,700 individuals are involved in the research enterprise. In any year, this institution trains about 800 postdoctoral fellows, many of whom are international scholars. In 2012, its clinical, basic, and translational research portfolio was valued at approximately $560 million. The BRI supports all investigators and all research and strives to support a culture of innovation and discovery. At BWH, science is part of the cure.

THE HARVARD–MASSACHUSETTS INSTITUTE OF TECHNOLOGY DIVISION OF HEALTH SCIENCES AND TECHNOLOGY

Joseph V. Bonventre

The Peter Bent Brigham Hospital and its evolutionary structure, the Brigham and Women's Hospital, have played a major role in the 1970 founding and development of the Harvard–Massachusetts Institute of Technology (MIT) Division of Health Sciences and Technology (HST). The HST Program is a successful experiment in cross-institutional collaboration and for many years was the only formal widely encompassing academic collaborative program of the two universities. In subsequent years, as its scope expanded, it was elevated from status as a program to a cross-institutional division.

In 1968, Robert H. Ebert, dean of Harvard Medical School (HMS), and Jerome B. Weisner, then provost of MIT, appointed Irving M. London, the first chair of medicine at the new Albert Einstein School of Medicine, as a consultant to aid in planning a program joining the two institutions. After working on this for two years, one of which was a sabbatical that he spent in Cambridge, he accepted the directorship of the HST program. He received a professorship at both MIT and Harvard, the latter at HMS, and an appointment to the Department of Medicine at the Brigham. London instilled in the HST his basic philosophies—an intense commitment to the integration of both medical and university education and interdisciplinary biomedical research, education, and medical practice. Thirty-eight years after he founded the HST, London was honored by having one of the five HMS societies (formerly the HST Society), to which

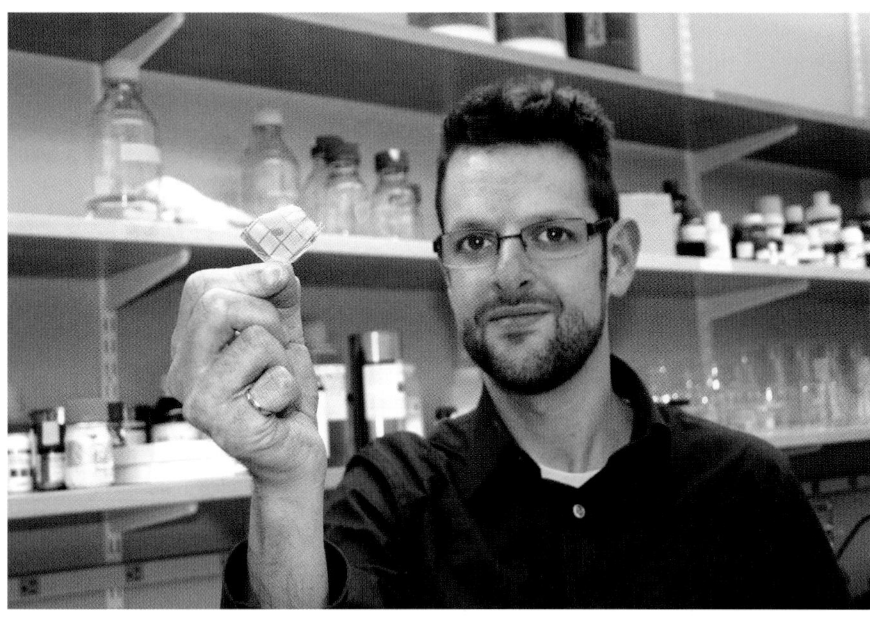

FIGURE 3-6 HST faculty member Jeff Karp, Co-Director at the Center for Regenerative Therapeutics at BWH.

all HST medical students belong, renamed the Irving M. London Society.

George W. Thorn, physician-in-chief at the Brigham during the planning and early years of the HST, supported and raised funds for the society. The curriculum for the first and second years of this program, and its instructors, were unique. For example, with the encouragement of Eugene Braunwald, the chair of medicine after Thorn, Brigham gastroenterologist Martin C. Carey, assumed the leadership of the HST Gastroenterology Pathophysiology course. He has maintained this position for 40 years, ceding it in 2011 to Chinweike Ukomadu, a Brigham hepatologist. Most HST students were also enrolled in an MD/PhD program, and many of these individuals obtained their PhD in a laboratory at the Brigham.

From the very founding of the HST, the Brigham became the site of the Introduction to Clinical Medicine (ICM) course for all HST students during the second half of their second year of medicals school, before entering their medical clerkships. This was also unique, combining quantitative sciences, fledgling engineering sciences, and fundamental aspects of medicine into an exciting introduction to physical diagnosis and history taking. The Brigham ICM faculty, led for many years by W. Hallowell Churchill, Jr., were also enthusiastic, as they ventured into this new world of medicine that the Brigham successfully taught in an innovative way. When HST students needed a re-entry ICM course because of years in a laboratory fulfilling their PhD requirements, the Brigham was the site for this refresher experience.

Over the years there were many HST graduates of the MD and PhD programs who were residents and fellows at the Brigham. These included such luminaries as physician Mark B. McClellan, who obtained his PhD in medical economics and public policy, was appointed commissioner of the national Food and Drug Administration (2002-2004), and became the director of the Centers for Medicare/Medicaid Services (2004-2006). Most HST students considered all Brigham residencies as strong programs that promoted their career development as physician-scientists. Among the many HST graduate physician-scientists who began these careers at the Brigham and are devoted to and leaders in clinical and investigative medicine are Dennis W. Choi, Alan S. Verkman, Barbara L. Smith, Jonathan M. Teich, Jeffrey D. Macklis, Stephen K. Burley, Barry P. Sleckman, Michael A. Weiss, and Vamsi K. Mootha.

In 2002, Joseph V. Bonventre, one of the two directors of the HST since 1997, moved to the Brigham from the Massachusetts General Hospital to lead the Renal Division. At his request, the current physician-in-chief,

Victor J. Dzau, committed resources to establish a Division of Biomedical Engineering, one of the very few divisions of biomedical engineering within a department of medicine in an academic teaching hospital. The faculty hired by Bonventre, at first four young individuals who had recently completed their PhDs or postdoctoral training, grew the program successfully and rapidly. In 2012, over 100 trainees participated in this program at the Brigham's Landsdowne Laboratories of Biomedical Engineering in Cambridge. The program attracts many MIT students as well as students and postdoctoral fellows worldwide and has added greatly to the culture of innovation at the Brigham. The activities and goals follow the tradition of the Brigham, which has been the site of groundbreaking translational technologies such as the development of the Brigham-Kolff dialysis machine, which ultimately led to the first successful therapeutic kidney transplantation worldwide at the Brigham in 1954.

David E. Cohen, now the Robert H. Ebert Professor of Medicine and Health Sciences and Technology at HMS, was recruited in 2007 to assume the co-directorship of the HST after Bonventre. A graduate of the internal medicine residency program and a former fellow in gastroenterology at the Brigham, he also heads its Section of Hepatology. Cohen has continued the strong association between what is arguably the most distinguished training ground for academic scientists in medical schools nationwide. Its productivity, through the essential relationship with the Brigham, an outstanding hospital with a long tradition of training physician-scientists, is superlative.

II. RESEARCH IN CARDIOVASCULAR MEDICINE

CARDIOVASCULAR MEDICINE AT THE BRIGHAM

Peter Libby

At the founding of the Peter Bent Brigham Hospital in 1913, the specialty of cardiovascular medicine was nonexistent. Nonetheless, Henry A. Christian, the first chief of medicine, was keenly interested in cardiovascular disease and was a careful thinker about the relationship between infections and cardiovascular disease. The specialty of cardiovascular medicine coalesced around the time that clinical electrocardiography debuted. Recording and interpreting an electrocardiogram required specialized expertise beyond the ken of traditionally trained internists. The advent of this new technology, and thus of new possibilities of understanding cardiovascular physiology and disease, created the specialty of cardiovascular medicine. Boston played an important role in this evolution.

At Massachusetts General Hospital (MGH), Paul Dudley White was a standard-bearer of this new specialty. The work of Samuel A. Levine at the Brigham was similarly instrumental. Levine was a keen observer, an authoritative clinician, and a masterful educator. Independently of the work of James B. Herrick in Chicago, Levine linked thrombosis to acute myocardial infarction in the 1920s. Levine also focused on valvular heart disease, resulting especially from rheumatic fever, which was epidemic in Boston's Mission Hill neighborhood during the first half of the twentieth century. His clinical expertise and focus on the physical examination, coupled with the emerging technologies of fluoroscopy and electrocardiography and the clinical problems of valvular heart disease encountered at the adjacent House of the Good Samaritan, provided stimuli for the first surgical approaches to valvular heart disease, pioneered by Elliott C. Cutler and later by Dwight Harken. Levine's collective wisdom about cardiovascular medicine, its practice, its integration with electrocardiography, and the role of the cardiologist as a consultant to other internists was crystallized in 1936 in his classic textbook, *Clinical Heart Disease*. The book, in its many editions, was a key nucleating factor for the entire specialty of cardiology.

Advances in cardiology proliferated during the mid-twentieth century. The Brigham's Lewis Dexter contributed immeasurably to the clinical application of invasive hemodynamic investigation, including cardiac catheterization. Dexter trained at Boston City Hospital with Soma Weiss (1938-1940) and in Argentina with Bernardo Houssay (1940-1941), developing his interest and expertise in vascular medicine. Returning to work with Weiss, now at the Brigham, he focused on renal hypertension, for which he attempted to catheterize human renal veins. One day, in late 1944, he ventured north of the diaphragm and to his terror saw his catheter penetrate the heart and enter the lung field. He asked the patient how he was faring, certain that he had punctured the right heart. According to Dexter, the patient replied, "I'm doing fine, Doc, but you don't look so good." Dexter, as he told it, did a little reading that night and realized that he had not perforated the heart but had crossed the pulmonic valve and entered the pulmonary arterial tree. At lunch in the doctors' dining room, Dexter told Harvard Medical School Dean C. Sidney Burwell of his exploit (or perhaps misadventure), and Burwell replied: "Young man, congenital heart disease is yours."

Dexter then redirected his research from the kidney to the heart and pulmonary circulation. He made the seminal observation, now employed routinely, that the pulmonary arterial wedge pressure—measuring capillary pressure in the lesser circulation—reflected the filling pressures on the left side of the heart, because it correlated with the left ventricular end-diastolic pressure. He described the pathophysiology of the pulmonary circulation in mitral stenosis, noting the greatly increased pulmonary resistance in some patients. Under his leadership, the hemodynamic and radiographic signs of pulmonary embolism were developed. Exploiting his approach to the outflow tract of the right ventricle, Dexter also simplified the measurement of variables from mixed venous blood that are required by the Fick principle for the calculation of cardiac output, an essential statistic of cardiac catheterization.

Dexter also supervised the research of one of his brilliant fellows, Richard Gorlin, to quantitate the degree of mitral stenosis. This was a major effort, because the availability of surgical approaches to alleviate valvular stenosis mandated accurate quantitation of the valve area. On a holiday at home, Gorlin mentioned this quandary to his father, a hydraulic engineer. His father suggested that the problem was a trivial one and, as the legend holds, wrote the equations on a dinner napkin. Gorlin returned to the Brigham with a method for calculating valve area, using data obtained at cardiac catheterization, which he quickly applied and validated. When he prepared to publish this finding, Dexter withdrew his name from coauthorship to ensure that Gorlin would receive the major credit for this innovation. The paper was ultimately published in 1951 with Richard Gorlin as the first author and his father as the senior author. After completing his fellowship with Dexter, who had exploited right heart catheterization, Gorlin turned his attention to the left side of the heart and coronary circulation. The left ventriculogram, standardization of the right anterior oblique view, and the terms *dyskinesis*, *akinesis*, and *hypokinesis*—used daily in cardiology worldwide—evolved from Gorlin's early work in left heart catheterization. Gorlin also helped to champion selective coronary arteriography and was an early student of myocardial metabolism using coronary sinus blood sampling. In their years together at the Brigham, through 1974, Dexter and Gorlin trained a generation of hemodynamically inclined cardiologists who populated many programs worldwide.

In 1972, Eugene Braunwald became the Hersey Professor of the Theory and Practice of Physic at the Brigham. At this time, the institution supported semi-autonomous groups focused on cardiovascular medicine: the Dexter group, the Gorlin group, the Coronary Care Unit and Arrhythmia Research group under the inspiring direction of Levine's successor, Bernard Lown, the cardiorenal unit under John P. Merrill, the research unit on myocardial metabolism and

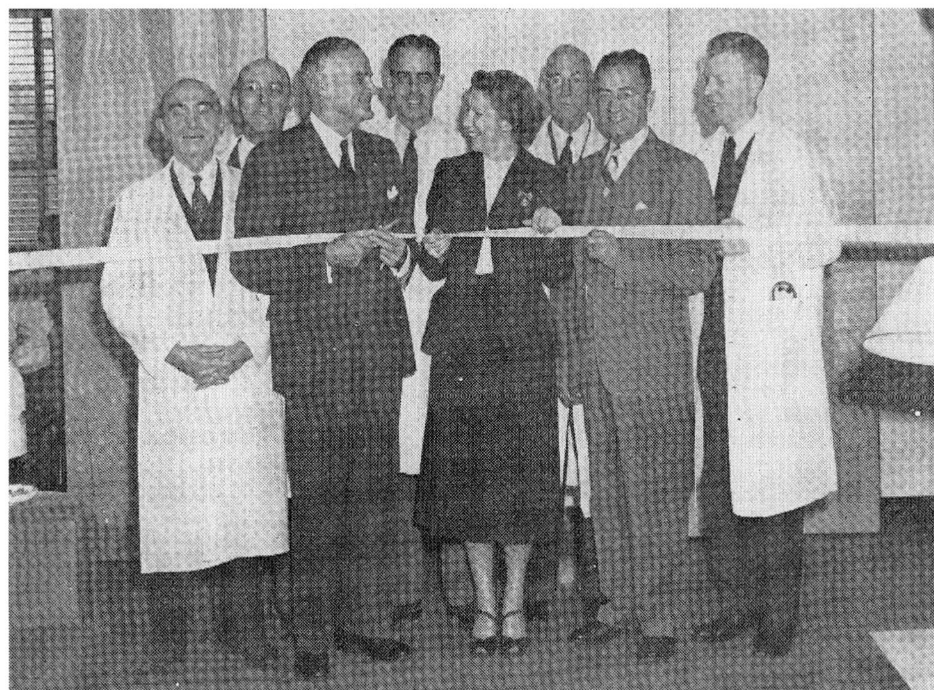

FIGURE 3-7 Opening of the Cardiovascular Unit in 1952. Left to right, front row: Samuel Levine, Robert Cutler, Claire McBride, N.A. Wilhelm, George Thorn. Back row: Harold Levine, Lewis Dexter, T. Sidney Burwell. Photo from the April 1952 *Brigham Bulletin.*

mechanics under Edmund Sonnenblick, Braunwald's former associate at the National Institutes of Health (NIH), and a research unit on the control of circulation in conscious animals, directed by Braunwald and Stephen Vatner. Braunwald shaped these groups into a cohesive whole over the first decade of his leadership. He recruited Thomas W. Smith, who had developed an immunoassay for digoxin at the MGH, to lead his amalgamated cardiovascular enterprise. Braunwald's energy, insight, and brilliance boosted cardiovascular medicine at the Brigham to new heights over many decades. The combined strength and breadth of this assemblage catapulted the Brigham cardiovascular training program to the top ranks and led to continued expansion of the basic research programs addressing myocardial disease.

Braunwald's personal research was focused on myocardial infarct (MI) size limitation. An MI was thought to lead irreversibly to loss of heart muscle until Braunwald, while at the NIH, was able to salvage ischemic myocardium by various maneuvers. He recruited Marc A. Pfeffer and his wife Janice M. Pfeffer, then just finishing their graduate and postdoctoral studies in Oklahoma, to establish a laboratory to focus on the pathophysiology of MI in animal models. Together, the Pfeffers and Braunwald discovered the phenomenon of myocardial remodeling after MI. They showed that interruption of the renin-angiotensin system could rescue the oxygen-starved heart from the hitherto inevitable ballooning of the heart's left ventricle after coronary artery occlusion. Marc Pfeffer then led a pilot study at the Brigham to show the feasibility of translating this laboratory finding to patients. He and Braunwald conceived and executed a large-scale clinical trial (the SAVE study) that has changed medical practice worldwide and saved countless lives, applying the principle that grew out of the experimental laboratory to large patient populations. The SAVE study provided the basis for the nearly routine treatment of survivors of MI with agents that block the renin-angiotensin system, such as angiotensin-converting enzyme (ACE) inhibitors.

This coalescence of interest in modifying the fate of the myocardium jeopardized by limited blood flow spurred Braunwald to found the Thrombolysis In Myocardial Infarction (TIMI) Study Group. Once again, a technical advance was key—the introduction of "clot busting" drugs enabled Braunwald to test the hypothesis that heart function could be rescued by breaking up the blood clot that Levine had implicated in heart attacks in the early part of the twentieth century. Braunwald's TIMI Study Group has completed some fifty trials, with many more currently in progress. The findings in many of these trials have contributed pivotally to clinical practice worldwide, decreasing the age-adjusted morality from ischemic heart disease, and have been incorporated into national guidelines.

While at the NIH, Braunwald pioneered the physiologic characterization of patients with hypertrophic cardiomyopathy. Smith and Braunwald recruited Christine E. Seidman to the Brigham with her husband, Jonathan G. Seidman, to apply the then-emerging advances in molecular genetics to cardiovascular disease. The Seidmans tackled heritable forms of hypertrophic cardiomyopathy and were the first to demonstrate mutations in the heart's contractile proteins, the machinery of the heart's pump, in this family of diseases. The Seidman laboratory has continued to lead and receive international recognition for many advances in applying molecular genetics and Mendelian principles to the unraveling of myocardial diseases.

Although alterations in the heart muscle itself cause many forms of cardiovascular disease, the myocardium itself is an innocent bystander in the majority of heart problems. Indeed, it is the events in the blood vessels—the circulation of blood, carrying oxygen and nutrients, to the hungry muscle of the heart—that cause heart attacks and many strokes. In the latter part of the 1970s, the time was ripe for launching studies on blood vessels and their relation to heart function. Ramzi S. Cotran came to lead the Department of Pathology at the Brigham, and his vision led to the establishment of one of the world's first Centers of Excellence in Vascular Biology. The work of Cotran, his early recruit Michael A. Gimbrone, and others in the Department of Pathology have led to a flourishing understanding of endothelial biology. Gimbrone, who has detailed his department's work on vascular biology in a separate essay in this publication, introduced the concept of endothelial "activation" that led to the first steps in the formation of atherosclerotic lesions—the fatty plaques that cause most heart attacks. He has also carried out molecular studies of the regulation of endothelial biology, and these have led to the concept of "atheroprotection," providing insights into why atherosclerotic fatty plaques occur only in certain areas of the circulation whereas risk factors such as high blood pressure or high cholesterol bathe the entire arterial bed.

These stories, although not all-inclusive, provide iconic illustrations of the advances in cardiovascular medicine that have emerged from the Brigham. Of the factors that led to this success, the first is partnership. Many of the advances took flight through multidisciplinary collaboration. Although the initial discoveries may have emerged from one laboratory, their expansion and clinical application required individuals with different expertise to come together. The Brigham has provided an incubator to foster such interactions and favored the rapid application to the clinic of advances in laboratory science. A second factor is the constant striving for innovation. Dissatisfaction with the status quo, coupled with patients' needs and new technological or scientific opportunities, has driven the Brigham's success in the cardiovascular arena. Another hallmark of successful cardiovascular research is the melding of clinical and laboratory work. Clinical investigators have brought patient materials and large populations to basic investigators, providing grist for their mills. Clinical investigators, in turn, have shown great alacrity to apply the advances in the laboratory to their populations. These principles have provided a foundation for much of the Brigham's success over its first century in advancing cardiovascular medicine.

VASCULAR BIOLOGY AT THE BRIGHAM: A BEACON FOR THE FIELD

Michael A. Gimbrone, Jr.

Serious diseases of the cardiovascular system—thrombosis and embolism, and atherosclerosis (and its complications, heart attack and stroke), which account for a majority of the morbidity and mortality in industrialized societies—are manifestations of dysfunction of blood vessels. Our knowledge of the cellular and molecular mechanisms underlying the function of blood vessels in health and disease comprises an expanding biomedical science: vascular biology. A synergistic congruence of people and ideas and a conducive environment in the Department of Pathology at the Brigham and Women's Hospital have contributed importantly, over almost four decades, to the emergence of this field worldwide.

In 1974, when Ramzi S. Cotran became the new chief of pathology at the Peter Bent Brigham Hospital, he brought with him a special interest in the mechanisms of acute and chronic inflammation and, in particular, the role of vascular permeability in those processes. His preferred scientific instrument was the electron microscope, which he skillfully exploited to visualize the pores and junctions of the gossamer-thin endothelial lining of small blood vessels. Using molecular probes, he traced the pathways of plasma leakage and the migration of white blood cells from the circulating blood across the endothelium into surrounding tissues—classic hallmarks of the inflammatory process. At this time very little was known about the vital functions of the endothelium—the single-cell-thick, continuous lining of the chambers of the heart and the body's blood vessels. Indeed, endothelium was viewed as "biological cellophane" that comprised a nonreactive container for blood.

This simplistic concept was challenged by a simple maneuver—the culture of human endothelial cells in sufficient quantities to enable the study of their metabolic activities. Experiments could now be designed to probe their *active* cellular and molecular interactions in various disease contexts. Utilizing discarded umbilical cords obtained from Boston Lying-In Hospital while a postdoctoral fellow with Judah Folkman and Ramzi Cotran, I devised a simple but reliable method for cannulating the umbilical vein, enzymatically harvesting a relatively pure sample of the endothelial lining, and culturing endothelial cells. In 1975, having further perfected vascular endothelial (and smooth muscle) cell culture while at the National Cancer Institute, I rejoined the Department of Pathology at the Brigham, first as a resident in training and subsequently as a junior faculty member. Working in a small laboratory cubicle, I began a systematic study of the vital properties of human endothelial cells. Over the next year, our laboratory hosted visits by scores of investigators who were anxious to adopt this new approach to enable their own studies. The publication of our early characterization of cultured human endothelial cells remains one of the most quoted papers in the vascular biology field.

In collaboration with Jordan S. Pober, another junior faculty member in pathology, we demonstrated that human endothelial cells stimulated with human gamma interferon expressed class II major histocompatibility antigens and thus were capable of presenting antigens to reactive T-lymphocytes. We observed that this property contributes to the vascular-directed immunological injury associated with solid organ transplantation and to delayed graft failure. Michael P. Bevilaqua, a pathology resident and postdoctoral fellow, then showed that the proinflammatory cytokine, interleukin-1, could induce human endothelial cells to express on their surfaces a novel adhesion molecule that mediated the attachment and transmigration of blood leukocytes. The molecule, endothelial-leukocyte adhesion molecule-1 (ELAM-1), was purified, its gene cloned, and a new family of cell–cell adhesion molecules important in inflammation and immunity thus was revealed—the Selectins. This discovery established the ability of the vascular endothelial lining to *inducibly* express, under stimulation by proinflammatory cytokines or bacterial products (such as endotoxins), cell surface adhesion receptors that would selectively attract circulating blood leukocyte to sites of inflammation. The endothelium is thus an *active*, rather than *passive*, player in the body's response to injury. Another postdoctoral fellow, Myron I. Cybulsky, extended this model of "endothelial activation" to the pathogenesis of atherosclerosis by the discovery of the "Athero-ELAM" (now called vascular cell adhesion molecule 1 [VCAM-1])—an inducible adhesion molecule that selectively recruits mononuclear leukocytes, from the circulation at sites of developing atherosclerotic lesions, to become cholesterol-laden "foam cells." VCAM-1 is now recognized as the earliest detectible molecular change in the vascular lining of "pro-atherogenic" areas and is being exploited as both a molecular target for the noninvasive imaging of early lesions and a surrogate marker of the progression/regression of atherosclerosis in clinical trial populations. Other members of the Vascular Research Division in the Department of Pathology, particularly the late Tucker Collins (who subsequently became the chair of pathology at Boston Children's Hospital), dissected the mechanisms of endothelial activation at the level of signaling pathways and nuclear transcription factors, pointing the way to discoveries and then to anti-inflammatory therapies. Other investigators in the group, notably Francis W. Luscinskas, Tanya Mayadas, Richard N. Mitchell, David Milestone, and Andrew H. Lichtman, have extended these studies in various areas of endothelial pathobiology.

Another area of investigation, initiated in the late 1970s at the Brigham and still actively pursued worldwide, assesses the effects of hemodynamic forces generated by blood flow on the vascular endothelium. It had long been appreciated that the earliest lesions of atherosclerosis tend to develop "predilected sites," defined by vascular branches and curvatures, presumably as the result of vascular injury induced by turbulent blood flow. In collaboration with Professor C. Forbes Dewey at the Massachusetts Institute of Technology, our laboratory recreated, for the first time in vitro, the fluid mechanical environment that is a constant fact of life for the endothelial cells that line blood vessels in vivo. We subjected cultured human endothelial cells to defined laminar and turbulent fluid shear stresses characteristic of different vascular geometries and examined the cell responses, from the intact cell to the whole genome. The results were astounding! Endothelial cells appear to *differentially* sense and respond to a spectrum of biomechanical forces and to adapt to these stimuli via the induction of genetic programs that are "atherosclerotic-prone" or "atherosclerotic-resistant." This has led to the identification of "master-switches" that may be promising targets for pharmacological interventions to prevent cardiovascular disease. These studies, involving multiple members of the Vascular Research Division of the Department of Pathology (Peter F. Davies, James N. Topper, and Guillermo Garcia-Cardena), in collaboration with colleagues at MIT, represent a vibrant example of the power of interdisciplinary collaboration in the biological sciences.

This spirit of interdisciplinary collaboration has also led to the formation of the Center for Excellence in Vascular Biology at the Brigham, which has joined the considerable expertise of members of the Cardiovascular Division of the Department of Medicine under Peter Libby with colleagues in the Vascular Research Division of the Department of Pathology. The basic, clinical, and translational research promise of this center was recognized by its selection, by Harvard Medical School Dean Joseph P. Martin, to be an anchor-program its New Research Building in which other internationally recognized vascular biologists conduct their work, including Joseph Loscalzo, the current chair of the Department of Medicine.

In June 2011, at a scientific celebration marking four decades of Vascular Biology at the Brigham and Women's Hospital, the lasting impact of our many initiatives was addressed by a "connectivity map," illustrating the seeding of dozens of epicenters for Vascular Biology worldwide that are currently led by prominent investigators. These individuals trace their scientific origins to the Brigham—truly a beacon for the field![9]

BIOGRAPHY

EVA J. NEER, 1937-2000

Christine E. Seidman, David E. Clapham, and Thomas M. Michel

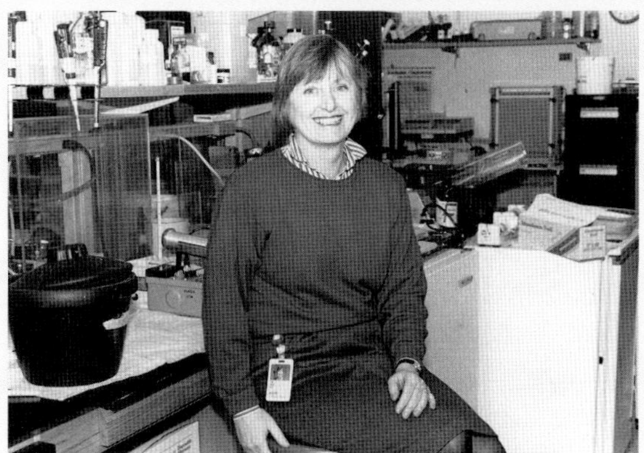

FIGURE 3-8 Eva Neer, 1992.

Eva Neer energized the campuses of Harvard College, Harvard Medical School, and the Brigham and Women's Hospital (BWH) for nearly twenty-five years with her enthusiasm for science and art, research, and teaching. Neer's family fled Nazi-occupied Warsaw in 1939, immigrating first to Brazil and then to New York. She graduated from Barnard College and then from Columbia University's College of Physicians and Surgeons in 1963. She pursued postgraduate research in Guido Guidotti's biochemistry laboratory at Harvard, studying signaling proteins and the universal second messenger cyclic adenosine monophosphate (AMP). Although her work had no obvious relationship to cardiac disease, Thomas W. Smith, the newly appointed chief of the Cardiovascular Division at the BWH, recruited her to the division, recognizing the major contributions that this brilliant biochemist with an interest in cell signaling would make to this discipline.

At the BWH, Neer spent her scientific career on the identification of proteins that modulate signals between cell surface receptors and adenylate cyclase (the enzyme that synthesizes cyclic AMP) and other effector proteins. Her rigorous biochemical approach led to the discovery of a new class of important modulator proteins in the brain. She also worked on this class of signaling proteins in cardiac cells by identifying their genes, producing transgenic mice with modified signaling protein function, and posing essential questions about the mechanisms of heart failure. Her early, seminal observations led to considerable scientific controversy, during which Neer displayed the highest principles of scientific integrity. Ultimately, her discoveries were totally accepted by the scientific world. Neer's scientific creativity and energy led to her becoming a tenured professor of medicine and biochemistry after only fourteen years, the second woman to achieve this rank at Harvard Medical School. Former Dean Daniel C. Tosteson noted that "she broke the glass ceiling for advancement in science faculties." She received a merit research award from the National Institutes of Health, election to the American Academy of Arts and Sciences and the National Academy of Science, and many other awards.

Neer's legacy reached beyond the research bench. She was a superb teacher of Harvard College undergraduates, Harvard Medical students, and her own research fellows. She nurtured their professional careers and personal lives. An important mentor for both women and men, Neer demonstrated what achievements were possible by pursuing science passionately, regardless of gender. She served on the Senior Advisory Committee on Women of Partners Healthcare, which defined problems impeding the advancement of women in academic medicine and constructed mechanisms for change.

Renowned for her intellect and achievements in science and teaching, Eva Neer taught her students to work hard, to care passionately about science and each other, and always to see the world with joy. Her passion, wit, and intellectual achievements live on to inspire all those colleagues and friends fortunate to have been touched by her.

THE TIMI STUDY GROUP

Eugene Braunwald

Reperfusion therapy to limit infarct size in patients with acute myocardial infarction is a concept based on animal experiments that I have carried out between 1968 and 1972. In 1984, the Thrombolysis in Myocardial Infarction (TIMI) Study Group, which was funded by the National Heart, Lung and Blood Institute, was established at the Brigham and Women's Hospital. The first TIMI trial compared two drugs for fibrinolysis—streptokinase, a well-established drug, and tissue plasminogen activator (t-PA), one of the first products of the then-new recombinant technique, developed by the earliest biotech company. The initial TIMI trial network consisted of thirteen hospitals. In addition to describing the superiority of t-PA in treating patients with acute myocardial infarctions (heart attacks), the first TIMI trial also showed that, however achieved, an infarct-related artery opened early in the course of acute myocardial infarction was associated with a better clinical outcome and longer survival than a closed vessel. This led to the "Early Open Artery Theory" of treatment of acute myocardial infarction, which has been central to most recent advances in care of patients with acute myocardial infarction.

Over the ensuing years (from 1984-2012), the TIMI Study Group grew into an academic research organization, beginning with six and growing to more than 200 employees. TIMI is administratively within the Cardiovascular Division of the Department of Medicine at the Brigham and Women's Hospital. The physicians who have led numerous trials are members of the Brigham's TIMI Study Group and its Department of Medicine.

The TIMI trials group has led and coordinated trials involving as many as 1,200 hospitals in forty-six countries on all six continents. In 2012, TIMI completed its fiftieth study, a drug trial of 26,449 patients that was led by David A. Morrow. TIMI began the REVEAL clinical trial in 2011, a study of heart attack prevention involving 30,000 patients, led by Christopher P. Cannon, and Stephen D. Wiviott. In addition to acute myocardial infarction, TIMI has studied patients with unstable angina (chest pain resulting from partially occluded coronary arteries) and chronic coronary artery disease. In 2010, TIMI began it first large trial, led by physicians Deepak Bhatt and Benjamin Sirica, in patients with diabetes mellitus.

Among the fifty completed TIMI trials, Christopher Cannon has demonstrated the clinical benefit of

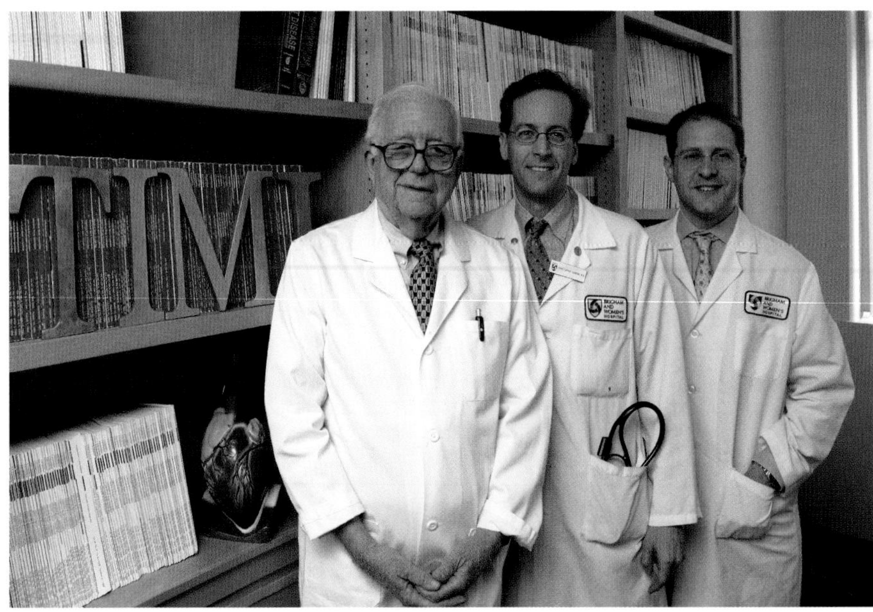

FIGURE 3-9 Three generations of TIMI investigators: Eugene Braunwald, Christopher Cannon, and Stephen Wiviott.

an early aggressive interventional strategy in the care of patients with unstable angina and related conditions, which are responsible for more than 1 million hospital admissions in the United States each year. Elliott M. Antman has also demonstrated the value of a special anticoagulant—low-molecular-weight heparin—in the treatment of these conditions.

One of the TIMI Group's most notable achievements is the *secondary* prevention in patients who have experienced an acute coronary syndrome (acute myocardial infarction and unstable angina). Christopher Cannon has demonstrated an improved clinical outcome with intensive lowering of low-density lipoprotein cholesterol—so-called "bad" cholesterol—by means of a high dose of a powerful statin drug. This finding has contributed to a sea change in the care of the many patients with this condition. In a trial that has just been completed, TIMI investigators, led by Jessica L. Mega, have demonstrated a reduction in mortality when rivaroxaban, a novel anticoagulant, was added to the postdischarge regimen of these patients.

Marc S. Sabatine has also studied drugs that reduce blood clotting by inhibiting platelets in patients with an acute myocardial infarction. Jessica Mega and Marc Sabatine have found that a common genetic variant interferes with the formation of the active form of clopidogrel, a platelet inhibitor. Patients with this variant require upward dose adjustment.

Led by David Morrow, TIMI has been studying novel biomarkers—chemicals released by damaged heart muscle—that play a critical role in selecting the proper treatment of patients with both acute and chronic coronary artery disease. In addition, the TIMI Study Group has used its databases of more than a quarter of a million subjects to understand the natural history of all varieties of coronary artery disease, which, despite many advances, still remains the most important cause of death in the developed world.

TIMI has been active in the education of Brigham medical residents and cardiology fellows. Indeed, almost all of the faculty members of TIMI became interested in cardiovascular clinical trials while spending elective rotations with the group. They have risen through the academic ranks at Harvard Medical School. Several have received national recognition for their work at TIMI.

I led the TIMI Study Group from its inception through 2010. Marc Sabatine has been its director since January 2011.

BIOGRAPHY

THOMAS W. SMITH, 1936-1997

Eugene Braunwald

In 1976, Thomas W. Smith took on an embryonic Cardiovascular Division at the Brigham and Women's Hospital (BWH), with seven faculty members, and led it to an astounding total of seventy staff (and 102 research and clinical fellows) at the time of his untimely death in 1997. He was a consummate leader of the Cardiovascular Division, encouraging staff to excel in the three limbs of the academic tripod—research, clinical care, and teaching. Personally, he was internationally known for his seminal work on myocardial cell biology and pharmacology. His research on digitalis included the development of a radioimmunoassay for measuring its concentration in blood and of a therapeutic antibody fragment ("Digibind") for the treatment of digitalis overdose, both in universal use.

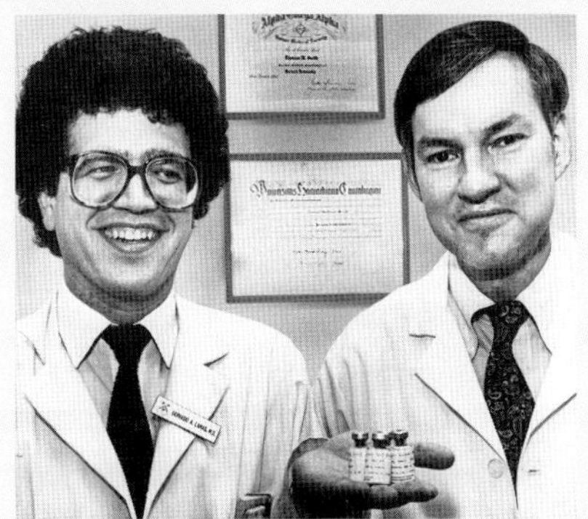

FIGURE 3-10 Gervasio A. Lamas and Thomas W. Smith, holding vials of the antibody for digitalis (digoxin) developed by Smith, 1982.

He led a large double-blind clinical trial of digitalis, which showed definitively that it reduced the composite end point of rate of hospitalization and death from congestive heart failure, thus resolving a centuries-old debate concerning the real efficacy of this drug.

For twenty-one years, Tom Smith provided exemplary leadership to the Cardiovascular Division at the BWH. He was a devoted mentor and friend of his faculty and trainees and put his personal stamp of excellence on all of the division's activities. He was a respected, consummate clinician who set the highest standards for clinical care. In addition to his own research, he encouraged the research of others in the division. Under his leadership, the Cardiovascular Division developed respected research programs in almost every area of cardiovascular science. Under his leadership, Brigham clinical cardiology also grew to be recognized nationally, including its training programs that are considered among the strongest worldwide. Tom played vital roles at Harvard Medical School, from which he graduated in 1965. He was active in the American Heart Association, from which he received its most prestigious awards: the distinguished Achievement Award and the James B. Herrick Award.

The many leaders in academic cardiology whose training Tom Smith nurtured are one of his most enduring legacies. His integrity; the high standards that he set for himself, his colleagues, and his trainees; and his enormous sense of responsibility to Harvard University, the Brigham, and its Cardiovascular Division serve as an inspiration to his friends, colleagues, and academic cardiologists worldwide.

III. RESEARCH IN KIDNEY MEDICINE

TISSUE TRANSPLANTATION

Nicholas L. Tilney

Against the advice of many of his surgical colleagues, Joseph E. Murray, a young plastic surgeon at the Peter Bent Brigham Hospital, transplanted a kidney between identical twins on December 23, 1954. Urologist Hartwell Harrison removed the normal organ from the donor, Ronald Herrick. In an adjacent operating room, Murray then placed it in the lower abdomen of the recipient, Richard Herrick, using a technique he had perfected in dogs and in human cadavers. The revascularized graft functioned

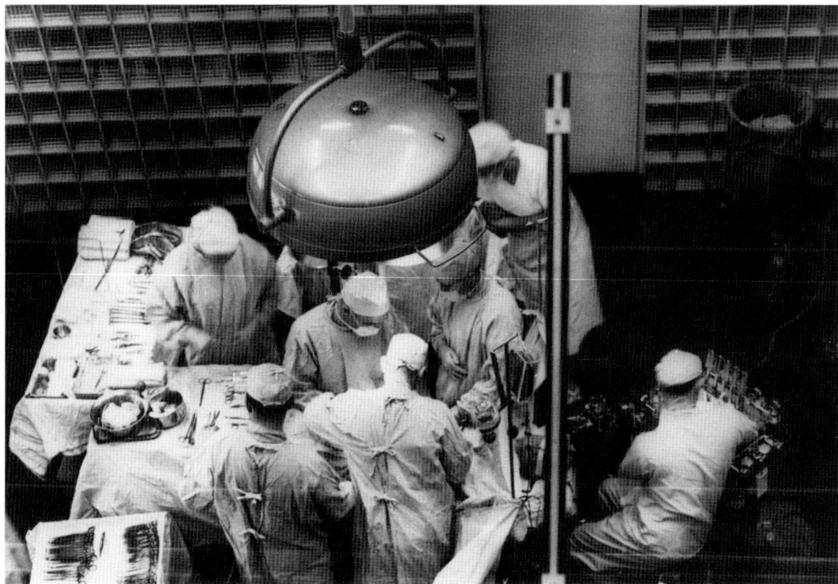

FIGURE 3-11 World's first successful kidney transplant, performed by Joseph Murray at the Peter Bent Brigham Hospital in 1954.

immediately, transforming the moribund patient to complete normalcy. Herrick married his nurse, fathered two children, and lived a full life for the next decade. The unprecedented success of this and subsequent identical-twin transplants performed at the 300-bed Peter Bent Brigham Hospital and then in a few other centers in the United States, Canada, and Europe over the ensuing years provided an unprecedented approach to the treatment of human disease. For his efforts, Murray received the Nobel Prize in Medicine in 1990, one of seven surgeons so honored.

Two reasons may explain this departure from accepted practice. First, kidney disease had been an enduring interest of the first Brigham physicians-in-chief, Henry Christian and Soma Weiss. Weiss's successor, George Thorn, studied hypertension, disorders of the kidney, and disorders of the adrenal gland. He also recognized, based on the experience with crush injuries in London during the Blitz, that some renal failure was reversible if water and electrolyte abnormalities of the afflicted patients could be normalized until the organs recovered. Second, this small institution had always supported research creativity. At that moment in history, the leadership, prescience, and enthusiasm of the departmental chiefs, Thorn and Francis D. Moore, created the correct environment for such a venture.

Although of vastly different personalities, the clinicians involved worked consistently as a cohesive team toward a common goal. Nephrologist John Merrill was an original thinker who supported radical new treatments for renal failure, both the unique entity of hemodialysis and the potential for substituting a functioning organ from a healthy donor for a failed organ. Hartwell Harrison was a patriarchal and empathetic figure, acutely aware of the responsibility of taking tissue from healthy patients, a startling digression of the ancient tenet to "do no harm." Joseph Murray combined his broad philosophical basis for pursuing transplantation with knowledge of its nascent biology and practical means of solving clinical conundrums. Pathologist Gustave Dammin was a careful scholar whose painstaking examination of relevant animal and human material provided objective scientific background for the whole enterprise.

The concept of organ substitution was not without precedent. Several European surgeons in the nineteenth and early twentieth centuries had attempted transplantation in animals and man, but ultimately understood that grafts placed in genetically dissimilar hosts were inevitably destroyed by a mysterious host process. Perhaps of more immediate relevance to the Brigham clinicians, however, were two events that occurred in the hospital in 1947. The first was introduction of the novel entity of hemodialysis. George Thorn had invited a Dutchman, Willem Kolff, to describe the dialysis machine that he invented during the Nazi occupation to treat individuals dying of renal failure. Thorn enlisted Merrill and Francis Moore recruited surgeon-engineer Carl W. Walter to work with Kolff to improve the device. The resultant Brigham-Kolff kidney, the prototype for all future dialysis machines, resides in the Smithsonian Institution.

At about the same time, a patient presented with renal shutdown after a septic abortion. Thorn suggested that if a normal kidney could be inserted transiently into her bloodstream, it might function long enough to allow her own organs to recover. Three surgeons connected the vessels of a kidney to those at the elbow of the patient. The revascularized graft immediately began to produce urine. Within three days, her own kidneys had recovered. Charles Hufnagel, a young staff surgeon and later chair at Georgetown, led the team; he was already creating a synthetic ball valve to be placed in the arterial circulation to normalize aortic insufficiency. Ernst Landsteiner, a urology resident and grandson of the physician who discovered the blood groups, was the second member. David Hume, another surgical resident, became an important principal in the new field as chair of surgery at Virginia Commonwealth University.

Stimulated by the surprising success of a kidney transplant in Chicago in 1950 and pressured by patients with renal failure seeking help at the Brigham, Hume transplanted unrelated kidneys into nine patients as a final and desperate recourse. All died of acute failure of the graft (in retrospect, irreversible rejection) except the final patient, whose new organ, by serendipity, supported him for nearly six months. This experience, coupled with similar data from a team in Paris, encouraged further attempts. Total body X-radiation was the only means then available to reduce the increasingly appreciated immune barrier. Both the Brigham and the French doctors transplanted twenty X-radiated patients. All died but two; these—one American, one French—not only survived but lived normally for many years.

It was clear, unfortunately, that the systemic effects of X-radiation were uncontrollable and usually lethal. Excitement built in 1959 when two hematologists from Tufts found that an anticancer drug, 6-mercaptopurine (6-MP), could reduce antibody titers in rabbits. In 1960, a young English surgeon, Roy Calne, joined Murray's laboratory group as a research fellow, trying chemical derivatives of 6-MP in canine recipients. It became quickly apparent that one of the agents, azathioprine, could increase graft survival significantly. Some clinical success followed, improved by the addition of corticosteroids, a combination that remained the linchpin of immunosuppression for nearly two decades.

In the late 1970s, Calne, now at Cambridge University, introduced a new and more effective substance, cyclosporin A. Clinician-scientists at the Brigham, Charles Carpenter, Terry Strom, and Nicholas Tilney, were the first to use the drug in North America. As its popularity grew throughout the world, transplantation became increasingly routine.

The role of the Surgical Research Laboratory at Harvard Medical School was of utmost importance in the evolution of transplantation. Initiated by Harvey Cushing, the first Brigham surgeon-in-chief, in 1912, the laboratory boasted an impressive list of innovations during its ninety-year existence. Although Hume had initially transplanted a few kidneys in dogs, Murray's subsequent experiments in this laboratory opened the emerging field. His initial studies showing that a kidney moved from one site in the body to another could function normally removed prior doubts and encouraged the transplants between identical twins. Results confirming that total-body X-radiation increased survival of skin grafts in mice and rabbits hastened initial clinical trials. The relative success of azathioprine in canine recipients solidified the new concept of chemical immunosuppression. Tilney and colleagues later explored the mechanisms of cyclosporin A and defined many of the intricacies of acute and chronic rejection.

The first heart transplant was carried out in 1967 in South Africa. Energized by this feat, cardiac surgeons worldwide undertook similar procedures. The result was so disastrous that professional bodies called a moratorium on heart transplantation. A few

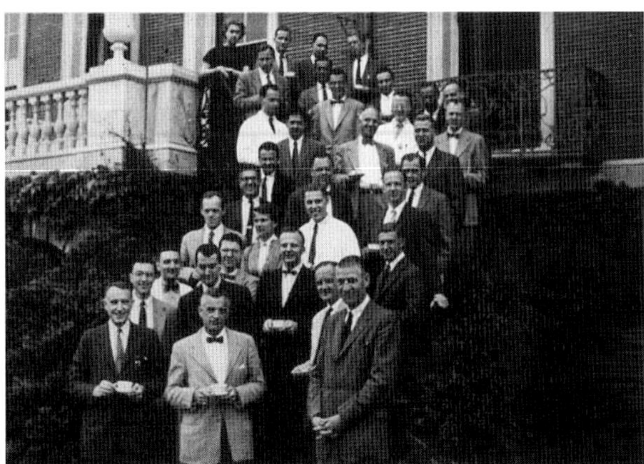

FIGURE 3-12 PBBH Transplant Staff, 1962.

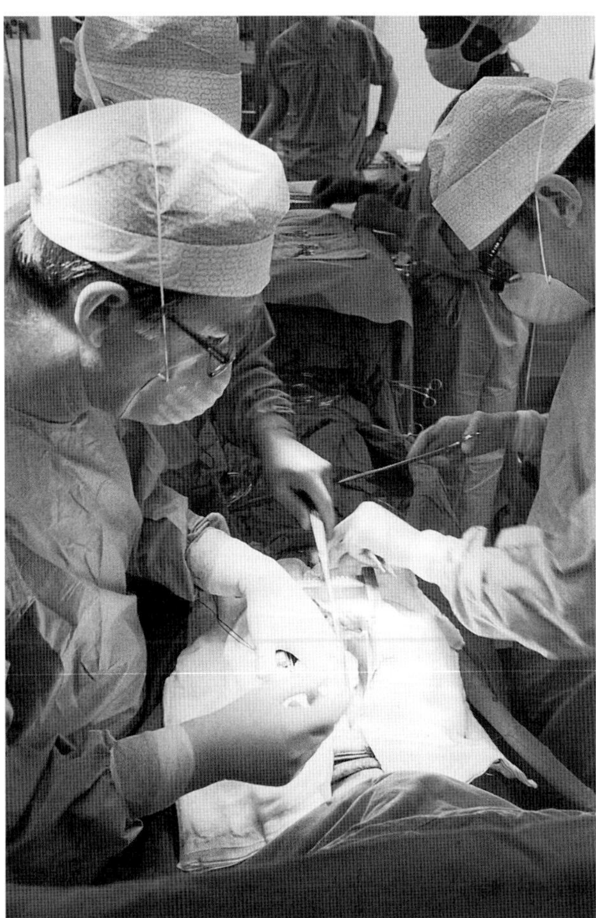

FIGURE 3-13 The first heart transplant in the Northeast, performed by John Collins and Lawrence Cohn in February 1984.

pioneers persisted in the laboratory, however, improving techniques and slowly accruing better results. The additional availability of cyclosporin A improved the possibilities further. Based on encouraging data from the laboratory and the clinic, John Collins and Lawrence Cohn successfully carried out the first heart transplant in New England in February 1984. Clinical results slowly increased to the point that heart transplantation has become a treatment of patients with intractable heart failure. Hundreds have been carried out at the Brigham and thousands over the world.

In similar fashion, transplantation of the lung became possible. A few centers led the way. Early in 1990, David Sugarbaker and his Brigham team performed the first single lung transplant in Massachusetts and then the first double lung transplant in New England (the second in the United States). Results have improved during the past decade with a spectrum of ongoing innovations. This engraftment of the lung, a notoriously difficult organ, has become a reality.

The transplantation of "composite" grafts, primarily hands and faces, has been a recent exciting departure. Pioneering work first came in 1998 from Jean-Michel Dubernard in Lyon, France, one of Murray's original research fellows and an enduring clinician-scientist in the field. A group of Brigham surgeons, led by Bohdan Pohamac, then carried out the first partial face transplant in New England in April 2009, the second in the United States and the seventh in the world. In recent months, this multidisciplinary group has also transplanted successfully several full face transplants (the world experience is currently four), a unique advance in a new field.

Beginning at the Brigham in the 1950s, organ and tissue transplantation has evolved throughout the world from a futile dream to a reality that has benefited tens of thousands of patients. Indeed, transplantation has been described as one of the most important scientific advances of the twentieth century. And the advances continue.[10]

BIOGRAPHY

JOSEPH E. MURRAY, 1919-2012

Peter V. Tishler

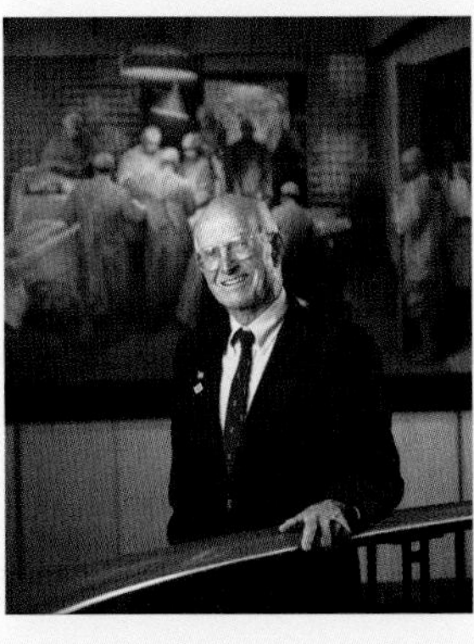

FIGURE 3-14 Joseph Murray.

Joe was an amazing person. He was a totally incisive, reflective, thoughtful person, characteristics that had been with him virtually all his life. He had limitless enthusiasm for his life (past, present, and future), for the factors that influenced his career and human path, and for the individuals whom he met. One walked away from him fully energized, ready to forget troubles and smile at everyone and everything. This ethic is certainly reflected in his autobiography, *Surgery of the Soul,* and in many other publications.[11]

Joe combined laboratory research with clinical practice of surgery for the majority of his professional life. Transplantation and plastic surgery became his interests when he cared for Charles Woods during his service in an army hospital in World War II. He pursued the science of transplantation by working in the Surgical Research Laboratory at the Harvard Medical School, where he had illustrious lab neighbors (e.g., Bernard Davis, Arthur Hertig, Clifford Barger), influential mentors (George Thorn, Francis D. Moore, David Hume), important associates (Sidney Farber, George Hitchings, Gertrude Elion, Paul Tessier), and incredible personal determination to master transplantation. His transplantation of a kidney from Ronald Herrick to his identical twin brother Richard Herrick, in 1954, with the team of John Merrill, J. Hartwell Harrison, and Gustave Dammin, was unique and remains legendary. Published in the *Journal of the American Medical Association* in 1956, this account was republished in 1984 as a *JAMA* landmark article.[12,13] His friend Thomas Starzl commented, "If gold medals and prizes were awarded to institutions instead of individuals, the Peter Bent Brigham

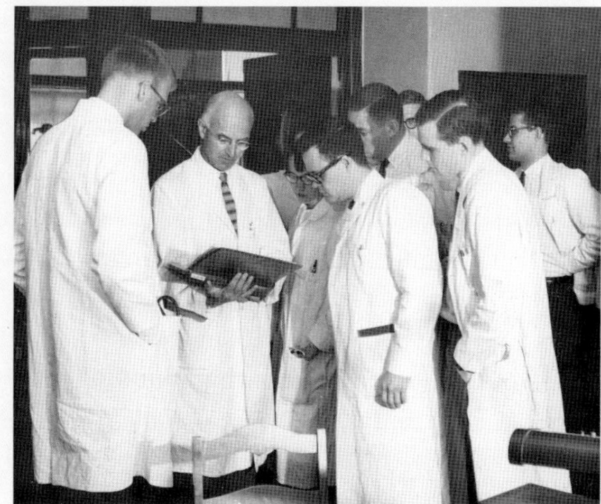

FIGURE 3-15 Joseph Murray on rounds.

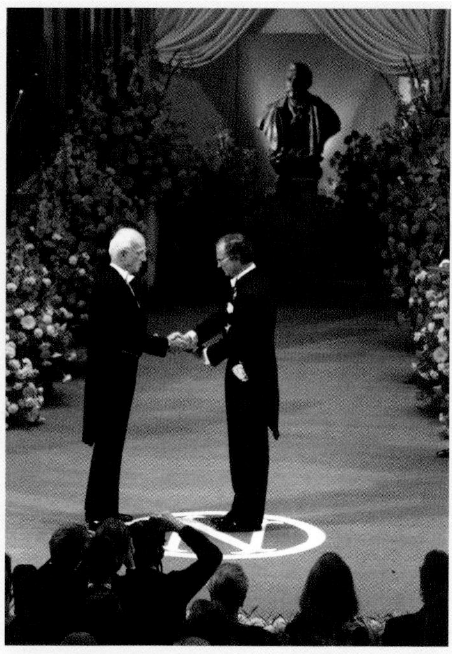

FIGURE 3-16 Joseph Murray receiving the Nobel Prize for Medicine or Physiology in 1990.

Hospital of 30 years ago would have qualified." Starzl specifically credited George Thorn and Francis D. Moore "with the qualities of leadership, creativity, courage and unselfishness that made the Peter Bent Brigham Hospital the unique world resource."[14] Murray subsequently led the team that performed the first successful sibling transplant in 1959 and the first successful transplant from a cadaver in 1962, opening the door for worldwide transplantation. In the process, Murray trained others in transplantation biology, including Sir Roy Calne of the UK, Max Dubernard of France (who performed the first successful facial transplant), and Nathan Couch (also on the Brigham staff for many years).

Simultaneously and subsequently, from 1951 to 1986, Joe Murray practiced as a plastic surgeon at the Brigham. He was also chief of plastic surgery at the Children's Hospital Medical Center (1972-1985), creating one of the first national centers for craniofacial reconstructive surgery. He created the first plastic surgery residency in Boston, involving the Brigham and Children's Hospital, in 1964. He donated his surgical expertise in India (1962), correcting hand and facial deformities in patients with leprosy, and in Iran (1974), where he cared for patients and trained Iranian surgeons and nurses, with a number of his colleagues.

Joe Murray's appraisal of the Brigham was that it is always an institution of inquiry, concern for and helpfulness to individuals, and preoccupation with humanity in general. He credited virtually all individuals with whom he interacted, during his lives in transplantation and plastic surgery, as noble individuals who had the best interests of humanity at heart. He lauded Francis D. Moore as a leader who recognized the core values of the Brigham, encouraging and facilitating its prospering as an institution of patient care, teaching, and research. He labeled the Brigham as a university, providing a locus in which people "come together to think freely and explore ideas and possibilities." This remains true today, in Joe's experience and observation, and is ever more reflected in the increased size of the institution. Joe predicted more of the same for the Brigham's future. The hospital's wonderful qualities will remain.

Francis D. Moore has stated "Only when the care of the sick is carried out with wisdom and mercy, will teaching and research also thrive."[15] Joe Murray personified this during his long tenure at the Brigham, and this governs his philosophies today. He often quoted the saying, "Service to society is the rent we pay for living on this planet." Members of his large family, some of whom are physicians, have inherited the same devotion to humanity. This all bodes well for humanity and the Brigham.

SOCIOLOGY AND RENEE FOX'S *EXPERIMENT PERILOUS*

Ann Conway

> *"The overall atmosphere of the hospital in which these pioneering days of dialysis, kidney transplantation, and nephrology took place was effervescent with enthusiasm, daring, optimism, determination, and tenacity."*
>
> —Renee Fox[16]

Many facets of today's call for health system reform center on a renewed awareness of the patient as a social being, a perception that has never been absent at the Brigham. An intriguing aspect of Peter Bent Brigham Hospital (PBBH) history in the 1950s and 1960s was its embrace of sociological inquiry. Physician-in-Chief George Thorn was a great champion of this viewpoint, noting the need to link medicine to what went on outside the hospital walls, particularly in regard to the increasing population of aging patients. Thorn even called for the establishment of a fourth branch of medicine, which would concentrate on social science in addition to the clinical realm.

The PBBH also embraced sociological investigation, examining the hospital operations from a social system perspective. This was the focus of sociologist Renee Fox's book *Experiment Perilous: Physicians and Patients Facing the Unknown*, a participant observation study of Ward F-second, the metabolic research unit.[17] Over the course of 1951-1954, Fox studied the desperately ill patients, physicians and other professionals who treated them, and the culture of the hospital in general. Her aim was to understand how physicians and patients alike coped with the ethical and emotional dilemmas and coping strategies presented by innovation—in this case, the pioneering development of organ transplantation.

Fox, now professor emeritus at the University of Pennsylvania, listed a number of new innovations for which success or failure was possible:

> *The major clinical research in which the physicians of the Metabolic Group were engaged, in collaboration with the Surgery and Renal Groups of the hospital, were associated with assaying what were at that time the newly synthesized steroids of ACTH cortisone, and compound F, which they were administering to patients with a wide variety of metabolic, endocrinological, cardiovascular, renal, and malignant diseases; investigating the effects of total bilateral adrenalectomy on patients with advanced hypertensive vascular disease, reactivated cancer of the prostate, and hyperadrenalism; studying the body water and electrolyte problems of patients who had undergone a mitral valvuloplasty that was then a pioneering form of cardiac surgery; and conducting studies on patients in acute renal failure, and with chronic renal disease, particularly end-stage glomerular nephritis who underwent hemodialysis on a stainless steel, rotating-drum artificial kidney built by the hospital.*[18]

Fox and medical historian Judith Swazey underscored the Brigham's "courage to fail" value system in undertaking these efforts for patients, noting in its culture a "death is the enemy" orientation" and "a relentless refusal to accept limits."[19] These themes are evidenced in the extraordinary PBBH 1954 kidney transplant from one identical twin to another, carried out by Joseph Murray and John Merrill, which led to a series of other milestone transplants and Brigham's legacy of success in this area. As Fox notes: "The continuous engagement of the Brigham during the 1950s and 1960s in striving to advance dialysis and renal transplantation through laboratory experimentation and clinical trials was shaped and energized by the social system of the hospital and its regnant value system."[20]

In many aspects, Fox's pioneering study of innovations at the Brigham was a precursor of other ethnographic observations, such as Charles Bosk's 1979 *Forgive and Remember: Managing Medical Failure,* which examined the ways in which surgical staff handle ethics and technical mistakes. Jerome Groopman's 2007 book, *How Doctors Think,* noted Fox's study of decision-making processes and their psychosocial effects. Her work was one of the major impetuses for a huge body of writing on medical practice and decision making, including subsequent work by Groopman, Jay Katz, JudyAnn Bigby, Donald Berwick, Atul Gawande, and many others.[21]

TRANSPLANTATION: THE EXPERIENCE OF BRIGHAM PATIENTS AND THEIR FAMILIES

Kristin DeJohn

The 1960s was a tumultuous decade for patients seeking kidney transplants. Joseph Murray, buoyed by the successful transplantation of a kidney between identical twins in 1954, knew the milestone would be only a footnote in history unless he could broaden transplantation to include nongenetic matches. Eventually, in 1959, he accomplished the first successful non–identical twin transplant between two brothers using X-radiation to suppress the immune system, but the dangerous protocol didn't work in another Brigham patient.

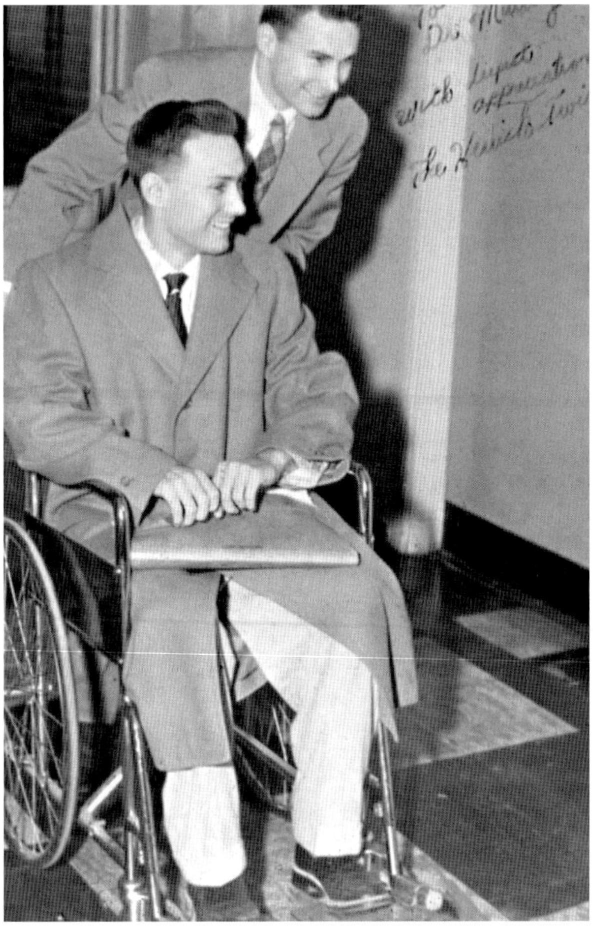

FIGURE 3-17 The Herrick brothers post-transplant, circa 1955.

The entrance of drugs to suppress the immune system offered new hope for patients. In 1962, Murray performed the first successful cadaver kidney transplant, using a derivative of the anticancer drug 6-mercaptopurine (azathioprine) and corticosteroids, which had the effect of suppressing the body's immune response. Still, the odds of survival were poor. "I arrived at the Brigham as a junior resident in 1964 and patients, who had no other options, were trying to stay alive, and we were trying to keep them alive,"

A HUMAN EXPERIMENT RESULTING IN TOLERANCE

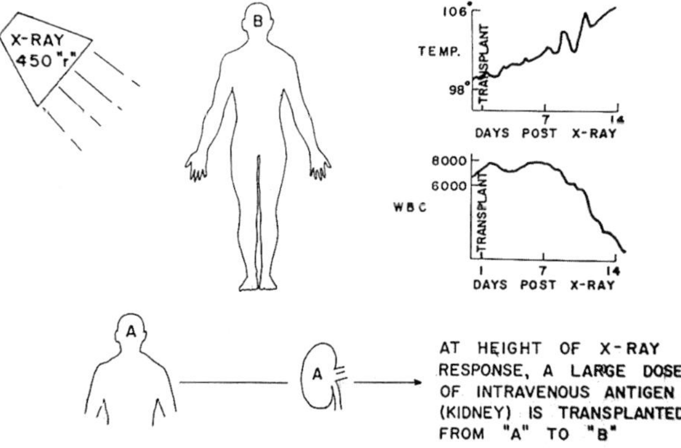

FIGURE 3-18 A Human Experiment Resulting in Tolerance, from the Riteris twins transplant, circa 1959.

recalls Nicholas Tilney, director of the Renal Transplant Program at the Peter Bent Brigham Hospital (and later the Brigham and Women's Hospital [BWH]) from 1976 to 1992, and author of *"Transplant: From Myth to Reality."* "Organ rejection remained an enormous problem, and the attempts to suppress the immune system involved very difficult drugs and protocols."

Despite this, families and patients desperate for any life-saving options flocked to the Brigham. "We all felt that we were part of an extraordinary mission," says Jodi Hartley, who had come to the Brigham in 1964 to support her brother. "My brother Stanley was 24 years old and had an incurable, hereditary disease that affected his kidneys, which he had been battling for years," she recalls. "He had been able to get his college degree, but over the next 6 months he had deteriorated, dialysis was no longer an option, and on New Year's Eve of 1963, he was at the end of his life." Fortunately, the family received some news. "The Brigham had been doing identical twin transplants, and that year, they were accepting parent-child cases," says Hartley. By the first week in January, the family made a rushed decision to test Hartley's mother to see if she was a match. "She was, so they performed the operation, and within 24 hours, Stan was sitting up and eating," notes Hartley. "It was a miracle. We were all ecstatic to watch his strength and health restored." Murray and colleagues, however, remained concerned. Stan's mother had been a carrier of the disease, and they had noticed the disease in the new kidney. Despite this, the new kidney remained functional for ten years. Gradually, the disease returned. But by then, Hartley's brother was able to receive a cadaver kidney, which gave him an additional ten years of life.

"Because of those surgeries, Stan was able to work a full time job, get married, have four children and live 20 years longer than we had expected," says Hartley. "My brother was on the tennis court after the second surgery when he stated, 'The difference between having had a transplant and being on dialysis is the difference between feeling like a real well person and not remembering you have kidney disease, and feeling ill. I'm back at work full time. I'm feeling like a normal, wonderful, healthy human being, and I can eat what

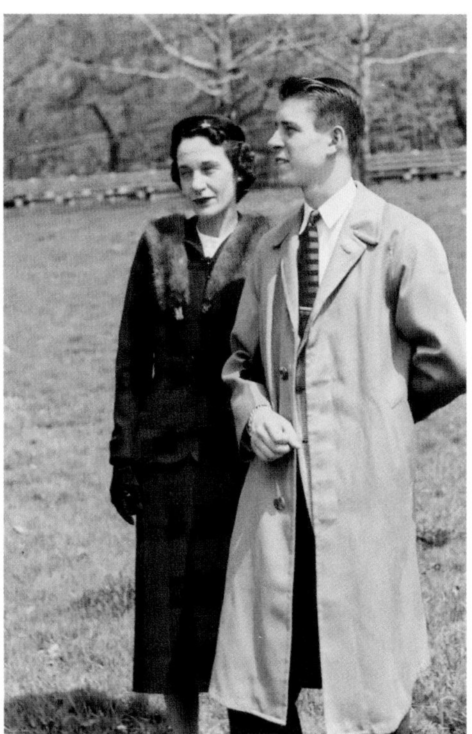

FIGURE 3-19 Stanley Williams and his mother Jessie Batson Williams, among the first mother-child kidney transplants in the world. Stanley Williams received his mother's kidney on January 8, 1964. The operation was performed by Joseph Murray.

I want instead of being on a restricted diet. I feel like a person who does not have an illness.'"

"When you had one case like Jodi Hartley's brother Stan, it was fantastic," recalls Tilney. "In the 60s, most patients did not survive. We were trying many approaches to dampen the immune response. Immunosupressive drugs were new and the drugs were toxic, so regimens were difficult and not exact. Other approaches included giving splenectomies or infecting patients with typhoid fever to trick their immune systems into accepting the new kidneys. It was pretty dire for many years." "They actually gave Stan typhoid fever, and I was told he was one of only two cases in which the approach worked, so he was very fortunate," says Hartley, whose family knew full well the extreme emotions patients and families faced. "My other brother, Jeffrey, who was 7 years younger than Stan, also had the same hereditary disease," says Hartley. "His progression was similar to Stan's; he had gone through numerous attempts to stay alive, including the radiation of his blood and removal of his spleen. By 1968, he was going downhill fast. I spent more than a week at the Brigham to see if I was a compatible match. I was, and on July 26, 1968, I donated my kidney. It seemed to be working fine, but Jeff did not survive the treatment regimen to suppress his immune system, and he died 8 weeks later."

The tenuous nature of transplantation during the 1960s made survival stories all the more inspiring for patients and their families. Jodi Hartley recalled a memorable event in the hours before her older brother Stan's surgery:

> *There had been five or six transplants that I knew of performed in 1963. Those patients who were well enough spent a lot of time at the hospital supporting each other. That evening of January 7th we were at the hospital all evening, visiting my mother, and then going over to the area where Stan was in holding prior to the surgery. We all were wide-eyed and terrified that night. Then a ruddy faced good-looking young man marched into the room and cheerfully said: "Hi!" He said he'd forgotten how hard the ice was; he'd been ice-skating with his daughter that afternoon. I thought: "Who let this lunatic in here? Doesn't he know Stan is very sick?" Then the man said: "Hi Stan, I'm Bob Canada!" We almost fainted, as he was one of the remarkable success stories we'd heard about. He had received a kidney from a parent, I believe, that prior summer. There are no words to describe what that moment did to all of us, including Stan. There WAS a life after being so close to death! Here was a gorgeous, healthy young man who had been ice-skating, and he'd had a transplant! It could all work!*

Although former transplant patients provided inspiration for those currently awaiting surgery, it was the daily support of family, friends, and staff that sustained many patients and their loved ones. During this period, families who had sought out the help of Murray as their last hope bonded due to a common sense of purpose. Hartley recalls the overarching sentiment at that time:

> *There was this feeling that we were part of something big. It was an amazing program. All the families knew each other. My parents bought and donated a tape recorder, and carried it back and forth for families who could not be together because loved ones were in isolation. Patients would come and stay in at the hospital for up to nine months. During that time, Dr. Murray was able to draw people together, and make this small group of people feel like they were part of a very, very extraordinary mission. They all felt it. And they all wanted to be a part of it.*
>
> *The whole environment was wonderful. Miracles were happening before our eyes. We had lived for six years knowing my brother Stan could not go any further in his life. There was nothing they could do for him. We all knew that it was only a matter of time. We give Joe Murray and all of them so much credit for allowing Stan to feel like a normal person. A great deal of love caring and interest sustained us all. And Joe was at the center of the wheel. He had the vision, the genius, skill, ability, and willingness to take the risk to make all this happen. And the nurses and other staff were so supportive. When I spent time in the hospital being tested to see if I was a match for my younger brother Jeff, we were trying to keep it quiet because we didn't want to raise his hopes if I wasn't a match. The doctors, nurses, all those bringing food and sweeping floors were part of the secret. As different people from the staff came by, they would give me news about Jeff. Everyone was very kind and very interested.*
>
> *Live kidney donation was still a very unusual situation. But through this period, Joe Murray created an atmosphere that helped us all. People were just so comfortable in his presence. Not only was he an excellent physician, but his personality was so caring; he was so interested in the families. You just felt really comfortable that you were in the right hands. And, he was so honest and understanding that you wanted to be involved. My parents both received several skin sample grafts on their arms for tissue matching of other possible transplant patients because they wanted to do anything they could to help.*

Colleagues credit Murray, who died November 26, 2012, at the age of ninety-three, for forging ahead and not giving up hope during a very dark time in transplantation history. "He was an incurable optimist," notes Tilney. "The glass was always half full with Joe. He caught onto an idea pushed by the Brigham leaders, and kept moving forward despite setbacks. And it's been a remarkable success story. It's been one of the most important advances of the 20th century. And he was very conscientious and kind to the patients; I can remember many times that someone would get sick or die and Joe would come in the middle of the night to talk to the patients or their families."

Murray would see increasing numbers of successful transplants and the gradual evolution of transplantation. By the 1970s and 1980s, new and better immunosuppressive regimens paved the way for the widespread transplantation of kidneys and other organs. Despite growing numbers of transplant patients coming through the doors of the Brigham, Murray maintained close contact with all his patients. "For Dr. Murray, staying in touch with patients was a life-long commitment," says Stefan G. Tullius, chief of Transplant Surgery at BWH and director of the Transplant Surgery Research Laboratory. "Dr. Murray had a story to tell about every patient, all close to him, and, not infrequently, he would fetch recent letters from his patients out of his many drawers and bookshelves." In 2010, Ronald Herrick, the man who had donated his kidney to his identical twin Richard in 1954 during the groundbreaking operation, died at the age of seventy-nine. Murray, his wife Bobby, and Tullius all attended the funeral in Maine. "It was very important to Dr. Murray that we were both there," adds Tullius. "I was there to show that the tradition of compassionate patient care continues at the Brigham. And, as Murray would have pointed out, the success of transplantation has rested on the shoulders of many. Nurses, support staff, and basic researchers made this possible. More than one million patients are estimated to have benefited from organ transplantation. Thus, all those who have made contributions have become heroes."

In 2011, Murray participated in the Brigham's celebration of the fiftieth anniversary of the kidney transplant he performed on the young Nightingale twins, who became the longest surviving donor and recipient, and returned to the Brigham to commemorate the anniversary of the 1960 transplant. "Both Johanna and Lana underwent procedures when they were 12 years old," marvels Tullius. "To be a donor at age 12, the young girls had to go through three courts

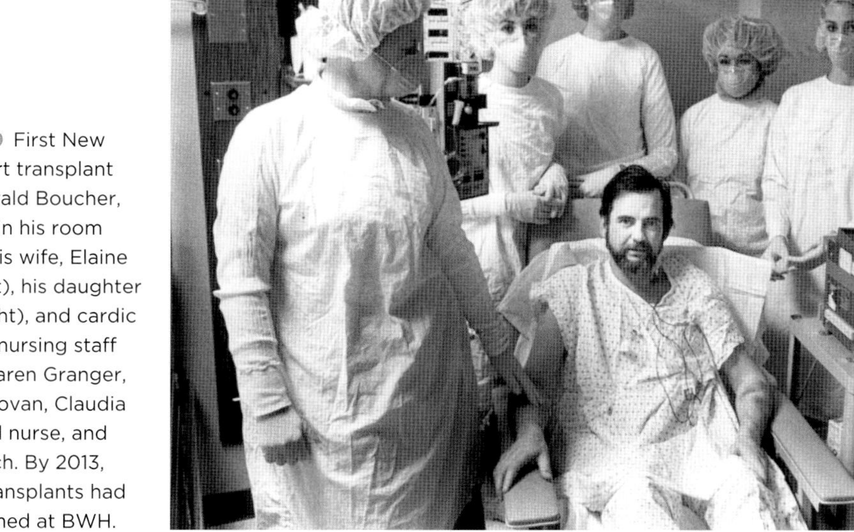

FIGURE 3-20 First New England heart transplant recipient Gerald Boucher, 43, is joined in his room at BWH by his wife, Elaine Boucher (left), his daughter Cindi (far right), and cardic surgery unit nursing staff (from left) Karen Granger, Barbara Donovan, Claudia Zirpolo, head nurse, and Barbara Hatch. By 2013, 600 heart transplants had been performed at BWH.

and the Supreme Judicial Court of Massachusetts to get permission."

The ethics surrounding transplantation did not deter Murray, who had received criticism before his first attempt to transplant. He was told it would never work; others brought up the ethical issues of operating on a healthy donor. "You don't worry about people's opinions if you have the proper motivation," said Joseph Murray, emeritus chief of Plastic Surgery at BWH. "We were just trying to help fellow humans."

More than five decades later, Murray again entered the ethics debate, this time on behalf of a young Brigham surgeon facing a similar challenge. In 2009, Bohdan Pomahac, now director of Plastic Surgery Transplantation at BWH, was a relatively unknown surgeon with a big goal. He had a patient whose face had been destroyed during an accident on an electrified subway rail. "I had seen that French surgeon Jean-Michel 'Max' Dubernard, who had trained under Murray as a fellow in 1965, had performed the world's first successful partial face transplant, and I knew this procedure could help my patient," recalls Pomahac. "There were ethical concerns, but Dr. Murray was highly supportive of what I was trying to do." At the time, the ethical issues surrounding facial transplants were being analyzed by the Catholic Church and Brigham leaders debated how to move forward. "Dr. Murray made a statement that influenced my decision-making," notes Elof Eriksson, chief of Plastic Surgery at BWH. "He said that the ethical discussions we were having were really no different than the ones he had about kidney transplants."

Once approval came, Pomahac recalls more helpful advice: "Before that first operation, I wondered if I had done as much as I could to prepare. Murray said: 'That feeling that you can be better prepared will never pass. You're ready. If you over-think it, it won't happen.'" Pomahac successfully completed the partial face transplant and then went on to perform the first full-face transplant in the United States in 2011, followed by additional face and hand transplants.

"When we were starting in the field after World War II, we never dreamed transplantation would expand so much," Murray said in 2012. He believed the Brigham

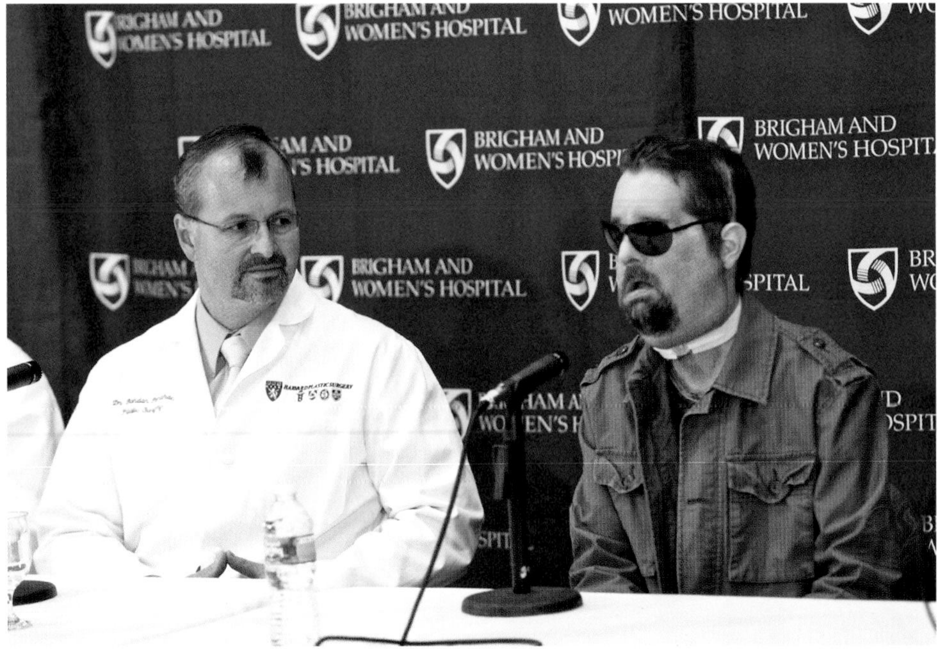

FIGURE 3-21 In April 2011, Dallas Wiens became the nation's first full face transplant recipient. A team of over 30 BWH physicians, nurses, anesthesiologists and residents, led by Bohdan Pomahac, a surgeon in the Division of Plastic Surgery and director of the Burn Unit, worked for more than 15 hours to complete the surgery. Pomahac also led the surgical team for the first partial face transplant at BWH, which was performed in April 2009.

provided a setting that bred innovation. "We always wondered, 'How can we do things better?'" he recalled. "We also used to say, 'If we can't do it, who will?'"

Pomahac sees parallels between his work and Murray's going forward. "In the 1950s, it took hard work and ten dark years to develop immunosuppressive medication," he notes. "Dr. Murray and his colleagues persevered and ultimately opened the gates to organ transplant. We believe if we can, once again, tweak the immune system and achieve better immune suppression, the transplant of faces, hands, legs, and other organs could become more common. It could really open the door to the replacement of any body part. And it could be historically similar."

IV. DEPARTMENTAL RESEARCH

DIVISION OF GLOBAL HEALTH EQUITY RESEARCH

DGHE Administrative Staff

Faculty at the Division of Global Health Equity (DGHE), in partnership with the nongovernmental organization Partners in Health, are engaged in research that seeks to understand and address the burden of disease in resource-poor settings. The department promotes the biosocial model of scholarship—understanding and addressing the interaction between the social determinants of disease and the disparities in health outcomes. As such, faculty research projects have emphasized infectious diseases such as human immunodeficiency virus/acquired immunodeficiency syndrome (HIV/AIDS), tuberculosis (TB), and, most recently, cholera, as well as noncommunicable diseases such as congestive heart failure and mental illness. The purpose of this research is to shape the provision of clinical services to serve the most vulnerable populations, both internationally and domestically. The growing body of knowledge obtained by DGHE researchers is shared and disseminated throughout the scientific community in an effort to improve the quality of and access to health care for all. Faculty members' research experience has translated directly to health policy in countries from Peru to Rwanda and at the World Health Organization.

DGHE research faculty members have backgrounds in a variety of disciplines. Insights from medicine and the social sciences are utilized to approach problems and evaluate findings from a number of different perspectives. By taking a multidisciplinary approach to the complex scientific and social roots of disease, DGHE researchers consider multiple aspects of prevention and treatment models.

Tuberculosis

DGHE faculty have long been involved in a number of sponsored and unsponsored research studies on tuberculosis, including a series of studies on molecular epidemiology and transmission dynamics of drug-resistant TB in Lima, Peru. The first of these, a National Institutes of Health (NIH) U01-funded study led by Mercedes Becerra, is designed to measure the transmissibility of multiple drug-resistant (MDR) and isoniazid-resistant *M. tuberculosis* strains compared with drug-sensitive strains to assess the impact of sociodemographic and clinical factors on transmission and to measure associations among specific resistance mutations and resistance. This study is linked to an NIH U19-funded project led by Megan Murray that also links three different studies focused on drug-resistant tuberculosis and one on the epidemiology and transmission dynamics of MDR/XDR (extensively drug-resistant) tuberculosis. To date, this project has recruited almost 4,000 TB patients and 12,000 household contacts. In related work, Ted Cohen is leading an NIH DP2-funded study to investigate the prevalence and consequences of mixed TB strain infection in this context and in a setting in South Africa where HIV prevalence is high. He is also studying surveillance strategies for monitoring the prevalence of MDR TB in Moldova and South Africa. Research in Lima involving a clinical trial of high-dose rifampin for drug-sensitive TB also is being funded by an NIH U01.

In Russia, DGHE faculty have been undertaking studies focused on treatment outcomes, risk factors for treatment failures, and community-based care delivery models. In an NIH R01-funded clinical trial led by Sonya Shin, the DGHE is assessing the effect of interventions in TB patients with alcohol disorders. Other research, funded through a grant from the Eli Lilly Foundation, focuses on care delivery models for TB, scale-up of the MDR program, and toxicities associated with the treatment of MDR TB. Attention is also being directed to improving TB transmission control through training programs and consultations provided by our faculty and staff. In South Africa, the DGHE is conducting studies using an innovative approach to measure the transmissibility of *M. tuberculosis*. An experimental ward has been constructed that vents air from patient rooms to a chamber where guinea pigs are exposed to airborne bacteria. In a National Institute for Occupational Safety and Health (NIOSH) R01-funded study, Edward Nardell is using this facility to study interventions to protect healthcare workers from airborne infections.

Human Immunodeficiency Virus

DGHE's HIV research agenda spans multiple sites. In Haiti, Louise Ivers is leading an NIH R01-funded study investigating the impact of a pilot nutritional intervention on HIV-positive individuals. In Peru, faculty members are studying the impact of social support on medication adherence among HIV/AIDS patients and conducting a pilot study on child development in households of HIV affected parents. In Boston, the Prevention and Access to Care and Treatment (PACT) project is conducting ongoing research to document the impact of service delivery on health outcomes and life expectancy for underserved HIV and diabetes patients and assessing the relative cost of community health worker interventions based on Medicaid data. PACT is also documenting the impact on a range of outcomes of a major collaborative initiative using Community Health Workers to help provide patient-centered medical homes to 2,500 chronically ill patients.

Primary Care

DGHE faculty are implementing and evaluating an integrated primary care program in the impoverished rural southeastern area of Rwanda. This project involves an analysis of changes in health indicators in intervention and non-intervention areas over the five years of the implementation project. It also includes a series of operational research projects that focus on economic analyses of health systems, ethnographic work on understanding barriers to accessing care, and the development of a rigorous monitoring and evaluation program capable of ongoing feedback and mid-course corrections.

School-Based Interventions for Child Health

DGHE faculty are leading the health component of a large randomized community trial of school-based interventions in impoverished urban neighborhoods in Santiago, Chile. Investigators are examining the impact of intensified case management within schools on outcomes including asthma frequency and school absenteeism.

Global Health Delivery

Global Health Delivery (GHD) is developing a series of case studies about how to develop and sustain large-scale HIV prevention programs and on the interaction between health systems and global health initiatives. In July 2011, GHD's library of twenty-one case studies and associated teaching notes were published at no cost by Harvard Business Press. With new funding, DGHE faculty is working to strengthen and study community-based primary healthcare services in rural Rwanda in partnership with Harvard Medical School, the Harvard School of Public Health, and Partners In Health. This consortium, led by DGHE faculty member Peter Drobac, is working with the Rwandan Ministry of Health to implement and study an innovative model of comprehensive, community-based health care in two rural districts in Rwanda. The funding will help expand health services beyond HIV/AIDS and tuberculosis to cover all primary healthcare needs and chronic diseases and measure the impact of these services on people's lives.

DERMATOLOGY AT THE BRIGHAM

Thomas S. Kupper

The Department of Dermatology at the Brigham and Women's Hospital was founded in 2000, after thriving for more than twenty-five years as a division of the Department of Medicine. Today, it is widely recognized as a leading dermatology department worldwide, as judged by its reputation, funding, clinical volume, and breadth and depth of faculty achievements. With more than forty full-time faculty, it is also one of the largest dermatology departments in the nation. Dermatology patients are seen at ten different clinical sites, and research is performed at three sites. The foundation for the rapid growth of the department to its current stature lies in a history spanning many decades.

Until the late 1960s, dermatology at the Peter Bent Brigham Hospital was primarily a consultative service, with consultants coming primarily from the Massachusetts General Hospital (MGH). In the early 1970s, research dermatologists Irma Gigli, Nicholas A. Soter, and Bruce U. Wintroub had a laboratory presence in K. Frank Austen's Robert Breck Brigham research group. When Harley A. Haynes became chief of dermatology at Peter Bent Brigham Hospital in 1976, a full-time on-site presence in the specialty was realized. He was also the Chief of Dermatology at the West Roxbury Veterans Affairs Medical Center, as well as consultant dermatologist at the Boston Hospital for Women and the Robert Breck Brigham Hospital. Inpatient consultation rounds often involved trekking to all of these in a single afternoon/evening. Haynes built and nurtured a first-rate consultative service during his tenure, with part-time faculty that included Richard F. Horan and Mitchell H. Rubenstein. By the mid-1980s, a small, high-quality outpatient service had started at the Brigham. In 1990, with funds raised for the Thomas B. Fitzpatrick endowed professorship at Harvard in place, a search was initiated for a physician-scientist to develop the dermatology research program. In 1992, Thomas S. Kupper became the Thomas B. Fitzpatrick Associate Professor of Dermatology and the director of dermatology research. His first appointee, cell biologist James G. Rheinwald, was recruited shortly thereafter. In 1994, Kupper and colleagues successfully competed for a National Institutes of Health Skin Disease Research Core Center, and the Harvard Skin Disease Research Center at the Brigham was founded. In 1995, Fitzpatrick Professor Thomas S. Kupper was appointed chief of dermatology, then a division of the Department of Medicine.

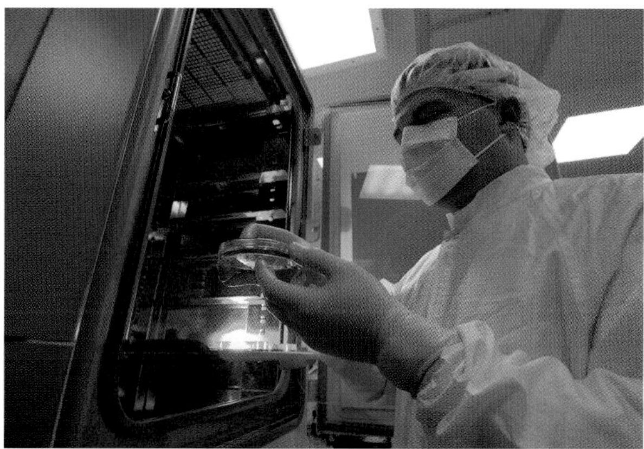

FIGURE 3-22 F. Stephen Hodi, Director, Melanoma Center, DFCI.

Dermatology at the Brigham in 1995 faced the fiscal and organizational challenges of all divisions and departments in Boston in response to healthcare reform initiatives introduced during the Clinton years. This led to the emergence of entities unthinkable only a few years before, including Partners Healthcare, the (then) unlikely union of the Brigham and the MGH. At this time, the MGH Dermatology Department, which began in the early 1900s, had more than 100 faculty members, a robust clinical program, more research space than any dermatology department nationally, and leadership of the combined Harvard residency program in dermatology. In spite of this considerable asymmetry, Kupper and the Brigham continued to recruit outstanding physicians and scientists, and clinical activities grew to include cutaneous oncology at the Dana-Farber Cancer Institute and Mohs surgery. In 2000, the Dermatology

Division had the requisite clinical, research, and educational resources and was granted departmental status. Kupper was named the first chair of the Department of Dermatology.

The next eleven years were characterized by rapid and expansive growth. Clinically, Brigham Dermatology increasingly became the home of both general dermatology and some twenty "specialty clinics," including rheumatology, infectious disease, melanoma, connective tissue disease, and many others. These clinics gave physicians an opportunity to increase their scholarship and expertise in specific, challenging diseases while maintaining practices of general medical and surgical dermatology. A new and innovative program, the Clinical Scholars program, offered postresidency dermatologists, who were recruited nationwide, formal and informal didactics and clinical experience in dermatologic specialties, and in addition provided forgiveness for medical school loans. This led to the development of a community of clinical scholars, led by physicians like Harley Haynes and Mitchell Rubenstein, and more recently by Abrar A. Qureshi, Andrew E. Wechniak, and Ruth Ann Vleugels. In addition, postgraduate fellowship programs in cutaneous oncology, dermatology/rheumatology, and Mohs surgery have successfully attracted high-performing graduates of dermatology residency programs who wish to increase their expertise in advanced medical dermatology and to become leading academic dermatologists.

Teaching Harvard Medical students and dermatology residents became an important function of the department as well. Haynes has for many years led the Department of Dermatology's efforts in educating students. Many Brigham dermatology faculty, including Elizabeth A. Buzney, Ruth Ann Vleugels, Andrew E. Werchniak, Arturo P. Saavedra, Adam Lipworth, and F. Clarissa Yang, are particularly active in giving lectures and leading group seminars.

On the research front, Brigham Dermatology and Kupper successfully competed for the first Specialized Program of Research Excellence (SPORE) in Skin Cancer from the National Cancer Institute. This $15 million, five-year grant solidified Brigham dermatology's position as a leader in translational research, a high priority for researchers in the department. A unique feature of Brigham dermatologic research is its multidisciplinary nature. Research faculty includes, among others, an oncologist/hematopoietic stem cell transplantation expert (Robert Sackstein), a pediatric rheumatologist (Robert C. Fuhlbrigge), investigative dermatologists (Rachael A. Clark and Abrar A. Qureshi), and basic scientists (Clare M. Baecher-Allan, James Rheinwald, Charles J. Dimitroff, Tobias Schatton, and others). Each investigator has recognized the skin as a unique model in which to test hypotheses involving not only skin disease but human disease in general. They have contributed a number of research "firsts," including 1) culture of human skin cells, termed keratinocytes (J. Rheinwald); 2) the discovery and characterization of immunological factors (cytokines) made by keratinocytes (T. Kupper); 3) elucidation of the structure of the molecules PSGL-1 and CD43 that permit T cells, which function in cell-mediated immunity, to enter skin cells (T. Kupper, R. Fuhlbrigge); 4) the discovery of the molecule, termed an E selectin ligand HCELL, that permits blood stem cells to enter the bone marrow (R. Sackstein); 5) the discovery and characterization of a population of memory cutaneous T cells, termed T resident memory cells (Trm), that live long-term in the skin (R. Clark); 6) the discovery that specific cutaneous T cell lymphoma subsets populate lymphomas of skin, that is, T_{RM} cells are causal of mycosis fungoides, and T_{CM} cells are causal of Sezary syndrome (J. Campbell, R. Clark, T. Kupper); 7) the appreciation that in mouse models of infection and human cancer patients, cutaneous T cells (T_{RM}) are the most potent infection-fighting T cells (T. Kupper, R. Clark); and 8) the discovery that surface markers on stem cells (and theoretically any cells) can be chemically modified and then intentionally directed to desired tissues (R. Sackstein). Breakthroughs in population science research and molecular epidemiology are being made by Abrar A. Qureshi and Jiali Han.

Dermatology at the Brigham has an illustrious history. It is safe to say that given its current trajectory, the best is yet to come.

TREATMENT OF BRONCHIAL ASTHMA: SOLVING THE INTRICACIES OF THE INFLAMMATORY RESPONSE

K. Frank Austen

In the 1950s, when I was a medical resident at the Massachusetts General Hospital (MGH), inflammation seemed a prominent aspect of many diseases. The role of inflammation in "innate immunity," by which the body generally responds to pathologic invasions, was somewhat understood. However, the link of inflammation to "adaptive immunity," by which cells recognize a foreign invader and organize a specific response, was largely unknown. In vitro systems for investigating most biochemical processes also were lacking. The interest I then developed in understanding the inflammatory process has focused my research and clinical interests over many decades at the Robert Breck Brigham (RBBH) and the Brigham and Women's Hospitals.

At the Walter Reed Army Medical Center from 1956-1958, in the immunochemistry laboratory of Elmer L. Becker, I was introduced to the complement system, a series of blood proteins involved in host defense and immune diseases. Research in immunology at the National Institute of Medical Research in London with John Humphrey from 1959-1961 solidified my commitment to exploring the inflammatory response, with a focus on allergy and asthma. I learned of the work of Walter Brocklehurst on "slow-reacting substance of anaphylaxis (SRS-A)," a substance released from sensitized guinea pig lung or human lung that had been removed from allergic patients because of a malignancy. The slow contractions induced by SRS-A were also observed in isolated human or guinea pig bronchioles. Antihistamines did not inhibit either these contractions or the airway constriction (bronchoconstriction) that occurs in asthma. Because this independent SRA-A–led pathway may contribute to the severe bronchoconstriction (bronchospasm) of asthmatic patients, I decided to investigate its origin, nature, and generation. I spent the bulk of my time in London defining the metabolic conditions needed for immunologic release of SRS-A from guinea pig lung fragments.

When I returned to the MGH in 1963, knowledge of the role of the immune system in diseases was expanding. My interest in the effector pathways of this system led to my taking on different clinical responsibilities, in infectious diseases and then pulmonary medicine. In 1966, supported by Harvard Medical School (HMS), Dean Robert Ebert, formerly my chief of medicine at the MGH, and George Thorn, chair of medicine at the Peter Bent Brigham Hospital, I became the physician-in-chief of the RBBH, dedicated to rheumatology and allergy.

My ongoing research has focused on three components of inflammation, one of which is the role of SRS-A. In collaboration with Kimishige and Teruko Ishizaka at Johns Hopkins, Robert Orange and I demonstrated in 1970 that activated specific human lung cells (mast cells) generate and release SRS-A and also release the stored chemical histamine. The finding of others of increased numbers of mast cells in a lung tissue (mucosa) of patients with asthma strengthened my belief that SRS-A was a mediator of human asthma. Jeffrey Drazen, a member of the Brigham Pulmonary Division and a former postdoctoral fellow, established in rats the in vivo pharmacologic action of SRS-A, which Robert Murphy at MIT and I had partially purified, on small peripheral lung airways. In 1978, Murphy, now at the University of Colorado School of Medicine, and Bengt Samuelsson at the Karolinska Institute in Sweden determined that SRS-A is a metabolic product of the chemical arachidonic acid that is linked by a sulfur moiety to a small peptide. E.J. Corey (Nobel laureate in chemistry, 1990) of the Harvard University Chemistry Department synthesized candidates for the chemical structure of SRS-A. Using parallel bioassays, we recognized that SRS-A was composed of three similar moieties. The three members of this family, derived from white blood cells (leukocytes), were termed the cysteinyl leukotrienes (LTC_4, LTD_4, LTE_4). Corey's synthetic chemicals provided a classic moment to determine whether my instincts had merit. When two colleagues and I injected each of the three cysteinyl leukotrienes under the skin in our arms, they potently induced the contraction of blood vessel muscles, thereby causing hives.

Drazen extended these findings in the 1980s, demonstrating that the cysteinyl leukotrienes, when inhaled, potently constricted human airways and elicited an "asthmatic" wheeze. Several pharmaceutical companies then screened and identified drugs that both block the biosynthesis of the cysteinyl leukotrienes or their action on smooth muscle and are successful therapies for bronchial asthma. Proving that the cysteinyl leukotriene pathway is an effector pathway that can be targeted as an intervention for bronchial asthma has validated my hopes. Today these drugs are widely used to treat millions of people who suffer from asthma. As an HMS graduate, I took special joy in being the 1998 recipient of the Warren Alpert Prize, awarded by HMS for laboratory discoveries with dramatic promise to improve human health.

We have also purified the leukocyte enzyme that is responsible for the synthesis of LTC_4, LTC_4 synthase. In 1994, after my colleague Bing Lam developed an immunoassay to detect LTC_4, we identified the gene coding for LTC_4 synthase, located on chromosome 5 (5q35). In early 2000, Yoshihide Kanaoka generated a mouse strain lacking LTC_4 synthase. Using these mice, Nora Barrett, a former BWH house officer who trained in both pulmonary medicine and allergy/immunology, showed that house dust mites, the most important allergen for asthma worldwide, elicited lung inflammation in mice through the cysteinyl leukotriene pathway. This response resulted from a signal by a sugar-like component of the dust mite to a specific receptor on allergen-presenting cells, thus stimulating the generation of cysteinyl leukotrienes. Thus we now have learned that the role of cysteinyl leukotrienes in human disease not only involves bronchoconstriction but also likely modulation of adaptive immunity.

The importance of basic science studies for medicine is highlighted by their unraveling disease processes, leading to the development of new targeted therapy. This is especially rewarding to those individuals who expanded their early initial findings, even if they had no clear vision of the ultimate application. Another joy is the lifelong friendships that are formed through this shared, intense, and often productive work. My highlight of the last three decades has been an annual reunion for members of my laboratory. These wonderful events, in which alumni discuss their experiences at the RBBH/BWH and their subsequent career successes, foster friendships among members of each laboratory generation. The graduates of this program, whether they have remained at the BWH or entered into faculty positions elsewhere, build on the training that they received here to advance the study of inflammation and its role in human disease.[22]

MILESTONES IN PSYCHIATRY

David A. Silbersweig

Psychiatry originated at the Peter Bent Brigham Hospital in 1939, when John Romano and his fellow George L. Engel established an inpatient consultation service while also studying delirium and unusual neurological and psychiatric disorders. In 1946, Henry M. Fox became the director of the Psychiatry Service, expanding its clinical and educational and research missions. He was succeeded in 1970 by Peter Reich, who led the division to prominence for its consultation-liaison service and education of Harvard Medical students. Jonathan F. Borus, a leading clinical educator, became director in 1990 and effected a major expansion of the educational, clinical, and research missions. In 1999, the service gained independent departmental status. An adult psychiatry residency training program was established in collaboration with the Beth Israel Hospital and the Massachusetts Mental Health Center. The department merged with the Department of Psychiatry at the Faulkner Hospital in 1998.

In 2008, David A. Silbersweig, a pioneering neuropsychiatrist and brain imaging scientist, assumed the chairmanship of psychiatry and the Institute for the Neurosciences. The department has become a leader in the transformation of psychiatry, identifying mechanisms of mind-brain disorders and enhancing evidence-based treatments. It is greatly immersed in patient care and research.

Consistent with its tradition, Psychiatry's focus is on problems associated with medical illness. The department is expanding its mission by initiating subspecialty programs with specific emphases and clinical research-educational integration. The focus, coordinated by Laura J. Miller, vice chair for Academic Clinical Services, and Arthur J. Barsky, vice chair for Research, is on the following areas:

Clinical Psychiatry

Medical Psychiatry

The Medical Psychiatry (Consultation-Liaison) Division, directed by David F. Gitlin, provides inpatient and emergency department diagnostic and management expertise to psychiatric problems that occur during other (e.g., medical and surgical) illnesses. A Complex Medical Psychiatric Diagnostic Clinic, headed by Michael J. Mufson, deals with the most difficult cases. It is a key site for medical student, residency, and fellowship training. In the Ambulatory Division, Brigham Psychiatric Specialties, directed by Jay W. Baer, provides evidence-based psychiatric evaluation and treatment and residency training. A multidisciplinary team includes psychiatry, psychology, nursing, and social work. It also includes a Center for Depression in Medical Illness, directed by Jane L. Erb. The center, a charter member of the National Network of Depression Centers, is leading a national task force addressing coexistent depression and medical illness. The Department is also developing and implementing new models of psychiatric care that are seamlessly embedded in primary and subspecialty medical care. These models will be increasingly important as health care shifts toward longitudinal and integrated, team-based comprehensive care.

Neuropsychiatry

The Neuropsychiatry Division, integrated with the Neurology Department's Division of Cognitive and Behavioral Neurology and its Neuropsychology program, has grown with Silbersweig and other dual psychiatrists/neurologists. Effecting the integrated approach of the Institute for the Neurosciences, it provides multidisciplinary, patient-centered care across the clinical neurosciences. This team (the Center for Brain Mind Medicine), led by Kirk R. Daffner, evaluates complex diagnostic dilemmas and therapeutic options at the interface of psychiatry and neurology. It trains physicians at all levels, including a neuropsychiatry/behavioral neurology fellowship.

Women's Mental Health

Directed by Laura Miller, psychiatrists, including members of the Women's Mental Health fellowship and the staff of the Department of Obstetrics/Gynecology, focus on perinatal psychiatry and perimenopausal and geriatric conditions across the reproductive lifespan. Expanded women's mental health services are operative at the Brigham's Fish Center for Women's Health, in the Outpatient Division and at the Faulkner Hospital.

Psychosocial Oncology

This program addresses the psychiatric conditions and needs of cancer patients, survivors and supporters. It is led by Susan D. Block, a pioneer and national leader in palliative care medicine. Specific areas include clinical, educational, and research aspects of psycho-oncology (directed by Ilana M. Braun).

Addiction Psychiatry

Psychiatry provides comprehensive addictions services for these prevalent clinical problems. Services include inpatient consultation, directed by Joji Suzuki; detoxification; partial (day) hospital treatment; and outpatient continuity of care at the Faulkner Hospital, led by physicians Erica Veguilla (psychiatry) and Carol V. Garner (medicine).

Geriatric Psychiatry

In the context of the medical focus and the aging population, Psychiatry has implemented a program to deal with geriatric depression, post-menopausal syndrome, late-life psychosis, and dementia. Physician leaders include Olivia I. Okereke, Geena K. Athappily, Catherine Gonzales, and Nancy Donovan.

Primary Psychiatric Illness

Patients with primary mood, psychotic, and anxiety disorders receive outpatient care at both the Brigham and the Faulkner Hospital. At the Faulkner, this includes a partial (day) hospital and an adult inpatient psychiatry clinical and teaching unit for acutely and severely ill psychiatric patients, directed by K.C. Potts.

Research

Three laboratory groups are dedicated to the neurosciences, studying brain circuitry and development in psychiatric disorders. The Functional Neuroimaging Laboratory, directed by Emily Stern and David Silbersweig, has performed groundbreaking work on several important psychiatric disorders, including localizing the brain fronto-limbic dysfunction circuitry that underlies the core features, developing biomarkers of diagnostic and therapeutic function, and studying the role of neuroinflammation. Martha Shenton, director of the Psychiatric Neuroimaging Laboratory, has demonstrated reduced volumes and disrupted connectivity among limbic and cerebral structures in schizophrenia. Jill M. Goldstein, also director of research for the Connors Women's Health Center, has led numerous studies of fetal antecedents to sex differences in normal brain and in schizophrenia and depression. Other researchers are investigating the application of transcranial magnetic stimulation to disordered volition in schizophrenia and Alzheimer disease, novel targets for deep brain stimulation in patients with refractory psychiatric illness, the efficacy of neuroprotective agents for depression, the genetics of subtypes of illness, neural stem cells, and neurogenesis.

In clinical and population research, Arthur J. Barsky established and expanded the concept of somatosensory amplification (a tendency to focus on unpleasant but benign bodily sensations and to misinterpret them as symptoms of serious disease). He delineated its role in the generation of unexplained symptoms and in contributing to the wide interindividual variability of symptoms among patients with the same disorder and has developed and documented the efficacy of cognitive-behavioral techniques. George E. Vaillant has continued his landmark, prospective cohort study of adult development and mental health. Researchers in the Center for Brain Mind Medicine are focused on early detection of Alzheimer disease and the role of psychosocial factors and the nature of executive dysfunction in dementias. Others have studied the process of normal bereavement, as distinguished from grief and major depression; the epidemiology of geriatric depression; psychophysiology; and the effect of light therapy on seasonal affective disorder.

Research in mental health services and treatment includes many studies. Among these are research on the development of cognitive-behavioral treatments for comorbid psychiatric and medical illness, detection and treatment of alcohol abuse in pregnancy, the treatment of opiate addiction in primary care practice, and the integration of mental health services into general medical care.

Education

Psychiatry offers clinical fellowships in psychosomatic medicine, psychotherapy, neuropsychiatry/behavioral neurology, women's mental health, and neuropsychology. Geriatric and addiction fellowships are offered in conjunction with the McLean and Massachusetts General Hospitals. The Harvard Longwood Psychiatry Residency Program, including the Department of Psychiatry at the Beth Israel Deaconess Medical Center (including the Massachusetts Mental Health Center), has received the American College of Psychiatrists Award for Creativity in Psychiatric Education. Known for its warm community and individualized environment, this expanding program was directed by William E. Greenberg for many years, and currently by Christie L. Sams and Charles W. Surber. Harvard Medical School (HMS) students who do their Principal Clinical Experience at the Brigham receive psychiatry clerkship training, overseen by Freemonta L. Meyer. Student electives include an integration with clerkships in neurology and neuroradiology. Departmental faculty work with others at HMS faculty to develop and teach first- and second-year courses.

In sum, although a relatively young department, Brigham psychiatry has grown substantially and has had a major impact on the hospital and the field of hospital-based psychiatry. Working closely with allied disciplines and departments, and with colleagues locally, nationally, and internationally, it is contributing to the transformation of mind-brain medicine, fighting the disorders of the most complex human functions of the most complex organ—the organ that make us who we are.

BIOGRAPHY

JOHN ROMANO (1908-1994) AND THE STUDY OF DELIRIUM

David M. Dawson

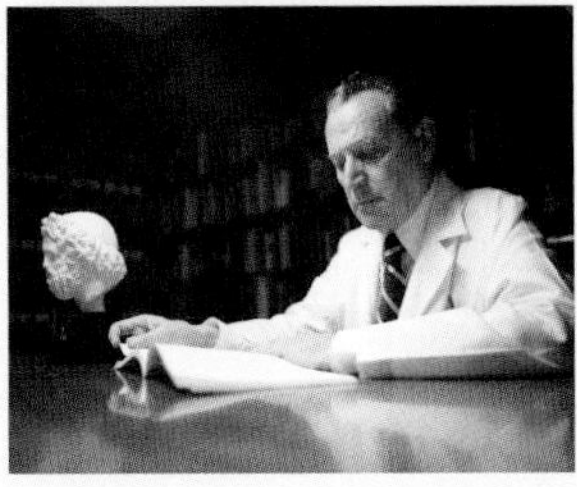

FIGURE 3-23 John Romano.

On September 1, 1939, new physicians joined the Peter Bent Brigham Hospital. Foremost among them was Soma Weiss, new professor of the Theory and Practice of Physic at Harvard Medical School (HMS) and chief of medicine. Weiss brought with him three assistants from the Boston City Hospital (BCH): Charles Janeway, Eugene Stead, and John Romano. Soma introduced them to the Brigham staff, stating "These are my three assistants. Please give them the opportunity to earn your respect."[23] Romano came as a neuropsychiatrist, the first of this discipline to be appointed to the Harvard faculty, to care for patients and to teach.[24] He was uniquely well equipped for this role. After training in outstanding neuropsychiatry in Colorado, he spent a year at the Neurological Unit of the BCH, at that time the premier academic neurological center in the United States. There he interacted with Tracy Jackson Putnam and H. Houston Merritt, two of the leading clinicians in the country, and observed the unfolding of the story of epilepsy and encephalography (EEG) under the aegis of William Lennox and Frederic Gibbs.

Romano embarked on a teaching program that exemplified his lifelong commitment to medical student and house staff education. His collected papers from that era, preserved in the University of Rochester Library, show a wealth of conferences and other didactic exercises, including bedside rounds that had been made famous by Soma Weiss. Most of Romano's clinical work at the Brigham was psychiatric. He made rounds and examined patients with his group of house staff and students. In the recent biography of Romano and George L. Engel, entitled *Their Lives and Work*, Engel is quoted:

> *I saw the attending, John Romano, a young psychiatrist, pull up a chair, and sit down with the patient and, in effect, invite him to tell his own story before the assembled group...The drama of Romano's "pulling up a chair" and listening to the patient, as he was accustomed to do on psychiatric rounds, changed my life forever.*[25]

Romano was also the neurologist for the hospital, exploiting his training by the eminent staff at the BCH Neurological Unit. He was assisted by weekly visits to the Brigham by H. Houston Merritt, considered the most expert and erudite clinical neurologist in Boston.

Romano and Engel, placed together by Soma Weiss, became a famous clinical and research team. They were famous for their work on psychosomatic medicine, that is, the impact of psychological processes on the clinical state of the patient. They studied carotid sinus sensitivity, syncope, and many other medical issues. Their studies of delirium, exploiting the newly developed EEG machine, were particularly exemplary. This machine had been developed in the early 1930s by Albert Grass, the BCH department engineer, and used in a number of pioneering studies. The Grass Model II was in use during World War II. In 1941, Romano and Engel borrowed their machine, probably this model, from HMS for their study. They studied forty-four patients with delirium of various causes. They were administered a neurologic examination,

EEG, and a battery of psychologic tests focusing on attention, memory, ability to abstract, and orientation. All patients showed some degree of abnormality. EEGs showed diffuse and nonspecific changes, but importantly, the degree of diffuse slowing closely paralleled the degree of abnormality on mental status testing. They were able to construct a system for overall wave frequency analysis, which also correlated well with the clinical state. They arrived at several findings and conclusions, which remain relevant today:

Delirium is accompanied by alterations in the function of the brain, as evidenced by slowing of the basic EEG rhythms.
Delirium can be accurately assessed by simple bedside tests of mental function (e.g., orientation, span of digit recall).
Delirium has many causes; the idea that there are specific defects with specific illnesses is incorrect.
Delirium can be recognized in patients who are somnolent or stuporous, not necessarily excited or hallucinatory.
Delirium is a serious medical condition with a poor prognosis.[26]

John Romano was recruited to be the head of the psychiatry department at the University of Cincinnati. After four years, he was recruited by the new medical school at the University of Rochester. His colleague George Engel accompanied him in both moves. According to his long-time colleague Robert Joynt, he was an engaging teacher and a leader in both establishing goals for student and resident education and devising means to attain these goals.[27] He was cited by the American Psychiatric Association, which named him as "the most influential voice in psychiatric education in [the twentieth] century." Fulfilling Soma Weiss's plea, John clearly earned universal love and respect.

THE CHANNING LABORATORY

Dennis L. Kasper and Julie B. McCoy

When the Channing Laboratory became a part of the Brigham and Women's Hospital in 1977, it was already a globally recognized facility for research on infectious diseases and chronic disease epidemiology. The laboratory's history dates from 1857, when Harriet Ryan founded the Channing Street Home for Sick and Destitute Women. Ryan (later Harriet Ryan Albee) first took poor women with tuberculosis into her own modest residence and then founded the home. Over the next century, the Channing Home evolved from a place of respite care into a nationally known center for the investigation and treatment of tuberculosis. When it closed in 1958 because of the advent of antituberculous drugs, its endowment remained intact. Through the efforts of Edward H. Kass, Maxwell Finland, and Theodore L. Badger of the Harvard Medical Unit at the Boston City Hospital (BCH), the endowment was channeled into the establishment of a new BCH-based laboratory for infectious disease research. Initially housed in the Mallory Institute of Pathology, under Kass's direction, this laboratory soon outgrew its space and moved to an adjacent new facility. When the Harvard Medical Unit left BCH In 1977, the Channing affiliated with the Brigham and relocated to a retrofitted Harvard Medical School–owned building at 180 Longwood Avenue, previously the Angell Memorial Hospital for veterinary medicine. The Channing moved in 1996 to its present custom-designed research facility at 181 Longwood Avenue. The activities of current investigators continue to reflect the objectives of the original Channing Home. Amalie M. Kass, widow of Edward Kass, has stated, "I sometimes wonder what Harriet Ryan Albee would think of [the Channing], but then I remember the words she herself spoke: 'The home has never done good by rule, but according to a present need.' Certainly there is a present need for the work going on here and now." Indeed, the Channing Laboratory today is a vibrant center for research in microbiology, virology, epidemiology, and most recently network medicine.

"No one ever really leaves the Channing" is a pervasive attitude at this institution. Although this obviously is not the case, many "Channingites" have spent substantial portions of their careers here. This includes the authors of this chapter, who arrived at the Channing in the early 1970s. At that time, a Channing tradition had already been established: the annual "Proc Soc," at which each investigator presented a capsule summary of ongoing work to the entire Channing community. Originally, ten minutes were allotted for each presentation, but Proc Soc lasted for eight hours! As the laboratory grew, each researcher exhibited a poster, a sampling of investigators gave oral presentations, and presenters and audience were rewarded with a Chinese buffet lunch. After nearly a half century, Proc Soc—a forum for bringing an ever-expanding laboratory together—remains emblematic of a certain spirit, originating with Ed Kass, that has made the Channing a distinct entity and an energetic workplace.

As a bacteriologist investigating the relationship between bacteriuria and hypertension, Kass collaborated with epidemiologists working in Jamaica and South Wales. He described this experience as his "12-year preceptorship in epidemiologic methods and approaches to the study of chronic diseases." As a result of this "training," Kass fostered research during the Channing's years at the BCH on bacteriology and chronic disease epidemiology. During these early years, the Channing attracted many brilliant young scientists, including Gustave A. Lorenzi, Leonard D. Berman, Gareth M. Green, and Elliott Goldstein. Mentored by Ed Kass and the legendary Max Finland, these investigators set the bar high for all who followed them and established the Channing internationally as a preeminent research hub. Kass's contributions to medical research were remarkable. For example, around the time of the Channing's move to the Brigham, Kass led urgent investigations into the newly recognized toxic shock syndrome, which was fatal to many young women. Kass discovered its etiology, implicating specific types of tampons. As important as his research, however, was Kass's inspired vision for the Channing, which, combined with his practical skills at organization and fund raising, left no room for mediocrity or failure.

The appointment of Dennis L. Kasper and Frank E. Speizer as associate directors of the Channing in 1982 and as codirectors on Kass's retirement in 1988 reflected the expanding scope of the epidemiology as well as the bacteriology group. These disciplines flourished after the Channing's consolidation with the Brigham. Bacteriology became Microbiology, reflecting specifically the addition to the Channing of a productive virology team led by Elliott D. Kieff, head of the Infectious Diseases Division at the Brigham. Speizer led the epidemiology research group. His landmark Nurses' Health Study of risk factors for chronic disease in women, and subsequent studies led by Graham A. Colditz, Susan E. Hankinson, and currently Meir J. Stampfer, are major efforts of the epidemiology group. The other arms, also extraordinarily productive, are the respiratory epidemiology component, now led by Scott T. Weiss; the pharmacological epidemiology component, led by Richard Platt; and the biostatistics component, led by Bernard A. Rosner.

Throughout his Channing career of more than four decades, current director Dennis Kasper has focused on two areas of investigation: glycoconjugate vaccine development, with group B *Streptococcus* (GBS) as a model, and immunologic development in relation to the population of microorganisms within the intestine (microbiota), with *Bacteroides fragilis* as a model. In 1976, Kasper and his Channing colleague Carol J. Baker purified and immunochemically characterized the GBS type III polysaccharide (GBSIII). They further documented that, whether or not she was colonized with GBS, a pregnant woman who had antibodies to GBSIII passed these antibodies to the fetus, with consequent protection of the baby from potentially fatal neonatal GBS infection. These findings prompted Kasper and Baker to develop a vaccine consisting of GBSIII antigens. Baker, now at the Baylor College of Medicine, and colleagues immunized adults with this vaccine, with moderate immunogenic success. Endeavors to improve the vaccine's immunogenicity led to a GBSIII–protein conjugate produced by a technology requiring years of work in the Kasper laboratory. By the late 1990s, Kasper's group, with key contributions by Lawrence Paoletti and Michael R. Wessels, had purified the five relevant serotypes of

GBS polysaccharide, and all types had been tested in humans. The next decade saw clinical trials, with antibodies measured by assays developed in the Kasper lab. Novartis Vaccines is now conducting clinical trials of this potentially life-saving vaccine, with phase 3 studies set for 2013.

Kasper's work on *B. fragilis* has established the essential role of a complex microbiota for normal immunologic development of the host. This line of investigation was prompted by his observation, with Andrew B. Onderdonk, that this encapsulated organism, which includes an unprecedented eight polysaccharides, was the intestinal anaerobe most commonly isolated from intestinal infections. Kasper and colleagues made a discovery that disproved the key immunologic paradigm, which had asserted that carbohydrates (including polysaccharides) were able to stimulate only the adaptive arm of the immune system—i.e., an antibody-associated immune response. They found that one polysaccharide, PSA, protected mice from intestinal abscess formation and that this resulted from the activation of T lymphocytes—that is, stimulation of the innate arm of the immune system. This finding raised the possibility of a new generation of carbohydrate-based vaccines against diseases such as inflammatory bowel disease. Subsequent studies are elucidating the mechanisms underlying T-cell activation by PSA and have highlighted the essential role of PSA in the development of the human immune system. These investigations demonstrate how the complex interactions of intestine-colonizing bacteria with the immune system critically affect human health and disease.

Other bacteriology research groups are making similarly notable contributions to human health. Gerald B. Pier leads a group that has carried out groundbreaking work on the pathogens *Pseudomonas aeruginosa* and *Staphylococcus aureus*. Laurie E. Comstock branched off from the Kasper group to study the mechanisms by which the bacterial intestinal flora express important molecules. Matthew K. Waldor, a former Brigham house officer who was recruited back to the Brigham in 2007, is an outstanding microbial molecular biologist with major interests in cholera and other enteric infections. Waldor is a Howard Hughes Investigator and the Edward H. Kass Professor of Medicine since 2011. Julia A. Wang has focused on anthrax vaccines, creating conjugates comprising the capsule of *B. anthracis* coupled to the Protective Antigen. The dozens of other exceptional scientists whose work meets the high bar set by Ed Kass and other Channing investigators include Robert S. Baltimore, Brian A. Cobb, Lawrence C. Madoff, Sarkis K. Mazmanian, Annalisa Pantosti, Peter A. Rice, and Arthur O. Tzianabos.

The able administrators, whose contributions have often exceeded day-to-day leadership, have contributed long-range planning and farsighted innovations. The efforts of Norman Stein, the administrator from 1980 to 2006, were essential to the Channing's stability and growth. This essential work is continued by the current, exemplary administrator, Sandra L. Hatten. Stein also negotiated and oversaw the establishment in 1990 of the Brigham and Women's Hospital Editorial Service. Founded by Jaylyn Olivo and Julie B. McCoy, this Service flourished at the Channing for two decades, editing hundreds of grant proposals, journal articles, book chapters, and other documents for Brigham faculty and staff.

From its conceptualization half a century ago at the BCH by Edward H. Kass and colleagues, the Channing Laboratory has evolved into powerful scientific groups with international reputations. In 2011, the laboratory consisted of 565 investigators, faculty members, fellows, and administrative staff members. During these decades, the team of Dennis Kasper and Frank Speizer (who retired in 2005) grew the Channing Laboratory from a $6 million-a-year institution to a nearly $75 million-a-year research giant. With this growth have come thousands of publications in the most highly regarded journals of medical science. This record of accomplishment at the Channing Laboratory is a remarkable tribute to the vision of Ed Kass and the Channing's outstanding leadership and faculty. Having successfully led this renowned scientific enterprise for more than twenty-five years, in July 2012, Kasper passed the baton of directorship on to Edwin Silverman, to continue to pursue his research in bacterial pathogenesis and vaccine development. Silverman has led the transition of the

Channing Laboratory into the Channing Division of Network Medicine in the Department of Medicine, in which epidemiologists, statisticians, network scientists, and systems biologists will endeavor to develop novel models of complex disease mechanism and treatment that takes into account the complex connectivity many goals and pathways that define pathophenotype. This goal is a laudable one that will, no doubt, continue to drive the influence and success of the Channing well into the future.[28]

V. INNOVATIONS

INNOVATIONS IN IMAGE-GUIDED THERAPY

Ferenc A. Jolesz

Image-guided therapy (IGT) describes any surgical or interventional procedure that uses advanced imaging to localize, target, monitor, and control procedures. Through the innovative use of imaging that complements direct visualization, IGT procedures are more targeted and less invasive and may have better outcomes. A neurosurgeon by training but having also completed a residency in diagnostic radiology and a fellowship in neuroradiology at the Brigham, I began research in IGT in the early 1990s in a new Surgical Planning Laboratory. An IGT program was also established at the Brigham in 1991, funded since 2005 by the National Institutes of Health as the National Center for Image Guided Therapy (NCIGT).

With research and clinical experience with intraoperative magnetic resonance imaging (MRI) and from the original concept of the "Operating Room of the Future," we developed and advanced our IGT program that during the years has introduced multiple integrated imaging and therapeutic modalities into operating rooms.[29] Some leading IGT innovations are discussed next.

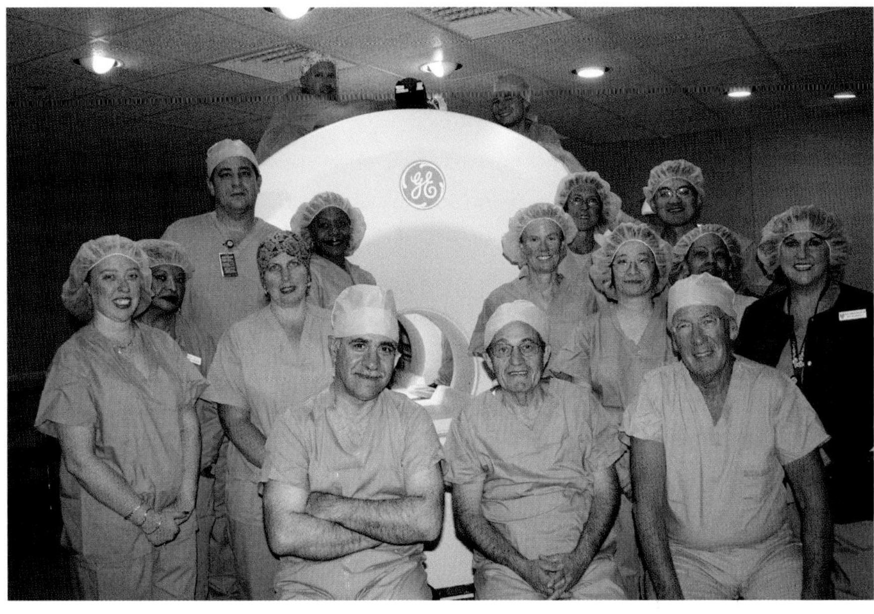

FIGURE 3-24 Image-guided therapy: Ferenc Jolesz (center) and team, 2006.

MRI-Guided Thermal Ablation

Heating and ablation of tumors with laser through a single fiber introduced by a needle can be monitored and controlled by both temperature-sensitive MRI and cryoablation.[30] Today, after two decades of the use of various MRI-guided thermal ablative methods, two commercial MRI-guided laser systems and one MRI compatible cryoablation system are approved by the Food and Drug Administration and used routinely in clinical settings worldwide.

Intraoperative MRI

The world's first intraoperative MRI, the famous "double doughnut," resulted from a collaboration with General Electric (GE) Healthcare. It had a 0.5 Tesla (field strength) MRI scanner with a vertically open configuration, with which patients were imaged in place during surgery or interventions. During its use, two physicians had full access to the patient.[31] The first application of intraoperative MRI was in neurosurgery in 1993.[32] Indeed, the use of intraoperative MRI in glioma surgery optimizes the extent of resection and lengthens survival. Brigham neurosurgeon Peter McL. Black and his colleagues performed more than 1,000 craniotomies, and all told, nearly 3,000 procedures, including endoscopic sinus surgery, cryo-, and laser ablations, have been carried out using intraoperative MRI. Brigham physicians Clare M. Tempany, the current co-principal investigator of the NCIGT, and Anthony V. D'Amico, have exploited this method for prostate brachytherapy. Today, more than 100 intraoperative MRIs are installed in operating rooms worldwide for neurosurgery, and hundreds of interventional MRI sites exist. Intraoperative MRI guidance and computer assistance greatly improve the capabilities of surgery.

Fast MRI Sequences

The development of Fast Spin Echo (FSE) and its three-dimensional (3D) version improved imaging speed in interventional MRI. Our team of physicists, Robert V. Mulkern, Koichi Oshio, Philippe S. Melki, and Stephen T. C. Wong, reduced acquisition times by factors of 1.4–16. FSE has become the most basic sequence in current diagnostic MRI.

MR-Guided Focused Ultrasound

After recognizing the advantages of MRI guidance for probe-delivered thermal ablations, I developed a method that deposits thermal energy without the insertion of a probe and distributes energy evenly regardless of tumor shape. The method, called high intensity focused ultrasound (HIFU) or, alternatively, focused ultrasound surgery (FUS), although not providing adequate imaging, did lead to procedures integrating MRI with therapeutic ultrasound. In collaboration with GE researchers and with Kullervo Hynynen, our group demonstrated the therapeutic potential of MR-guided FUS (MRgFUS) in 1991. Subsequently, GE developed the world's first MRgFUS clinical system, used early on for treating benign breast tumors. After further development by Israel company Insightec and studies at the Brigham, this technology was approved by the Food and Drug Administration in 1994. Since then, MRgFUS has been applied to treat benign and malignant tumors (breast, liver, prostate bone metastasis). Today, nearly 100 MRgFUS therapy delivery systems are installed worldwide, and more than 10,000 clinical cases have already been treated.

Use of Focused Ultrasound Surgery in the Brain

The ultimate clinical application of FUS is the treatment of the brain, but it initially lacked the ability to focus an acoustic beam through the bony skull. Work in our group primarily by Hynynen and Gregory Clement, using computed tomography data on skull thickness and a hemispheric phased array, solved this problem. Insightec then developed the first clinical brain treatment system, and several brain tumors have been treated noninvasively with this method at the Brigham. Other central nervous system diseases may be best treated with drugs administered intravenously, but drugs with large molecular sizes cannot penetrate the intact blood–brain barrier. Based on the work of Hynynen and Nathan McDannold, our group developed the method of FUS-induced transient and reversible disruption of the blood–brain barrier that can be used for targeted drug delivery. We have demonstrated the applicability of this method to the localized delivery of target antibodies and chemotherapeutic agents to the brain. In a similar vein, Krisztina Fischer showed that with FUS one can modify the ultrafiltration function of the kidney, thus facilitating the clearance of toxic drugs and toxins.

Integrated Multimodality Operating Suite

The Advanced Multimodality Image-Guided Operating Suite (AMIGO), developed in our division, opened at the Brigham in 2011. It is a unique IGT-oriented operating suite that is integrated with multimodal imaging (MRI, positron-emission tomography [PET], computed tomography [CT], 3D ultrasound, X-ray fluoroscopy, angiography, optical imaging), all of which (especially PET) enrich the anatomical and functional guidance provided by MRI. These advances in molecular imaging are being used primarily to improve oncologic surgery. To facilitate the use of complex imaging, the Surgical Planning Laboratory developed an image processing software platform, called 3D Slicer, open-source software that is used by thousands of investigators worldwide.

OPTICAL COHERENCE TOMOGRAPHY

Mark E. Brezinski

Attacking disease at a reversible early stage benefits both patients and society. Treating disease at later stages is usually less effective and more costly. The optimal therapy requires identifying abnormalities at early stages. Magnetic resonance imaging (MRI) and ultrasound are powerful medical technologies, but limits in magnification prevent their detecting early disease. The imaging technology Optical Coherence Tomography (OCT) addresses this limitation by yielding much greater resolution. I have been pioneering the birth and development of this technology for almost eighteen years. Exploiting OCT patient scans, whether they are uniquely revealing early collagen breakdown or dangerous coronary plaques less than 100 layers thick, has become routine. OCT has received Food and Drug Administration approval for assessing coronary artery disease, and regulatory evaluation is underway across a spectrum of medical specialties.

OCT grew out of unusual origins. In the early 1990s, finishing my cardiology fellowship at Massachusetts General Hospital and anticipating a successful career in biochemistry, I attended a lecture at which the chief (Arthur E. Weyman) stated "the biggest problem in cardiology is that most heart attacks are caused by plaques that are too small to be detected by current imaging modalities." I thought that there must be some way to address this with light- or infrared-based technologies, which have extremely high resolutions. For the next several weeks I read literature, ranging from geology to telecommunication, looking for some theory or technology that could be transformed to address this problem. Six weeks later, sitting with a friend in an Atlanta restaurant, I articulated my plans for changing my career and attacking early disease imaging with OCT.

OCT is analogous to ultrasound or radar, except that it measures back-reflection infrared light rather than sound or radio waves. The technology is more complex because of higher infrared light frequencies and speed of propagation. The resolution in OCT approaches 4 μm, twenty-five times higher than the next highest-resolution imaging technology (high-frequency ultrasound). It runs at a super-video rate, with some systems at 120 frames/sec (video is 30 frames/sec), thus yielding many more images. Because it is fiberoptic-based, catheters and endoscopes are extremely small—as small as the size of a human hair. With OCT, one can watch nuclei divide in living tissue, an amazing phenomenon! The machine is compact and portable. It can be combined with a range of spectroscopic techniques to examine special anatomy.

In 2000, while OCT was undergoing clinical trials in cardiology, I was recruited to the Department of Orthopedics at the Brigham and Women's Hospital by Chair Thomas S. Thornhill. This recruitment was strongly supported by Scott D. Martin, an internationally recognized sports medicine orthopedic surgeon, a longtime friend, and collaborator. Thornhill saw the need, particularly as the lifespan often extended well beyond eighty, to prevent the development of osteoarthritis (OA), a leading cause of chronic disability. OA in elderly individuals was often treated with joint replacement. Several major issues clouded the treatment of OA at earlier stages, when cartilage and bone injury were minimal. First, symptoms are primarily related to inflammation and soft tissue swelling, which does not correlate well with structural damage. Second, imaging techniques at that time were only capable of identifying structural changes at relatively late, irreversible stages. Third, a plethora of therapeutic approaches to late-stage OA was effective in animals; but without high-resolution imaging, their effectiveness could not be assessed in humans. To focus on this challenging problem, I established the center for Optical Coherence Tomography and Optical Physics in the Department of Orthopedics.

OCT can assess cartilage on a micron scale as well as small breaks in subchondral bone, which is not achievable in patients with other technologies. However, the technique in which OCT is combined with the spectroscopic approach polarization-sensitive OCT (PS-OCT) has had the greatest impact on early-stage OA, as well as in other musculoskeletal diseases. PS-OCT, which detects early collagen breakdown, is performed using OCT first with polarized light and then after rotating the polarization state. Healthy tissue is polarization-sensitive: when the tissue has highly organized structure, like the collagen matrix, the image changes with the polarization. When cartilage becomes diseased, long before thinning, the collagen network becomes disorganized. This early OA, even before cartilage thinning, loses its polarization sensitivity. Clinical trials are assessing the ability of PS-OCT and OCT to predict the development of OA, based on abnormalities that are detected. In year 1, patients received OCT/PS-OCT, MRI, and arthroscopy assessments. The areas normal by MRI and arthroscopy but abnormal by PS-OCT are being followed subsequently. If in year 3 MRIs of areas with abnormal PS-OCT findings detect gross cartilage erosion, whereas MRIs of areas with normal PS-OCT demonstrated no erosion, then we may have established the first early in vivo marker of OA. Additional musculoskeletal studies of OCT include the assessment of possible early therapeutic targeting in rheumatoid arthritis (and early treatment failures) and the ability to predict rotator cuff surgery failure.

From the beginning, when I met with interested individuals at a local McDonalds and drew designs on napkins, the OCT has been a story of translation from concept and benchwork to the patient. Essential research collaborators have included Scott D. Martin, James G. Fujimoto, Eric Swanson, Xing de Li, James Southern, and Gary J. Tearney. Several of us founded Lightlab Imaging, which manufactures the apparatus for OCT. I have had mentoring and prominent insights from Brigham leaders Marshall A. Wolf, Eugene Braunwald, Charles N. Serhan, and Joseph Loscalzo. The OCT system has created more than 10,000 jobs, is used in thirty-seven countries, and saves lives.

BIOGRAPHY

CARL W. WALTER, 1905-1992

Nicholas L. Tilney

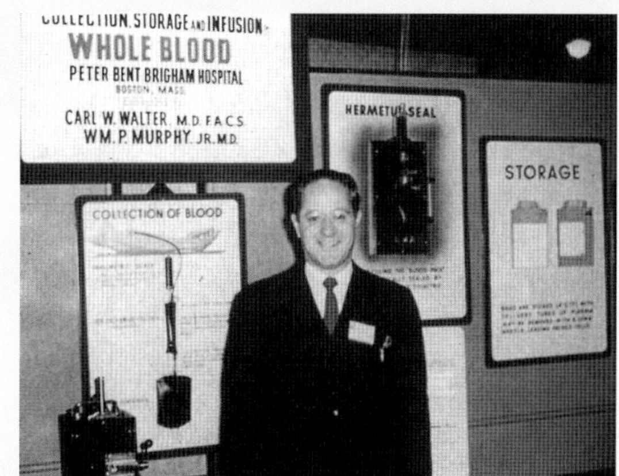

FIGURE 3-25 Carl Walter, circa 1950.

Elliott Cutler, Harvey Cushing's successor as Brigham surgeon-in-chief, populated departments of surgery throughout the United States with his innovative and imaginative surgical trainees during the 1930s and 1940s. Carl Walter was one of the distinguished members of this pantheon of talent. A colorful and iconoclastic figure during his four decades at the Brigham, Walter held many medical patents, headed the hospital fracture service, and pioneered significant advances in blood banking, hospital engineering, autoclave design, and the hemodialysis machine. He founded and directed a renowned biomedical company and was a pioneer in improving aseptic technique and control of infection in surgical patients. A master fundraiser at Harvard Medical School (HMS), he endowed two academic chairs. Medical students and faculty attend lectures in the Carl Walter Auditorium.

Despite his accomplishments during an extended professional career, many residents were unaware of his talents and accomplishments. His clinical presence was relatively sparse and the importance of his contributions, long accepted as routine in many institutions, inadequately appreciated. Aloof, outspoken, and authoritarian, he was viewed as an engineer rather than as a surgeon by his departmental colleagues. Yet, he trained generations of surgeons in aseptic technique and was responsible for standardizing and insuring the safety of many operating room activities.

Walter quickly developed an antipathy with the Brigham administrators during his residency in the 1930s when he discovered that the hospital-produced parenteral fluids were primarily responsible for a high incidence of complications. Indeed, the fever, chills, and severe malaise that developed in many patients after intravenous infusions became so severe that the departmental chairs forbade their use. Tracing the problem to its source, the young resident quickly discovered that both the distilled water and the dry chemical constituents of the fluids prepared in the hospital pharmacy contained endotoxin. Not only was the water stored for prolonged periods in inadequately sterilized glass containers, but the pharmacy still, not cleaned for years, was packed with mud and debris. He refined the process so effectively that intravenous treatment ultimately became a ubiquitous practice. However, his chief, Elliott Cutler, had to defend him on several occasions to preserve his hospital position, particularly after Walter shocked the administration by demonstrating a connection between the clean water intake and the sewer line.

This experience piqued Walter's interest in the autoclave. Despite routine steam sterilization of instruments between cases, the incidence of wound infections remained high. In studies on the existing autoclave, he could routinely culture pathogens from the instruments after sterilization. Furthermore, and again to the disgust of the hospital administration, he demonstrated that ice cubes placed at the back of the horizontal autoclave cylinder never melted despite allegedly accurate settings of temperature, time, and cycle. Steam circulated correctly throughout much of the space but apparently never made it to the back corner. He also noted that the readings of the improperly located and inaccurate thermostats had little relevance to temperatures throughout the cylinder. The presentation of his findings to a surgical audience at a major conference drew such ire that the autoclave manufacturers initiated two major lawsuits—later dropped. Walter improved the designs so effectively that the ancillary creation of the technique of "flash sterilization" subsequently entered routine use. Fifty years later, the Surgical Research Laboratory at HMS continued to use one of his large autoclaves to sterilize instruments for the student course in aseptic technique. His prototype of an improved thermostat became so popular that it was used in many commercial jet engines after World War II.

Carl Walter made significant improvements in hitherto rudimentary blood banking technology. Because both HMS and the Brigham trustees considered the storage and use of human blood to be "immoral and unethical," Walter formed a clandestine blood bank in a basement room. In addition to devising methods to prevent clotting, bacterial contamination, and red cell lysis in the storage container, he discovered that the sterilization techniques he had developed for parenteral fluids were equally effective in preserving blood. So successful were the improvements in typing, cross-matching, and storage that he founded the Blood Bank at the Brigham in March 1942, collecting 84,000 units for the war effort.

Fully satisfactory methods to preserve and store blood remained unsolved, however, until Walter introduced the plastic blood bag in 1948. In this novel departure, he incorporated hemorepellent tubing and administrative ports into a completely closed system. He solved complications that included fungal contamination and fracture of frozen plasma-filled containers by employing a plasticized polyvinyl material and improving the sterilizing techniques. The plastic blood bags were used successfully during the Korean War and remain in commercial use in all blood banks. Walter's company, Fenwall Laboratories, later to become part of the Baxter-Travenol Company, did much to aid in the research and development of this important advance. He offered both the Brigham and Harvard the patent rights to his spectrum of blood bank inventions. Both institutions eschewed the opportunity, considering any infusion of commercial money contrary to their ideals.

The original hemodialysis machine was developed in Nazi-occupied Holland and consisted of sausage casing, a semipermeable membrane that was wrapped around a frame made of pieces of wooden herring barrels. When the apparatus was placed in a water bath and blood circulated through the tubing, uremic toxins and abnormally elevated levels of electrolytes would move from the blood to the bath. Several patients with terminal renal failure were sustained by this treatment for some time. Walter and John Merrill, a young nephrologist, were assigned to work with the inventor, Willem Kolff, to perfect the existing apparatus. The resultant design, the Brigham-Kolff kidney, became the prototype for all future dialysis machines.

One of the most enduring of Carl Walter's legacies was the course in aseptic technique, given each year to the Harvard Medical students. Initiated by Harvey Cushing in 1912 and based on the course he had given at Hopkins, this became such an important curriculum in many teaching hospitals and medical schools throughout the country. At HMS, students performed standard surgical procedures on dogs that mimicked operations carried out in patients. They organized and packed supplies, selected and sterilized instruments, administered anesthesia, operated, made rounds on the animals postoperatively, and carried out a postmortem examination if necessary. The instructors—usually staff surgeons, anesthesiologists, and nurses—emphasized the accurate recording of an ether chart and the keeping of full notes and records. An exacting taskmaster, Walter taught the students and residents the intricacies of proper scrubbing before the procedure using lampblack and how to gown and act correctly in the operating room. The course remained a popular part of the medical school curriculum until the 1980s. Mary Graves Tilney, the long-time laboratory supervisor, organized the annual six-week course for many years. She, our research fellows, and I taught it. About forty students attended; many were stimulated to pursue surgical careers.

The Brigham Hospital has produced a spectrum of nationally and internationally recognized innovators and original thinkers throughout its century-old history. Carl Walter was one of the most important. It has been said that his improvements in the safety of the surgical patient rank only second to those of Joseph Lister and his principles of asepsis and antisepsis. Hyperbole or not, Walter's contributions continue to endure unscathed as the decades pass. They have affected hundreds of thousands of lives.

THE TREATMENT OF PERNICIOUS ANEMIA

H. Franklin Bunn and Martin A. Samuels

> *"Now sick people came to the Peter Bent Brigham Hospital in extremis, absolutely at the end of their tether. They came with their blood ten times thinner than it should be. They came in with next to no blood at all. . . Now Minot and Murphy sat by their beds. They poured fresh liver down them through stomach tubes. They kept pouring it down them that way for two, three, four, five days. They didn't give up though this fellow's breathing was so faint you could hardly detect it. . . . They stayed by those bedsides feeding liver and liver and more liver and saw life come back into those lost ones whose eyes opened, whose lips began moving, at last, to whisper that they felt a little better . . . . In a week they were sitting up clamoring for something to eat. In less than two weeks they were wanting to walk."*
>
> —Paul de Kruif, *Men Against Death*

In 1855, Thomas Addison reported "a very remarkable form of general anemia, occurring without any discoverable cause whatever. . . Its approach is slow and insidious....The patient can hardly fix a date to his earliest feeling of that languor that is to become so extreme...The countenance gets pale... There is increasing indisposition to exertion with an uncomfortable feeling of faintness and breathlessness on attempting it."[33] Over the next thirty years, it became apparent that this was a potentially fatal, generalized disease, involving the blood and the lining of the stomach (i.e., atrophy of the gastric mucosa). In 1880, Paul Ehrlich reported that occasional patients had large circulating nucleated erythrocytes with abnormal histologic characteristics.[34] In 1900, Russell et al. described the severe spinal cord involvement in this syndrome, termed pernicious anemia (PA), labeling it "subacute combined degeneration of the spinal cord."[35]

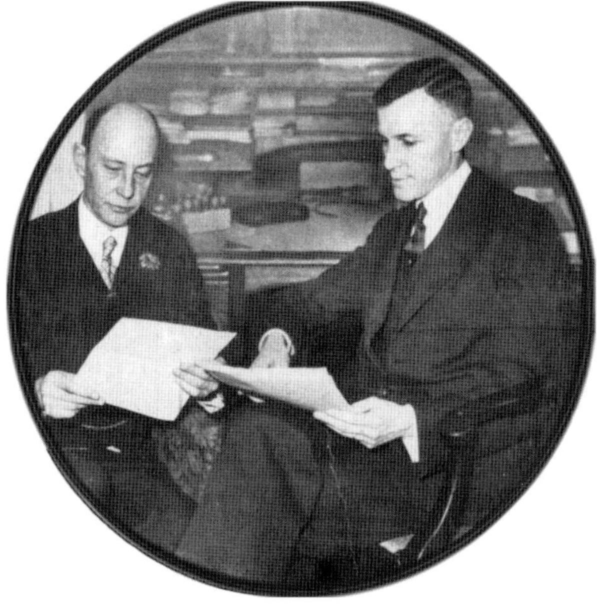

FIGURE 3-26 Minot and Murphy.

In 1908, Richard Cabot, a physician at Massachusetts General Hospital, reported on 1,200 patients with PA.[36] About 10% of them had sensory abnormalities in the hands or feet and/or spinal cord damage resulting in an ataxic and/or spastic gait. Most patients survived only one to three years after onset of symptoms. Full recovery was observed in only six patients. Samuel A. Levine, a young physician at the Peter Bent Brigham Hospital , established the nearly universal absence of acid in the stomach (gastric achlorhydria) in patients with PA.[37]

PA intrigued two other prominent Boston physicians, Francis Weld Peabody and George Richards

Minot, who were friends and associates.[38] Peabody, at the Brigham since its opening in 1913 and also chief of the medical service at the contiguous Huntington Memorial Hospital, became the head of the Harvard Medical Unit and Thorndike Memorial Laboratory at Boston City Hospital (BCH) in 1921. Minot succeeded him at the Huntington Hospital, devoted primarily to the care of cancer patients, and became a staff physician at the Brigham in 1925. Peabody and Minot shared a deep appreciation of the importance of cell morphology in the diagnosis and monitoring of blood disorders.

In 1927, Peabody published posthumously his definitive observations (made several years earlier) on bone marrow biopsies of PA patients that led him to conclude that red blood cell production was disordered and ineffective. They both were impressed with the research of George Whipple at the University of Rochester, demonstrating the efficacy of diet, including liver, in the regeneration of red blood cells in dogs following periodic phlebotomy.[39] Whipple's observations prompted Peabody and Minot to initiate dietary trials (independently of each other) in patients with PA.

Discovery of the Cure

From his early training, Minot was inculcated with the importance of taking a comprehensive dietary history on all patients. He noted that his patients with PA often excluded meat from their diets. He also began to follow his PA patients with frequent blood counts and discovered that when a few went into spontaneous partial remission, there was a transient increase in immature red blood cells (reticulocytes). This observation proved crucial in objectively assessing the efficacy of subsequent dietary manipulations.

In planning his study of diet therapy, Minot joined forces with an equally motivated colleague to reap the benefit of a second observer. He chose well in selecting William P. Murphy, a young member of the medical staff at the Brigham. Murphy, seven years Minot's junior, came to Boston in 1922 to complete a residency at the Brigham. Like Minot, Murphy had a strong interest in hematology and in the judicious application of blood tests. Minot found in Murphy a like-minded zealot who combined extraordinary thoroughness both at the bedside and in the laboratory with the conviction that Whipple's results in dogs made liver the key component of their dietary regimen. The two investigators were meticulous in applying uniform protocols for the study of their patients. As their studies progressed, there was a considerable time lag before they shared results with each other. This informal "blinding" greatly enhanced confidence that their positive findings were reproducible.

In 1926, Minot and Murphy published a landmark paper reporting studies on forty-five PA patients treated at the Brigham with "a special diet" consisting of 120-240 grams of seared (nearly raw) liver per day along with 120 grams of beef or mutton and 250-500 grams of fresh fruit.[40] By the end of the first week of treatment, a striking increase in the number of reticulocytes was accompanied by a clear improvement in well-being. Within two to four months, the red blood cell count rose to normal levels in virtually all patients who were able to adhere to the prescribed diet. To achieve their stunning success, Minot and Murphy applied a heavy dose of constant coaxing to get their sick and often discouraged patients to adhere to their barely palatable diet. Moreover, by closely monitoring reticulocyte counts, Minot and Murphy were able to detect early hematologic responses that justified the continuation of the diet. A follow-up report on 150 patients contains a very convincing graph depicting the characteristic pattern of the reticulocyte response, peaking at about day seven after initiation of therapy.[41] Importantly no reticulocyte response was seen when liver or "liver pulp" was administered to either normal individuals or to those with other types of anemia. In collaboration with Edwin Cohn, a chemist at Harvard Medical School, Minot and Murphy were able to test the efficacy of purified liver extracts in patients with PA, a strategy that eventually led to the isolation of vitamin B_{12} (cobalamin). The subacute combined degeneration described by Russell et al., a white matter disease, usually begins in the posterior columns of the lower cervical and upper thoracic spinal cord and then spreads caudally and rostrally, ultimately producing similar changes in the white matter of the brain. It is characterized by a subacutely worsening

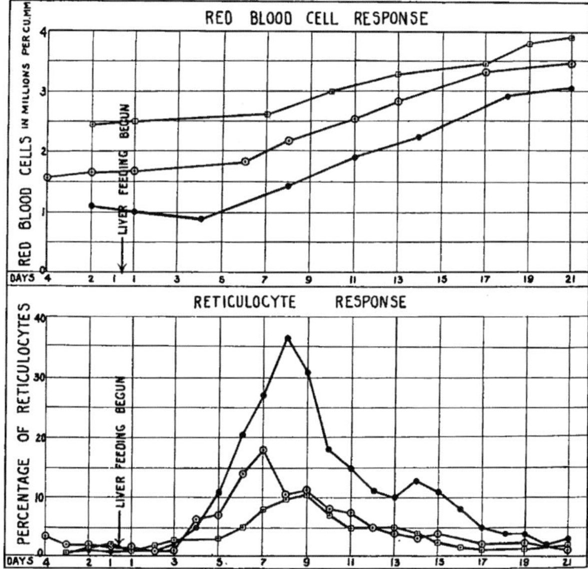

FIGURE 3-27 Changes in the bed blood cell and reticulocyte counts of three patients with PA after initiation of liver therapy. Note that the most anemic patient has the most robust erythropoietic response. Chart from Minot GR, Cohn EJ, Murphy WP, Lawson HA, "Treatment of pernicious anemia with liver extract: effects upon the production of immature and mature red blood cells." *American Journal of the Medical Sciences,* 1928;175:599-621, p. 584.

gait disorder, with spasticity and ataxia of the legs. In advanced cases, blindness, deafness, and dementia may ensue. Remarkably, the liver treatment of PA usually led to dramatic improvement of these neurological manifestations. The lesions were caused by a metabolic disorder that was potentially reversible. The discovery by Minot and Murphy is one of the best examples of what is now called translational research.

The 1934 Nobel Prize in Medicine or Physiology

On December 10, 1934, the Karolinska Institute in Stockholm awarded the Nobel Prize in Physiology or Medicine to Minot, Murphy and Whipple "in recognition of their discoveries respecting liver therapy in anaemias." Two days later, Murphy delivered the Nobel Lecture and in the concluding paragraph stated, "Rather than enlarge further upon the details and results of the treatment of pernicious anemia, I shall now present, with your permission, a motion picture which will illustrate many points more clearly than I could discuss them here." This film, made at the Brigham, described progress in optimizing the treatment of PA, emphasizing the superiority of parenteral liver extract to oral liver or its extract.

Aftermath

Fractionation of liver eventually led to the isolation and purification of vitamin B_{12} and its widespread use as a therapeutic agent. Understanding the mechanism underlying the assimilation of vitamin B_{12} began with William B. Castle's discovery of intrinsic factor and culminated in the cloning and characterization of this gastric protein along with others responsible for binding vitamin B_{12} and transporting it to cell receptors. Research by others worldwide has also led to the awarding of Nobel Prizes.

In 1928, George Minot succeeded Peabody as professor and head of the Harvard Medical Unit and Thorndike Memorial Laboratory at the BCH. He remained in that position until 1948, when he was succeeded by William Castle. Minot, who had insulin-dependent diabetes mellitus since 1921, died two years later. William Murphy published *Anemia in Practice: Pernicious Anemia* in 1939 and remained on staff at the Brigham as a senior associate in medicine and consultant in hematology until 1958. He died in 1985 at the age of ninety-seven.

This brief historical account conveys both the severity and significant prevalence of PA during the century, bookended by its initial description and the discovery of its cure. During the last several decades, there has been a marked decline in the incidence of PA as well as gastric cancer and peptic ulcer disease. This may result from the parallel decrease in infection of the gut by the bacterium *Helicobacter pylori*, the primary cause of gastric atrophy in aging individuals.

BIOGRAPHY

GUSTAVE J. DAMMIN, 1911-1991

Michael A. Gimbrone, Jr.

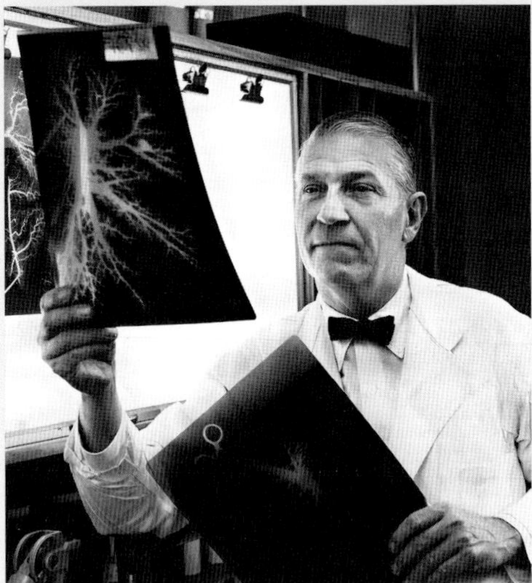

FIGURE 3-28 Gustave Dammin.

Gustave J. Dammin served as the pathologist-in-chief of the Peter Bent Brigham Hospital from 1952 to 1974. Dammin was born in the Bronx, New York, in 1911. He received his undergraduate and medical degrees from Cornell University, the latter in 1938. While in medical school, he became interested in infectious disease and did postgraduate study in parasitology and tropical medicine at the University of Havana, Cuba. His initial residency training was in internal medicine, first at Johns Hopkins and then at the Peter Bent Brigham Hospital under Soma Weiss (1940). He then began his training in pathology at Columbia, but soon was called to active duty as an Army medical laboratory officer. His assignments took him to Walter Reed Army Hospital, the Armed Forces Institute of Pathology, the Army's Caribbean area laboratory in Puerto Rico, and the India-Burma and European theatres. In these environments, he began a very productive career-long study of the epidemiology, pathophysiology, and pathology of acute diarrheal diseases, malaria, schistosomiasis, and hookworm disease, for which he was to receive international recognition. In 1946, he returned to academic pathology at Washington University of Medicine in St. Louis, where he rapidly rose through the ranks to become professor of pathology and pathologist-in-chief at the Barnes Hospital. He then was recruited here to the Peter Bent Brigham Hospital to serve as its pathologist-in-chief, succeeding William Councilman and Bert Wolbach. He laid the cornerstones for what was to become one of the major academic departments of pathology in the world.

In addition to his many contributions in the field of infectious disease and tropical health, Gus Dammin is known for the identification of the tick vector for Lyme disease. He was a key member of the team that first successfully accomplished the transplantation of a human kidney—which was recognized by a Nobel Prize, accepted on behalf of the team and this institution by Joseph Murray. A painting of this surgical event, including the figure of Dammin, is on permanent display at the Countway Library.

A young pathologist has written the following memory of his first encounter with Dammin:

> *I met him first in 1960, when he came to a research seminar I gave as a young faculty member at Harvard Medical School. I was working on pyelonephritis with the late Ed Kass and although I felt well prepared, the appearance of Dr. Dammin in the room was distinctly unsettling because he was an expert in both renal pathology and infectious disease. However, as I came to learn, I needn't have been perturbed because he gave a typical "Gus performance"—tall, handsome, very impressive in his white lab coat; he sat in the front row and listened attentively, took copious notes, and was the first to get up after I had finished. He made a few gracious remarks to put me at ease, asked an incisive question, and then explained why he asked it. Graciousness, helpfulness, and intense scientific curiosity marked his entire career.*

That young person was Ramzi Cotran, who was to become Dammin's successor as chair of the department.

OURGENES, OURHEALTH, OURCOMMUNITY

Nicole L. Mayard, Elizabeth W. Karlson, and Christine E. Seidman

OurGenes, OurHealth, OurCommunity is an innovative research initiative at the Brigham and Women's Hospital that aims to lead the future of biomedical research and transform the practice of medicine. Founded in 2007, OurGenes is collaborating with the Partners Biorepository for Medical Discovery to create a state-of-the-art tissue and data bank of genetic and health information from Brigham patients. The principal goals are to enable researchers to conduct studies on causes, prevention, and treatment of diseases. To achieve these goals, OurGenes integrates multiple data sets so that researchers can examine factors affecting human health, including genetics, environment, behavior and lifestyle, family history, and one's personal medical history. In so doing, investigators can uncover the relations of an individual's genetics and genomics, family history, and environment to the development of disease. Importantly, all genomic data in OurGenes samples remain permanently in bank, so that the value of OurGenes will expand over time. Ultimately, we anticipate that discoveries made using this unique resource will advance preventive personalized medicine.

Members of the Partners Biomedical Research Institute's Human Genetics Working Group conceived the OurGenes project. This committee envisioned creating a research project that would involve the Brigham's clinical faculty, who are expert in all areas of clinical medicine, a state-of-the-art electronic medical record, and a patient population that is committed to research to advance human health. With these resources, OurGenes' goals align closely with that of the hospital—to provide forward-looking compassionate clinical care, educate the next generation of physician scientists, and transform the future of health care through better understanding of the causes of disease and the factors that affect treatment responses. Christine Seidman and Elizabeth Karlson, members of the Brigham Research Oversight Committee's Genetics Working Group, are the co-leaders and principal investigators of OurGenes. Both are clinical research scientists. Seidman's lab uses genetic and genomic approaches to study the molecular basis of human cardiovascular disease, with particular focus on the cardiomyopathies and congenital heart defects. Karlson's group investigates the epidemiology and outcomes of rheumatic diseases and has identified genetic and environmental interactive determinants of risk for developing these debilitating illnesses.

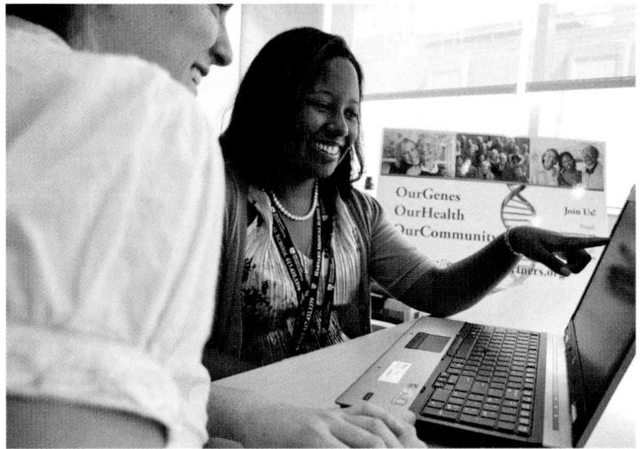

FIGURE 3-29 Senior Research Assistant Nicole Mayard Allen (right) explains the benefits of the grounbreaking OurGenes, OurHealth OurCommunity study to a potential participant.

OurGenes is invested in educating patients, physicians, and all Brigham healthcare professionals in both contemporary genetics and genomics and how to integrate this emerging science into clinical medicine. To achieve this goal, an OurGenes website has been created to define the vocabulary used by geneticists, identify opportunities and challenges of genetic research, and address its impact on personal, family, and social issues. The OurGenes team also participates in broader education programs, including National DNA Day, to expand outreach both at the Brigham and to the broader Boston community.

OurGenes, OurHealth, OurCommunity is one of seventeen large-scale population biorepositories worldwide. Although the goal of all biorepositories is to support future biomedical research and facilitate genome-wide association studies, each differs in the population targeted, the information and samples collected, and the use of the samples. OurGenes, unique in a number of aspects, seeks to enroll all Brigham patients, healthy or ill, into the biorepository. Having samples from patients with disease to compare with healthy control subjects is essential for identifying genetic determinants of health and thus ultimately to finding cures for diseases. OurGenes also gathers comprehensive health, behavioral, environmental, and family history data on all participants, thus facilitating diverse research on the multifaceted causes of health and disease. Finally, OurGenes obtains broad-based consent for the use of subjects' samples and information. Instead of limiting the areas of research, OurGenes plans to advance all fields that can improve human health. As an academic medical center, the Brigham has leveraged incredible collaborations among patients, physicians, and researchers to make this project possible.

Since the groundbreaking start of the acquisition of material from patients in July 2010, more than 5,000 patients have been enrolled in this research initiative. Although every Brigham patient aged eighteen and older is eligible for the OurGenes study, patients are approached as focused subgroups. Subjects were recruited initially at six participating pilot clinics: Rheumatology, Cardiology, Neurology, the Jen Center for Primary Care, the Fish Center for Women's Health, and the Maternal-Fetal Medicine department. Recruitment has since been expanded to additional outpatient clinics and will in the near future include high-throughput clinical locations such as the Emergency Department. The major efforts in recruiting and re-contacting subjects, maintaining and updating protocols, and obtaining approvals from the Partners Committee for the Protection of Human Subjects is carried out by Nicole Mayard, the OurGenes project manager, and a "small army" of research assistants. Prior to a scheduled, upcoming clinic visit, OurGenes research assistants mail eligible patients a letter from the principal investigators and the patient's physician, an OurGenes brochure, and an opt-out card. At the clinic visit, patients who do not opt out are engaged by a research assistant, who provides additional information and asks for participation. Patients who volunteer for the OurGenes project sign the consent form permitting researchers to link health information from their medical record over time with biomarker and genetic results, complete a brief health survey, and contribute a small sample of blood. Subjects are also asked (and almost always respond positively) if they are willing to be re-contacted for additional questioning or a follow-up blood draw if additional information is needed by a researcher. OurGenes keeps its consented patient population abreast of any revolutionary findings via an annual newsletter.

The issue of communicating the results of studies that are of clinical relevance to participating subjects was initially a source of considerable debate. One physician scientist has addressed this issue by distributing a survey to consented subjects about their interest in receiving genetic research results. The four-question survey assessed participants' interest in receiving personal research results, their perceived importance of receiving these research results, with whom they would discuss these research results, and what they want to be done with the research results when they die. Prior to this survey, the OurGenes protocol did not permit the return of any genetic research results, similar to other biorepositories. The overall response of subjects to the survey was an overwhelmingly positive support for the return of genetic research results that had immediate health consequences. Thus OurGenes worked with the Partners ethics committee to include the ability to return actionable research results to consented patients. All OurGenes subjects will now receive any research results that a team of expert physicians and scientists deem important to future health care. This incredible progression of the OurGenes project occurred because of an engaged patient community, a forward-thinking leadership, and an ethics committee that strongly considers patient rights as the first priority.

OurGenes, OurHealth, OurCommunity will continue to engage key clinicians and investigators Brigham-wide to build the biorepository and generate productive research. The name of this project summarizes its mission and future goals. OurGenes refers to the biobank of consented BWH patient samples linked to patients' longitudinal medical record, supplemented with family history and personal health data; OurHealth addresses the mission of improving health by accelerating fundamental discoveries and promoting clinical translation; and OurCommunity speaks to how the Brigham will use the results of this research to increase our understanding of genetics, ensure privacy, and engender collaborative relationships of members of our community.

POSTSCRIPT: BRIGHAM RESEARCH IN THE FUTURE

Joseph Loscalzo and Peter V. Tishler

Predicting that research to improve the treatment of patients with diseases that defy current therapeutics will be a major effort at the Brigham seems obvious. The research possibilities are infinite and beyond the scope of this essay, except for a few predictions. Surgical focus on organs that must be restored or replaced will continue, utilizing advanced and less invasive techniques, newer methods of creating immunological tolerance to grafts from unrelated individuals, and new tissues and organs created from stem cell research. Medical research additionally will focus increasingly on several relatively new endeavors. Further enrichment of the understanding and knowledge of our genetic underpinning has seemingly limitless possibilities in its application to medicine. Currently, several institutions worldwide, including the Brigham, are banking DNA samples from patients or other populations, and these samples can be used to delineate the correlations between physiologic or pathophysiologic parameters, however subtle, and genotype. Similarly, correlating genotype with efficacy or adverse effects of pharmacotherapy is potentially an efficient way of identifying newer therapeutic agents and applying them within the appropriate genetic milieu. The ultimate result, which is already gaining public recognition, is diagnostic and therapeutic personalized medicine. Whether this approach will extend the lifespan is uncertain, but that it will increase healthy living is likely.

A second new scientific endeavor at the Brigham and elsewhere is termed network medicine. This discipline stems from the fact that although the conventional scientific approach—experimental reductionism followed by inductive generalization—has been effective in understanding and advancing biomedicine, it is inconsistent with biological reality. Most biological systems respond to multiple inputs that vary simultaneously and can interact, that is, they are complex systems and thus require different experimental and analytical approaches to predict their behavior optimally. Systems biology is defined as the science of integrating genomic, proteomic, metabolomic, biochemical, cellular, physiological, and clinical data to create a network that predicts biological phenomena. Systems biology and network modeling can now be applied to human pathobiology, redefining human disease in its preclinical stage, and used for predicting disease prognosis and tailoring individualized therapies. The application of these systems principles to human disease defines the new field of network medicine. It will be an area of growing emphasis to Brigham investigators as they lead the way in creating novel approaches to understanding and treating the broad range of complex illnesses that plague our species.

PART 2: EVOLUTION OF CLINICAL CARE

VI. INTRODUCTION

THE EVOLUTION OF CLINICAL CARE

Peter Tishler

The Peter Bent Brigham Hospital opened in 1913 with a small but talented group of clinicians in surgery and medicine. The initial leaders, Harvey W. Cushing in surgery and Henry A. Christian in medicine, advocated that the Brigham patients receive both excellent care and observational research. Their major mission was to integrate new clinical and research findings, and by this to provide improved patient care. Cushing, an international leader in innovations in surgery, emphasized in parallel patient care and the education of his juniors. Because of his attention to detail, his operative results were substantially better than those of his peers, and he taught his techniques to his trainees, who ultimately gained positions of prominence. He recruited staff surgeons with similar philosophies and interests in patient care and teaching, including David Cheever, Elliott C. Cutler, John Homans, Francis C. Newton, and William C. Quinby. His development of the new field of neurosurgery was perhaps his greatest contribution. Christian, a leader in the creation of the hospital physically and administratively, provided the conditions in which the full-time staff physicians in his department delivered superb patient care and teaching while conducting research. Christian himself focused and wrote extensively, describing many clinical phenomena and their natural histories. He insisted that the workup of patients by members of his full-time and resident staff be meticulous, well recorded, and well communicated. His associates, including Joseph C. Aub, Reginald Fitz, George R. Minot, Cyrus C. Sturgis, and Francis Weld Peabody, were well known for integrating research findings into patient care. Clearly, these physicians were influential in establishing the Brigham as a site of modern, concerned patient care.

The tradition was continued by successors Elliott C. Cutler in Surgery (1932-1947) and Soma Weiss in Medicine (1939-1942). Cutler was a charismatic, enthusiastic individual of protean interests who was always teaching—at the bedside, in the operating room, and at numerous sessions with the house staff. His teaching emphasized providing the best care for the patient. A number of his trainees, including J. Engelbert Dunphy and Robert M. Zollinger, populated the United States as professors of surgery. Weiss was legendary in his clinical acumen and research productivity, and their integration at the bedside or in the classroom. He loved to see patients and to conduct bedside rounds, which were immensely popular. He exploited his acumen and personality to motivate trainees to provide the absolute best patient care. Although his tenure was short, his trainees (e.g., Eugene A. Stead, Jr., Charles A. Janeway) also became leaders in American medicine.

The beginnings of subspecialty training and certification began during the Cutler–Weiss era, although certainly some specialists, such as Samuel A. Levine and Harvey Cushing, had been in subspecialty practice earlier. Nonetheless, the clinical and investigational nature of the Brigham, as well as its bed census (Table 3-1), remained relatively constant. Although the hospital was established to and did provide care for indigent people, it also focused on patients who were admitted for research on specific pathophysiological processes. The medical demands of World War II ultimately fostered both further evolution of subspecialization and also a change in the basis of admissions to the Brigham and other academic hospitals. Larger numbers of students were graduated from medical schools and caring with minimal postgraduate training for wounded soldiers. As exemplified by Brigham trainee Joseph E. Murray, who was an intern for nine months in 1944 before serving in the military, these physicians learned from their military experiences

TABLE 3-1 The Brigham: Patient Load

		INPATIENTS			
YEAR	BEDS	ADMISSIONS	MEAN PATIENTS/DAY	OUTPATIENTS TOTAL VISITS	EMERGENCY ROOM VISITS
1914	225	2,843	135+	30,434	
1915	-	3,417	165+	36,523	
1927	-	4,607	216	60,671	
1935	247	4,422	187	77,728	
1938	-	4,584	192+	84,365	
1950	~300	5,169	208	48,360	
1963	311	7,930	248	50,957	14,528
1976	330	10,437	394	135,111	27,734
1982	698	28,201		131,830	28,583
1988	720	35,136	640	179,596	44,510
2009	777	46,432	713	396,000	59,323
2010	793	45,995	662	406,210	58,466

and returned to their postgraduate training with both additional expertise and preferences for specialization. The marked increase in governmental funding of medical research and training that began during the war continued, leading to further training opportunities for medical graduates. Similarly, therapies that were developed shortly before or during the war (e.g., penicillin, streptomycin) made the application of research findings to patient care ever more relevant.

This growth and impact of medicine and medical care that really began during the World War II era has continued unabated. For the Brigham, the postwar changes led to a marked increase in the number of staff physicians, who profited from the availability of liberal research funding and of patients to study. The major chiefs, Francis D. Moore (1948-1976) in surgery and George W. Thorn (1942-1972) in medicine, were both forceful, magnetic personalities who emphasized patient care while also creating large, patient-related, and patient-profitable research enterprises. Facilities for the intensive care of seriously ill patients were developed. New disciplines in both surgery (e.g., transplantation, cardiac surgery) and medicine (e.g., invasive cardiology, nephrology) reflected the continuing rise and influence on patient care of subspecialization. The integration of the Peter Bent Brigham with the Robert Breck Brigham Hospital (specializing in rheumatological and immunological diseases) and the Boston Hospital for Women (specializing in obstetrical and gynecological medicine) in the late 1970s created the most profound change in the nature of hospital admissions and in the number of hospital beds. Led by chiefs John A. Mannick, (1976-1994) and Eugene Braunwald, (1972-1996), the hospital was now a general hospital, doubled in bed size and in service to patients (Table 3-1). Both surgery and medicine embraced the growing spectrum of specialties, divisions, and clinical advances (e.g., minimally invasive surgery, new, and potent pharmacological therapies).

Today, primary care physicians provide the majority of care for individuals and populations. Even so, hospital growth continues. Patients are admitted solely for medical care and may secondarily participate in medical research. Admission is medical need-based. Socioeconomic status may reflect the number of individuals seeking medical attention at the Brigham, but it does not affect the decision to admit. The tradition of revered super clinicians remains.

SOCIAL AND ECONOMIC TRENDS SHAPING THE CONTEXT FOR LEADERSHIP IN CLINICAL CARE

Arnold M. Epstein and David W. Bates

Societal changes in the role of hospitals, availability of insurance coverage, growth of health technology, and the expanding role of the public sector shape the context for continuing excellence and leadership in clinical care at the Brigham and Women's Hospital now and into the future.

When the Peter Bent Brigham Hospital was founded in 1913, hospitals were most commonly independent institutions almost solely devoted to inpatient care. The services that hospitals provided differed from those offered today. Inpatient management focused on diagnosis, treatment, and convalescence, whereas today it is now common for patients to be discharged home under the guidance of a visiting nurse or to a rehabilitation facility where convalescence can be completed. In recent years, length of stay has decreased dramatically nationwide from an average of 7.8 days in 1970 to 4.9 days in 2009.[42] Today hospitals often provide both ambulatory as well as inpatient care. For example, ambulatory care in 1990 accounted for 23% of hospital revenue versus 42% in 2010.[43] Whereas once most hospitals were independent, today many are integrated horizontally as part of multihospital chains or affiliates and integrated vertically in partnership with ambulatory practices and long-term care institutions. The Brigham reflects all these developments with its affiliation to five other hospitals through Partners Healthcare and a Physician Organization with more than 1,650 doctors. All these trends seem likely to continue.

Another important factor setting the context for hospital care has been the spread of insurance. Health insurance was rare indeed early in the twentieth century. Private insurance did not emerge until the 1930s, and then in the form of the nonprofit Blue Cross and Blue Shield plans.[44] Commercial insurers began to follow suit, once it became clear that Blue Cross plans were viable. Between 1940 and 1960, the number of persons with private health insurance increased from approximately 20 million to 140 million. In more recent years, we have also seen the development of the public health insurance programs, Medicare and Medicaid. Adoption of "universal coverage" in Massachusetts has led to further expansion of coverage in the state, with the number of uninsured adults decreasing from 13% of the population in 2006 to approximately 6% in 2010.[45] The increased availability of insurance has reduced the Brigham's concern about bad debt from self-pay patients (the cost of free care provided by the hospital decreased from $47 million to $38 million between 2006 and 2011), but in turn has increased the importance of negotiations with private payers and meeting the regulatory requirements imposed by Medicare and Medicaid.

Changes in the insurance market have interacted with growth of new technology and more specialized care to alter the content of hospital care. Today 22% of the Brigham's revenue comes from caring for Medicare beneficiaries. Since 1983, Medicare has paid hospitals per case based on prospectively set prices related to the patient's "diagnosis-related group" (DRG). That mode of payment has provided incentives for hospitals to provide care as efficiently as possible, with ever shortening lengths of stay. Length of stay at the Brigham has decreased from 9.4 days in 1980 to 5.8 days in 2011. In the last thirty-five years, patents for pharmaceutical and surgical innovations have increased roughly six-fold, leading to more intensive care during shortened hospital stays and greater ambulatory services. It is not surprising that Medicare expenditures have increased by 9% annually in the last twenty-five years, certainly greater than the 5% annual increase in the gross domestic product.[46] Tertiary and quaternary care hospitals like the Brigham have led the way in these critically important advances.

The increasing outlays for Medicare coupled with the growing budget deficit have focused legislative attention on Medicare payments. The Patient Protection and Affordable Care Act, passed in 2010, includes multiple programs to address Medicare expenditures that will likely have a substantial impact on care and practice at the Brigham. These include the following:

- Financial incentives tied to achievement of quality metrics, also known as "value based purchasing"
- Financial incentives tied to adoption of certain forms of information technology
- Refusal to pay additional medical expenses for patients suffering avoidable complications
- Penalties for hospitals with high rates of readmission
- Incentives for hospitals and other providers to take payment for a bundled set of services around a hospital admission
- A program for accountable care organizations (ACOs), constellations of hospitals and physicians that will undertake care of a defined population and receive shared savings for achieving quality targets and lowering utilization below historical trends.

Of note, to be successful under the latter three programs—lowering readmissions, providing bundled services efficiently, and undertaking care for a defined population—requires effective management and close coordination between the hospital and an array of ambulatory and post-acute care providers. It is a change in orientation toward thinking about populations as opposed to the individual patients and a focus on care across the continuum rather than just in the hospital. The Brigham, with its closely affiliated physician organization, is well positioned to take on these challenges. As part of Partners Healthcare, it has volunteered to join thirty-one other organizations nationwide as one of the initial "Pioneer" ACOs.

The federal government is not alone in emphasizing cost control—all the private payers are joining in. For example, Blue Cross, the largest private insurer in Massachusetts, has initiated its own ACO-like program, called the Alternative Quality Contract. Like the federal program, it provides for shared savings with providers who meet quality targets and achieve cost control compared with historical trends. As of 2012, approximately 13% of the Brigham's revenue was related to capitation-like programs, a number that now seems likely to grow rapidly.

The Center for Medicare and Medicaid Services (CMS), which oversees Medicare, has not focused solely on cost control. Since the latter part of 2003, CMS has conducted a national program of publicly reported quality measures for hospitals. The program began with process indicators for acute myocardial infarction, pneumonia, and congestive heart failure, such as whether patients with congestive failure had an assessment of their left ventricular ejection fraction. Steadily the battery has expanded to include a broader array of process measures, risk-adjusted rates of mortality and readmission, patient reported outcomes, and safety measures. The Brigham has performed at a very high level. For example, in a current report issued online by the U.S. Department of Health and Human Services, the Brigham scored higher than the national average on thirteen of seventeen reported process measures for acute myocardial infarction, pneumonia, and congestive heart failure.[47] Reflecting these numbers, the *US News and World Report* has rated the Brigham among the top ten hospitals in the nation for four of the last five years. The Brigham also went 150 days without a catheter-related bloodstream infection, a statistic that was not even tracked until recently. Publicly reported quality measurement and accountability for quality of care is likely to be an important feature of our health care going forward.

To address external demands as well as to address internal needs to make care better, the Brigham has developed the Center for Clinical Excellence, which includes about thirty employees. They focus on areas ranging from performance improvement to quality, safety, efficiency, and satisfaction. In 2012, the hospital will have approximately $47 million at risk based on its performance in these areas, and that figure seems certain to increase.

When the Peter Bent Brigham Hospital was founded early in the twentieth century, health care was a cottage industry. Today the industry has become much more consolidated with large-scale payers and affiliated provider organizations. Hospitals are intimately involved in care that takes place outside their walls and is delivered by providers who may provide predominantly or only outpatient services. Large private payers and the federal government are likely to set the future context for hospital policy. With its Partners affiliation and closely allied staff, the Brigham seems well-positioned to meet the challenges going forward.

PATIENT SAFETY RESEARCH AT BRIGHAM AND WOMEN'S HOSPITAL

David W. Bates and Tejal K. Gandhi

The magnitude and scope of the problem of patient safety in health care has been recognized only since the 1990s. Many of the studies describing both how big the issue is inside and outside the hospital and how safety can be improved have come from Brigham and Women's Hospital.

The seminal 1991 Harvard Medical Practice Study, led in part by Troy Brennan and Howard Hiatt of the Brigham, demonstrated that injuries to patients caused by hospitalization were common and often preventable. Drug injuries, wound infections, and technical complications were the most frequent types of injuries. This study served as a backdrop for the Institute of Medicine's formative report, "To Err Is Human: Building a Safer Health System," which brought the problem of patient safety into the public eye in 2000. Following this study, David W. Bates and Lucian L. Leape formed the Adverse Drug Event Prevention Study Group to evaluate and reduce the incidence of adverse drug events in academic hospitals. This Study Group brought together multiple disciplines, including physicians, pharmacists, and nurses, which has been a key to its success. The Brigham's William W. Churchill, executive director of the pharmacy, and Mairead Hickey, director of nursing research and of outcome measurement, played important roles in the Study Group's activities. It found that 28% of adverse drug events were preventable, that most of the errors occurred at the ordering stage, and that wrong dosages were a major problem. Another study determined that the mean national cost for each injury was $2,500 and $4 billion annually, thus motivating hospitals to invest in adverse drug event prevention. Subsequently, the Study Group investigated a method of potentially improving medication safety. Using computerized physician order entry and a clinical team intervention, it found that computerizing ordering reduced the rate of serious medication errors by 55%, even with limited decision support. This was a landmark study that has influenced the national push toward the use of computerized order entry. Indeed, computerized order entry has been identified by a coalition of the nation's largest employers, including General Electric and General Motors (the Leapfrog Group) as one of three changes that most improve safety in hospitals. The following year (1999), the Study Group determined that including pharmacists in rounds in the hospital intensive care unit with resident physicians, attending physicians, and nurses reduced the rate of harm dramatically.

Later studies addressed specific populations and different aspects of patient safety. A study in the pediatric inpatient setting demonstrated that the rate of potentially adverse drug events was three times higher in this setting than in comparable adult settings. Adverse drug events occurred most frequently in neonates, with the most common error being medication dosing. Another study reported that adverse events occurring after discharge from an adult medical service occurred in nearly 20% of discharged patients, two-thirds of which were drug-related. In community-dwelling primary care patients in Boston, Gandhi et al. found that 25% had experienced one or more adverse drug events. Of these adverse drug events, 20% were preventable. The medications most frequently involved in adverse events included drugs for depression, high blood pressure, and arthritis. To assess the impact of fatigue on error rates, a study compared medical errors made by first-year residents on different work schedules. Interns working traditional hours (80-100 hours weekly) made 36% more serious medical errors than those in the intervention group, who worked fewer hours. This study has had a major impact on national regulations of resident work hours. The causes of missing or delayed diagnoses were investigated by Gandhi et al., using malpractice claims as the primary data source. Errors in judgment, impaired memory or vigilance, handoffs, and patient-related factors contributed to the majority of missed diagnoses. These primary causes led to failures to order appropriate diagnostic tests, create

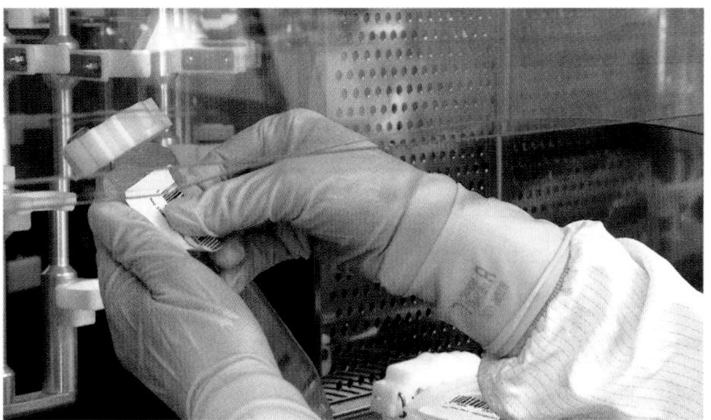

FIGURE 3-30 Barcode placement.

proper follow-up plans, obtain accurate histories and physicals, and correctly interpret tests.

More recently, a series of evaluations of surgical safety have been carried out by Atul Gawande and his colleagues. Their major innovation was the development of a checklist, which must be completed with total agreement by the surgical team in the operating room before surgery. The impact of this checklist was evaluated in patients undergoing noncardiac surgery at eight hospitals worldwide. Using the checklist decreased the death rate from 1.5% to 0.8% and inpatient complications from 11% to 7%. Although all sites experienced significant reduction in overall rates of inpatient complications, the rates of death at low-income sites fell by more than 50%! This study has lead to worldwide adoption of the World Health Organization surgical checklist.

The impact of bar coding, which has not been widely used in medicine, has been assessed by Poon and colleagues, who carried out a study of the impact

TABLE 3-2 Timeline of Selected Key Patient Safety Research Studies from BWH

YEAR	AREA COVERED	MAIN FINDINGS
1991	Adverse events in hospitalized patients	Adverse events are common and often preventable
1995	Adverse drug events (ADEs) in hospitalized adults	Injuries caused by drugs are common and often preventable
1997	Costs of ADEs in hospitalized adults	Costs are $2,500 per drug injury
1998	Computerized Physician Order Entry and serious medication errors	Computerizing ordering greatly improves medication safety
1999	Pharmacist intervention in physician rounds	Pharmacist rounding improves medication safety
1999	"To Err Is Human" report released by the Institute of Medicine	Patients are injured regularly by the care they receive, and much of this can be prevented with safer systems
2001	Inpatient pediatric medication error study	Many serious medication errors occur in pediatrics, especially in neonates
2003	Postdischarge adverse events	Nearly 20% of discharged patients suffer an injury after discharge
2004	Work hours	First-year residents made 36% more serious medical errors than a group with fewer work hours
2005	Tests pending at discharge	A tenth of patients discharged from hospital with pending results have results that could change management
2006	Impact of bar coding in the pharmacy	Bar coding reduces the error rate in the pharmacy
2007	Missed or delayed diagnoses in outpatients	Errors in judgment, memory, vigilance and handoffs contributed to many missed diagnoses
2009	Safe surgical checklist	Use of a checklist in the operating room improved outcomes worldwide
2010	Bar coding and eMAR at the point of care	Bar coding of drugs improves safety of administering drugs by about half

of the Brigham's pairing its bar code technology with an electronic medication administration record to track what medications had been given. Strikingly, rates of medication administration error were reduced by 41% and of potential adverse events by 51% . This study is likely to advance the adoption of bar code technology worldwide.

The last twenty years have demonstrated that injuries caused by medical care are a leading cause of death and disability, that they are expensive, and that much can be done to prevent them, both inside and outside the hospital. Many of these studies were carried out by investigators linked to the Center for Patient Safety Research and Practice and the Division of General Medicine at the Brigham, which have played an internationally important leadership role in patient safety research, especially in medication safety, work hours, and surgical safety.[48]

NURSING RESEARCH AND SCHOLARSHIP

Patricia C. Dykes, Patrice Nicholas, Jackie Somerville, and Mary Lou Etheredge

The foundation for nursing research at Brigham and Women's Hospital dates from Carrie Hall, who joined the nascent Peter Bent Brigham Hospital in 1912 as head of the School of Nursing and superintendent of nursing. Today, nurses conduct research to both improve patient care and advance nursing and medical science. The Department of Nursing has several signature research programs, well-supported through the generosity of major benefactors. Selected investigators and their research programs that have brought the institution recognition and advanced the profession are highlighted herein.

Anne Bane is the director of Clinical Systems Innovations and a national leader in patient safety. For nearly a decade, Bane has worked with interdisciplinary team members to develop and implement an electronic Medication Administration Record with bar code scanning (eMAR) and to study its impact on nursing function and patient care. Initially, she and her research team documented nurses' satisfaction with the new eMAR.[49] The use of eMAR also led to an increase, albeit modest, in the time nurses spent providing direct patient care.[50] The team has also studied the impact of bar code technology on the number of medication errors, and found a 41% reduction in non-timing errors.[51]

Patricia C. Dykes is a scientist in the Haley Nurse Scientist Program, established by Steven and Kathleen Haley in 2009 to advance the care of patients and families through the mentorship of nurse researchers. In this role she mentors clinical nurses who conduct nursing, informatics, and patient safety research. Dykes and her team were funded by the Robert Wood Johnson Foundation to develop a fall prevention toolkit, a program that leverages health information technology to improve fall prevention communication among all care team members, patients, and family caregivers. They found that the toolkit reduces falls significantly in acute care hospitals.[52] They have expanded this research and are currently studying the use of technology to provide essential information to care team members, including patients and family caregivers, for safe patient care.[53] Dykes has received the prestigious 2012 Nurse.com Nursing Spectrum National Excellence Award for Advancing and Leading the Profession.

Linda A. Evans, a perioperative nurse with more than thirty years of experience in clinical practice, education, and research, is currently developing an investigative program dealing with facial transplantation.[54] Evans has led a qualitative study, based on earlier ethical consideration by former surgical chief Francis D. Moore,[55] to explore the ethical acceptability of the facial transplantation procedure to healthcare team members who participated in early procedures. The participants believed that the

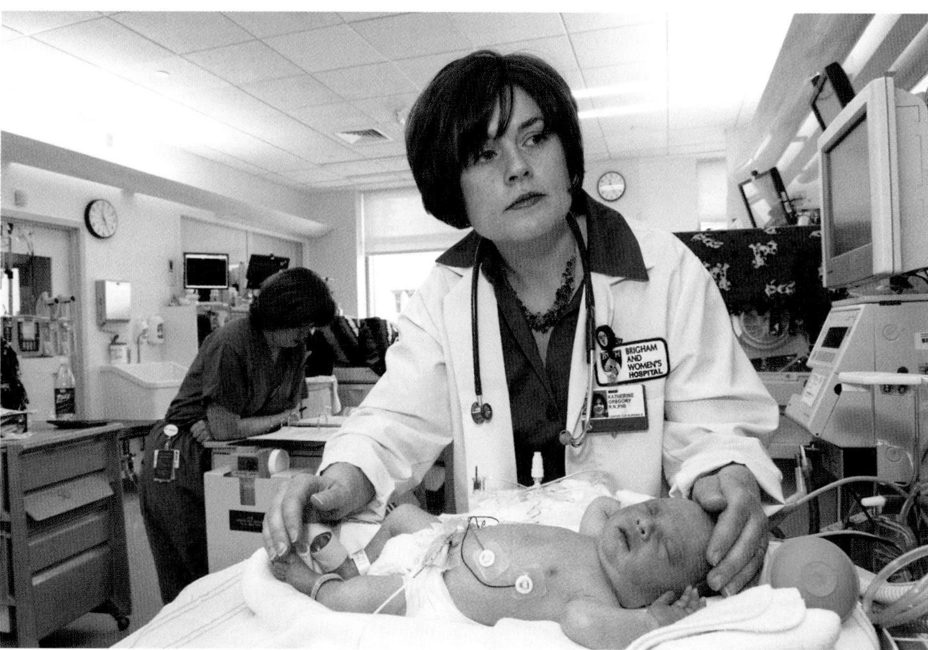

FIGURE 3-31 Katherine Gregory with infant.

risk-benefit ratio of facial transplantation favored proceeding with the surgery, expressed personal fulfillment as a result of involvement in the extraordinary transformation of a human being's life, and documented the highly effective team work, esprit de corps, and superior leadership.

Katherine Gregory is a neonatal intensive care nurse and a Haley Nurse Scientist. Collaborating with clinical nurses, she focuses her research on disease prediction strategies, nutrition, growth, and development of preterm infants. Her current investigation aims to identify biomarkers of necrotizing enterocolitis, a gastrointestinal disease common to premature infants, and the relationship of the microbiome (all microbes, their genes, and environmental interactions) to prematurity and development of this disease.[56] She intends her research findings to assist in early identification of infants at risk of this disease and to lead to treatment interventions.

Ann C. Hurley, a senior nurse scientist emerita in the Center for Nursing Excellence, has had an extensive career in healthcare research at the Brigham and the Veterans Administration. Hurley has mentored nurses while publishing on a wide range of topics, including Alzheimer disease.[57] In recent years, she has mentored a new generation of nurse researchers in developing instruments to measure the impact of health information technology, medical error recovery, and fall prevention nursing self-efficacy.[58]

Lichuan Ye, a Haley Nurse Scientist, focuses her research on understanding the experience of sleep, sleep disturbing factors, and perceptions of the influence of sleep on healing in the context of inpatient hospitalization.[59] Her findings will lay a foundation to develop strategies to improve sleep in the hospital. In 2011, Ye launched the Sleep Interest Group, including bedside nurses from various clinical departments, whose goal is to promote sleep in patient populations. In addition to mentoring these nurses as they conduct research, Ye works with them on a campaign to promote sleep for patients in the hospital.

Patrice Nicholas is director of Global Health and Academic Partnerships in both the Center for Nursing Excellence and the Department of Medicine's Division of Global Health Equity. Nicholas investigates symptoms and their effects on quality of life in patients with HIV/AIDS and chronic illness, with a primary focus on painful sensory neuropathy and its symptom management. She is a member of the International HIV/AIDS Nursing Research Network and, with other members, has conducted numerous research studies on adherence to anti-HIV medications[60] and to anti-tuberculosis medications,[61] and symptom management in HIV/AIDS.[62]

Mary Lou Etheredge is executive director for Nursing Practice Development and interim executive director of the Center for Nursing Excellence. Her research at the Brigham, entitled *Finding and Defining the Good*, is a qualitative study documenting the characteristics of excellent nursing care, as described by nurses known for giving excellent care. This study has provided the framework for department-wide change.

Jackie Somerville, chief nurse and senior vice-president for Patient Care Services, studies patients' perceptions of feeling known by their nurses. Somerville's doctoral dissertation described the development of an instrument for quantitative psychometric analysis, called the Patients' Perception of Feeling Known by Their Nurses (PPFKN) Scale. Her first qualitative study of patients who were known by their nurses during an acute, surgical admission yielded four findings. The patients felt recognized as unique human beings, beyond their reasons for hospitalization; had a meaningful, mutual and personal connection with their nurses; felt safe (e.g., their nurses "had their backs"); and were empowered by their nurses to participate in their care. These findings were used to guide the development of the reliable and valid forty-eight-item PPFKN Scale, which is currently being utilized in replication studies in the Department of Nursing.

Annie Lewis-O'Connor is director for nursing practice in the Connors Center for Women and Newborns. Her research program is focused on violence against women, specifically intimate partner violence and sexual assault . Her main objective is focused on the intersection of health and violence, and the response of the healthcare system to violence. She has served as a co-investigator on grants funded by the National Institutes of Health and National Institute of Justice.

Our goal as BWH nurses is to advance the state of nursing science, in service to our patients and families. In 2012, we proudly launched a Doctoral Nurse Forum, a think-tank for doctorally prepared nurses who come together to share their research and advance the state of nursing science at the Brigham. We look forward to launching a Nursing Research Committee, whose purpose will be to engage clinical nurses in critiquing evidence and advancing its application at the bedside.

THE BRIGHAM EMERGENCY DEPARTMENT

J. Stephen Bohan and Katherine Wei

From its opening on May 21, 1913, the Peter Bent Brigham's Out-Door Department, as it was called, was available from 6:00 am to 8:00 pm daily. Individuals were evaluated as either medical or surgical patients, a practice that was maintained until 1994. By 1916, a major increase in patient visits and overcrowding became major challenges that have persisted to the present day. Patient care in the Out-Door Department was provided by trainees in medicine and surgery, without supervision by qualified attending physicians. These trainees worked long hours and provided marginal care, provoking Henry A. Christian to lament in 1921 that "their...work is makeshift, not satisfactory... and [using them] should be abandoned as soon as possible."[63] He presciently suggested making the Out-Door Department a "diagnostic machine...one which is not subdivided into services...but one in which all work with the common end of diagnosis."[64]

In 1942, a generous benefactor funded the enlargement and renovation of the newly renamed Emergency Ward. This new ward (renamed the Emergency Department in 1957 and Emergency Service in 1961) had six beds and a central nursing station. Despite being "staffed" twenty-four hours daily by residents,

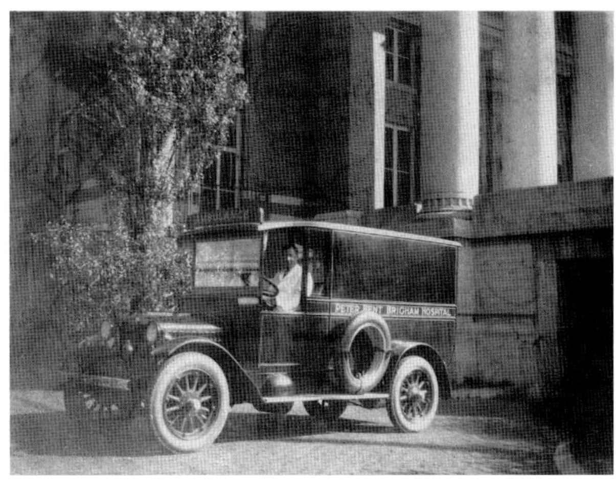

FIGURE 3-32 Peter Bent Brigham Hospital ambulance, 1924.

the unit was neither open for twenty-four hours nor supervised by qualified attending physicians. Patients seeking care at night rang a bell at the Emergency Department entry. This was answered by the switchboard operator, who determined which resident—medical or surgical—to summon. The number of patient visits to the ward doubled from 1953 to 1957, prompting the director of the Out-Patient Department, Roe E. Wells, to advocate enlarging the Emergency Department. In 1960, frustrated by inaction, surgeon-in-chief Francis D. Moore declared that the department should be tripled in size, to serve as "a haven for the acutely ill, a resort for those who cannot find a doctor at night, a place for special treatments and small operations...consultative diagnosis and special X-ray examinations, [and] where the severe emergencies of surgical illness and trauma may begin their definitive treatment."[65]

In 1965, the Board of Trustees authorized the construction of "an up-to-date, beautiful, absolutely necessary new Emergency Service,"[66] intended to "eliminate a primitive emergency set-up that is more of a barrier than an entrance to the Hospital."[67] A building to accommodate a new Emergency Service was constructed in the courtyard in front of the Administration Building. The new facility opened in 1967, preparing the hospital for the influences of Medicare and Medicaid, both of which encouraged "diagnostic work to be done as an outpatient rather than in the Hospital." However, modern facilities brought modern problems, and the chief of radiology, Herbert L. Abrams, complained in 1969 that "Virtually every patient who enters the emergency room with a superficial scalp laceration is subjected to 'a complete skull series'.... Every pain...now requires a radiologic examination with the malpractice lawyer looking over the physician's shoulder. The question might well be asked as to whether exposing patients to multiple x-rays unnecessarily is not equally in the category of malpractice."[68]

In 1971, the Department of Medicine opened a new "Holding Unit" adjacent to the Emergency Service to reduce the number of admissions to inpatient units. Certain patients, particularly those with equivocal manifestations, were admitted to this ten-bed unit for maximally seventy-two hours, after which inpatient admission was mandatory. Also in 1971, the Emergency Service incorporated a General Practice Unit for patients with "urgent but not truly emergent complaints." Additionally, service leaders, recognizing the need for twenty-four-hour coverage for laboratory studies and X-rays, made these resources available.

Throughout the 1980s, the Emergency Service was run by residents, loosely overseen by a small cadre of attending physicians with variable backgrounds, usually in internal medicine. A desire to improve patient care and outcomes for high-risk patients with acute, severe illness or injury pointed toward adopting the well-established national model of specialist emergency physicians. Adopting this great advance in the care of emergency patients, in 1993 Brigham and Women's Hospital created the Department of Emergency Medicine. Ron M. Walls, then the chair of a new department of emergency medicine at the Vancouver General Hospital, was appointed the first leader.

Walls, an expert in resuscitation and emergency airway management, quickly set about to establish national leadership in Emergency Medicine. He led the most extensive redesign of the department and its functions, partnering with nursing leaders and newly recruited specialist emergency physicians to re-engineer virtually every aspect of emergency care. The new forty-two bed department included a unit for patients with every conceivable acute emergency and a ten-bed Observation Unit, directed by J. Stephen Bohan, for complex diagnostic evaluation and treatment. For the first time, specialist emergency physicians directly oversaw the care of each patient, who was triaged according to acuity and immediacy of need. The first residency in emergency medicine at a Harvard hospital, led initially by Richard E. Wolfe, was established in 1996 in partnership with Massachusetts General Hospital. Subsequently, the Harvard Affiliated Emergency Medicine Residency expanded to include the Boston Children's and the Mount Auburn Hospitals. Fifteen residents trained in each of the four postgraduate training years, becoming board certified in emergency medicine.

In addition to the Observation Unit, additional landmark innovations by other clinical services transformed clinical practice in the Emergency Department. Under the guidance of M. Stephen Ledbetter, the Radiology Department established a Division of Emergency Radiology. A specialized emergency psychiatry consult service was created and staffed by fully qualified psychiatrists. Patient care is supported by on-site social services, pharmacists, and medical interpreters. With new nursing leaders, the nursing staff advanced greatly in expertise and professional development. Nurses achieved certification as certified emergency nurses and in courses in trauma and advanced cardiac life support, which they then taught to national and international audiences. Introducing these new clinical models and establishing robust emergency medicine teaching and training programs for medical students and residents were accompanied by exponential growth in clinical and population-based research. Richard C. Wuerz partnered with Nursing Educator Nicola Gilboy to develop an entirely new emergency triage system, the Emergency Severity Index, which was subsequently adopted by the U.S. Department of Health and Human Services Agency for Healthcare Research and Quality as the national standard triage system. Wuerz died unexpectedly in 2000 at age thirty-nine, and a memorial research fund bearing his name has seeded the careers of several widely published young scientists. Through a series of innovative internal grants, the department fostered research

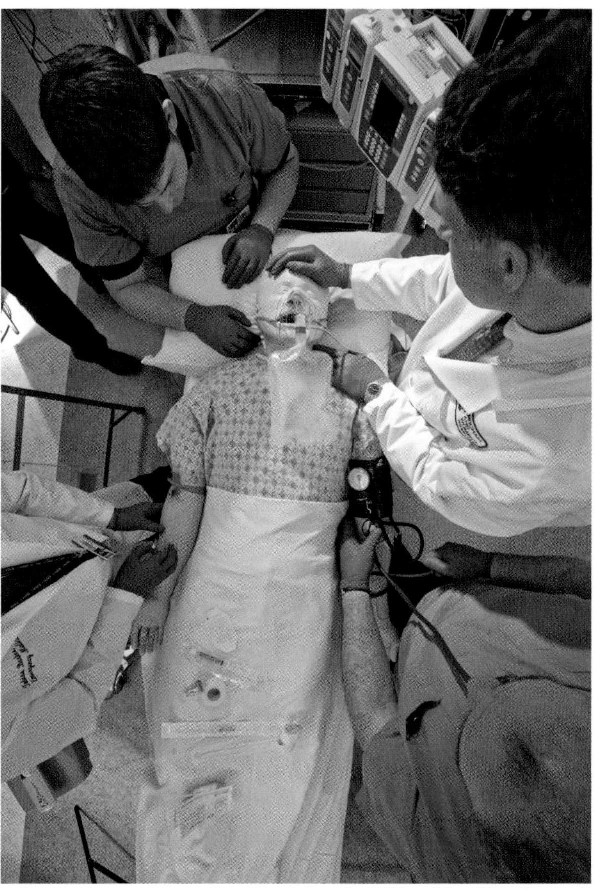

FIGURE 3-33 Simulation training.

development and soon was supporting externally funded projects. Research productivity grew, with investigators focusing on emergency resuscitation, infectious disease, shock, emergency ultrasound, cardiac disease, health services, and health policy.

In 2004, the department established the Neil and Elise Wallace STRATUS Center for Medical Simulation, a high-fidelity simulation center that enriched the training of emergency medicine residents and students. Led by Charles Pozner, STRATUS expanded in 2008 to incorporate training in surgical and medical procedures, competency assessment, and research. In the same year, Michael J. VanRooyen became the first chief of the new Division of International Health and Humanitarian Programs. The division became the seed for the interfaculty Harvard University Humanitarian Initiative, led by VanRooyen and Jennifer Leaning, another early department member. Under VanRooyen's leadership, the division grew rapidly to encompass seven faculty researchers and soon was recognized as the leading academic and research unit of its type in the world. In 2006, Walls became a professor at Harvard Medical School, the first in the specialty of emergency medicine; VanRooyen became the Brigham's second emergency medicine professor in 2012. Also in 2012, the department created the Division of Health Policy Translation, under the leadership of Jeremiah D. Schuur, and the Division of Emergency Ultrasound, under the leadership of Michael B. Stone.

In 2009, with volume having grown from 36,000 to almost 60,000 visits over the fourteen years since its previous renovation, the department faced crushing patient demand and a shortage of space, beds, and resources. With a major expansion derailed by the economic downturn, department leadership committed to a complete re-engineering of every aspect of operations, process, and staff roles. After an exhaustive journey of lean process redesign, led by Clinical Director Joshua M. Kosowsky and Nursing Director Heidi Crim, the department launched its new process of care. The new space and system debuted in May 2011, with its remarkable success particularly manifest in three crucial facts: the median time from patient arrival to initial physician evaluation fell from over an hour to about ten minutes, length of stay decreased by an astounding 20%, and patient satisfaction rose from the 30th percentile nationally to the 99th percentile. Not yet satisfied, department leaders embarked on an ambitious team training program to ensure that all staff worked harmoniously to provide superior patient care and reduce the opportunity for medical error.

The Brigham's Department of Emergency Medicine is the fruition of many ideas of its founders regarding research, efficiency, service to the community, patient-centeredness, teaching, clinical practice, and partnership with nursing and social services. Although we have greater resources than were available to our founders, and our technology and administration are more advanced, we can only hope that our vision is as prescient as was theirs as we plan for the future.

THE HISTORY OF PRIMARY CARE

Lori Wiviott Tishler

Although the Brigham has always had outpatient medicine, the term "primary care" as we think of it today became part of the hospital's core services in the second half of the last century. As we look to the past, we find that many of the challenges and joys of generalist medicine remain unchanged.

The ambulatory arm of the hospital was called the Out-Door Department until 1940. It served mainly as a conduit for admitting the sickest (or most interesting) patients to the hospital wards. It was not until the 1920s that the Out-Door Department added the concept of appointments, followed by ancillary support such as laboratory staff and nursing, and then by a social worker who made home visits, clearly avant-garde for this era in academic medicine. In these early years, those responsible for the Out-Door Department struggled with issues that contemporary physicians would find familiar: space, salaries for physicians, and continuity of care. Acting Chief of Medicine Cyrus C. Sturgis, in the hospital's annual report of 1926, commented thoughtfully on the role and stature of out-door medicine:

> *In the evolution and development of hospitals in this country, it is an obvious fact that the facilities for the care of ambulatory patients have been the last to receive proper attention. Most of the interest, teaching, and research have centered about the hospital wards, and it has been there that the better trained and more experienced clinicians with higher hospital and academic rank, have devoted their time, thought and efforts.*[69]

He urged that outpatient care at the Brigham be considered on a par with inpatient medicine. Over the next twenty years, the number of patients grew and the name changed, but the department did not provide continuity of care. Its status remained secondary for most physicians, for whom "real work" was on the wards.

The 1960s heralded much change for both the United States and academic medicine. Medicare was born. The number of women physicians began to increase. Community health centers and health maintenance organizations (HMOs) dotted the landscape of Boston. Healthcare planners now thought about maintaining health in addition to treating disease, and physicians planned for this expanded role. Primary care, as we think of it today, really began in this decade.

In 1961, a major reorganization of the outpatient department occurred. Lamenting the decline of the family doctor, hospital Director F. Lloyd Mussels wrote in his annual report that "a whole new concept of patient care was evolved in the clinic." The leadership of the clinic created a new policy whereby "each patient is under the guidance of one physician, who is responsible for the patient's total care."[70] This was the first time that patients in a Brigham clinic had continuity of care by a specific physician. Several years later, George W. Thorn described the changes in the clinic and the support given to its physicians as "the envy" of comparable institutions.[71] Patients came in great numbers. Legislative change helped the public to be "freed of economic constraints in the purchase of medical services." The Brigham Clinic provided comprehensive support for patients in a comfortable setting. The governmental changes in the 1960s that made health care more accessible led to the development of two Brigham-sponsored community health centers: Brookside and Southern Jamaica Plain Community Health Centers, which opened their doors in the early 1970s. The Brigham also initiated comprehensive adult services at the Martha Eliot Health Center and created a Spanish Clinic at the hospital. In keeping with the Brigham's commitment to research, the Office of Ambulatory Research was founded in 1967, with Robert C. Buxbaum as its first director.

Concurrently with these novel developments outside the hospital, the medical clinic inside the hospital was struggling to define its role. Members of the medical clinic questioned the need for in-house primary care when there were so many new community settings. Should primary care be internal to the hospital, provided by affiliates outside the hospital, or both? The answer soon became clear as numbers of patients in health centers, Harvard Community Health Plan (HCHP), and the community clinics soared. Clearly the public felt that primary care was a good idea, and a significant subset preferred to get care at the hospital.

Eugene Braunwald, who became chief of medicine in 1972, felt strongly that those house officers who ultimately practice as generalist physicians should be specifically trained for this central role. A Brigham-based primary care residency track began. The Brigham affiliated with the HCHP, the first Boston-based HMO, and an HCHP-based primary care training program was also initiated. The Brigham Medical Clinics made a new leap with the opening of an additional primary care setting, the Pearl Primary Care Center. Staffed by two recent graduates of the Brigham and Women's Hospital (BWH) residency, Arthur J. Siegel and John Witherspoon, the Pearl Center was a full-time primary care practice committed to team-based continuity of care and provider-patient relationships. After only three years, in 1973, the Pearl Center accounted for a third of the general medical visits in ambulatory services. An article written about the Pearl Center experiment reported greater patient satisfaction and relatively improved outcomes compared with the general medical clinic. Plans began to exploit this model to implement a larger primary care center. In 1975, H. Richard Nesson became the first division chief of General Medicine and Primary Care. One of the first divisions of its type in the country, its mission was "to look at the patient as a whole" and develop a comprehensive program of patient care, education, and research. A new primary care center opened in 1977 following the Pearl Center model. As primary care physician Anthony L. Komaroff has explained, "Dick Nesson spotted talent." Although the research mission was growing, he ensured a "shared responsibility" to teach and care for patients.[72]

In 1982, Nesson became president of the Brigham and Komaroff became division chief of General Medicine and Primary Care, remaining in that position until 1997. The number of primary care faculty members increased nearly ten-fold. Komaroff ensured protection of clinician-educators, making the unit a cohesive place for generalists and leaning away from the exclusive "up or out" policies of most academic divisions. From 1982 to 1997, the division produced more than 1,000 peer-reviewed publications covering many generalist disciplines. During this period, primary care and general medicine gained what Komaroff calls "intellectual legitimacy." Although specialists inside and outside the institution viewed generalist medicine with some skepticism, both Dick Nesson and Marshall A. Wolf, director of the Housestaff Program, proudly identified themselves as generalists. Primary care practice became a focus of continuous improvement, and medical directors such as Phyllis Jen led the Brigham charge to improve quality of life for both patients and physicians.

New opportunities and challenges faced BWH primary care and general medicine in the 1990s as the hospital grew and developed offsite practices in Brookline, Newton Corner, Norwood, and elsewhere. Primary care suffered growing pains as it struggled to find a shared sense of belonging for all members of the division, intensifying what the current vice chair of Medicine for Primary Care, Joseph P. Frolkis, calls "the town-gown divide."

Today, David W. Bates, the current division chief, leads a huge research program that has moved rapidly to involve a team of researchers using the latest techniques to improve knowledge, care, and practice. The program highlights, but is not limited to, medical informatics and patient safety. The clinical program, lead by Frolkis, encompasses fourteen primary care practices, including the Phyllis Jen Center on the hospital's Nesson Pike, the neighborhood health centers, and more distant centers ranging west to Newton and south to Foxborough. It is a time of tremendous growth for primary care practices as they work toward a five-year goal of transforming into Patient-Centered Medical Homes, a care model aimed at strengthening coordination of team-based care. Leveraging the art of patient care with both data provided by research and the tools of business and information technology, these practices aim to

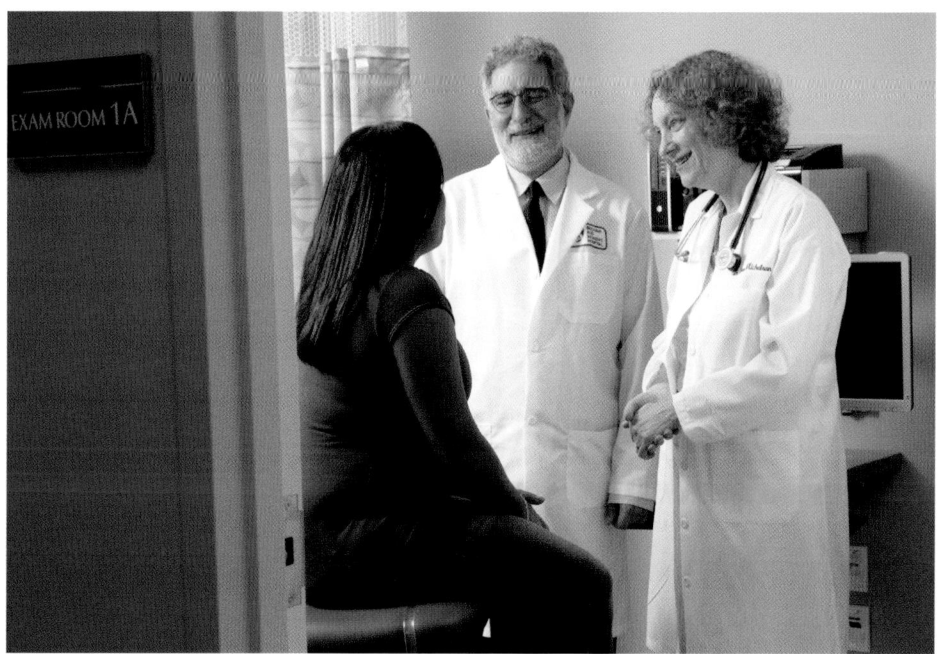

FIGURE 3-34 Mitchell Medow and Donna Michelson talk with a patient.

provide the best care possible for the most people in the right setting at the right time. We have come far in primary care and yet we struggle today with the same core issues: compensation, space, and the roles of generalist care and research in an academic center. Most primary care doctors, however, would argue that the rewards of caring for our patients and communities outweigh all the challenges!

BIOGRAPHY

PHYLLIS JEN, 1948-2009

Thomas H. Lee, Jr.

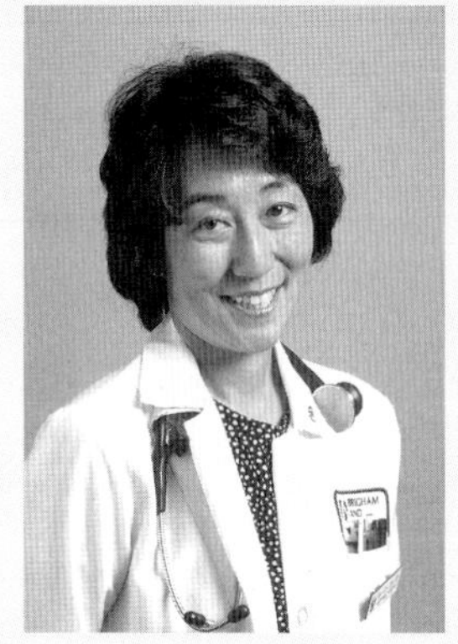

FIGURE 3-35 Phyllis Jen.

The portrait of Phyllis Jen that hangs on the Brigham Pike outside the primary care center may one day seem just part of the background, one of many details that collectively convey the message that the Brigham is a great institution with a rich history. But that portrait and the woman it portrays still give people reason to pause. In preparation for this essay, I twice stood in the Pike to study it. Both times, every minute or so, a clinician, administrator, or patient would slow down and stop, look at the painting, and say something like, "I still cannot believe it," or "She was amazing, wasn't she?"

In a Brigham and Women's career that spanned more than thirty years, Phyllis Jen provided an affirmative answer to the question of whether an institution can love a person. Her death in an automobile accident on April 21, 2009, precipitated an outpouring of grief that will be difficult to understand for future generations of Brigham and Women's Hospital personnel. That grief was followed by institutional and individual efforts to honor her memory—none of which could adequately fill the hole that she left.

Phyllis was the daughter of Chinese immigrants, one of four sisters. She was born in Cambridge, Massachusetts, and raised in Silver Spring, Maryland. During the turbulent 1960s and within that brilliant family, Phyllis developed a set of sensibilities that integrated traditional Chinese values, fierce idealism, and deep emotional intelligence with a sense of humor that included appreciation of both irony as well as practical jokes. She made her way to Boston medicine slowly. After her undergraduate years at Brown University, she worked at the National Institutes of Health as a laboratory technician and then attended medical school at the State University of New York's Downstate Medical Center in Brooklyn. During those years, she met her future husband, Robert Schlauch, who would become a respected Boston psychiatrist. Phyllis went to Stanford for her internship in internal medicine, but then came to Boston in 1976 for the rest of her training and to marry Schlauch. They bought a home in Needham on the bank of the Charles River, and it quickly became a social hub for an enlarging subset of Brigham physicians and trainees.

After the completion of her residency in 1978, Phyllis practiced primary care, becoming the medical director of Brigham Internal Medicine Associates (BIMA) in 1982. It was an era in which the term "primary care" was still new, and the notion that primary care physicians might be leaders at a major academic medical center was novel at best. In the late 1970s, however, the Brigham was the perfect place for Phyllis Jen and several other physicians who had "come of age" during the Vietnam and Watergate era to define excellence for the emerging discipline.

Eugene Braunwald, chair of the Department of Medicine in 1972, and Marshall A. Wolf, the director of the residency training program, were early advocates of primary care and created one of the first primary care residency training programs in the country. They and nephrologist H. Richard Nesson, the founding director at the time of a new Division of General Medicine, helped create the context in which primary care physicians could become central to the life of a great academic medical center. The early members of Nesson's Division of General Medicine included physicians who would go on to be leaders and role models, including William T. Branch, Jr., Arnold M. Epstein, Lee Goldman, Matthew H. Liang, and Beverly Woo. And, in the middle of photographs and other records of that era, there was always Phyllis Jen.

As the medical director for the Brigham's primary care teaching clinic, Phyllis had a daunting task. BIMA provides primary care to any and all patients, regardless of insurance status, and thus the population was then (and now) predominantly drawn from Roxbury, Dorchester, Mattapan, and other poorer neighborhoods of Boston. The interns and residents who provided much of the care needed training as well as emotional care themselves. Most of the faculty physicians practiced for only one or two sessions per week. They frequently did not know the names of their supporting staff, most of whom lived in the same neighborhoods as the patient population. Somehow, though, Phyllis turned BIMA into one of the best places in the city for primary care. The care became consistently at or near the top on all the publicly reported measures of quality, thus defying the conventional wisdom that excellent and reliable patient care could not be achieved in disenfranchised patient populations. For both trainees and staff, BIMA was a happy place in which to work. With time, patients who could have gotten their care anywhere started to show up in BIMA waiting rooms. The mayor of Boston, Harvard professors, and corporate chief executive officers determined that the wonderful BIMA physicians delivered excellent medical care.

One of those physicians was, of course, Phyllis Jen, who became a "doctor's doctor," one of those physicians to whom other physicians turn when they themselves need medical care. Phyllis set a good example for other physicians. She taught me, for example, that every time a patient has a needle pierce the skin for a laboratory test, that patient should receive the test results. This practice is common today, but I am embarrassed to say that this thought had not occurred to me or many other physicians until Phyllis suggested it in the 1980s.

Phyllis did not transform BIMA just by setting a good example. She worked relentlessly to create systems to improve care. Gaps in quality simply drove her crazy. Phyllis could not rest until she could rectify such problems, including abnormal laboratory results that had slipped through the cracks or patients who did not receive the preventive care they needed. She knew that the solutions to problems often lay in systems. She became an enormous influence on Partners' information systems, particularly its electronic longitudinal medical record (LMR). She was relentless in using (and suggesting improvements in) the LMR to better patient care. She was one of about 25,000 individual users of the LMR, but accounted for 5% of the enhancement requests submitted by LMR users. Her real impact may have been even greater, because Phyllis sometimes asked others to submit requests for enhancements in their own names. She would say, "I am worried that the LMR people are getting sick of me." She had no reason for concern, because the LMR team adored her.

Phyllis' relentlessness was at the core of her personal and professional greatness. She never stopped trying to make BIMA better, to improve life for her husband and three children, or to make a greater contribution to society. She became the clinical leader of the Brigham and Women's Hospital volunteer program that enlists physicians to provide care to Native Americans in New Mexico. She won numerous awards, including the Samuel O. Thier Physician Leadership Award, a prize given annually to a single physician at Partners HealthCare System who epitomizes resilience, creativity, and integrity in the pursuit of better health care.

Phyllis never sought such attention. She surely drew greater satisfaction from the friends and colleagues who made their way to her door every day to share news, seek advice, and make connections. At the memorial service, one former Brigham resident described how she thought of Phyllis as her best and most important friend and how, even though she had left the Brigham a decade earlier, she always returned to discuss with Phyllis the most important questions arising in her life. She looked at hundreds around her, many of whom were telling similar stories, and said, "I had no idea that she was playing this role for so many others."

After her death, her family, friends, patients and colleagues struggled to understand how she had managed to touch so many lives so deeply. The answer seems to have been simple—one at a time. At her funeral service, her son Michael recounted how she had told him many times, "Try to be the kindest, most generous person you know." For many people, Phyllis Jen was exactly that.

THE HARVARD COMMUNITY HEALTH PLAN AND HARVARD VANGUARD MEDICAL ASSOCIATES

Joseph L. Dorsey

Robert H. Ebert, dean of Harvard Medical School (HMS), was the driving force behind the creation of Harvard Community Health Plan (HCHP), a prepaid staff model, not-for-profit health maintenance organization (HMO). (See Chapter 6 in this volume for more information.) Joining him in the planning were healthcare economist Jerome Pollack, finance administrator Henry C. Meadow, and Sidney Lee, all associate deans at HMS. Although other medical schools set about making primary care services available for poor, inner city residents in neighborhood health centers, Ebert and his colleagues made the deliberate decision to develop a healthcare delivery system that would integrate care for patients of all social classes, compete in the private healthcare marketplace, and function independently of government subsidies. When these diverse patients required hospitalization, they were to be admitted to "private services" and cared for by house staff working side by side with senior attending physicians.

HCHP opened its doors in the Kenmore Center in October 1969, in collaboration with the Peter Bent Brigham Hospital, Children's Hospital, and the Boston Hospital for Women (with Joseph L. Dorsey as medical director) and the Beth Israel Hospital (with H. Richard Nesson as medical director). HCHP was the nation's first medical school–sponsored managed care organization. Strong support for this exciting venture came from the Brigham's Board of Directors, under the leadership of Chair F. Stanton Deland, Jr., and Department Chairs George W. Thorn in medicine, Francis D. Moore in surgery, Duncan E. Reid in obstetrics and gynecology, and Clement Sledge in orthopedics. Many of the initial physician recruits were already members of these departments.

In the early years, patients had either private insurance or Medicaid, resources that are considerably expanded in 2012. Membership grew to 30,000 individuals by 1972 and to 75,000 by 1979, coincident with the acquisition of the Brigham-affiliated Hospital at Parker Hill for providing secondary-level inpatient care. Outgrowing this facility within a few years, HCHP began a close long-term relationship with the Brigham that epitomized how HMOs and hospitals could establish mutually beneficial partnerships. Over the ensuing years, fifteen additional health centers were established in Boston and its suburbs. In 1985, HCHP became one of the first national health plans to contract with the federal government to provide comprehensive care for Medicare beneficiaries. In 1986, a merger increased membership to 295,000, leading to an HCHP–Brigham and Women's Hospital contract to provide hospital care at a discounted rate. HCHP merged with the medical insurance company Pilgrim Health Care in 1995 to form Harvard Pilgrim Health Care. In 1998, after insurance functions were separated from healthcare delivery, the medical group practice component of the former HCHP was renamed Harvard Vanguard Medical Associates. In 2004 and 2005, Harvard Vanguard merged with four other ambulatory group practices to form Atrius Health, a nonprofit alliance that now serves almost 700,000 patients.

In 1992, HCHP and HMS established the Department of Ambulatory Care and Prevention, the first medical school department to be housed in and sponsored by an HMO. This department serves as a focal point for outpatient house staff training, HMS student education, and health services research. Harvard Pilgrim Health Care provides major funding for this department, which is now called the HMS Department of Population Medicine.

Although changes in the financial climate led in 2011 to HVMA's contracting with another hospital, patients are still admitted to the Brigham. Trainees in the HVMA-Brigham primary care medical residency program, established in the early 1970s, continue to rotate to the Brigham. Over these many years, the potentially enriching effects of the HVMA-Brigham relationship are clearly demonstrable. This is exemplified by the inter-relationship of a number of outstanding clinicians and administrators who have been role models for members of both institutions, including but not limited to Donald M. Berwick, formerly a pediatrician at the HCHP serving as vice-president for quality care measurement, and now a national leader in healthcare improvement; Joseph L. Dorsey, a Brigham trainee in Medicine who led many HCHP/HVMA programs both in-house and at the Brigham and the Faulkner Hospitals; Jennifer Leaning, who served for many years as a clinician and executive at HCHP and is now a professor at the Harvard School of Public Health; Gene Lindsay, a Brigham trainee and staff cardiologist who is currently the HVMA-Atrius Health chief executive officer; Richard Platt, the executive director of the Harvard Pilgrim Health Care Institute, Chair of the HMS Department of Population Medicine, and a Brigham staff member; Lawrence N. Shulman, an oncologist who practiced for more than ten years at the HCHP and is now a clinician-executive the Dana-Farber Cancer Institute; and Gordon Vineyard, a Brigham trainee and staff surgeon who was an early HCHP surgeon and former chief executive officer.

Gene Lindsay noted: The history of our organization has always been about the future—about the search for better ways to care for all patients...We have honored their boldness and courage with our own continued belief in the centrality of the patient, and with our relentless quest to find new and better ways to make it easier for our patients to be healthy.

ANESTHESIOLOGY AT THE BRIGHAM

Monica M. Sa Rego, Robert W. Lekowski, Daniel F. Dedrick, and Sukumar P. Desai

The Department of Anesthesiology, Perioperative and Pain Medicine at Brigham and Women's Hospital began within the Department of Surgery. Harvey Cushing appointed Walter M. Boothby, a graduate of Harvard Medical School, as the first supervisor of anesthesia (1913-1916). Thereafter, surgery was without a physician anesthesiologist until William S. Derrick joined the Brigham in 1948 and established a residency program. Leroy D. Vandam, who became the anesthetist-in-chief in 1954, took the Division of Anesthesia to new heights in patient care, teaching, academic contributions, and leadership. Harvard Medical School recognized these achievements and complexities and in 1969 granted Anesthesiology a Department status, a change that allowed anesthesiologists and surgeons to work in a renewed partnership. The merger of the three hospitals to form the Affiliated Hospital Center and later the Brigham and Women's Hospital brought about major increases in personnel and academic output. Vandam was succeeded by Benjamin G. Covino in 1980, under whose leadership the residency program expanded to include an incoming class of thirty residents and fifteen fellows. Covino was succeeded by Simon Gelman in the mid-1990s and by our current Chair Charles A. Vacanti a decade later. The department is ranked amongst the best nationally for academic activity, as measured by research publications and success in obtaining extramural research funding. The department currently employs 143 full-time faculty members, fifty-four of whom are women, and 104 residents, fifty-five of whom are women.

Patient Care

Our involvement with patient care usually begins at the Weiner Center for Preoperative Evaluation, a creation of Angela M. Bader that has become a national and international model for patient assessment and management. Our ambulatory anesthesia team, led originally by Beverly K. Philip, and currently by McCallum R. Hoyt, aims for rapid recovery with minimal side effects from anesthetic drugs. The operating rooms, directed by Hugh L. Flanagan, Jr., are a major focus. Thoracic anesthesiologists, led by Philip M. Hartigan, administer some of the most difficult anesthetics, including inserting thoracic epidural catheters and managing lung isolation, for procedures ranging from bronchoscopy and lobectomy to extra-pleural pneumonectomy or lung transplantation. Cardiac anesthesiologists, led by Stanton K. Shernan, care for patients who often have little cardiovascular reserve while also performing intraoperative transesophageal echocardiographic examinations. Obstetrical anesthesiologists, led by William R. Camann, are expert in the care of high-risk pregnancies. Lawrence C. Tsen edits a leading textbook in obstetrical anesthesia. The Neuroanesthesia Service has developed expertise in intraoperative neuromonitoring during complex neurosurgical procedures. The Division of Regional Anesthesia, developed initially by Mercedes A. Concepcion and currently led by Kamen V. Vlassakov, utilizes the latest technological advances to promote safe regional analgesia, for example, in orthopedic procedures. Members of our department also provide anesthesia coverage in locations outside the operating rooms. Ramon F. Martin and Wendy L. Gross lead our efforts in these areas—the endoscopy suite, the electrophysiology laboratory, the cardiac catheterization laboratory, the interventional neuroradiology suite, the angiography and radiation therapy suites, and most recently the state of the art Advanced Multimodality Image-Guided Operating Suite. Several members of our department provide comprehensive care for patients suffering from chronic pain, whereas others are intensivists who staff and codirect the surgical intensive care units.

Research

Among their many research efforts, members of the Center for Regenerative Medicine, headed by Piero Anversa, study cardiac stem cells—their role in health and disease and their therapeutic potential. Data from a phase I clinical trial, which utilizes autologous cardiac stem cells to treat patients with ischemic cardiomyopathy, are encouraging. Anversa's group has also identified and isolated human lung stem cells. Simon C. Body leads the Coronary Artery Bypass Grafting Genomics Program, a study conducted jointly by the Brigham and the Texas Heart Institute, examining how genomic factors influence adverse cardiac and noncardiac outcomes after coronary artery bypass graft surgery. He also co-leads the Bicuspid Aortic Valve Genetics Program, a multinational consortium of researchers investigating the genetic causes of this developmental anomaly. Gregory Crosby and Deborah J. Culley established the Laboratory for Aging Neuroscience to focus on the effect of aging on the brain and the impact of general anesthesia on cognitive dysfunction, a postoperative disability common in the elderly. Two decades ago, Charles N. Serhan established the Center for Experimental Therapeutics and Reperfusion Injury to elucidate novel molecular mechanisms and endogenous receptor-ligand interactions that occur during inflammation and to understand cellular and biochemical pathways of resolution and anti-inflammation. His group discovered and characterized resolvins, small-molecule chemical signals made by the body during the natural resolution of inflammation. The resolvins are potent anti-inflammatory, pro-resolving, and pain-controlling mediators in a wide range of experimental animal models of disease. These resolvins are now in clinical trials. Department Chair Charles A. Vacanti, who also heads the Center for Tissue Engineering, seeks to introduce tissue-engineered cells and scaffolds into the human body to allow tissue regeneration. Researchers in the Pain Research Center investigate both basic biological and clinical aspects of pain and its management. Gary R. Strichartz is exploring the role of endothelin receptors in cancer pain, inflammation, and tissue injury. Ging-Kuo Wang is electrophysiologically mapping the local anesthetic receptor within the sodium channel. Igor Kissin studies the neurobehavioral pharmacology of anesthetics and analgesics and the role of preemptive analgesia. Robert N. Jamison, Robert R. Edwards, and Ajay D. Wasan study the role of psychiatric factors in pain treatment response. Christine N. Sang evaluates novel potential analgesics in clinical trials to target and treat pain that occurs via selective mechanisms. Others in the department are studying aspects of excitation-contraction coupling in the myocardium (Paul D. Allen), the usefulness of nanotechnology to deliver chemotherapy to tumors (Omid C. Farokhzad), and molecular mechanisms regulating immune and inflammatory events during organ failure (Hongwei Gao). Every Division within our department is also actively involved in clinical research and the development of educational programs and guidelines for the optimal care of our patients.

In conclusion, Cushing, Boothby, and Vandam would be most pleasantly surprised by the wonderful metamorphosis of anesthesia over the past century.[73]

BIOGRAPHY

LEROY DAVID VANDAM, 1914-2004

John A. Fox, Andrew D. Miller, Ramon F. Martin, and Sukumar P. Desai

The arrival of Leroy David Vandam (or LDV as he was known to his colleagues) at the Brigham in 1954 was a return to Harvard, but could hardly be termed a déjà vu. He had begun surgical training at Beth Israel Hospital in 1940, after which he enlisted in the Army. Uncle Sam accepted him even though he had experienced visual disturbances due to a scotoma in his left eye. Later, a progressive deterioration in his vision ended his surgical career. Surgery's loss was anesthesiology's gain, as he became a giant in the field and served the Brigham in one capacity or another for almost half a century.

A native of New York and the son of second-generation immigrants, LDV always had a strong work ethic. Excelling in studies, he entered Brown University at age sixteen, and after graduation studied medicine at New York University Medical School before commencing his surgical training in Boston. After an honorable discharge from the Army, he undertook research training at Johns Hopkins Hospital, working with Bing, Thomas, Blalock, and Taussig, and moved to Philadelphia to train in anesthesiology. As a subsequent faculty member at the University of Pennsylvania, he developed a very close relationship with his chair, Robert Dripps, and also with his colleague, James Eckenhoff. The three of them authored the first American textbook of anesthesiology (*Introduction to Anesthesia*), a work that went through nine editions and was the first text for generations of American trainees. Additionally, while at Penn, LDV began a research effort examining neurological complications of spinal anesthesia, a task that involved examining more than 10,000 anesthetics. This seminal work verified the safety of spinal anesthesia and revived its popularity—a feat that was subsequently recognized as a landmark effort.

As a young lad, LDV was very artistic, and in medical school he drew sketches of cadavers just as Leonardo Da Vinci had done centuries earlier. He illustrated his text generously with line diagrams. This interest continued throughout his life as he became a very prolific painter, favoring watercolor as his medium. Four of his works were featured on the cover of the *Journal of the American Medical Association*. He painted historically significant structures, such as the Bulfinch Building where the Ether Dome is located and a series of homes occupied by William Thomas Green Morton, the person most credited with the discovery of modern anesthesia. His love of painting took him to New Hampshire and Nantucket during summer vacations. He bestowed his paintings very selectively to friends and admirers, and many of us remember being summoned to his office and being told: "I hear you wished one of these! Sift through that pile (of art) and choose one you like." The feeling of being given a "Vandam" by Vandam was indescribable, and the watercolor immediately earned a place of honor in one's home or office.

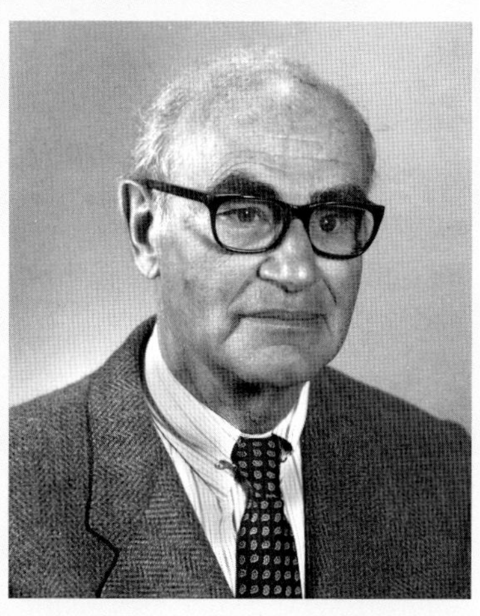

FIGURE 3-36 Leroy David Vandam.

In 1954, Vandam accepted Surgeon-in-Chief Francis D. Moore's offer to head the Division of Anesthesia at Peter Bent Brigham Hospital (the Brigham). LDV knew that he would only have limited autonomy, because the Division of Anesthesia remained tightly bound within the Department of Surgery—an arrangement that was common throughout the nation. The anesthesiology service when LDV started consisted of three residents, several nurse anesthetists, and one other physician who was ready to leave for private practice. Gradually, a cadre of physician anesthesiologists and residents were added, with staggered starting dates for new residents so that each neophyte could be thoroughly indoctrinated into the "Vandam method." He worked tirelessly to develop his division. He waited for fifteen years before Harvard granted department status to his chosen specialty. By this time, he had transformed a service-oriented division into one of the finest academic departments in the country.

The Brigham motto, "Patient Care, Teaching, and Research," resonated mightily with LDV, and he never doubted that this was their relative order of importance. He felt and taught that the preoperative interview with the patient was a very special time, an opportunity not only for obtaining relevant medical information, but also a time for the patient and physician to assess one another psychologically during this vulnerable period in the patient's life.

Trained as a surgeon in the Halstedian tradition, LDV was a demanding taskmaster. Individuals who were not enthusiastic about the specialty or did not display sufficient interest in learning would be at the receiving end of the "full Vandam treatment." He set very high professional standards for himself and for others in his department, and he would often react ferociously to slipshod or inadequate efforts by his team. One such errant house officer remarked, "It took me some time to realize when I met his gaze under these circumstances, the eye with the kindly expression was the glass one!"

As chair, Vandam knew that anesthesiology would never take its place among respected subspecialties unless anesthesiologists became involved in basic research. Faculty members were encouraged to seek out projects related to cardiovascular physiology, regional anesthesia, or neuromuscular blocking agents and to publish their research and clinical experiences. In 1963, Vandam became editor-in-chief of the journal *Anesthesiology*, and in the ensuing decade it became the preeminent journal for the specialty.

During his clinical career, Vandam saw the birth of open heart surgery at the Brigham, and he administered the anesthetic during Joseph Murray's first successful kidney transplantation in 1954. The American Society of Anesthesiologists (ASA) conferred its highest award, the Distinguished Service Award, on him in 1977.

After a quarter century as chief, he stepped down as chair in 1980 and became senior statesman in Benjamin G. Covino's new department. His practice moved off campus to the Harvard Community Health Plan Hospital, where senior residents rotated with him to learn "The Vandam Way." He would still cajole residents and staff to improve, often commenting to individuals "You need to write more" or "I would not do the anesthetic that way." These comments meant that LDV saw potential in the recipient and was ready to help if asked.

After a few years, he retired from clinical practice but continued to attend departmental meetings, offering guidance and mentoring into the 1990s. When topics of interest were brought to him, he would offer to assist junior faculty members in writing a paper. He would be merciless in his editing, but one knew that the work was enriched and also felt the thrill of having collaborated on an academic endeavor with Roy Vandam.

At the age of ninety, Leroy David Vandam died in Westwood, Massachusetts. Everyone who interacted with him carries on his tradition and ensures that it is passed on to current trainees. Roy Vandam was committed to excellence in everything he did. This commitment continues to this day in the Department of Anesthesiology, Perioperative and Pain Medicine.

CARDIAC SURGERY AT THE BRIGHAM

Lawrence H. Cohn

Harvey Cushing, the first chief of surgery at the Peter Bent Brigham Hospital and known for his development of neurosurgery, also showed early interest in cardiac surgery. As a Johns Hopkins general surgeon in 1908, he published "Experimental and Clinical Notes on Chronic Valvular Lesions in the Dog and their Possible Relation to a Future Surgery of the Cardiac Valves," in which he examined the pathophysiology of mitral stenosis and predicted a surgical solution to this problem.[74]

In 1913, in his first year at the Brigham, Cushing accepted Elliott Carr Cutler as surgical house officer. A 1913 graduate of Harvard Medical School (HMS), Cutler was an excellent surgical resident, a volunteer military surgeon during World War I, and a Brigham staff member thereafter. In the early 1920s, with Cushing's encouragement, Cutler began experiments on the heart. He developed the median sternotomy incision and recorded basic physiological observations on the manipulation of the heart during surgery. Clinically, he pursued an approach to treat stenosis of the mitral valve from rheumatic fever, affecting thousands of young Bostonians. Cutler invented an instrument, the cardiovalvulotome, to alleviate mitral stenosis by removing a section of the diseased valve. In 1923, while waiting for this instrument to be manufactured, he was referred a comatose twelve-year-old girl with severe mitral stenosis. Cutler performed a median sternotomy, entered the left ventricle through its apex using a neurosurgical tenotomy knife, and opened both fibrotic commissures of the mitral valve. The child woke up the next day, was presented at Brigham Surgical Grand Rounds five days postoperatively, and was reported in the *Boston Medical and Surgical Journal* four weeks postoperatively. In his surgeon-in-chief report of 1923, Cushing said, "Unless all fails we are on the eve of a new surgical specialty of great promise, dealing with chronic disorders of the heart." Unfortunately, all did fail, as Cutler's surgery on seven additional patients (with his cardiovalvulotome) led to their deaths from severe mitral regurgitation. He abandoned this approach in 1929, acknowledging that this was not the way to treat mitral stenosis. He did become the second department chair in 1932. Cutler served in World War II as a Brigadier General, becoming head of the European Theatre Medical Operations.

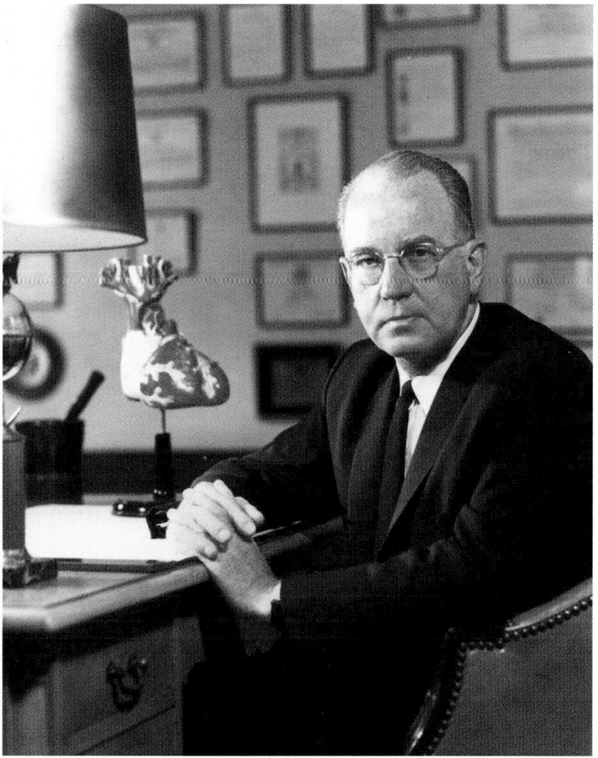

FIGURE 3-37 Dwight Harken.

Another World War II surgeon was Dwight Harken from Iowa, who reported the safe operative removal of shrapnel and bullet fragments from the lungs, great vessels, and heart muscle of wounded soldiers.[75] After Cutler passed away in 1947, the third chief of surgery at the Brigham, Francis D. Moore, appointed Harken in 1948 as the first chief of cardiothoracic surgery. Harken pioneered the surgical treatment of mitral stenosis, using finger dilation and subsequently mechanical dilation of the valve that was accessed through the left atrium. Operating on hundreds of patients with rheumatic valve disease, he and his cardiologic colleague Lawrence B. Ellis published early actuarial life table analyses documenting "the natural history" of the surgical therapy of mitral stenosis. In 1951, he also established the first cardiac surgical intensive care unit.

In the late 1950s, Harken developed a ball-and-cage valve to replace the diseased aortic valve and in 1959 was the first to insert this device in a patient. This valve had limited use because it could be inserted only in a very large aorta. In the late 1960s, with the development of the coronary artery bypass operation, Harken's research team developed the concept of arterial counterpulsation.[76] Developed to treat cardiogenic shock and heart failure by increasing coronary artery blood flow, counterpulsation was produced in a patient by withdrawing blood during

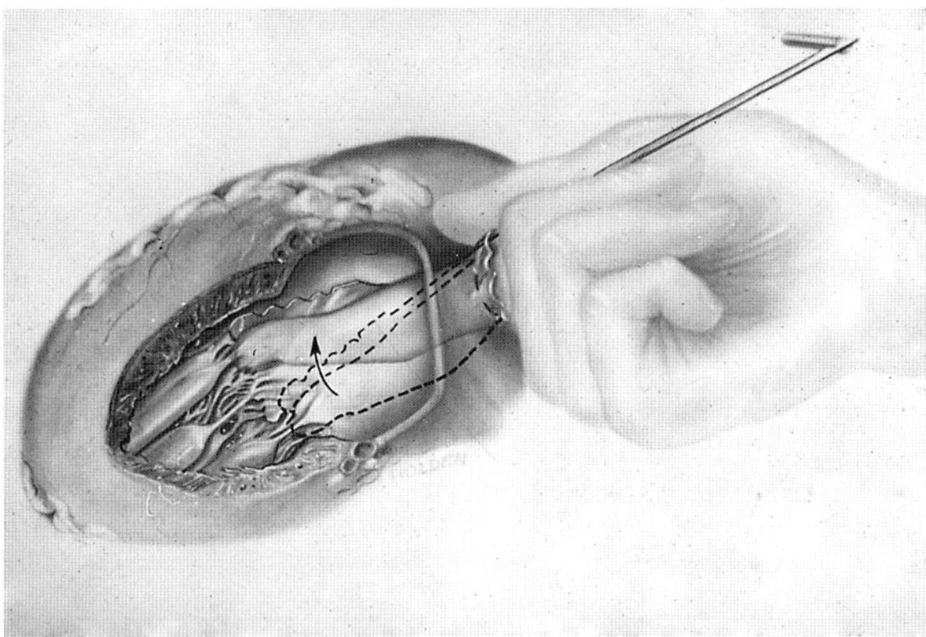

FIGURE 3-38 Harken mitral valve surgery.

systole and re-infusing it in diastole. This cumbersome pump was used in only a few patients at the Brigham, but the physiologic observations led to the development of a less invasive and ultimately widely used counterpulsation balloon pump. In 1966, Harken implanted the first demand pacemaker, which he had helped to design.

In 1970, Harken retired. His trainee and practice partner John J. Collins, Jr., was appointed chief of cardiothoracic surgery. Collins was an excellent technical surgeon, especially interested in the field of coronary artery bypass surgery, and did some of the first coronary bypass operations in New England. In 1971, Collins hired Lawrence H. Cohn, after his cardiothoracic training at Stanford University under Norman Shumway, who developed the cardiac transplant operation. Cohn helped Collins to transform Peter Bent Brigham cardiac surgery to a modern system, including withdrawing coronary artery perfusion during bypass, introducing local cardiac hypothermia for myocardial protection, and using new methods of valve repair and replacement. In 1972, Cohn and Collins implanted both porcine and human valves for the first time in New England. The Brigham surgical team was also one of the first to use the internal mammary to left anterior descending bypass, now a standard procedure. A landmark paper by Cohn and associates, also presented at a meeting of the New England Surgical Society in 1972, described the first results of surgical treatment of acute myocardial infarction by emergency coronary artery bypass grafting.[77] This soon became the standard procedure nationwide. During this decade, considerable advancement was also made in the treatment of dissecting aortic aneurysms by performing surgery immediately without extensive preoperative cardiac catheterization and by using aortic valve-sparing procedures during dissection repair.

In 1983, Cohn began doing mitral valve repair surgery in patients with not only rheumatic heart disease but also valve prolapse. His series became one of the largest and longest followed accounts of repair of mitral valve prolapse.[78] In 1984, Collins and Cohn performed the first heart transplant in New England. Currently, the Brigham has the longest running and busiest cardiac transplant service in New England, with more than 750 heart transplants. In 1987, Cohn succeeded Collins as chief of cardiothoracic surgery. John Mannick, the fourth chief of surgery at the Brigham, established separate divisions for the subspecialties of cardiac and general thoracic surgery led,

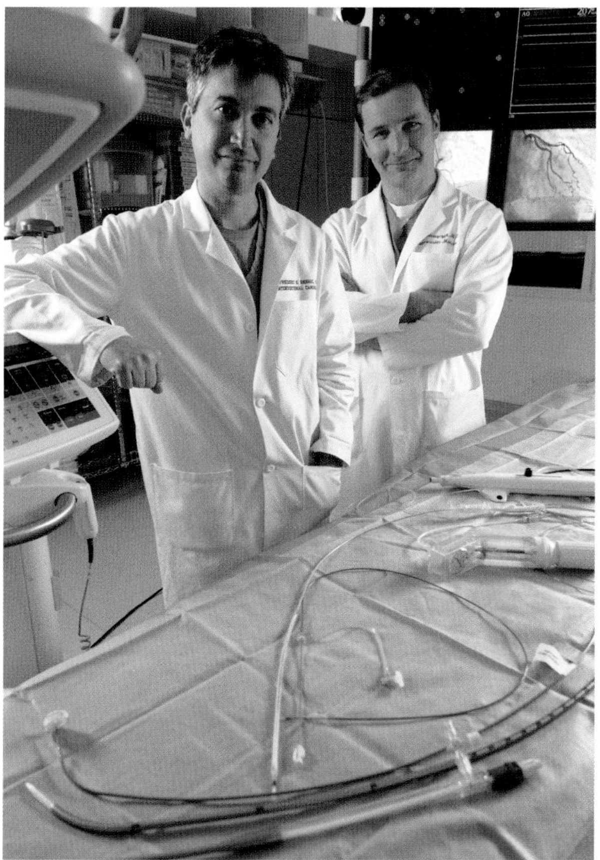

FIGURE 3-39 Fred Resnic, former director of the Cardiac Catheterization Lab at BWH, and Piotr Sobieszczyk, Associate Director of the Cardiac Catheterization Lab.

respectively, by Cohn and David Sugarbaker, a former Brigham surgical resident.

With the spotlight on cardiac transplantation, many landmark events took place at Brigham and Women's Hospital in the 1990s: implantation of the first left ventricular assist device (LVAD) in 1991 by Gregory S. Couper, the first heart-lung transplant in New England in 1992 by Sary F. Aranki, a single-patient donation of heart and lungs to three organ transplant recipients in 1995, and discharge of a patient after implantation of an electrical LVAD in 1997 by Couper. In 1996 Cohn's group began performing minimally invasive heart surgery, one of two hospitals in the world to do so. Their early series of patients undergoing minimally invasive valve surgery, presented at a meeting of the American Surgical Association in 1997, suggested that this approach was clinically equal to the standard median sternotomy but yielded faster postoperative recovery.[79] Cohn was elected president of the American Association for Thoracic Surgery in 1999 and was named the Virginia and James Hubbard Professor in Cardiac Surgery in 2000, the first endowed chair in cardiac surgery at HMS.

Early in the new millennium, robotic surgery was performed in several patients with mitral valve disease as part of a Food and Drug Administration trial validating the approach. This approach is now used in many centers throughout the world. Laboratory research continued. Frederick Chen, in charge of laboratory research, has published many papers on nontransplant operations for heart failure. In addition, a number of papers were published by the Brigham Outcomes Research group using a sophisticated computerized database extending back twenty years. In 2005 Cohn stepped down as chief of cardiac surgery, and R. Morton Bolman III was appointed the fourth chief of cardiac surgery. In 2008, the first percutaneous aortic valves were implanted with the help of Michael Davidson, who was cross-trained in cardiac surgery and cardiac catheterization.

The success of any academic program depends in large part on the success of its trainees. Since 1970, the Division of Cardiac Surgery has trained more than 200 residents: 77% are in full-time academic positions, forty-four of these hold an academic rank of associate or full professor, and a significant number are chief of a division or a department of cardiothoracic surgery. The success of the Brigham's Division of Cardiac Surgery also depends on the leadership for its success. Both the surgical and administrative chiefs have supported many important innovative research and clinical programs since the beginning of cardiac surgery in 1923. With their support, this division has revolutionized adult cardiac surgery at the Brigham and throughout the world.

THE CORONARY CARE UNIT AT THE BRIGHAM

Bernard Lown

The original Coronary Care Unit (CCU) at the Peter Bent Brigham Hospital (PBBH) was but a four-bed unit, yet it exerted a profound impact on cardiology worldwide. Foremost, it drew attention to the formidable and prevalent problem of sudden cardiac death. Hospitalizing patients with acute heart attacks in CCUs markedly reduced this early mortality, from about 30% to 10%. The improved outcome related primarily to the introduction of innovative technologies, such as direct current defibrillation, cardioversion, electronic monitoring for disordered heart rhythms, and arrhythmia prevention.[80]

The Introduction of Direct Current (DC) Defibrillation and Cardioversion

My first preoccupation with electricity was compelled by a dying patient who had survived several heart attacks and recurring bouts of rapid ventricular tachycardia. Initially these episodes responded to antiarrhythmic agents, but ultimately these drugs failed. I recalled that a few years earlier, Paul Zoll at the Beth Israel Hospital had used alternating electrical current (AC) delivered across the intact chest to resuscitate unconscious patients experiencing ventricular fibrillation. Luckily, the PBBH possessed an AC defibrillator, which was unused. Although many questions arose concerning how best to use the machine and what adverse effects might be anticipated, we could not reach Zoll for guidance. This was the first time an electric shock was to be used on a living patient to normalize the heart's rhythm. After obtaining both approval for this procedure from his wife and rebutting the objections of the director of the PBBH medical services, we anesthetized the patient and administered a single electric shock. Normal heart rhythm resumed. Never before had a *lub-dub* sounded so exhilarating to my ears. When the tachycardia recurred, we proceeded confidently with our once-tried method, but the AC induced irreversible ventricular fibrillation.[81]

I searched the literature but found nothing describing adverse effects of AC on the heart. We thereupon began a systematic study of AC shock in experimental animals in our laboratory at the Harvard School of Public Health. Even a single discharge, delivered across the closed chest, induced disordered rhythms, including irreversible ventricular fibrillation. Repeated AC discharges permanently injured the heart. We concluded that AC should not be employed as a therapeutic device.

I nonetheless remained impressed with the power of electricity to normalize a disordered heartbeat. We postulated that direct current (DC) could be therapeutic without being injurious. After one year of studies in experimental animals, we discovered a monophasic waveform that was consistently effective. Even numerous transthoracic shocks produced no demonstrable myocardial injury. Subsequent experiments, however, indicated that this "safe" DC waveform could provoke occasional ventricular fibrillation, for a specific reason. Each heartbeat is followed by a very brief "ventricular vulnerable period," and when an electric impulse coincides with the vulnerable period, it can trigger ventricular fibrillation. This was remedied with an electronic timer to avoid the vulnerable period. DC cardioversion, using a cardioverter, was now safe for treatment of arrhythmias.[82] The PBBH was now flooded with patients with arrhythmias craving a normal heart rhythm.

Sudden Cardiac Death

In the late 1950s, I constructed a CCU for animals in my laboratory, to my knowledge the first such unit anywhere. Dog cages were equipped with cardiac monitors and a standby DC defibrillator. We observed that surgically induced coronary artery occlusions provoked immediate disordered heart rhythm and death from ventricular fibrillation. Animals that were resuscitated immediately and remained arrhythmia-free for the twenty-four hours usually recovered, proving that sudden cardiac death in animals was not only reversible but survivable. We now prepared to extend this to the human heart.

The Brigham's own Soma Weiss was among the first to suggest that a deranged heart rhythm in humans caused sudden death.[83] Approximately 70% of patients dying from an unanticipated heart attack and arrhythmia never reached a hospital.[84] If patients in the earliest throes of this event could be expeditiously hospitalized in a specialized unit with trained personnel, equipped with monitoring technology and DC defibrillators, their chances of survival might be enormously improved. Such a unit had already been organized in the early 1960s by Hughes Day, a general practitioner in Bethany, Kansas.[85]

The Brigham Takes an Unexpected Leap

Even though the innovations of DC defibrillation and cardioversion were first employed at the PBBH, there was little initial support for a CCU. Richard Gorlin, the head of cardiology, needed no convincing, but was not optimistic that George Thorn, the physician-in-chief, would support it. When I spoke to Thorn, he termed a CCU a foolhardy luxury in a hospital already focused excessively on cardiology. Subsequently, I asked Thorn what his response would be to a personal heart attack. Looking puzzled, he replied, "Of course I would be rushed to the Brigham." "But why?" I questioned. He surely would have much less noise and invasion of privacy, more rest and loving care, and a better chance for recovery at home. I continued that because the greatest threat from an acute coronary thrombosis is ventricular fibrillation, for which we could do little, "You would be much wiser staying at home." He let out a nervous chuckle. "Strange that you should be talking about this subject. Just this morning I heard from my good friend Bob Williams in Seattle, who had a cardiac arrest and was successfully resuscitated with your contraption." Thorn then suggested that I create a CCU in the semiprivate room next to the nurses' station on Ward A2. I thanked him profusely but made an additional request for the unused solarium at the other end of that ward. He promptly concurred without questioning this seemingly bizarre request.

I then met with the hospital director, Bill Hassan, to review Thorn's approval of the CCU and its location on both ends of ward A2. Hassan was upset that the hospital would lose eight beds for a four-bed unit. "Do you realize what a CCU entails?" I asked. I expounded on its merits, the favorable publicity it would garner, its fund-raising potential, and its minimal cost to the PBBH. After listening with mounting interest, he arranged a meeting with architects, and we were off flying.

I had to shape nearly every facet of this enterprise, including creating the design, obtaining and installing the novel electronics, and devising the operational plan. I obtained funding from Samuel A. Levine's Research Foundation, a special campaign waged by the PBBH Ladies Auxiliary, and the American Optical Company, with which I had worked to develop the defibrillator and cardioverter. The fourteen Brigham nurses whom we recruited were given a three-week course in electrocardiography, arrhythmia recognition, emergency cardiovascular medicine, and cardiopulmonary resuscitation, taught by Samuel A. Levine, Paul Dudley White, Dwight Harken, Lewis Dexter, Richard Gorlin, and others. I have never since encountered a brighter, more committed, and more enthusiastic group of nurses.

The CCU-LCU

We named the CCU the Samuel A. Levine Coronary Care Unit, or the LCU, at the opening ceremony held on February 16, 1965. It was the first CCU in New England and the fifth in the United States. Having the CCU named after my great clinical teacher was a life-fulfilling experience. The unit was honeycombed with futuristic technologies, while also projecting a homey feel of human proximity. It emphasized patient individuality and privacy, but did not limit visibility from the nurses' central station. From the very outset, we shifted the focus from resuscitation, which may injure the heart, to prevention. The preventive strategy was made possible by the discovery in my laboratory that the anesthetic drug lidocaine, when administered intravenously, abolished all ventricular arrhythmias with few adverse effects. We began to use lidocaine prophylactically in the LCU in response to ventricular arrhythmias or extrasystoles. Prevention of arrhythmic death required not only this treatment but also meticulous attention to other issues such as pain, apprehension, insomnia, uncertainty, and hopelessness. Discussion in front of the patient was couched in encouraging phraseology, with emphasis on signs of improvement. Patients were encouraged to spend most time out of bed in a comfortable chair and to be an active participant in the healing process.[86] Nurses assumed a major role in patient management. They participated in morning rounds and invariably had much to contribute. They alerted physicians to significant heart rhythm changes and instituted prompt lidocaine prophylaxis.[87] They were the first responders to cardiac arrest. To combat depersonalization that might be brought on by cutting-edge technology, nurses related interpersonally to the patients. In addition, nurse-led weekly family rounds explored the social dimensions of a patient's illness.

During the first year, 248 patients were admitted to the LCU. Of these, 130 had a heart attack, confirmed by sequential electrocardiographic changes or a rise in cardiac enzymes. This was an unusually sick population, in whom 88% exhibited ventricular arrhythmias, 59% developed left ventricular heart failure, and 19% had cardiogenic shock, the most dire complication. Nonetheless, the mortality of patients in the LCU that first year was only 11.5%.[88] Not a single patient developed primary ventricular fibrillation with the prophylactic use of lidocaine. CCUs from around the United States, on the other hand, were at the time reporting an incidence of ventricular fibrillation ranging from 14% to 22%! Thus we proved that "the focus of management in the coronary care unit should be altered from resuscitation to the prevention of the need for resuscitation."[89]

Hopefully, if future medical historians encounter this remarkable experience, they will not miss one important aspect of this pioneering CCU, namely that it was possible to maintain a humanitarian focus in the heartland of the advanced technology of its day.

ORTHOPEDIC SURGERY AT THE BRIGHAM

James H. Herndon

"Everyone is against specialization except the patient. The patient always seeks the most expert care."

—Francis D. Moore, 1977

Orthopedic surgery began in the second decade of the twentieth century at both the Peter Bent Brigham Hospital and the Robert Breck Brigham Hospital (RBBH). As a division in the Department of Surgery, the service remained small at the Peter Bent Brigham. However, it became a major service at the RBBH because of the strong influence of one of its founding trustees, Joel E. Goldthwait, an orthopedic surgeon whose major interest was in disabilities.[90] With the hospital's mission of treating Boston citizens who were unable to work because of physical disability, Goldthwait convinced the RBBH trustees to focus on the care of patients with arthritis. This new arthritis specialty hospital achieved major advances in the research and treatment of chronic arthritis, especially rheumatoid arthritis, with the specialties of rheumatology and orthopedic surgery. Goldthwait became chief of orthopedics in 1917, remaining in that position until 1935.

In 1962, Theodore A. Potter was appointed chief of orthopedic surgery at the RBBH.[91] A talented and innovative reconstructive surgeon, he brought many new pain and deformity-relieving procedures to severely affected arthritis patients. During the 1950s and early 1960s, the orthopedic surgeon's armamentarium for the treatment of destroyed joints was limited (to arthrodesis or resection arthroplasty with or without a fascial interposition) and often failed. Potter published early reports with use of a nylon membrane for knee arthroplasty (1953). Later (1972) he began using metal tibial implants (the McKeever partial knee prosthesis) with improved results and newer improved knee prostheses. Postoperative patient care at this time was comprehensive and multidisciplinary. Patients remained in the hospital for long periods and were discharged after they had become independent and their wounds usually fully healed. Physical and occupational therapy was essential for satisfactory results after these early attempts at major joint arthroplasty. Patients received these therapies seven days a week while in the hospital and were managed by both orthopedic surgeons and rheumatologists.

When the Peter Bent Brigham Hospital opened in 1913, Edward H. Bradford, the Dean at Harvard Medical School, strongly desired that this new hospital become the major teaching hospital for the medical school. Previously the first professor of orthopedic surgery at HMS, at the nearby Children's Hospital, he was responsible for establishing orthopedics as a separate, although small, discipline from general surgery. The first orthopedic patient, a nine-year-old girl with cerebral palsy and bilateral hip dislocations, was treated by Harvey W. Cushing, with adductor tenotomies.[92] Most patients admitted for orthopedic care during its infancy had fractures and dislocations and were treated at this time by the general surgeons John Homans and David Cheever. Frank R. Ober, chief of orthopedics at Children's Hospital, and his associates began seeing orthopedic consultations at the Peter Bent Brigham in about 1932. Later, Carl W. Walter developed an interest in treating fractures and dislocations and in 1938 was asked to organize a fracture division in the Department of Surgery.[93] A clinician/scientist, he developed the first external fixator for the treatment of Colles fractures of the wrist.[94] He also demonstrated the effect of electricity on bone healing in rabbits, probably the first research publication in orthopedics from the Peter Bent Brigham.[95] In 1946, when William T. Green became chief of orthopedics at Children's Hospital, he was asked to organize a division of orthopedic surgery in the Department of Surgery at the Brigham and to include the already established fracture service.[96] The clinical staff, including Green's associates at Children's Hospital, were Walter and Thomas (Bart) Quigley, who later became a popular physician for athletes at Harvard University.

As the Division of Orthopedics grew at both the Peter Bent Brigham and the Children's Hospital, Albert B. Ferguson, Jr., was asked by Green as he completed his residency to become the first full-time orthopedic surgeon at the Brigham. He accepted the position in 1951. In 1953, he left the Brigham for the University of Pittsburgh, and was replaced four months later by Henry H. Banks. Banks remained the full-time orthopedic surgeon at the Brigham until 1970, becoming chief of the service in 1968 when Green retired.[97] At the encouragement of Francis D. Moore, the chair of surgery, Banks developed an amputee clinic with Richard Warren and a hand clinic with Joseph E. Murray. Moore also encouraged Banks to conduct research in orthopedics. After receiving grant support from the National Institutes of Health (NIH) and funds from patients and Moore, Banks developed the first research laboratory for orthopedics. He focused his research on fracture healing, especially intracapsular femoral neck fractures (in humans and animals), and collaborated with Moore and others in studies on metastatic bone disease, calcium metabolism, and the effects of immunosuppressives on the musculoskeletal system.[98]

Orthopedic surgery at both Brigham hospitals underwent major changes in 1969. Clement B. Sledge was recruited from the Massachusetts General Hospital (MGH) to head orthopedic surgery at both the Peter Bent Brigham and the RBBH. Sledge was a clinician/investigator, having spent three years as a graduate student studying embryonic cartilage under Honor B. Fell in the Strangeways Laboratory in Cambridge, England.[99] He was subsequently appointed the John Ball and Buckminster Brown Chair of Orthopedic Surgery, originally a chair at Children's Hospital. Orthopedics involving both Brigham hospitals was subsequently named a department, and Sledge merged the orthopedic surgeons into this new unit. Sledge recruited J. Drennan Lowell to serve as the clinical chief of Brigham orthopedics. He added to the staff by hiring recent academic-and research-oriented graduates of the residency program who had research expertise: Richard D. Scott, who studied collagen while at the NIH; Stephen J. Lipson, who carried out research in the laboratory of Helen Muir in England; Thomas S. Thornhill, who studied cartilage immunology at the University of Hawaii with Eugene Lance and viral immunology at the NIH; Donald T. Reilly, who worked with several eminent investigators on knee and total knee replacement biomechanics; and Barry P. Simmons, who studied hand surgery in France with Raoul Tubiana. When the two Brigham hospitals and the Boston Hospital for Women merged physically in 1980, orthopedic surgery became an independent department.

Comprehensive care of the arthritic patient continued at Brigham and Women's Hospital, with rheumatology and orthopedic surgery working closely together. Clinical growth in the new Department of Orthopedic Surgery was remarkable. In addition to the major emphasis on the surgical care of the arthritic patient, the orthopedic subspecialties expanded to include adult reconstruction (replacement of hip and knee joints), hand and upper extremity, foot and ankle, spine, sports, and oncology. Operating room capacity was exceeded, requiring the orthopedic staff to obtain privileges at the New England Baptist Hospital for additional surgical cases. Sledge's research interests expanded to include, with his staff, the effect of growth hormone on articular cartilage, the biology of cartilage and synovium, the effect of radiation on synovium, cartilage breakdown in rheumatoid arthritis, and joint replacement of the knee, hip, shoulder, and elbow. Many new implants, especially for the knee and hip, were developed initially by Sledge and other members of the arthroplasty division. Frederick C. Ewald designed a new total elbow prosthesis. All patient outcomes were documented in a total joint registry under the direction of Robert Poss, one of the first hospital registries in the United States. In addition, Sledge was involved in creating the Harvard Combined Orthopedic Residency Program in the early 1970s that included the Brigham, MGH, the Brigham-affiliated Veterans Administration, Beth Israel, and Children's Hospital. Sledge retired in 1997, after almost thirty years at the Brigham.[100]

Modern-Day Orthopedics

Thomas Thornhill succeeded Sledge as the John Ball and Buckminster Brown Professor and chair of orthopedic surgery. With the retirement of Henry J. Mankin as chief at the MGH, leadership of the newly formed Partners Healthcare System recruited James H. Herndon, as chair of the Partners Orthopedic Department, including both hospitals. Thornhill and Herndon worked together over the next five years,

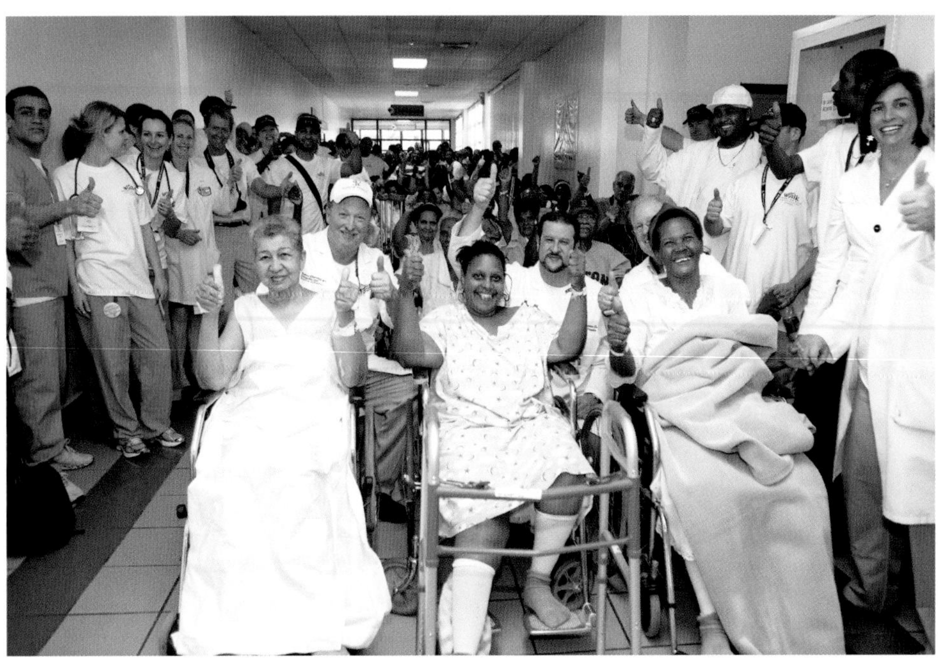

FIGURE 3-40 Operation Walk patients. Operation Walk Boston, established in 2007 by Thomas Thornhill and Richard Scott from the Department of Orthopedics at Brigham and Women's Hospital, provides free joint replacement and rehabilitation services every spring to patients in the Dominican Republic.

also in conjunction with the HMS Orthopedic Executive Committee, expanding educational and clinical programs in all adult subspecialties and both clinical and basic research.[101] Herndon retired in 2003. His administrative duties were assumed by Thornhill and Harry E. Rubash at the MGH, facilitating continued clinical and research growth.

Herndon and Thornhill, with the Executive Committee, augmented teaching in the Harvard Combined Orthopedic Residency Program, an important integrating factor for Partners orthopedics. Grand Rounds at BWH and MGH were combined for all residents and staff. Grand Rounds was followed by a four-hour core curriculum, the centerpiece of the teaching program for residents at each hospital. At the beginning of the academic year, anatomy was taught with cadaver dissections at the Medical School, recently led by Scott D. Martin at BWH. Faculty and resident retreats were held to improve the teaching program and comply with the evolving Core Requirements of the Accreditation Committee on Graduate Medical Education. Outstanding residents continue to train in the program. Many graduates of this program continue to advance orthopedics and hold major positions in academic medical centers and professional organizations throughout the United States.

Clinically, the adult reconstruction program remained a major strength of the department, and Dan M. Estok was recruited to head a program of revision hip surgery for complex cases. Tom Minas established an international center of cartilage transplantation. Mark S. Vrahas was appointed to head orthopedic trauma for Partners, the most successful clinically integrated specialty division in orthopedics at BWH and MGH.[102] Mitchell B. Harris was recruited as the chief of trauma at BWH. The shoulder service was also integrated and directed by Peter J. Millett. By 2000, the number of surgical cases had increased by 8%. With the merger of Faulkner Hospital with Brigham and Women's Hospital, orthopedic clinical volume grew by 13%.[103] A foot and ankle center was established at the Faulkner, under Michael Wilson, who later became its chief of orthopedics. Sheila A. Dugan, physiatrist, joined to treat overuse problems and back pain. Total surgical volume grew by 39% by 2002. At the same time, the percentage of patients whose surgery was conducted on an outpatient basis increased from 28% in 1998 to 43% in 2002. Office visits during the same period increased by 31% and total surgical procedures grew 39%.[104] Currently, the department includes ten clinical specialty divisions (and chiefs): Adult Reconstruction (Dan Estok), the Cartilage Repair Center (Tom Minas), Foot and Ankle (Christopher Chiodo), Hand and Upper Extremity (Barry Simmons), Oncology (John Ready), Trauma (Mitchel B. Harris with Mark Vrahas as Partners Chief), Podiatry (James Ioli), Sports Medicine (Lawrence D. Higgins), Spine (Christopher M. Bono), and Shoulder (Lawrence Higgins). Elizabeth Matzkin is the surgical director for Women's Musculoskeletal Health in the Center for Excellence in Women's Health. Tamara L. Martin assumed the position of chief of the orthopedic service at the VA Boston Healthcare System, following John Ready.

Basic research is now focused in five laboratories (with chiefs): Optical Coherence Tomography (Mark E. Brezniski; an essay on this endeavor is included in this volume), Nanotechnology and Polymer Science (Anuj Bellare), Skeletal Biology (Julie Glowacki), Proteomics and Genomics (Keith D. Crawford), and the Orthopedic and Arthritis Center for Outcomes Research (Jeffrey N. Katz and Elena Losina). Research funding from the NIH and industry continues to increase.

Orthopedic surgery at Brigham and Women's Hospital is a large, mature surgical specialty department that includes all the adult specialties, staffed by an outstanding faculty with national and international reputations. Its research program is a national leader in extramural support in orthopedics and the department has a large, diverse clinical and research faculty. It has continued its major strength, begun by Potter at the RBBH, in adult reconstructive surgery, and remains an active collaborator in the Robert B. Brigham Arthritis and Musculoskeletal Disease Clinical Research Center. The department has recently added a new important focus, assessing patient outcomes in the Orthopedic and Arthritis Center for Outcomes Research, setting the stage for the department's continued leadership in the new healthcare paradigm in the United States.

EXCELLENCE FROM OUT OF THE SHADOWS: A CENTURY OF BRIGHAM RADIOLOGY

Bryan Murphy and Steven E. Seltzer

The rich history of excellence in radiology at the Brigham and Women's Hospital was shaped primarily and permanently during three distinct eras and the tenures of four chairmen. In the first era, Merrill C. Sosman established the standard for clinical excellence that defines the department to this day. In the second, Herbert L. Abrams and a team of talented researchers and educators made Radiology an academic department of national prominence. In the third era, B. Leonard Holman, who sadly passed away in the midst of a flourishing career, and his successor, current chair Steven E. Seltzer, built on the strengths of the department in positioning it to respond to a rapidly changing healthcare landscape.

A First-Rate Clinical Service

Merrill C. Sosman accepted the position as chair of Brigham radiology in 1922. He thus began a tenure that would last for thirty-four years, and for nearly thirty years, he was the hospital's sole radiologist. He displayed voluminous clinical knowledge, a sharp wit, and a commitment to first-rate service on arrival, all of which quickly gained him equal footing with the chairs of the other, larger departments. As founding Physician-in-Chief Henry A. Christian wrote in his annual report for 1922, "Sosman has maintained the best traditions of his predecessors and brought a new skill, so that the medical and surgical services feel that... in the rapid strides of progress in this branch, our patients are being ever better served."

With radiology still in its formative years, Sosman's vision for the department focused primarily on establishing unequivocal standards for clinical service excellence. Despite being understaffed and belabored with an ill-lit and poorly ventilated location in the basement of the Brigham, Sosman consistently met the X-ray needs of the hospital's steadily increasing patient caseload. Working alone, he managed his

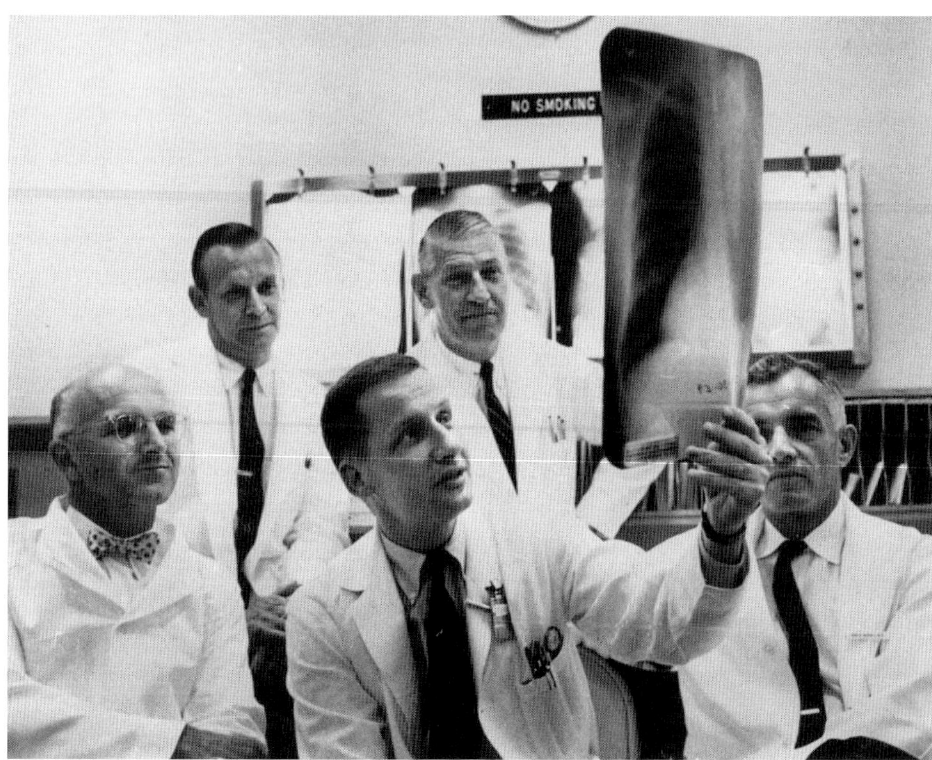

FIGURE 3-41 John Merrill reviews an x-ray with Joseph Murray, Gustave Dammin, and others.

department's own annual growth in X-ray volume, revenue, and operating costs. Reports from hospital leadership during this time offer glowing assessments of his work. This focus on clinical work was complemented by equally demanding research and training responsibilities. In 1924, he wrote the first two of his 130 lifetime papers, editorials, and annual reports on his department. In 1925, he persuaded hospital administrators to add a second radiology resident to his department, and this ultimately led to more than sixty alumnae from Sosman's years as chair. Most alumnae had successful careers of their own, both in private practice and academic radiology.

When he retired in 1956, Merrill Sosman had succeeded in establishing the standard for excellence in patient care that remains a driving force of the Department of Radiology. By the end of Sosman's tenure, although most radiology was performed at the Brigham, small radiology services had also begun at the Robert Breck Brigham Hospital and the Boston Hospital for Women. Compared with the clinical service, the research and education programs that Sosman seeded were less developed, but poised to flourish. It was under the leadership of chair Herbert L. Abrams, another towering figure in American radiology, that radiology research and education at the Brigham ascended to excellence.

A Fully Academic Department

When he arrived at the Brigham in September 1967, Herbert L. Abrams was sixteen years into a career that saw him achieve successes in all aspects of academic radiology: clinical, research, and teaching. As chair of diagnostic radiology at Stanford Medical School, he had built an impressive track record of funded research that gave him not only knowledge of the intricacies of grant writing, but also the authority to negotiate commitments from the hospital to support his efforts to expand these programs.

Abrams' first priority was to relocate the department's clinical services and add salaries for hiring new staff. Radiology still occupied the same basement site that Sosman had found inadequate forty-five years earlier. A new building was constructed to accommodate the initial staff of seventeen full-time radiologists, six residents, eighteen radiologic technologists, thirty support staff, and the twelve trainees of the technologist training program. The hospital leadership also agreed to designate three floors of the Shields Warren Radiation Laboratory for radiology research and to fund the procurement of innovative research equipment. This space eventually housed cardiovascular, pulmonary, and renal physiologic research programs. Abrams' appointment as radiology's first full professor at Harvard Medical School also established the resources to revitalize the sagging residency and fellowship programs.

With the assets necessary for a strong academic department in place and a leadership team comprised of trusted colleagues, Abrams turned his attention to what was the centerpiece of his vision for Brigham Radiology: a bid for a Radiology Center Grant from the National Institutes of Health (NIH). By the 1970s, most other medical disciplines had received large grants from the NIH and other funding agencies to establish research centers for the physiological and pathological study of diseases afflicting specific organs and systems. As increasingly specialized and research-oriented as radiology was becoming, no academic department had yet received one of these center grants, but Abrams and Brigham Radiology succeeded in being a unique recipient. The Center Grant was initially a commitment by the NIH of $1 million for three years. It enabled the recruitment of dozens of bright young physicians and scientists with basic research interests and skills, funded equipment and travel, and provided an untouchable base for research activities. The clinical innovations that emerged from the center grant were deemed so vital that it was renewed continuously over the next two decades.

A Modern Department for Modern Times

B. Leonard Holman, a member of the residency class that entered in 1970, saw firsthand the benefits the Center Grant brought to the department. A nuclear medicine specialist, Holman spent his career at the Brigham compiling an admirable portfolio of published research and a reputation as a brilliant clinician. As Abrams neared retirement, he mentored Holman to be his successor and began teaching him the finer points of running a thriving academic radiology department.

Holman was appointed the department's acting chair in 1986 and the official chair in 1988. Those were changing times for radiology. Technological advances had led to the development of multislice computed tomography scanners and high-field strength magnetic resonance imaging magnets, powerful devices that were widely sought, even if their clinical utility was not yet fully understood. The pace of subspecialization in radiology, which had begun during Abrams' chairmanship, was picking up, and the advent of digitization and web-based information technology systems provided radiologists and technologists with more complicated sequencing protocols and larger data sets than ever before. Under Holman, the department deftly incorporated the sweeping changes in radiology. As professional subspecialization continued, reorganization of technical services led to a new Division of Ambulatory Radiology and a comfortable, convenient facility for examining outpatients. A new Information Technology Division was formed, one of the first in academic radiology, and its members began to harness the power of the worldwide web to improve productivity and efficiency. As the 1980s drew to a close, Holman remarked in a note to the department members that the Brigham radiology was strong, with outstanding staff in all areas of its function.

Sadly, Holman became seriously ill in 1997, in the midst of a brilliant career that was just reaching its prime. He passed away the following year. In the spring of 1997, Steven E. Seltzer was named acting chair and became the permanent chair later in the year.

Picking up where Holman, his friend and mentor, left off, Seltzer continues to shape the department in proper response to emerging trends and the needs of patients. Brigham Radiology has grown to include community-based locations throughout southeastern Massachusetts that offer patients access to Brigham quality closer to home. Tireless work to enhance the information technology infrastructure has resulted in applications that both assist referring doctors in selecting the best imaging test and deliver images and reports to their computers with the press of a button. Building on work that began under Holman, the first decade of the new millennium was marked by major departmental advances in molecular imaging, the construction and opening of an on-site cyclotron, and the August 2011 opening of the Advanced Multimodality Image Guided Operating (AMIGO) suite, created by department member Ferenc A. Jolesz.

As the staff of the Department of Radiology welcomes a new century, they do so knowing that sustained excellence will be the result of daily renewed commitment to the clinical, research, and teaching mission of the Brigham and Women's Hospital.

STEREOTACTIC RADIOSURGERY AT THE BRIGHAM

Edward R. Laws, Jr.

In 2011, stereotactic radiosurgery has become a standard part of the treatment of a variety of disorders affecting the brain and the nervous system. These include the noninvasive treatment of many brain tumors, benign, malignant, and metastatic; vascular malformations of the brain; trigeminal neuralgia; and a number of experimental applications.

The concept of stereotaxis is one of localizing precisely specific areas within the brain based on the anatomy as demonstrated by radiographic techniques. This concept dates back to the beginning of the twentieth century and was vastly enhanced by the recent development of computed tomography and magnetic resonance imaging.

The development of the gamma knife in the early 1950s marked the advent of the modern era of radiosurgery. This device was based on a number of radioactive cobalt sources precisely focused on a single point within the head and guided by imaging that included skull radiographs and pneumoencephalography. Subsequent applications of the concept were developed in Boston and in California, using high-energy particles produced by a cyclotron. The deposition of energy from these particles could be carefully directed to precise areas within the brain where the radiation, as with the gamma knife, produced destructive lesions at the center of the target. The great expense of the underlying technology (cyclotron, Gama Knife with 201 Cobalt 60 sources) and the dedication of the methods to neurosurgical conditions hindered the widespread use of these modalities. These technical platforms were uncommon, whereas the linear accelerator, used for many forms of standard radiotherapy was ubiquitous. Although there were some sporadic attempts to modify the commonly available linear accelerator-derived radiotherapy for radiosurgical treatment, none had been found to be practical, effective, and safe enough for general use.

Attempts to develop a practical radiosurgical system were always a collaborative effort. Commonly, they involved a neurosurgeon, a radiation oncologist, a radiation physicist, and the appropriate engineering necessary to modify and optimize the equipment. This concept came to fruition in the late 1980s at the Brigham when the Joint Center for Radiation Therapy was initiated, involving members of various specialties from the Brigham and the Children's Hospital. An inspired team led by Ken R. Winston, a neurosurgeon, and Wendell Lutz, a radiation physicist, worked together to develop the first truly practical radiosurgical instrument. The criteria they used included accuracy of the anatomic focus and target planning, accuracy in the nature and distribution of the radiation dose, and safety to the surrounding brain and radiosensitive structures such as the optic nerves. Their methodologic approach utilized a newly developed stereotactic frame that was fixed to the skull, a "phantom" device that would accurately approximate the brain and the target area, and specifically designed collimators for the radiation beam. The "phantom" consisted of the stereotactic frame within which a mock target point was placed according to the calculations based on each individual patient's cerebral anatomy. This allowed for precise pretreatment confirmation of the radiosurgical plan. They also developed systematic methods for verification of all the mathematical calculations and for analyzing errors in measurements and targeting.

"Linear Accelerator as a Neurosurgical Tool for Stereotactic Radiosurgery" by Winston and Lutz was a landmark paper,[105] heralding the safe and evolving widespread use of this exciting modality.[106] From 1988 on, and for the next decade, the Brigham performed more radiosurgical procedures than anywhere else in the United States. This perhaps was related to the legacy of Harvey Cushing and his pioneering work on brain tumors and also on the work and reputation of Donald Matson, who pioneered the field of pediatric neurosurgery at the Children's Hospital.

With the help of Jay Loeffler from Radiation Oncology and others, outcome data regarding the usefulness of stereotactic radiosurgery for treating a variety of brain tumors and vascular malformations of the brain were published and established the Brigham as the national leader in this important area of treatment and research.[107] More recently, these principles have been utilized with dramatic effect in the treatment of multiple metastatic tumors in the brain. Some exciting examples of newly developing indications, currently under study, are psychiatric disorders, movement disorders, and epilepsy. Presently, virtually every academic neuroscience and neuro-oncology program has the capability of offering radiosurgery as part of its armamentarium. The majority of these units are based on the linear accelerator as the radiation source, and are direct descendants of the pioneering work at the Brigham.

NEUROLOGY AT THE BRIGHAM

Martin A. Samuels

When the Peter Bent Brigham Hospital opened in 1913, Harvey W. Cushing was named the surgeon-in-chief. During the Cushing era (1913-1932), Physician-in-Chief Henry Christian never appointed a neurologist to the staff. Cushing functioned as both a neurosurgeon and neurologist and even served a term as the president of the American Neurological Association. Among his many contributions, he incorporated X-ray into the evaluation of neurological illnesses only a short time after Roentgen's discovery. He also commissioned an engineer, W.T. Bovi, to create a coagulation device for intraoperative use. He introduced the recording of careful intraoperative measurements. The rise in blood pressure caused by increased intracranial pressure is still known as the Cushing reflex. Cushing pioneered surgeries for tic douloureux, vestibular schwannomas, meningiomas, and pituitary tumors. Tumors that secreted corticosteroids are still known as Cushing disease. The syndrome imitating the tumor, but caused by exogenous use of therapeutic steroids, is known as Cushing syndrome.

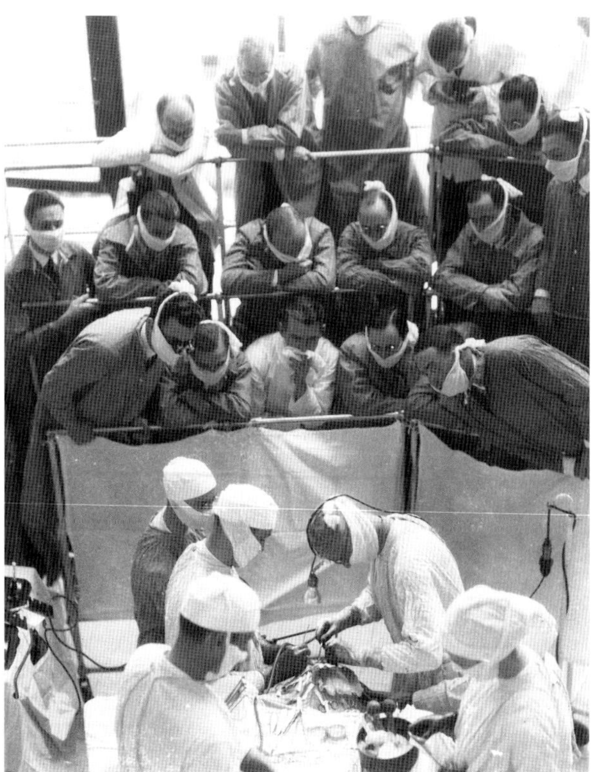

FIGURE 3-42 Harvey Cushing operating on a patient.

When Soma Weiss succeeded Henry Christian in 1939 as the Hersey Professor and physician-in-chief at the Brigham, he brought with him from the Boston City Hospital physicians John Romano, Eugene A. Stead, and Charles Janeway as his full-time faculty: Romano for neurology and psychiatry, Stead for general medicine, and Janeway for infectious diseases. For the next three years, H. Houston Merritt, also from the Boston City Hospital, made Tuesday afternoon rounds with John Romano on all the neurological patients identified during the week. Studies on delirium and syncope, initiated in 1941 by Romano and George L. Engel, led to the birth of psychosomatic medicine, further developed by Romano and Engel at the University of Cincinnati and then the University of Rochester.

Throughout the rest of the 1940s and early 1950s, neurological consultations at the Brigham were performed by a number of distinguished neurologists, including physicians Augustus Rose, Derek Denny-Brown, and Raymond Adams, all based at the Boston City Hospital. Roy Swank, a specialist in multiple sclerosis, based most of his practice at the Brigham until the mid-1950s and is still known for his introduction of a low fat diet (the Swank diet) for the treatment of multiple sclerosis. In 1956, Physician-in-Chief George Thorn recruited H. Richard Tyler to be the first truly full-time neurologist at the Brigham. Tyler had completed his internship at the Brigham followed by neurological training under Denny-Brown at the Boston City Hospital. Tyler made numerous contributions, particularly in the area of medical neurology, including describing the neurological aspects of congenital heart disease, renal failure, and dialysis. Tyler was one of the first to study the physiology of asterixis, the characteristic movement disorder of many metabolic encephalopathies, most notably portosystemic (hepatic) encephalopathy. Neurologist David M.

Dawson, also a City Hospital trainee, joined Tyler shortly thereafter, followed by H. Harris Funkenstein in stroke and Mark Hallett, the founding director of the clinical neurophysiology laboratories. Dawson had many interests, including neuro-rheumatology (he was the neurological consultant to the Robert Breck Brigham Hospital), cancer neurology (he was the first neurological consultant to the Dana-Farber Cancer Institute), multiple sclerosis, and neuromuscular diseases. Dawson discovered the isoenzymes of creatine kinase, the elevation of which were characteristic of cardiac muscle (CK-MB) and skeletal muscle (CK-MM) disorders.

During the Tyler era, the neurology division remained in the department of medicine but grew impressively with the addition of major basic research programs led by Dennis Selkoe in Alzheimer disease and Howard Weiner in multiple sclerosis. Selkoe is perhaps the leading proponent of the amyloid hypothesis as the cause of Alzheimer disease. Weiner has created the most comprehensive center for the treatment of multiple sclerosis and the search for its cause. From the early 1960s onward, the Brigham was part of the Harvard Longwood Neurology Training Program. This program graduated many physician leaders of academic neurology, including Dennis Choi, Michael Moskowitz, Howard Weiner, Dennis Selkoe, Michael Goldberg, Steven Sergay, Marc Dichter, Stuart Lipton, Arnold Kriegstein, Stefan Pulst, Jeffrey Buchalter, Bruce Korf, Jeffrey Saver, Steven Warach, and Orla Hardiman.

In 1988, Martin A. Samuels succeeded Tyler as neurology division chief and in 1995 became chair of the independent Brigham Department of Neurology. Partners HealthCare system was created in 1995 with its anchor academic medical centers the Brigham and the Massachusetts General Hospital. The Partners Neurology Training Program began shortly thereafter, graduating its first cadre of residents in 2000. In 2007, Allan H. Ropper joined the department as the executive vice chair of Neurology. Ropper, well-known worldwide and the Raymond D. Adams Distinguished Professor of Neurology at the Brigham, developed the field of neurological intensive care. Other notable contributions include the use of plasma exchange to treat Guillain-Barré syndrome, and descriptions of the mechanism of herniation from increased intracranial pressure, the clinical features of chronic inflammatory demyelinating polyneuropathy, and many other phenomena. Samuels is widely considered the leading expert in the interface between neurology and the rest of medicine. Samuels and Ropper are the coauthors of the *Adams and Victor's Principles of Neurology* and coeditors of *Samuels's Manual of Neurological Therapeutics*, two of the most widely utilized neurology books in the world.

Today the Department of Neurology is a very large and complex entity with more than 400 faculty members divided into twelve divisions and a major basic, clinical, and translational research program. The research program occupies about 50,000 square feet of laboratory space and is funded by more than $42,000,000 in total modified direct costs annually, mostly from the National Institutes of Health. Operating programs include a very active acute neurology inpatient service (about 1,500 discharges annually), a twenty-bed neurological intensive care unit, a busy consultation service (about 2,000 inpatient and emergency department consultations annually), and a full array of subspecialty ambulatory programs, including stroke, multiple sclerosis, epilepsy, sleep, headache, movement disorders, neuromuscular disease, neuro-ophthalmology, cancer neurology, and behavioral neurology. The Brigham Department provides the neurology services for the Faulkner Hospital, the South Shore Hospital, and the Dana-Farber Cancer Institute and maintains a close relationship with the Department of Veterans Affairs Medical Center, where department member Michael Charness is the current chief of staff. A close liaison is maintained with the Children's Hospital's Department of Neurology, which provides pediatric neurology coverage to the Brigham's busy neonatal intensive care unit. Current Brigham Department of Neurology division chiefs, all of whom are leaders in their respective fields, are physicians Steven K. Feske (Stroke), Galen V. Henderson (Critical Care), Anthony A. Amato (Neuromuscular Diseases), Barbara A. Dworetzky (Epilepsy and Sleep), Patrick Y.Wen (Cancer Neurology), Kirk R. Daffner (Cognitive and Behavioral Neurology), Don

C. Bienfang (Neuro-ophthalmology), Joshua P. Klein (Hospital Neurology), Thomas M. Walshe (General Neurology), Elizabeth W. Loder (Headache), Lewis R. Sudarsky (Movement Disorders), Howard L. Weiner (Multiple Sclerosis), Michael T. Hayes (South Shore Hospital), David M. Pilgrim (Harvard Vanguard Neurology & Faulkner Hospital), and Dennis J. Selkoe (Neuroscience).

Nervous system diseases have been at the core of the Brigham's mission over its first century. As the founding surgeon-in-chief, Cushing established the Brigham as the leading institution for the diagnosis and treatment of neurological and neurosurgical disorders and for the training of the next generation of academic neuroscientists. Over the century, neurology has grown from a few visiting physicians into an enormous department with an international reputation for groundbreaking basic and translational research, superb clinical care, and training of future leaders.

BIOGRAPHY

H. RICHARD TYLER

Peter V. Tishler

Rick Tyler, a veteran at the Brigham, created and was chief of the Neurology Division from 1955 until 1988. He came to the Brigham initially in 1951 as a medical intern. He then trained at the outstanding neurology unit at the Boston City Hospital (BCH), run by Harvard Professor Derek Denny-Brown. He returned as the Brigham's first full-time staff neurologist (1956), at a time when neurology was considered a medical stepchild. He continued his friendship and association with Denny-Brown, who sent senior residents to Tyler at the Brigham for a complementary neurological experience. He developed the neurology inpatient and consultation service, employing outstanding neurologists whom he often paid with his personal funds. One such person, David M. Dawson, was also a Brigham intern and a BCH/Denny-Brown trainee. He joined the neurology staff in 1967 and remains active to this day. Another neurologist, Mark Hallett, also interned in medicine at the Brigham and was a staff associate from 1976-1984. He is currently a leader at the National Institute of Neurological Disorders and Stroke. Rick created a training program for residents in neurology, in affiliation ultimately with the Children's and the Beth Israel Hospitals (the "Longwood Area neurology program"). He carried out research with associates who were either already medical statesmen (e.g., George Thorn) or destined for this role (Eugene Robin, who spent his subsequent professional life at the University of Pittsburgh).

After resigning from his leadership position and leaving the Brigham (1988), Rick entered private practice, which continues to this day at a venue within walking distance of the Brigham. He maintains his interest in the history of both the Brigham and neurology. A prolific writer, he has recently coauthored an article (with his son Kenneth L. Tyler) on Derek Denny-Brown for the book entitled *The Cradle of American Neurology: The Harvard Neurological Unit at the Boston City Hospital*, edited by D.M. Dawson and T.D. Sabin (2011). He has donated numerous artifacts and records of historical importance to the Countway Center for the History of Medicine. Three of his four children are physicians, and the fourth is a doctor of education. Son Kenneth continues the family tradition. After making rounds with his father on Sundays as a child, he trained in medicine at the Brigham before entering neurology. He is as currently chief of neurology at the University of Colorado. Full circle!

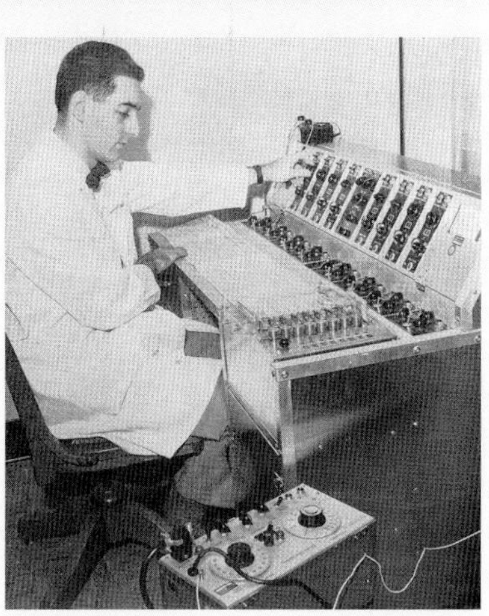

FIGURE 3-43 Rick Tyler and EEG machine, 1957.

PATHOLOGY AT THE BRIGHAM

Michael A. Gimbrone, Jr.

The Department of Pathology at the Brigham and Women's Hospital traces its roots to the founding of the Boston Lying-In Hospital in 1832, the Free Hospital for Women in 1875, and the Peter Bent Brigham Hospital in 1913. The situation of the Peter Bent Brigham Hospital in close proximity to the newly constructed Harvard Medical School (HMS) set the stage for a coevolution of the two institutions and the discipline of pathology in the Harvard medical community. The Brigham Department of Pathology thus has a long-standing tradition as an academic department defined by its commitment to excellence in clinical care, teaching and training, and research.

William Thomas Councilman, chair of the department at HMS, was also appointed the first pathologist-in-chief in 1913. Councilman was an expert in the study of amoebiasis, diphtheria, smallpox, and yellow fever. His vivid morphologic description of changes seen in the liver of yellow fever lives on today as "Councilman bodies." S. Burt Wolbach served as Shattuck Professor, pathologist, and chair from 1916 to 1947. Among Wolbach's numerous research contributions, his discovery of the causative agents (rickettsial organisms) of Rocky Mountain spotted fever and typhus remains the most significant. Wolbach also served simultaneously as the chair of pathology at HMS, where he spent most of his time conducting research. He came to the Brigham daily to mentor the chief resident who then taught other junior residents. He reportedly personally supported the Brigham Pathology Department financially during frequent fiscal crises.

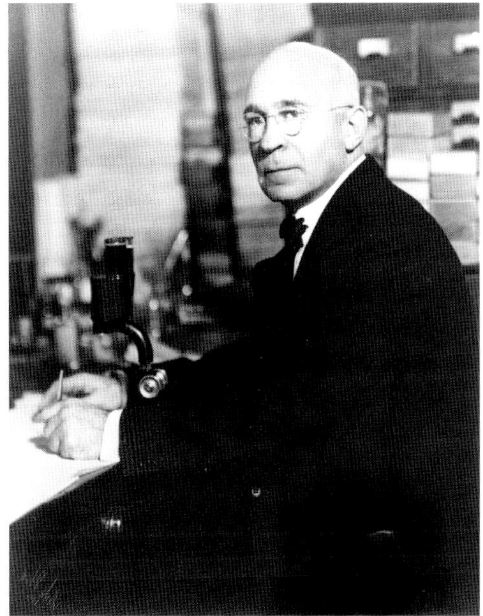

FIGURE 3-44 S. Burt Wolbach, Chief of Pathology at the Peter Bent Brigham Hospital, 1916-1947, and pathologist at the Boston Lying-In Hospital.

Postwar Era

Gustave (Gus) J. Dammin became the pathologist-in-chief in 1952. Gus made seminal observations in the early days of organ transplant pathology, including contributing to the understanding of the mechanisms of organ and tissue rejection. He was an important member of the team, led by Joseph Murray, that performed the first successful kidney transplant in 1954. Building on his interests in tropical parasitic diseases, which he studied during his World War II service, he studied many infectious diseases, including Lyme disease and babesiosis. Dammin was awarded one of the very first National Institutes of Health (NIH) Institutional Research Training Grants in Pathology in 1958 (which has remained funded continuously to the present), led a departmental NIH-funded program project (on transplantation), and graduated a large number of academic leaders, including several departmental chairs. The late Piero Paci and some of the senior members of the current department, including Mac Corson, Franz von Lichtenberg, Geraldine Pinkus, William Schoene, and Nora Galvanek, all joined Brigham Pathology during his tenure.

The Women's and Perinatal Division

The Pathology Services at the Boston Lying-In Hospital and the Free Hospital for Women, the forerunners of the Women and Perinatal Division, made major contributions in both gynecologic and obstetric pathology.

These early achievements included the detailed morphologic descriptions of early human development (by Arthur T. Hertig, a student and mentee of Wolbach), the first classifications of trophoblastic neoplasia (Arthur Hertig, Hazel Gore, Shirley G. Driscoll), detailed descriptions and documentation of placental development (Kurt Benirschke), classification of premalignant cervical intraepithelial neoplasia (CIN; Ralph M. Richart), and establishing the association between a human papillomavirus and high-grade CIN (Christopher P. Crum). In the last sixty years, directed in the separate facilities and their merged hospital (Boston Hospital for Women, 1966-1982) by Arthur T. Hertig, John Craig, and Shirley Driscoll, and in the consolidated Brigham by Shirley Driscoll and currently Christopher P. Crum, the division has trained many past and future leaders in the field.

The Legacy of Ramzi Cotran

Ramzi S. Cotran, the Frank Burr Mallory Professor of Pathology, succeeded Dammin in 1974. By current standards, the department was small, with thirteen faculty members conducting clinical service, teaching, and research in cramped, outdated facilities. The merger of the Peter Bent Brigham Hospital with the Robert Breck Brigham Hospital (1977) and the Boston Hospital for Women (1982), with the resultant major expansion of facilities, and the enormous growth of clinical and research activities in the 1980s precipitated an explosive growth in pathology under Cotran's stewardship. Ramzi was a visionary leader who saw great value in interdisciplinary collaboration and believed in the importance of bridging clinical service and research. Exploiting his charisma, leadership, warmth, skills, intellect, and devotion, he established a truly integrated academic pathology department. His deliberate early recruitment of young investigators, including Venkatachalam, Abbas, Rennke, Gimbrone, Madara, Pober, Davies, Bevilacqua, and Collins, established the Brigham's leadership in experimental pathology, and, especially the new field of vascular biology. Cotran was a tireless and legendary mentor to all his staff, trainees, friends, and colleagues. He established a standard that everyone associated with our department will forever try to model. With more than twenty past and current departmental chairs, deans, and other leaders of academic medicine counted among his former Brigham trainees and associates, his spirit and legacy endures.

Brigham Pathology Today and Tomorrow

Michael A. Gimbrone, Jr., the first Ramzi S. Cotran Professor of Pathology, became chair of pathology at BWH in 2001. Trained as a resident in pathology at this institution, he has been a member of the staff since 1974. His research interests in endothelial pathobiology were developed under the mentorship of Judah Folkman and Ramzi Cotran. Michael is an internationally recognized researcher in vascular biology and has served as the director of the Brigham Center for Excellence in Vascular Biology since 1998. A committed teacher and longtime leader of the MD student research Honors Thesis Program at Harvard Medical School, he continues to play an active role in both the HMS and Harvard-MIT Health Sciences and Technology (HST) undergraduate medical curricula.

During Gimbrone's tenure as chair, the department has grown considerably, implementing new clinical and research endeavors. It currently consists of some 120-plus faculty members, fifty-eight residents and clinical fellows, and fifty-five research fellows; examines more than 74,000 surgical specimens and 56,000 cytologies annually; runs a modern Molecular Diagnostics Laboratory, including a large academic cytogenetics program; occupies some 89,000 sq. ft. of clinical space and more than 51,000 sq. ft. of research space; and attracts more than $15 million in research funding annually. The department emphasizes translational molecular pathology as a vehicle for realizing the potential of pathology to facilitate the practice of personalized medicine. The Center for Molecular Oncologic Pathology, an effort of the Dana-Farber/Brigham and Women's Cancer Center dedicated to translational research, was formed in 2007. The Center for Advanced Molecular Diagnostics, which opened in 2008 in the new Shapiro Building, has become the hub of a major collaborative effort between the Dana-Farber Cancer Institute and the Brigham in the area of the molecular genetics of cancer. This partnership has launched

"Profile," a study that will create a huge database of genomic analyses of malignancies. Profile aims to identify genetic causes of cancers, afford affected patients access to targeted therapeutics, and develop sophisticated molecular diagnostics. In 2011, total laboratory automation for the Clinical Laboratories was implemented, followed by a complete redesign of the Anatomical Pathology facilities. The "capstone" of this ambitious project was the dedication of The Ramzi Cotran Conference Center in January, 2012, the intellectual center of this forward-looking department.

In March, 2012, Jeffrey A. Golden succeeded Michael Gimbrone as the chair of Brigham Pathology and the second Ramzi S. Cotran Professor of Pathology at HMS. Recruited from the Children's Hospital of Philadelphia, where he was chair of the Department of Pathology, he is an internationally recognized translational neuropathologist who brings special expertise to the emerging neurosciences initiative at the Brigham.

In 1947, Burt Wolbach stated how pleased he was by the major academic achievements of his pupils and trainees, including academic stars Ernest Goodpasture, Monroe Schlesinger, Sidney Farber, Arthur Hertig, Frank Horsfall, and Robert Gross. He also stated, with some modesty, that "the list is presented not as a proof of the superiority of the Brigham Hospital Department or training, but as evidence that the Department and the Hospital attracted individuals of ability, who found here adequate opportunities for development." This remains as true today as it was then, and preserving these opportunities for academic pathologists remains the department's commitment.

BIOGRAPHY

RAMZI S. COTRAN, 1932–2000

Peter V. Tishler

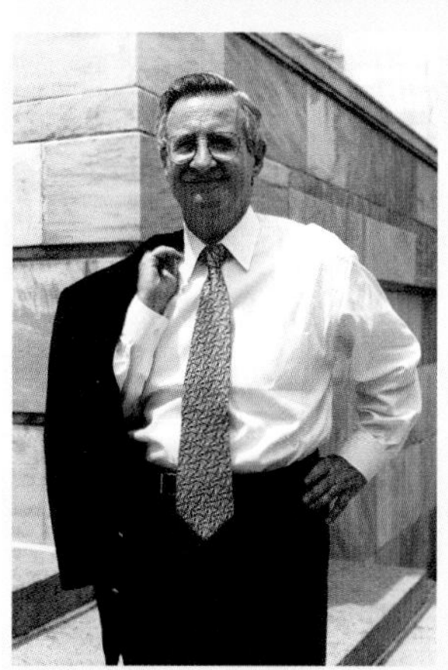

FIGURE 3-45 Ramzi Cotran.

Ramzi Suliman Cotran (pathologist-in-chief, 1974-2000) was a distinguished scientist, mentor, and seminal leader who set a pervasive tone for what Frederick J. Schoen has called the "top-to-bottom Departmental ethos of opportunity, program flexibility and mentorship." He introduced the Gross Conference, whereby all autopsies were reviewed by senior faculty to augment teaching. Cotran and his colleague Stanley L. Robbins (initially at Boston City Hospital, joining the Brigham and Women's Hospital faculty in 1980) authored what has been for many decades the world's leading general pathology textbook, *Pathologic Basis of Disease* (Robbins and Cotran, editors, currently in its seventh edition). As stated by Barry Bienner, "In teaching and mentoring in pathology, Cotran was without peer in his influence and legacy. In his many years of contact with students, residents, fellows, and junior faculty at Harvard, Cotran directly guided hundreds of talented individuals."[108]

Early in my house staff days on the Harvard Medical Unit at the Boston City Hospital, I met Ramzi. He had come recently to the Mallory Institute of Pathology as a fellow. Simultaneously, he was working in the Channing Laboratory with Edward H. Kass on recurrent urinary tract infections and their importance in the pathogenesis of chronic pyelonephritis. This was the beginning of his lifelong interest in diseases of the kidney, leading to his international recognition as a clinical investigator. Also at the same time, when we house officers needed expert pathological consultation, we went to Ramzi, who was a Harvard appointee even then. With this interaction, we became friends. Later, after I joined the Channing, we talked together, joked together, and did some research (tapping his expertise in electron microscopy) together. Ramzi was a very bright person, a wonderful fellow, an expert pathologist, and just the right researcher for me. His appointment as the Frank B. Mallory Professor of Pathology at Harvard Medical School in 1972, while still at the Mallory (the sole Harvard Pathology representative), was totally consistent. I was not surprised but did feel bereft when he left for the green pastures of the Peter Bent Brigham Hospital, to succeed Gustave Dammin as pathologist-in-chief in 1974.

Ramzi inherited a small department (thirteen faculty members) in a small area of the Tackaberry Building on Shattuck Street. Adding the elixir of Cotran to the mix led to a department of more than seventy faculty (eleven with professorial rank) and an equal number of residents and fellows. The department's many functions grew commensurately. Research expanded to become the second largest effort of all departments at the Brigham, and his role as investigator and mentor permeated this phenomenon throughout his tenure. He committed to major advances in the education of pathologist trainees, who populated academic pathology worldwide, including two dozen departmental chairs, institute directors, and deans. He took great delight in helping young physicians navigate the uncertain waters of academic medicine and showed true joy in their accomplishments. Ramzi was expert in listening to what a young person said, and then, in a gentle but direct fashion, he provided simple reality testing and constructive advice. Michael Gimbrone, his successor as chair of pathology, learned to write scientific papers from Ramzi. "Ramzi would patiently sit with me over handwritten drafts, and with the help of a sharp red pencil and his wonderful talent for gentle persuasion, he taught me the art of scientific writing—with an emphasis on clarity of both thought and expression." He played a pivotal role in the politics of medical care at the Brigham, and even at the VA Hospital in West Roxbury, where he developed a working plan, enthusiastically accepted, for the integration the faculty and training programs of Boston University School of Medicine and Harvard Medical School. He became the chair of pathology at the Children's Hospital Medical Center in 1990.

Ramzi's efforts were recognized by numerous awards, including The Gold Headed Cane of the American Society for Investigative Pathology, the Distinguished Service Award of the Association of Pathology Chairs, and (at Harvard Medical School) the lifetime Achievement Award in Mentoring and the Dean's Award for Support and Achievement of Women Faculty. He had numerous illustrious friends and associates, from his early days (Guido Majno, Morris Karnovsky, Arthur Hertig), later days (Judah Folkman, Helmut Rennke, Michael Gimbrone, Franz von Lichtenberg, Stanley Robbins, whom he succeeded as editor of Robbins' classic pathology text, and others), and long term (Ernest Barsamian, chief of surgery then chief of staff at the West Roxbury VA Medical Center). He had a wonderful family (daughter Nina is a physician at the Brigham). His early death was such a blow to all. Michael Gimbrone notes: "To this day, I treasure the time he so generously shared with me." I agree; Ramzi is still with us.

HUMAN IMMUNODEFICIENCY VIRUS (HIV) CARE AND RESEARCH AT THE BRIGHAM: PROGRESS BEYOND PROGRESS

Paul E. Sax

In December 1979, a forty-eight-year-old gay male was admitted to the Peter Bent Brigham Hospital with a nine-month history of diarrhea and weight loss. In a stormy hospital course lasting more than three months, he ultimately died of wasting and respiratory failure. Notable microbiologic diagnoses included intestinal cryptosporidiosis and cytomegalovirus pneumonitis—both uncommon human pathogens for which there was no effective therapy. Today, the clinical details of this case—vividly detailed in a paper published by Louis Weinstein and colleagues—are instantly recognizable as consistent with advanced acquired immunodeficiency syndrome (AIDS).[109] Indeed, this patient may have been the first person to die from human immunodeficiency virus (HIV)–related complications at the Brigham. However, the first descriptions of cases of AIDS were still almost two years in the future, and the authors could only speculate that "immunologic incompetence, although suspected, could not be proved in the patient described in this paper."

In the more than three decades since this case, enormous progress in the prevention, diagnosis, and treatment of HIV infection has been made worldwide. Many Brigham faculty have played a major role in moving the field forward through their work in both basic and clinical research, and the hospital has become a well-known center for excellence in HIV care.

The Early Years of the HIV Epidemic (1981-1990)

The prognosis for patients with AIDS in the 1980s was poor. In the late 1980s, the median survival of patients after an AIDS-related complication was twelve to eighteen months. Long lengths of stay and challenging issues regarding end-of-life care frequently characterized HIV-related hospitalizations. Although AIDS-related hospital admissions steadily increased, outpatient care was relatively limited. Discharges from the Brigham were often to the nearby Hospice at Mission Hill, a dedicated inpatient hospice for people with AIDS. (A reflection on this hospice appears in Chapter 5.)

The most active infectious disease clinician in HIV care at the Brigham during this period was James (Jamie) H. Maguire. Despite the poor outcomes described in the preceding paragraphs, clinical expertise in identifying and managing HIV-related complications was critical, and judicious use of opportunistic infection prophylaxis prolonged survival. Typical patients from this period included gay men, people with hemophilia (the Brigham has the largest adult hemophilia center in New England), injection drug users, and foreign-born individuals from the Caribbean—including many heterosexual women with no history of drug use and often only one sexual partner. The formal collaboration in 1986 with the Harvard Community Health Plan (HCHP), which had added a population of young adult, single male patients, markedly increased the Brigham HIV inpatient population. This large ambulatory population was cared for by hematologist Joan H. Goldberg and a team of four nurses.

Conspicuously absent from the Brigham's HIV-related activities during the 1980s was research. This was in stark contrast to the other major Harvard teaching hospitals, which had begun major programs in both laboratory-based and clinical research. That the Brigham, with its growing research portfolio, close contact with Harvard Medical School, and a diverse patient population would have no research program in HIV through the first decade of the epidemic was a surprising omission that would soon would be corrected.

The Next Ten Years (1991-2001): Progress at the Brigham and Elsewhere

Faced with an increasing number of HIV-related admissions, many with prolonged lengths of stay, inconsistent outpatient follow-up, and frequent readmissions, the Division of Infectious Diseases created a team of HIV providers to manage the HIV population. Under the direction of Powel Kazanjian, Jr., the original team in 1991 also included infectious diseases fellow James Breeling, a nurse, and social worker Susan Larrabee, who remains a key member of the HIV team. I joined the HIV team in 1992 and was immediately impressed with the dedication of the providers and the cohesiveness of the group. Virtually all inpatients with HIV were seen in consultation by the HIV team. Every such inpatient was also seen by Ms. Larrabee or other social workers who later joined her, to address issues such as benefits, arranging outpatient care, disclosure of diagnosis to family or friends, workplace discrimination, treatment of addiction, or end-of-life decisions. Office hours of the HIV clinic were increased to accommodate all patients. In addition, in weekly team meetings that continue today, the team discussed active medical and psychosocial problems of all the inpatients and active outpatients. The results of having a dedicated HIV team were tangible for both patients and providers. Patient satisfaction increased, length of stay decreased, readmissions were prevented, and emergency room utilization declined. In addition, given the often tragic outcomes of these cases in the pre-antiretroviral therapy era, the HIV team provided much-needed peer support to all providers, many of whom might have otherwise burned out.

Clinical outcomes began to improve. Newly developed drugs were now administered in combination, with an incremental but significant effect of reducing AIDS complications. Most importantly, in the early 1990s, a clinical study demonstrated that zidovudine given to pregnant women with HIV and to their newborns at the time of birth led to a three-fold reduction in the risk of HIV transmission.[110] This multicenter clinical trial, led at the Brigham by Ruth Tuomala, in the Department of Obstetrics and Gynecology, was the first major HIV-related clinical trial to enroll study subjects at the Brigham. The study results immediately made zidovudine treatment standard-of-care for all pregnant women with HIV, and pediatric HIV cases plummeted nationally. The study also provided evidence that the Brigham could conduct HIV-related clinical research. As a result, Powel Kazanjian and I both actively sought clinical trials opportunities.

These HIV clinical research opportunities expanded greatly with the formation of Partners Healthcare in 1994. The Brigham had a diverse patient population, including a high proportion of women and racial and ethnic minorities. Because the HIV epidemic had broadened to increasingly include these groups, Martin S. Hirsch, who directed a large clinical trials unit at Massachusetts General Hospital (MGH), believed that including the Brigham's patients would fulfill an important mission of the national HIV research agenda. One of our first joint clinical trials, in 1995, was of the efficacy of the investigational protease inhibitor indinavir. Patients with the greatest HIV-related immunosuppression (those who had CD4 cell counts <50 cells/mm^3) were selected for this study. The results of this and other studies evaluating combination antiretroviral therapy were revelatory: subjects receiving triple therapy that included a protease inhibitor improved dramatically in clinical status, with sharp increases in their CD4 cell counts, and in many cases durable virologic suppression. For HIV specialists, witnessing this therapeutic miracle first-hand was a thrilling clinical experience.

Combination antiretroviral therapy, a remarkably successful treatment, became the standard of care in 1996 and changed the practice of HIV medicine nationally. At the Brigham, annual HIV-related hospital admissions fell from 400 in the early 1990s to 150 in 1998. Deaths from AIDS plummeted, and the Hospice at Mission Hill closed in 1997. As the number of patients living with HIV increased, the demand for outpatient services increased. The Division of Infectious Diseases now ran twenty-seven scheduled outpatient sessions weekly, a major change from the two to three outpatient sessions in 1992.

The effective HIV treatment drew the attention of Paul Farmer, a Brigham staff member and a former fellow in Infectious Diseases. Paul and collaborator, Jim Kim, had founded Partners in Health, an organization to improve the health for people, initially in Haiti, living in poverty. Paul and Jim recognized the disparity of HIV treatment between the United States and Haiti. In 1998, with guidance from Howard H. Hiatt, Partners in Health launched an initiative to treat Haiti's sickest patients with this new therapy. Using their experience treating tuberculosis with community-based directly observed therapy, the leaders enlisted the help of community-based *accompagnateurs* to ensure adherence to treatment and provide social support and other functions to optimize recovery.[111] The high levels of adherence and positive treatment responses in this nation, among the poorest in the world, demonstrated that HIV treatment could be expanded globally, a critical effort since the epidemic was worse in developing countries than in the United States. Farmer and Kim's work also attracted numerous physicians to the Brigham for training in both internal medicine and infectious diseases. Many of them have gained renown for similar work done in resource-limited settings, including Heidi L. Behforouz in Boston, Peter Drobac, in Rwanda, Sonya S. Shin, in Peru, and Louise Ivers, also in Haiti.

2001-Present: Building on Strength

HIV research at the Brigham took a substantial leap forward in 2001, with the recruitment of Daniel Kuritzkes. An internationally known virologist and laboratory scientist with expertise in HIV drug resistance and clinical trials, Dan was also Vice Chair of the AIDS Clinical Trials Group (ACTG), the largest consortium of HIV-related clinical trials sites worldwide, sponsored by the National

Institutes of Health. When he joined the Brigham, he became its first director of AIDS research and head of the Section of Retroviral Therapeutics. In 2010, he became chair and principal investigator of the ACTG. Dan's contribution to the HIV research environment at BWH was transformative, through both his own work and his mentorship. With his leadership position within the ACTG and his knowledge of both basic science and clinical trial methodology, he was able to offer Brigham faculty new opportunities in clinical and translational research. I was one of the beneficiaries of this connection, cochairing a major ACTG clinical trial[112] and conducting analyses on several others. Similar opportunities have arisen for junior faculty members Jonathan Li, Timothy J. Henrich, Athe M. Tsibris, and Florencia M. Pereyra.

Other members of the Infectious Diseases Division have been leading major HIV research programs. Shahin Lockman, who was a fellow in this division in the late 1990s, has focused on clinical trials and epidemiologic research related to the prevention of mother-to-child HIV transmission, circumcision to prevent sexual transmission, and the use of antiretroviral therapy in the developing world in general. In collaboration with Max Essex, at the Harvard School of Public Health, and with the ACTG, she has led or collaborated on pivotal clinical trials, some of them truly practice-changing. Shahin has definitively shown that single-dose nevirapine given for prevention of mother-to-child transmission reduces that woman's subsequent response to nevirapine-based therapy, largely due to the selection of a drug-resistant HIV.[113] Lindsey R. Baden, another Infectious Diseases Fellowship graduate, leads a large clinical trials effort focused on HIV vaccine. Working with Raphael Dolin and Dan H. Barouch, at the Beth Israel Deaconess Medical Center and Bruce D. Walker, at the MGH, his research group is enrolling study subjects into a wide range of preventive HIV vaccine trials.

The outpatient HIV practice at the Brigham currently follows more than 800 patients. The primary members of the clinical HIV team, in addition to me, include Sigal Yawetz, Jennifer Johnson, Florencia Pereyra, Lisa A. Cosimi, Cameron D. Ashbaugh, Daniel Kuritzkes, a fellow in infectious diseases, registered nurses Charles Dewan and William Theisen, and social workers Susan Larrabee and Carrie A. Braverman. Of the patients, 39% are women and 66% are nonwhite, both consistent proportions over the years. The median age has increased significantly, to forty-eight years, in response to effective HIV treatment. Three patients are in their eighties. The two most common non-English spoken languages are Spanish and Haitian Creole. Hospitalizations for patients with HIV today are largely for non–HIV-related problems. Remarkably, opportunistic infections, such as those described by Weinstein and colleagues in 1979,[114] occur only in patients not receiving antiretroviral therapy. Among patients treated in our clinic, 85% have undetectable HIV ribonucleic acid (RNA), an indication that they are being treated successfully. Ongoing clinical challenges include the management of reproductive options for serodiscordant couples, reducing non–HIV-related complications (evidence suggests that HIV accelerates the aging process) and the ongoing care of patients with significant psychosocial issues.

HIV at the Brigham (and elsewhere) has indeed become largely a stable, chronic disease, and research efforts today are focusing on strategies for cure of the disease—a goal that would have been unimaginable a decade ago.

PHYSICIAN REFLECTIONS ON CHANGES IN PATIENT CARE

Medical care has changed a great deal in the course of the twentieth and early twenty-first centuries. Here, several Brigham and Women's Hospital (BWH) physicians with long careers at the institution reflect on changes in their specialties over the past thirty to forty years. This is, of course, a very incomplete list of both doctors and changes. What might be similar across BWH's departments and divisions, however, is the increasing use of technology for diagnosis and treatment, the availability of new drugs for use in treatment, and a move toward less paternalistic and more patient-centered care. Another similarity would be increased ability to effectively treat and cure more conditions than in prior decades as well as greatly increased understanding of the biology, mechanism, and progress of disease, with many discoveries and innovations coming from BWH faculty research.

—Christine Wenc

CHANGES IN GASTROENTEROLOGY

Jerry S. Trier

Senior Physician, Brigham and Women's Hospital
Professor of Medicine, Emeritus, Harvard Medical School

In 1961 when I began my subspecialty fellowship, gastroenterology was largely a cognitive specialty. Gastroenterologists spent the vast majority of their patient care time talking with and listening to patients. Relatively little time was spent performing procedures. Endoscopy was performed with rigid endoscopes. Only the esophagus, part of the stomach, and the distal 25 cm of the rectum and distal sigmoid colon could be visualized with these instruments. Interventional endoscopy was largely limited to removal of small polyps from the rectum and distal sigmoid and dilatation of esophageal strictures. A few brave souls also sclerosed esophageal varices. Some organs including the pancreas and the biliary ducts could not be reliably imaged and could only be well visualized at surgery.

When I joined the Department of Medicine at the Peter Bent Brigham Hospital twelve years later, care of patients with digestive diseases was already undergoing dramatic change. Functional, flexible fiberoptic upper endoscopes, sigmoidoscopes, and colonoscopes had been developed and refined during the previous decade. Although thicker, less flexible, and less versatile than endoscopes used today, they allowed visualization and biopsy of the entire mucosal surface of the upper gastrointestinal tract including the duodenum, as well as the entire colon and distal ileum. Techniques and tools facilitating colonoscopic polypectomy, which would revolutionize the treatment of colonic polyps and the approach to colon cancer surveillance, had been recently described. Likewise, endoscopic retrograde cholangiopancreatography, which allowed visualization of the pancreatic and biliary ductal systems and which would transform the approach to the diagnosis and management of biliary and pancreatic diseases, had just been developed.

At that time, in 1973, the Division of Gastroenterology did not have a large footprint at the Brigham. During the previous several years, there had been only two staff gastroenterologists in the division. No clinical space had been assigned to the division, and there were no clinical support personnel. Endoscopic procedures were performed in the operating room, often in the late afternoon after the scheduled surgical cases had been completed or at the bedside with the help of ward nurses. Within a few weeks of my arrival, a dedicated endoscopy room and a dedicated fluoroscopy room had been identified and equipped and an endoscopy technician had been hired. Within fifteen months, three additional senior staff gastroenterologists were on board, increasing the faculty to six, and within two years, a National Institutes of Health–funded academic digestive diseases training program was established. The Brigham's first dedicated endoscopy suite became available on completion of Ambulatory Services Building 1 in 1978.

Fast forward to 2012. The Gastroenterology, Hepatology and Endoscopy Division at Brigham and Women's Hospital is now staffed by twenty-three full-time and seven part-time physicians. Dedicated endoscopy facilities include twelve procedure rooms with a support staff that includes thirty-three registered nurses and nine technicians. Endoscopy volume has increased from less than 400 procedures in 1974 to more than 17,000 in 2011. But far more significant than the numbers is the impact many of these procedures have on patient care and well-being. In the early 1970s, patients with major gastrointestinal bleeding, stones obstructing the common bile duct, large colonic and gastric polyps, and biliary duct and colonic strictures required surgical treatment. Now bleeding can be controlled, biliary duct stones can be extracted, polyps excised, and strictures stented by endoscopic intervention in the majority of patients, circumventing the need for surgery, with its attendant longer recovery period and higher cost. Universal screening for colon cancer of the general population starting at age fifty years with removal of significant polyps has been shown to reduce colon cancer mortality and morbidity. Patients at Brigham and Women's Hospital have access to these and other advances for the treatment of digestive diseases.

Additionally, advances in our understanding of the biology of digestive diseases that have had an enormous impact on patient care during the past forty years are numerous. For example, identification of *Helicobacter pylori* as the major cause of peptic ulcer disease together with the development of H_2-receptor blockers and proton pump inhibitors have transformed our understanding of and our treatment of acid peptic disease. Similarly, identification of the hepatitis B and hepatitis C viruses has led to the development of antiviral regimens that treat effectively and, in many, cure these devastating diseases.

The members of the Gastroenterology, Hepatology and Endoscopy Division at Brigham and Women's Hospital have been at the forefront in the development of innovative new treatment options for our patients. For example, gastroenterologists at the Brigham were among the first to drain pancreatic pseudocysts endoscopically. In recent years they have performed and modified the technique of endoscopic necrosectomy for patients with infected necrosis caused by severe pancreatitis, substantially reducing complications and mortality associated with this life-threatening condition that, before, required surgical debridement. Not only is the Brigham interventional endoscopic team expert at endoscopic repair of bariatric surgical procedures that are no longer effective, they are now refining endoscopic endoluminal suturing to reduce gastric volume as a primary bariatric therapeutic procedure.

Now, unlike forty years ago, gastroenterologists spend much of their day performing procedures. However, adequate time to converse unhurriedly with patients is still essential if the gastroenterologist is to be an effective consultant and contribute maximally to overall patient care. Since 1973, more than 140 fellows have been clinically trained at Brigham and Women's Hospital in our digestive diseases training program in which comprehensive patient care has always been emphasized. Some are now members of our divisional senior staff, contributing directly to patient care at the Brigham; most are at other medical centers around the country and in foreign lands contributing to patient care at their institutions.

CHANGES IN ONCOLOGY

Lawrence N. Shulman

Lawrence N. Shulman, is chief of staff, senior vice-president for medical affairs, and chief, Division of General Oncology, Department of Medical Oncology, at Dana-Farber Cancer Institute (DFCI). He is also director of the Center for Global Cancer Medicine and director of the Department of Regional Strategy and Development, where he oversees DFCI ambulatory oncology units at regional sites throughout New England, and physician leader for the development of clinical information systems at DFCI. A specialist in the treatment of patients with breast cancer, his research includes development of new cancer therapies. He works closely with Partners in Health, where, as senior advisor of oncology, he is helping to lead the development of structured cancer programs for resource-limited healthcare sites in Rwanda, Malawi, and Haiti.

I came to Harvard Medical School (HMS) in 1971, just before President Nixon had declared his War on Cancer. Cancer care was in its embryonic stages, and there was tremendous excitement about the potential of new treatments being developed, curing many patients with acute lymphoblastic leukemia, Hodgkin disease, large-cell lymphoma, and testicular cancer. By the end of my second year at HMS I had made a decision to enter the field of hematology and oncology. At that time the Peter Bent Brigham Hospital (PBBH) was well known for innovation, having pioneered renal transplantation and many other important areas. It became the first Boston center of excellence for the treatment of adult acute leukemia under the direction of William Moloney, and many of the early successes emanated from his work. Soon thereafter the hospital became the first center in New England to perform bone marrow transplantation, and today remains one of the largest and most successful transplant programs in the world. The PBBH was, though, an old and antiquated clinical facility, out of a different and bygone era, and behind the other Harvard hospitals in this regard. But it was a time of great and rapid change. Eugene Braunwald arrived and transformed the Department of Medicine, establishing not only the premier cardiology program in the country, but also strong divisions in other specialties. And in 1980 we saw the opening of a new clinical facility and the formation of the Brigham and Women's Hospital.

Shortly thereafter, Dick Nesson became president of BWH, and the hospital truly entered the modern era as a national leader in health care. In the meantime, the Dana-Farber Cancer Institute (DFCI) opened its doors to adult cancer care in 1976. I was in the first house staff group to care for patients there. When I was recruited as clinical director of the hematology-oncology division at BWH in 1989, the relationship between BWH and DFCI was as competitive as it was collaborative. It remained that way until 1997, when the hematology and oncology services of the two institutions were merged, and I was asked to lead both the consolidation of services and the new joint clinical service. DFCI inpatient beds were moved to BWH, and BWH ambulatory cancer services were moved to DFCI. Joining physician and nursing services from two excellent but competitive programs was a challenge.

In 2012, looking back, the Dana-Farber/Brigham and Women's Cancer Center has created one of the premier hematology and oncology programs in the United States. In almost all areas—bone marrow transplantation, leukemia, lymphoma, myeloma, breast cancer, sarcoma, lung cancer, genitourinary cancer, gastrointestinal cancer, and others, we have programs that are leading the field, playing key roles in scientific discovery and the development of new and more effective treatments for our patients with cancer. As an example, in the 1970s, patients with chronic myelogenous leukemia and gastrointestinal stromal tumors could look forward to a short and painful life. The "targeted" agent imatinib, in which investigators at BWH and DFCI played a leading developmental role, has revolutionized the treatment of patients with these two diseases, dramatically improving the quality as well as the duration of these patients' lives.

CHANGES IN HEMATOLOGY

Robert Handin

Robert Handin is a senior physician in the Hematology Division and a professor of medicine at Harvard Medical School. After graduating from the University of California San Francisco School of Medicine in 1967, he came to the Peter Bent Brigham Hospital as an intern and medical resident. He joined the faculty in 1972, establishing a practice and a research program specializing in coagulation disorders. He served as chief of the Hematology Division for twenty-seven years, from 1980 to 2007. He maintains an active hematology practice, helps to train future hematologists, and now studies blood cell and blood vessel development in zebrafish to further our understanding and develop new treatments for human blood disorders.

Shortly after the opening of the Peter Bent Brigham Hospital (PBBH) in 1913, Minot and Murphy revolutionized hematologic care by demonstrating that force-feeding large quantities of liver could cure patients with the then-fatal blood disorder pernicious anemia. Minot and Murphy subsequently received the Nobel Prize for this work. Within a few years, the key ingredient, vitamin B_{12}, was isolated, and the important role of intrinsic factor secreted by the ileum was worked out by another Harvard physician William B. Castle. When I arrived at the PBBH in 1967, William Murphy practiced general internal medicine in Brookline and still administered injections of liver extract to his patients, although most practitioners had moved on to the use of purified vitamin B_{12}.

In 1967, medical oncology was in its infancy, and the hugely successful adult oncology program that has developed at the Dana-Farber Cancer Institute did not exist. During my internship year I took care of at least a dozen patients with acute leukemia and remember, quite clearly, that none of them left the hospital. The same was true for patients with advanced Hodgkin's disease as well as most other lymphomas and for patients with diseases such as thrombotic thrombocytopenia purpura, which are now readily treated.

After a two-year hiatus for military service, I returned to the Brigham as a hematology fellow under the late William Moloney and was privileged to watch the inception of a revolution in hematologic oncology. With the introduction of new chemotherapeutic agents such as the anthracyclines and cytosine arabinoside, 50% of patients with acute leukemia entered remission and left the hospital. Some of them survived for several years, although the disease returned in most patients. Combination chemotherapy was introduced for both Hodgkin's and non-Hodgkin's lymphomas, with excellent cure rates. Similar positive results were reported for young men with disseminated testicular tumors.

I remember feeling that I was entering an amazing, dynamic field and that, in short order, we would work out therapy for most forms of cancer. Sadly, progress has been much slower than I had anticipated and, at present, the majority of patients with advanced cancer are not cured. Ironically, we still use slight variations of treatment regimens for many of the hematologic malignancies that were pioneered four decades ago.

Although getting chemotherapy is still not easy, the logistics of chemotherapy administration were daunting forty years ago. The Brigham did not have any dedicated infusion unit space and no trained chemotherapy nurses. We gave chemotherapy in a small office just off the old PBBH lobby. We had a shortage of intravenous (IV) poles and equipment, and I remember mixing chemotherapy myself and hanging IV bottles on the drawer pulls of office file cabinets. The potent antinausea medications we now take for granted were not available, and all of our patients developed severe, refractory nausea and vomiting. At times, we resorted to office wastebaskets to help patients with waves of nausea and vomiting.

Patients with bleeding disorders, such as hemophilia, had to come to the emergency room for the treatment of bleeding episodes. They waited for hours, with excruciating joint pain, for medical assistance. In the early 1970s, the hemophilia community championed the concept of self-administered home infusion. The idea was greeted with skepticism and downright hostility but, in time, revolutionized hemophilia treatment. Forty years ago, the major treatment material for hemophilia was cryoprecipitate, a product derived from fresh-frozen plasma, which had to be stored in –20° freezers or relatively crude concentrates that, unfortunately, were contaminated with HIV and hepatitis B and C viruses. A large number of our patients were infected, and many died during the early days of the AIDS epidemic. We are still treating hemophilia patients with hepatitis C–induced liver failure. Now, thanks to the work of the biotechnology and pharmaceutical industry, we have highly purified and recombinant factor VIII and IX concentrates that are shipped as lyophilized powders and reconstituted in a small volume of diluent. Pediatric patients receive prophylactic treatment several times a week and may reach adulthood with no significant joint damage and a normal life expectancy. The first clinical gene therapy has been successfully concluded, and patients with hemophilia can look forward to a near normal and productive life.

A NEUROLOGY PATIENT—NOW, OR FIFTY YEARS AGO

David M. Dawson

David Dawson was a member of the Harvard College class of 1952. He attended medical school in Michigan and came back to Boston as an intern in medicine under Thorn in 1956. After a tour in the Army, he returned to the Brigham for a year and then went to Boston City Hospital for neurology training. In the 1960s he did biochemical research at Brandeis, Boston City Hospital, and the Peter Bent Brigham Hospital. He and Howard Weiner started a multiple sclerosis clinic at the Brigham that has slowly transformed into a large, successful neuroimmunology program, where his role has been purely clinical. Dawson was also the residency director for the neurology program at the Brigham, Children's, and VA hospitals and Beth Israel for some years.

Let us imagine a sixty-five–year-old woman with a small stroke causing a weakness of the right side, nowadays called a lacunar stroke. Comparing what it would be like for her in 2012 versus 1962, here is what she would have experienced:

In 2012, she would be in a double room. Her roommate, more than likely, would be unconscious most of the time. At the nursing station, no more than twenty feet away, as many as twenty people would be present during the day and four or five all night. The ward would be very noisy most of the time, from conversations, beepers, monitors, alarm systems, and telephone calls. In 1962, she would be in a common ward, with twenty other women, and with partitions between the beds. She would get to know a lot of the people if she stayed a few days. If she needed to use the bathroom, she would have to walk, or be wheeled, to the end of the ward where the bathroom was located, or use a bedside commode.

In 2012, she would spend a lot of time in radiology, undergoing magnetic resonance imaging (MRI) scans, a computed tomography (CT) angiogram, and maybe a bubble study looking for a hole in the heart. The author has seen situations in which a patient was admitted for a stroke, spent a major portion of her or his time in radiology, and then was discharged without getting into an inpatient bed! In 1962, no imaging studies of the brain were available. In 1962, she would have been evaluated and cared for by one staff physician (whom she might have known as her personal doctor), an intern, and a resident. In 2012, endless numbers of teams provide these services. Team members would know ten times more about her, but she would not know them!

In 2012, her total hospital stay at the Brigham might be three or four days, after which she would go to a rehabilitation facility. In 1962, she would have stayed for nearly two weeks, have had some physiotherapy, and be already partially recovered when she went home. She would know her caregivers. If her family members visited, she might have gone with them to the gift shop or the cafeteria for a snack.

Her outcome from the stroke would be approximately the same. However, one difference is that in 1962 there was no proven treatment to prevent another stroke. Importantly, in 2012 her doctors would put her on an intensive program for what is called secondary stroke prevention: careful control of blood pressure, an antiplatelet agent to prevent clotting in blood vessels, and a cholesterol-lowering drug. Her chances of a recurrent stroke would be far less.

THE CULTURE OF MEDICINE

Julian Seifter

Julian Seifter is associate professor of medicine at Harvard Medical School, senior physician at Brigham and Women's Hospital, and a chair of the Human Subjects Research Committee at Partners Hospitals. He graduated from the Albert Einstein College of Medicine in 1975, completed his internal medicine residency and chief residency at Bronx Municipal Hospital Center, and completed his renal fellowship at Yale School of Medicine before coming to the Brigham and Women's Hospital in 1982. He is the author of numerous scientific papers, journal articles, and textbook chapters on renal physiology and clinical nephrology, and the author of Concepts in Medical Physiology *(Lippincott Williams & Wilkins, 2006). He recently won the Neil Duane Award for Distinction in Medical Communication for his book* After the Diagnosis: Transcending Chronic Illness *(Simon & Schuster, 2011) and the inaugural Award for Patient- and Family-Centered Care given by the Brigham & Women's Professional Organization in 2011.*

The more things change, the more they stay the same. Some aspects of medicine are immutable and eternal: We are here to take care of patients, to understand and treat their diseases, and to help them, psychologically, spiritually, emotionally, recover from, or live with, illness. Yet, still the world turns, and in another sense, we're living in a different medical world each generation. The culture of medicine has changed over the thirty years of my career, with consequences good, bad, and (sometimes) simply ironic.

Take, for example, a recent conversation I had with a medical student on rounds. We were examining a patient, and the student turned to me, thrilled, when he heard a loud systolic murmur. "Isn't it amazing that you can actually hear on exam something that you can see on the echocardiogram?" That gave me a moment's pause. "I think it's the other way around: it's amazing you can see on echo what you heard on the exam." The point is, technology often comes first these days, and the body itself—including the patient who owns the body—is sometimes almost an afterthought. In past years, we didn't have anything like the toolbox that is available now, and we mostly had to rely on the time-honored inspect, auscultate, palpate, percuss. Which meant we had to approach the person, and touch the person.

Another story about how doctors think, or, rather, used to think: I was a young attending when, one Saturday morning, we were evaluating a patient with a fever of unknown origin, and I suggested that it might be a drug reaction. The resident told me very definitively that you never see a drug fever without a rash. "Where did you hear that?" I asked. He said, "That's what a dermatologist told me." And I said, "One thing is for sure; the dermatologist never saw a drug fever without a rash." Back then, and still, to some extent, we learn by cases, examples, or, as they say, "anecdotes." Our minds open up as we see more and more. But now, it's more about the evidence gleaned from large clinical trials, and residents on rounds are likely to be checking their PDAs for the latest statistics on whatever it is we're looking at. There are fewer funny stories about mistaken first impressions and odd conceptual maps.

Statistics rule these days, sometimes quite reliably. We were rounding recently on the Intensive Teaching Unit with two attendings—one a specialist (me) and the other a hospitalist, very knowledgeable about the evidence in the literature. After seeing a patient with deep vein thrombosis in the lower leg, I asked if the house staff had looked for Homans' sign—pain or resistance in the calf when the patient dorsiflexes the foot with the leg extended. The hospitalist explained to me that Homans' isn't useful anymore, because it lacks both positive and negative predictive value. I waited a beat or two. "But," I said, "it's free."

Which brings me to another massive change in the way we do business as doctors: the huge emphasis on cost-effectiveness, time, billing, and management issues. When I first heard the phrase "risk management," I thought we were talking about managing the patient's risks of complications. It took me a while to catch up to the fact that we were usually talking about the risk to hospitals and clinicians of legal consequences.

Full disclosure is another change in medical practice. Thirty years ago, it was common not to tell patients the whole story, particularly in cases of terminal illness. We were paternalistic, looking out for what we thought were the patients' best interests, certainly, but also protecting them from despair, or from needless confusing detail when we were the ones who knew best. Now, though, full disclosure is one of the bedrocks of medicine—a good thing, obviously, though not without its own complications. As an example, a diabetic patient with schizophrenia, fifty years old, approaching end-stage renal disease, was asked whether he wanted life-saving dialysis. The patient quickly said yes. The intern told me that he wanted to get a psychiatry consult because he wasn't sure the patient could reliably make that decision given the question of competency. I did a double take. "I don't think it works like that. He's choosing to live—is there a different plan he should accept?"

Then there is the necessity to enter prescribed information into the electronic medical record, leading to lengthy notes or prefabricated "smart phrases" such as "I have seen and examined the patient with the resident and agree with the resident's findings and plan." I remember presenting to a medical attending physician when I was a resident, and the bedside discussion covered the gamut of metabolic interconnections, but with no conclusive diagnosis. Ultimately, the attending wrote in the chart a single phrase: "There is something wrong with this man's Krebs cycle." I longed for the day when I could write such a succinct note. That day has never come. Now the attending is responsible for a complete review of organ systems, including a checklist of a dozen items, to be entered into the computer. It's one thing, to be thorough, but checklists and paperwork mean less time for actual patient care and teaching.

HIPAA and all the regulations governing privacy and confidentiality are also a good thing that nonetheless brings a backwash of complexity. When I ride the elevator, I see signs that say, in two languages, that there be no public discussion of patients—though still, you'll hear things like "the interesting case of pheochromocytoma." No names, at least. But while we're protecting the patients, we're also ever so slightly dehumanizing the practice of clinical care. "No names, sign here, here are the statistics, here are the results." We focus on checklists, on evidence, and, importantly, on precautions—masks, gowns, and gloves. We do the procedures correctly but sometimes forget the person.

In a visit to see a simulated patient with my medical team, I and the other attending evaluated the response of the trainees to a cardiopulmonary crisis. All the available technology was in the room with us, as well as a weak voice seemingly coming from the mannikin: "Help me Doc, I'm dying." The house staff did an A+ job. I said the medical care was superb, but nobody acknowledged the emotional distress of the person. I noted that only the third-year student made any attempt to offer comfort, by placing a hand on the knee of the "patient." "Oh," she said, "I was just looking for something to lean on."

The information explosion has put a huge burden on trainees to try to master everything, a sheer impossibility, and it's a natural consequence of so much cognitive demand to push emotions aside and focus on what you have to do to get it right. Given the state of the art, there are innumerable things that you *can* do, and maybe *should* do—but maybe not.

A young lawyer had a possible ovarian mass on pelvic exam, and her gynecologist scheduled a pelvic ultrasound. Her ovaries were ok, but while they were in the neighborhood, why not image the kidneys? Seemed there was something, possibly, on the kidneys—a cyst? Next, a CT scan. The cyst was benign, but, wait, what was that mass on the pancreas? Unknown to the doctors, the lawyer's father was currently dying of pancreatic cancer, so this was a devastating possibility. On a Friday afternoon, after she had seen the best pancreas expert in town, she got the biopsy results: benign. This is not an unusual occurrence: to begin with something that's probably nothing and end with something that's nothing, with a round of costly tests and a world of worry in between.

We know a lot but not everything, despite our tests and statistics. And communication is a tricky thing: the language we use with patients, as we're (quite properly) informing them, can create huge emotional distress unless we frame, translate, and contextualize. A phrase like "end-stage renal disease" can cause nightmares if you don't explain what you can do next. I remember when a patient was terrified after she'd been told she had terminal ileitis. Now patients can Google their diagnoses on the internet and will occasionally suggest some reading for the doctor. TV ads for various drugs end with "Ask your doctor," and then there's the whole world of over-the-counter and herbal remedies and supplements that can wreak all kinds of havoc.

We're doing better, true—progress is always a good thing—but we're also facing all these new problems involving the explosion of information, costs, and complexity. Training has become more fragmented as more is handled in the emergency department, hospital stays are briefer, rotations are shorter. A lot is about the handoff and the discharge, and for the clinician, number of patients seen, length of office visit, and rate of reimbursement. But some things are immutable in medicine: the sense of responsibility, the sense of professionalism, and the sense of relationship. We need to help our patients and to accompany them in their illnesses, even if we can't always cure them. We need to keep the personal encounter between doctor and patient central, even in the swirl of facts and regulations that surround us.

How do we retain the human heart of medicine? Remember the person, not just the disease. Involve the family—the people whose love will be a central part of the patient's care. Be honest, but hopeful. Remember that, for all of us, we're alive until we're dead—which, to me, means that our job as doctors is to treat everyone with respect and to help sustain meaning even as time runs out. I always say we need a lecture in medical school on how to give *good* news, not just bad.

Recently a patient of mine came for an office visit, terribly anxious that her renal disease was progressing. I took her hands and looked into her eyes. "I want you to know that it's my belief that you are not going to have kidney failure. But, we've known each other for a long time and you know that I am an optimist. If you want a second opinion, I know many pessimists I could send you to." Doctors offer not only expertise and knowledge, but company, support, humor, and hope. The more things change, the more they stay the same.

REFERENCES

1. Kenneth M. Ludmerer, *Time to Heal: American Medical Education from the Turn of the Century to the Era of Managed Care* (Oxford: Oxford University Press, 1999), pp. 18-19.
2. Kenneth M. Ludmerer, "The Rise of the Teaching Hospital in America," *Journal of the History of Medicine and Allied Sciences* 38 (1983), pp. 389-414.
3. Edward H. Ahrens, "The Birth of Patient-Oriented Research as a Science (1911)," *Perspectives in Biology and Medicine* 38, (1993), pp. 548-553.
4. Ludmerer, "The Rise of the Teaching Hospital in America," pp. 389-414.
5. Charles E. Rosenberg, *The Care of Strangers: The Rise of America's Hospital System* (New York: Basic Books, 1987), p. 150.
6. A. McGehee Harvey, *Science at the Bedside: Clinical Research in American Medicine, 1905-1945.* (Baltimore: Johns Hopkins University Press, 1981), p. 80.
7. Oglesby Paul, *The Caring Physician: The Life of Dr. Francis W. Peabody* (Boston: The Francis A. Countway Library of Medicine, 1991).
8. Charles E. Rosenberg, *Our Present Complaint: American Medicine, Then and Now* (Baltimore: Johns Hopkins University Press, 2007).
9. References for this essay include: Michael A. Gimbrone, Ramzi S. Cotran, and Judah Folkman, "Human Vascular Endothelial Cells in Culture Growth and DNA Synthesis," *The Journal of Cell Biology* 60, no. 3 (1974), pp. 673-684; Guohao Dai, Mohammad R. Kaazempur-Mofrad, Sripriya Natarajan, Yuzhi Zhang, Saran Vaughn, Brett R. Blackman, Roger D. Kamm, Guillermo García-Cardeña, and Michael A. Gimbrone, "Distinct endothelial phenotypes evoked by arterial waveforms derived from atherosclerosis-susceptible and-resistant regions of human vasculature," *Proceedings of the National Academy of Sciences of the United States of America* 101, no. 41 (2004), pp. 14871-14876.
10. References for this essay include: David M. Hume, John P. Merrill, "Homologous Transplantation of Human Kidneys," Journal of Clinical Investigation 31 (1952), p. 640; John P.Merrill, Joseph E. Murray, J. Hartwell Harrison, and Warren R. Guild, "Successful Homotransplantation of the Human Kidney Between Identical Twins," *Journal of the American Medical Association* 160, no. 4 (1956), pp. 277-282 (note that Merrill misuses the term homotransplantation; it should be isotransplantation); Joseph E. Murray, J. P. Merrill, G. J. Dammin, J. B. Dealy Jr, C. W. Walter, M. S. Brooke, and R. E. Wilson, "Study on transplantation immunity after total body irradiation: clinical and experimental investigation," *Surgery* 48 (1960), p. 272; Joseph E. Murray and J. Hartwell Harrison, "Surgical management of fifty patients with kidney transplants including eighteen pairs of twins," *The American Journal of Surgery* 105, no. 2 (1963), pp. 205-218; Joseph E. Murray, John P. Merrill, J. Hartwell Harrison, Richard E. Wilson, and Gustave J. Dammin. "Prolonged survival of human-kidney homografts by immunosuppressive drug therapy," *New England Journal of Medicine* 268, no. 24 (1963), pp. 1315-1323; Nicholas L. Tilney, Terry B. Strom, Gordon C. Vineyard, and John P. Merrill, "Factors contributing to the declining mortality rate in renal transplantation," *New England Journal of Medicine* 299, no. 24 (1978), pp. 1321-1325; Francis Daniels Moore, *Give and Take: The Development of Tissue Transplantation.* (Phildelphia: Saunders, 1964); Nicholas L. Tilney, *Transplant: From Myth to Reality* (New Haven, CT: Yale University Press, 2003).
11. Joseph E. Murray, *Surgery of the Soul: Reflections on a Curious Career* (Canton, MA: Science History Publications, 2001).
12. John P. Merrill, Joseph E. Murray, J. Hartwell Harrison, and Warren R. Guild, "Successful Homotransplantation of the Human Kidney Between Identical Twins."
13. John P. Merrill, Joseph E. Murray, J. Hartwell Harrison, and Warren R. Guild, Landmark Article: "Successful Homotransplantation of the Human Kidney Between Identical Twins," *Journal of the American Medical Association* 1984; 251, pp. 2566-2571.
14. Thomas E. Starzl, "The Landmark Identical Twin Case," *The Journal of the American Medical Association* 251, no. 19 (1984), p. 2572.

15. Victor Lane, "Peter Bent Brigham Hospital, 1913–1963: Report on Golden Jubilee Meetings," *Irish Journal of Medical Science* (1926-1967) 39, no. 1 (1964), pp. 37-41.

16. "From Dialysis, to Transplantation, to Palliative Care: A Trajectory." Presentation for the Care of the Renal Patient Towards the End of Life Conference, Royal Society of Medicine, October 14, 2009. Renée C. Fox, p.3. http://www.renal.org/pages/media/TsarFiles/EoL_141009_ReneeCFox.pdf, accessed August 1, 2012.

17. Renee Fox, *Experiment Perilous: Physicians and Patients Facing the Unknown* (Glencoe, IL: The Free Press, 1959). Paperback edition, Philadelphia: University of Pennsylvania Press, 1974. Republished, with a new epilogue by the author, New Brunswick, NJ: Transaction Publishers, 1998. (Participant observation is a qualitative data collection method derived from traditional ethnography. The researcher participates in the social system that he/she is studying in order to answer the research questions he/she has about it.)

18. Ibid., p. 2.

19. Ibid., p. 2.

20. Ibid., p. 4.

21. For an excellent annotated bibliography, see Jerome Groopman, *How Doctors Think* (New York: Houghton Mifflin, 2007), pp. 283-6.

22. References for this essay include: K. Frank Austen and Walter E. Brocklehurst, "Anaphylaxis in Chopped Guinea Pig Lung III. Effect of Carbon Monoxide, Cyanide, Salicylaldoxime, and Ionic Strength," *The Journal of Experimental Medicine* 114, no. 1 (1961), pp. 29-42; Robert P. Orange, Robert C. Murphy, Manfred L. Karnovsky, and K. Frank Austen, "The Physicochemical Characteristics and Purification of Slow-Reacting Substance of Anaphylaxis," *The Journal of Immunology* 110, no. 3 (1973), pp. 760-770; J. W.Weiss, Jeffrey M. Drazen, Nancy Coles, E. R. McFadden Jr., Peter F. Weller, E. J. Corey, Robert A. Lewis, and K. F. Austen, "Bronchoconstrictor Effects of Leukotriene C in Humans," *Science (New York, NY)* 216, no. 4542 (1982), p. 196; Bing K. Lam, John F. Penrose, Gordon J. Freeman, and K. Frank Austen, "Expression Cloning of a cDNA for Human Leukotriene C4 Synthase, an Integral Membrane Protein Conjugating Reduced Glutathione to Leukotriene A4," *Proceedings of the National Academy of Sciences* 91, no. 16 (1994), pp. 7663-7667; Yoshihide Kanaoka, Akiko Maekawa, John F. Penrose, K. Frank Austen, and Bing K. Lam, "Attenuated Zymosan-induced Peritoneal Vascular Permeability and IgE-dependent Passive Cutaneous Anaphylaxis in Mice Lacking Leukotriene C4 Synthase," *Journal of Biological Chemistry* 276, no. 25 (2001), pp. 22608-22613; Nora A. Barrett, Opu M. Rahman, James M. Fernandez, Matthew W. Parsons, Wei Xing, K. Frank Austen, and Yoshihide Kanaoka, "Dectin-2 Mediates Th2 Immunity Through the Generation of Cysteinyl Leukotrienes," *The Journal of Experimental Medicine* 208, no. 3 (2011), pp. 593-604.

23. William Hollingsworth, Taking Care: The Legacy of Soma Weiss, Eugene Stead, and Paul Beeson. Medicine Education & Research (San Diego: Medical Education and Research Foundation, 1994), p. 62.

24. Sharon R Kaufman, *The Healer's Tale: Transforming Medicine and Culture* (Madison, WI: University of Wisconsin Press, 1993), p. 208.

25. Jules Cohen and Stephanie Brown Clark, *John Romano and George Engel: Their Lives and Work* (Rochester, NY: Meliora Press/University of Rochester Press, 2010).

26. John Romano and George L. Engel, "Delirium: I. Electroencephalographic Data," *Archives of Neurology and Psychiatry* 51, no. 4 (1944), p. 356.

27. Robert J. Joynt, "John Romano, MD November 20, 1908, to June 19, 1995," *Archives of General Psychiatry* 52, no. 12 (1995), p. 1076.

28. Some information presented in this essay is adapted from a lecture presented by Amalie M. Kass entitled "A Brief History of the Channing Laboratory" on October 31, 1996.

29. Ferenc A. Jolesz, "1996 RSNA Eugene P. Pendergrass New Horizons Lecture. Image-Guided Procedures and the Operating Room of the Future," *Radiology* 204, no. 3 (1997), pp. 601-612.

30. Alan R. Bleier, Peter D. Jakab, Paul W. Ruenzel, Kalman Huttl, and Geza J. Jako, "MR imaging of laser-tissue interactions," *Radiology* 168, no. 1 (1988), pp. 249-253; Silverman, Stuart G., Kemal Tuncali, Douglass F. Adams, Kelly H. Zou, Daniel F. Kacher, Paul R. Morrison, and Ferenc A. Jolesz, "MR Imaging-guided Percutaneous Cryotherapy of Liver Tumors: Initial Experience 1," *Radiology* 217, no. 3 (2000), pp. 657-664.

31. John F. Schenck, Ferenc A. Jolesz, Peter B. Roemer, Harvey E. Cline, William E. Lorensen, Ronald Kikinis, Stuart G. Silverman, Christopher J. Hardy, William D. Barber, E. Trifon Laskaris, Bijan Dorri, Robert W. Newman, Catherine E. Holley, Bruce D. Collick, Douglas P. Dietz, David C. Mack, Maureen D. Ainslie, Patrick L. Jaskolski, Michael R. Figuerira, John C. von Lehn, Steven P. Souza, Charles L. Dumoulin, Robert D. Darrow, Richard L. St. Peters, Kenneth W. Rohling, Ronald D. Watkins, David R. Eisner, S. Morry Blumenfeld and Kirby G. Vosburgh, "Superconducting Open-Configuration MR Imaging System for Image-Guided Therapy," *Radiology* 195 (1995), pp. 805-814.

32. Peter McL. Black, Thomas Moriarty, Eben Alexander III, Philip Stieg, Eric J. Woodard, P. Langham Gleason, Claudia H. Martin, Ron Kikinis, Richard B. Schwartz, and Ferenc A. Jolesz, "Development and Implementation of Intraoperative Magnetic Resonance Imaging and its Neurosurgical Applications," *Neurosurgery* 41, no. 4 (1997), pp. 831-845.

33. Thomas Addison, *On the Consitutional and Local Effects of Disease of the Suprarenal Capsules* (London: Samuel Higley, 1855), pp. 1-43; Paul De Kruif, *Men Against Death* (New York: Harcourt, Brace and Co., 1932).

34. Paul Ehrlich, "Über Regeneration und Degeneration rother Blutscheiben bei Anämien," *Berl Klin Wochenschri* 17 (1880), p. 405.
35. J.S. Risien Russell, F. E. Batten, and James Collier, "Subacute Combined Degeneration of the Spinal Cord," *Brain* 23, no. 1 (1900), pp. 39-110.
36. Cabot, Richard C, "Pernicious and Secondary Anemia, Chlorosis and Leukemia," *Modern Medicine: Its Theory and Practice*, Vol IV (Philadelphia: Lea & Febiger, 1908), pp. 612-639.
37. Samuel A. Levine and William S. Ladd, "Pernicious Anemia: A Clinical study of One Hundred and Fifty Consecutive Cases with Special Reference to Gastric Acidity," *Bulletin of the Johns Hopkins Hospital* 32 (1921), p. 254.
38. Francis Minot Rackemann, *The Inquisitive Physician: The Life and Times of George Richards Minot* (Cambridge: Harvard University Press, 1956).
39. George Washington Corner, *George Hoyt Whipple and His Friends: The Life-Story of a Nobel Prize Pathologist* (Philadelphia: J. B. Lippincott, 1963).
40. George R. Minot and William P. Murphy, "Treatment of Pernicious Anemia by a Special Diet," *Journal of the American Medical Association* 87, no.7 (1926), pp. 470-476.
41. George R. Minot, William P. Murphy, and Richard P. Stetson, "The Response of the Reticulocytes to Liver Therapy: Particularly in Pernicious Anemia," *The American Journal of the Medical Sciences* 175, no. 5 (1928), p. 581.
42. Centers for Disease Control and Prevention. "Number, Rate and Average Length of Stay for Discharges from Short-Stay Hospitals by Age, Region, and Sex: United States, 2009." National Hospital Discharge Survey, selected tables. 2009. www.cdc.gov/nchs/nhds/nhds_products.htm, accessed April 14, 2012
43. American Hospital Association, "Chartbook: Trends Affecting Hospitals and Health Systems," 2011, www.aha.org/research/reports/tw/chartbook/index.shtml, accessed April 14, 2012
44. David Blumenthal, "Employer-Sponsored Health Insurance in the United States – Origins and Implications," *New England Journal of Medicine,* 2006; 355, pp. 82-88.
45. Sharon K. Long, Karen Stockley, Heather Dahlen, "Massachusetts Health Reform: Uninsurance Remains Low, Self-Reported Health Status Improves as State Prepares to Tackle Costs," *Health Affairs* 2012; 31, pp. 444-451.
46. The Henry J. Kaiser Family Foundation, "Medicare Spending and Financing, a Primer," 2011, www.kff.org/medicare/upload/7731-03.pdf, accessed April 14, 2012
47. U.S. Department of Health and Human Services. Hospital profile. Brigham and Women's Hospital. 2012. www.hospitalcompare.hhs.gov/hospital-profile.aspx?pid=220110&lat=42.3399&lng=-71.08989&#POC, accessed April 14, 2012
48. A series of articles incorporating these studies have appeared in *The New England Journal of Medicine, Journal of the American Medical Association*, and the *Annals of Internal Medicine*. Authors of these papers include David W. Bates, Tejal K. Gandhi, Troyan A. Brennan, Lucian L. Leape, Nan M. Laird, and Eric G. Poon.
49. Ann C. Hurley, Anne Bane, Sofronia Fotakis, Mary E. Duffy, Amanda Sevigny, Eric G. Poon, and Tejal K. Gandhi, "Nurses' Satisfaction with Medication Administration Point-of-Care Technology," *Journal of Nursing Administration* 37, no. 7/8 (2007), pp. 343-349.
50. Carol A. Keohane, Anne D. Bane, Erica Featherstone, Judy Hayes, Seth Woolf, Ann Hurley, David W. Bates, Tejal K. Gandhi, and Eric G. Poon. "Quantifying Nursing Workflow in Medication Administration." *Journal of Nursing Administration* 38, no. 1 (2008), pp. 19-26.
51. Eric G. Poon, Carol A. Keohane, Catherine S. Yoon, Matthew Ditmore, Anne Bane, Osnat Levtzion-Korach, Thomas Moniz, et al, "Effect of Bar-Code Technology on the Safety of Medication Administration," *New England Journal of Medicine* 362, no. 18 (2010), pp. 1698-1707.
52. Patricia C. Dykes, Diane L. Carroll, Ann Hurley, Stuart Lipsitz, Angela Benoit, Frank Chang, Seth Meltzer, Ruslana Tsurikova, Lyubov Zuyov, and Blackford Middleton, "Fall Prevention in Acute Care Hospitals: A Randomized Trial," *Journal of the American Medical Association* 304, no. 17 (2010), pp. 1912-1918.
53. Christine A. Caligtan, Diane L. Carroll, Ann C. Hurley, Ronna Gersh-Zaremski, and Patricia C. Dykes, "Bedside Information Technology to Support Patient-Centered Care," *International Journal of Medical Informatics* (2012), p. 442.
54. Linda A. Evans, "A Historical, Clinical, and Ethical Overview of the Emerging Science of Facial Transplantation," *Plastic Surgical Nursing* 31, no. 4 (2011): 151.
55. Francis D. Moore, "Ethical Problems Special to Surgery: Surgical Teaching, Surgical Innovation, and the Surgeon in Managed Care," *Archives of Surgery* 135, no. 1 (2000), p. 14.
56. Katherine E. Gregory, "Microbiome Aspects of Perinatal and Neonatal Health," *Journal of Perinatal and Neonatal Nursing* 25, no. 2 (2011), p. 158.
57. Ann C. Hurley and Ladislav Volicer, "Alzheimer disease: 'It's okay, Mama, if you want to go, it's okay.'" *Journal of the American Medical Association* 2002; 288, pp. 2324-2331.
58. Patricia C. Dykes, Diane Carroll, Kerry McColgan, Ann C. Hurley, Stuart R. Lipsitz, Lisa Colombo, Lyubov Zuyev, and Blackford Middleton, "Scales for Assessing Self-Efficacy of Nurses and Assistants for Preventing Falls," *Journal of Advanced Nursing* 67, no. 2 (2011), pp. 438-449.
59. Lichuan Ye, "Factors Influencing Daytime Sleepiness in Chinese Patients With Obstructive Sleep Apnea," *Behavioral Sleep Medicine* 9, no. 2 (2011), pp. 117-127.
60. Busisiwe P. Ncama, Patricia A. McInerney, Busisiwe R. Bhengu, Inge B. Corless, Dean J. Wantland, Patrice K. Nicholas, Chris A. McGibbon, and Sheila M. Davis, "Social

Support and Medication Adherence in HIV Disease in KwaZulu-Natal, South Africa," *International Journal of Nursing Studies* 45, no. 12 (2008), p. 1757.

61. Inge B. Corless, Dean Wantland, Busi Bhengu, Patricia McInerney, Busi Ncama, Patrice K. Nicholas, Chris McGibbon, Emily Wong, and Sheila M. Davis, "HIV and Tuberculosis in Durban, South Africa: Adherence to Two Medication Regimens," *AIDS Care* 21, no. 9 (2009), pp. 1106-1113.

62. Busisiwe R. Bhengu, Busisiwe P. Ncama, Patricia A. McInerney, Dean J. Wantland, Patrice K. Nicholas, Inge B. Corless, Chris A. McGibbon, Sheila M. Davis, Thomas P. Nicholas, and Ana Viamonte Ros, "Symptoms experienced by HIV-infected individuals on antiretroviral therapy in Kwazulu-Natal, South Africa," *Applied Nursing Research* 24, no. 1 (2011), pp. 1-9.

63. Henry A Christian, "Report of the Physician-in-Chief," Eighth Annual Report of the Peter Bent Brigham Hospital For the Year 1921 (Cambridge, MA: The University Press, 1922), p. 129.

64. Henry A Christian, "Report of the Physician-in-Chief," *Thirteenth Annual Report of the Peter Bent Brigham Hospital for the Year 1926* (Cambridge: The University Press, 1927), p. 125.

65. Francis D. Moore, "Report of the Surgeon-in-Chief," *Forty-Seventh Annual Report of the Peter Bent Brigham Hospital for the Fiscal Year Ended September 30, 1960* (1960), pp. 54-55.

66. Charles B. Barnes and Alan Steinert, "The Joint Report of the Chairman of the Board and of the President," *Fifty-Third Annual Report, Peter Bent Brigham Hospital, 1965-1966* (1966), p. v.

67. Charles B. Barnes and Alan Steinert, "The Joint Report of the Board and of the President," *Fifty-Fourth Annual Report, Peter Bent Brigham Hospital, 1966-1967* (1967), p. x.

68. Herbert L. Abrams, "Report of the Radiologist-in-Chief," *Fifty-Sixth Annual Report, Peter Bent Brigham Hospital, 1968-1969* (1969), p. 135.

69. Henry A. Christian, "The Out-Door Department: Report of Dr. Sturgis," in "Report of the Physician-in-Chief," *Thirteenth Annual Report of the Peter Bent Brigham Hospital for the Year 1926* (Cambridge: The University Press, 1927), pp. 137-138.

70. F. Lloyd Mussels, "Report of the Director," *Forty-Eighth Annual Report of the Peter Bent Brigham Hospital for the Fiscal Year Ended September 30, 1961* (1961), p. 10.

71. George W. Thorn, "Report of the Physician-in-Chief," Fifty-Third Annual Report, Peter Bent Brigham Hospital, 1965-1966 (1966), p. 6.

72. Anthony L. Komaroff, interview with author, September 2011.

73. References for this essay include: Roberto Bolli, Atul R. Chugh, Domenico D'Amario, John H Loughran, Marcus F Stoddard, Sohail Ikram, Garth M Beache, Stephen G Wagner, Annarosa Leri, Toru Hosoda, Fumihiro Sanada, Julius B Elmore, Polina Goichberg, Donato Cappetta, Naresh K Solankhi, Ibrahim Fahsah, D Gregg Rokosh, Mark S Slaughter, Jan Kajstura, and Piero Anversa, "Cardiac Stem Cells in Patients with Ischaemic Cardiomyopathy (SCIPIO): Initial Results of a Randomised Phase 1 Trial, *The Lancet* 2011; 378, pp. 1847-1857; Piero Anversa, Jan Kajstura, Annarosa Leri, and Joseph Loscalzo, "Tissue-Specific Adult Stem Cells in the Human Lung," *Nature Medicine* 2011; 17, pp. 1038-1039; Charles N. Serhan, "Inflammation: Novel Endogenous Anti-inflammatory and Proresolving Lipid Mediators and Pathways," *Annual Review of Immunology*, 2007; 25, pp. 101-137.

74. Harvey Cushing and J.R.B. Branch, "Experimental and Clinical Notes on Chronic Valvular Lesions in the Dog and their Possible Relation to a Future Surgery of the Cardiac Valves," *Journal of Medical Research* 1908;17, pp. 471-486.

75. Dwight E. Harken, Paul M. Zoll, "Foreign Bodies in and in Relation to the Thoracic Blood Vessels and Heart, III. Indications for the Removal of Intracardiac Foreign Bodies and the Behavior of the Heart During Manipulation," *American Heart Journal* 1946;32, pp. 1-19.

76. Roy H. Clauss, William Clifford Birtwell, George Albertal, Steven Lunzer, Warren J. Taylor, Anna M. Forsberg, and Dwight E. Harken, "Assisted Circulation. I. The Arterial Counterpulsator," *Journal of Thoracic and Cardiovascular Surgery* 1961;41, pp. 447-458.

77. Lawrence H. Cohn, Richard Gorlin, Michael V. Herman and John J. Collins Jr., "Surgical Treatment of Acute Coronary Occlusion," *Journal of Thoracic and Cardiovascuar Surgery*, 1972; 64, pp. 503-513.

78. Daniel J. Dibardino, Andrew W. Elbardissi, R. Scott McClure, Ozwaldo A. Razo-Vasquez, Nicole E. Kelly, and Lawrence H. Cohn, "Four Decades of Experience with Mitral Valve Repair: Analysis of Differential Indications, Technical, Evolution and Long-term Outcomes," *Journal of Thoracic and Cardiovascular Surgery* 2010;139, pp. 76-84.

79. Lawrence H. Cohn, David H. Adams, Gregory S. Couper, Sary F. Aranki, David P. Bichell, Donna M. Rosborough, and Samuel P. Sears, "Minimally Invasive Cardiac Valve Surgery Improves Patient Satisfaction while Reducing Costs of Cardiac Valve Replacement and Repair," *Annals of Surgery* 1997;226 (4), pp. 421-428. (Oct 1997)

80. From the 1930 to 1960, many innovative observations by Wiggers, Kouwenhoven, Ferris, and Zoll in the United States, Gurvich and Yuniev in the USSR, and Peleska in Czechoslovakia focused on ventricular fibrillation as the arrhythmia of sudden death and introduced electrical devices for defibrillating the heart.

81. Bernard Lown, *The Lost Art of Healing* (New York, NY: Ballantine Books, 1996), pp. 188-201.

82. Bernard Lown, Raghavan Amarasingham, Jose Neuman, "New Method for Terminating Cardiac Arrhythmias,"

Journal of the American Medical Association, 1962;182, pp. 548-555.
83. Soma Weiss, "Instantaneous 'Physiologic' Death," New England Journal of Medicine, 1940; 223, pp. 793-797.
84. Lewis Kuller, Abraham Lilienfeld, and Russell Fisher, "Epidemiological Study of Sudden and Unexpected Deaths due to Arteriosclerotic Heart Disease," *Circulation* 1966;34:1056-1068; Eve Weinblatt, Sam Shapiro, Charles W. Frank, and Robert V. Sager, "Prognosis of Men after First Myocardial Infarction: Mortality and First Recurrence in Relation to Selected Parameters," *American Journal of Public Health,* 1968;58, pp. 1329-1347.
85. Hughes W. Day, "An Intensive Coronary Care Area," *Chest* 1963;44, pp. 423-427.
86. Samuel A. Levine, Bernard Lown, "'Armchair' treatment of acute coronary thrombosis," *Journal of the American Medical Association,* 1952;148, pp. 1365-1369.
87. Bernard Lown, Ali M. Fakhro, William B. Hood, and George W. Thorn, "The Coronary Care Unit: New Perspectives and Directions," *Journal of the American Medical Association,* 1967;199, pp. 188-198.
88. Ibid.
89. Ibid.
90. Robert Breck Brigham Hospital. Records, 1889-1984. Center for the History of Medicine, Francis A. Boston, MA: Countway Library of Medicine, Harvard Medical School.
91. "Dr. Theodore Potter, 83. Taught, Practiced Orthopedics," *Boston Globe,* December 11, 1995, p. 25.
92. H.H. Banks, Osgood Lecture. Delivered at Massachusetts General Hospital, 1983
93. Ibid.
94. Nicholas L. Tilney, *A Perfectly Striking Departure: Surgeons and Surgery at the Peter Bent Brigham Hospital 1912-1980* (Sagamore Beach, MA: Science History Publications, 2006), p. 159.
95. Henry H. Banks, "Orthopaedic Surgery at the Peter Bent Brigham Hospital 1913-1970," Osgood Lecture, Massachusetts General Hospital, May 21, 1983.
96. Henry H. Banks, "Memoirs." Unpublished manuscript.
97. Henry H. Banks, interview with author, July 14, 2009.
98. Henry H. Banks, "Memoirs."
99. C.B. Sledge. Interview with author, September 18, 2009.
100. Ibid.
101. James H. Herndon, " Chairman's Corner," *Orthopaedic Journal at Harvard Medical School* (1999, vol 1, pp. 5-9; 2000, vol 2, pp. 5-8; 2001, vol 3, pp. 11-17; 2002, vol 4, pp. 11-18; 2003, vol 5, pp. 8-13); T.S. Thornhill, "Brigham and Women's Hospital." *Orthopaedic Journal at Harvard Medical School* (1999, vol 1, pp. 17-20; 2000, vol 2, pp. 11-13; 2001, vol 3, pp. 20-23; 2002, vol 4, pp. 22-26; 2003, vol 5, pp. 17-26)
102. James H. Herndon, "Chairman's Corner," *Orthopaedic Journal at Harvard Medical School* (1999, vol 1, pp. 5-9; 2000, vol 2, pp. 5-8; 2001, vol 3, pp. 11-17; 2002, vol 4, pp. 11-18; 2003, vol 5, pp. 8-13)
103. T.S. Thornhill, "Brigham and Women's Hospital." *Orthopaedic Journal at Harvard Medical School* (1999, vol 1, pp. 17-20; 2000, vol 2, pp. 11-13; 2001, vol 3, pp. 20-23; 2002, vol 4, pp. 22-26; 2003, vol 5, pp. 17-26)
104. Ibid.
105. Ken R. Winston and Wendell Lutz, "Linear Accelerator as a Neurosurgical Tool for Stereotactic Radiosurgery," *Neurosurgery* 1988; 22, pp. 454-464.
106. Wendell Lutz, Ken R. Winston, and Nasser Maleki, "A System for Stereotactic Radiosurgery with a Linear Accelerator," *International Journal of Radiation Oncology Biology Physics,* 1988; 14, pp. 373-381.
107. Jay S. Loeffler, Eben Alexander III, Robert L. Siddon, William M. Saunders, C. Norman Coleman, and Ken R. Winston, "Stereotactic Radiosurgery for Intracranial Arteriovenous Malformations using a Standard Linear Accelerator," *International Journal of Radiation Oncology Biology Physics* 1989;17, pp. 673-677.
108. Barry M. Brenner, "In Memoriam Ramzi S. Cotran: December 7, 1932 - October 23, 2000," *Journal of the American Society of Nephrology* 2001; 12(4), p. 635.
109. Louis Weinstein, S. Miguel Edelstein, James L. Madara, Kenneth R. Falchuk, Bruce M. McManus, Jerry S. Trier, "Intestinal Cryptosporidiosis Complicated by Disseminated Cytomegalovirus Infection," *Gastroenterology* 1981; 81, pp. 584-891.
110. Edward M. Connor, Rhoda S. Sperling, Richard Gelber, Pavel Kiselev, Gwendolyn Scott, Mary Jo O'Sullivan, Russell Van Dyke, Mohammed Bey, William Shearer, Robert L. Jacobson, Eleanor Jimenez, Edward O'Neill, Brigitte Bazin, Jean-Francois Delfraissy, Mary Culnane, Robert Coombs, Mary Elkins, Jack Moye, Pamela Stratton, and James Balsley for the Pediatric AIDS Clinical Trials Group Protocol 076 Study Group, "Reduction of Maternal-Infant Transmission of Human Immunodeficiency Virus Type 1 with Zidovudine Treatment," *New England Journal of Medicine,* 1994;331, pp. 1173-1180.
111. Paul Farmer, Fernet Léandre, Joia S Mukherjee, Marie Sidonise Claude, Patrice Nevil, Mary C Smith-Fawzi, Serena P Koenig, Arachu Castro, Mercedes C Becerra, Jeffrey Sachs, Amir Attaran, Jim Yong Kim, "Community-Based Approaches to HIV Treatment in Resource-Poor Settings," *Lancet* 2001; 358, pp. 404-409.
112. Paul E. Sax, Camlin Tierney, Ann C. Collier, Margaret A. Fischl, Katie Mollan, Lynne Peeples, Catherine Godfrey, Nasreen C. Jahed, Laurie Myers, David Katzenstein, Awny Farajallah, James F. Rooney, Belinda Ha, William C. Woodward, Susan L. Koletar, Victoria A. Johnson, P. Jan Geiseler, and Eric S. Daar

for the AIDS Clinical Trials Group Study A5202 Team, "Abacavir-Lamivudine versus Tenofovir-Emtricitabine for Initial HIV-1 Therapy," *New England Journal of Medicine* 2009; 361, pp. 2230-2240.

113. Shahin Lockman, Michael D Hughes, James McIntyre, Yu Zheng, Tsungai Chipato, Francesca Conradie, Fred Sawe, Aida Asmelash, Mina C Hosseinipour, Lerato Mohapi, Elizabeth Stringer, Rosie Mngqibisa, Abraham Siika, Diana Atwine, James Hakim, Douglas Shaffer, Cecilia Kanyama, Kara Wools-Kaloustian, Robert A Salata, Evelyn Hogg, Beverly Alston-Smith, Ann Walawander, Eva Purcelle-Smith, Susan Eshleman, James Rooney, Sibtain Rahim, John W Mellors, Robert T. Schooley, and Judith S Currier, "Antiretroviral Therapies in Women after Single-Dose Nevirapine Exposure," *New England Journal of Medicine* 2010; 363, pp. 1499-1509.

114. Weinstein et al., "Intestinal Cryptosporidiosis."

CHAPTER 4

A HISTORY OF WOMEN'S HEALTH RESEARCH AND SERVICES

BIOMEDICAL RESEARCH ON WOMEN IN THE HISTORY OF BRIGHAM AND WOMEN'S HOSPITAL

Lara Freidenfelds

The birth control pill. In-vitro fertilization. The epidemiology of breast cancer. Diet, exercise, and smoking cessation as preventive measures against heart disease. Diethylstilbestrol (DES). "Women's Health" as a meaningful scientific, clinical, cultural, and political category. Developments in health care for women have crucially shaped American culture over the past century. And Brigham and Women's Hospital holds a central place in the research that enabled each of these innovations.

This is not by any means a complete list of the record of Brigham and Women's investigators in areas related to women's health. However, these highlights give a sense of just how central a place the Brigham holds in the history of women's health research and, by extension, in the history of American society.

RESEARCH AT THE FREE HOSPITAL FOR WOMEN

The history of Brigham and Women's accomplishments in women's health research begins in its antecedent institutions. The Free Hospital for Women, long a valuable service institution, became an important site of women's health research in the 1930s and 1940s. The most famous of the Free Hospital's researchers was John Rock, an infertility specialist who eventually collaborated on the development of the birth control pill. In 1926, Rock took leadership of the sterility clinic.[1] At the time, physicians could offer little in the way of effective therapies for infertility. While he offered patients what assistance he could as a clinician, Rock began his research by tackling

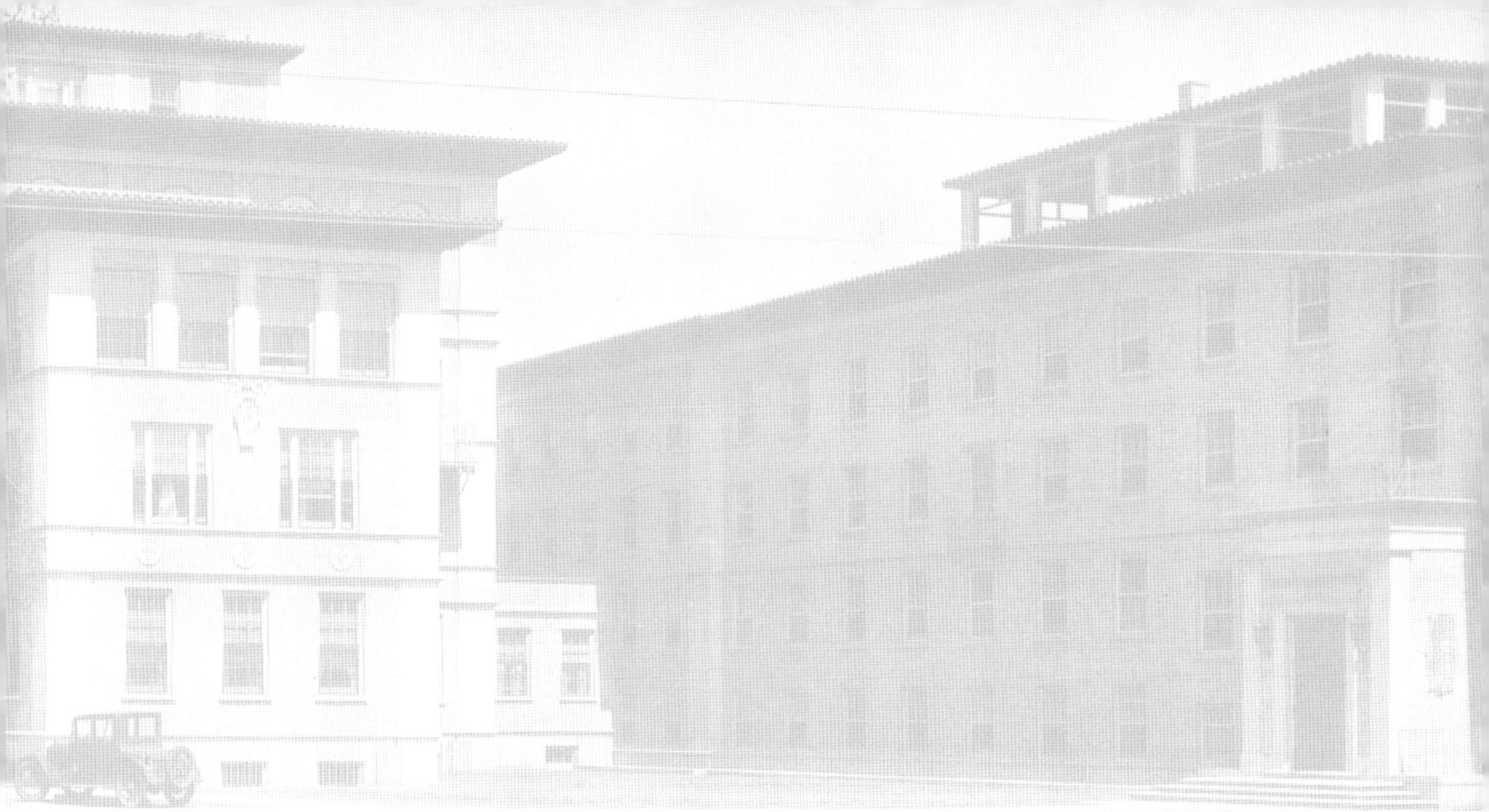

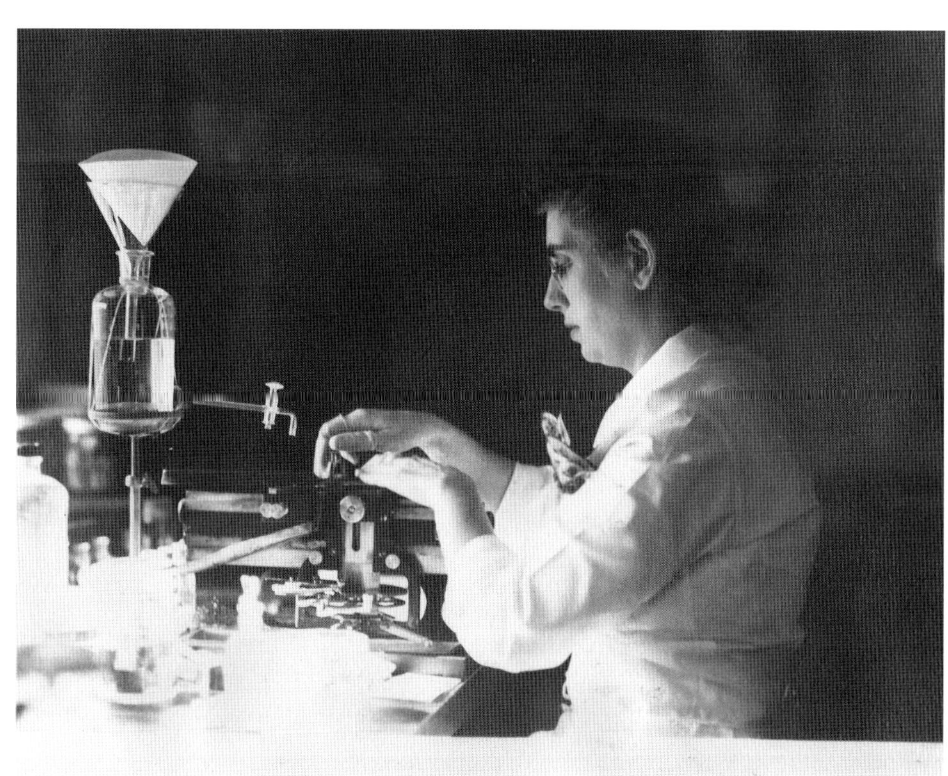

FIGURE 4-1 Technician Sara Danziger (listed as an author with Arthur Hertig on several of his published embryo studies), Free Hospital for Women pathology lab, circa 1940.

the problem of determining when in the menstrual cycle a woman was ovulating and how to tell whether in fact she was ovulating. He studied endometrial tissue, correlating its characteristics with the time in the menstrual cycle, and was able to characterize day-by-day endometrial changes as well as the signs that indicated that ovulation had occurred. Although this information did not allow physicians to tackle infertility directly, the knowledge and techniques he developed at least allowed clinicians to diagnose whether fertility issues were due to a failure to ovulate.[2]

A decade later, Rock began an ambitious research program to characterize the very early development of human embryos, and, he hoped, to someday grow embryos outside the womb. First, with Arthur Hertig, Rock began a study designed to recover fertilized eggs and very early embryos from hysterectomy patients. From a twenty-first-century perspective, the study they designed appears tremendously controversial: women waiting for nonurgent hysterectomies were asked to have unprotected sex with their husbands during their most fertile period in the weeks before the surgery. Then, after the surgery, Hertig spent an entire day examining the excised uterus and fixing any specimen that might be found. In the course of the 211 hysterectomies performed as part of the study, Rock and Hertig found thirty-four fertilized eggs and embryos, representing the first seventeen days of human development. They, and the women who participated in the study, were careful to schedule the unprotected intercourse and the surgery in such a way that it would be done before an anticipated menstrual period might be missed. However, it seems clear that the women, most of them Catholic patients from the clinic Rock ran advising women on the rhythm method of birth control, understood that the point of the study was to interrupt pregnancies in a very early stage. In these years before the passionate and divisive abortion debates of the later twentieth century, researchers and study participants alike focused on the potential of the study to help infertile women bear children. As a result, Rock and Hertig were able to document never-before-seen stages of human development, and, importantly to clinicians, demonstrate that the time of ovulation is in predictable temporal relationship to the following menstrual period, not the preceding one.[3]

Building on his enhanced understanding of early development, Rock and collaborator Miriam Menkin next decided to tackle in vitro fertilization of human embryos. Gregory Pincus had already succeeded with rabbits, so the concept was not far-fetched, even if it might remind contemporaries of Aldous Huxley's dystopian novel *Brave New World*, published in 1932, only about five years before Menkin and Rock began their work. The first challenge was obtaining eggs. Rock retrieved ovarian tissue from women undergoing various surgeries involving ovarian resection or removal, and with their permission, eventually attempted to fertilize 138 eggs from forty-seven women. The eggs were not easy to find; these 138 ova were the result of nearly a thousand surgeries. Sperm was a different story: in the procedure Menkin developed, she used the leftovers from patients attempting artificial insemination. Between 1938 and 1944, Menkin patiently tweaked her procedure, until one day a few accidental changes to the routine resulted in a fertilized egg. She was able to repeat her success with three more ova, but life circumstances pulled her away from her work with Rock, and no one else seemed to have her magic touch. Menkin and Rock had performed the first human in vitro fertilization; it would take three more decades for others to develop their beginning into modern in vitro fertilization.[4]

The capstone of Rock's career was the development of the birth control pill, in collaboration with Gregory Pincus. Rock had spent much of his career trying to help infertile women get pregnant, but he also had long directed the Rhythm Method clinic at the Free Hospital. In Massachusetts, this was the only legal method of birth control at the time, and it was also sanctioned by the Catholic Church, a consideration for many of his patients. Rock himself was a faithful Catholic, and he envisioned a birth control pill that would regulate a woman's cycles so that she could essentially use the rhythm method very successfully and in good conscience.

Rock had initiated research on the pill while he was director of the Free Hospital's Fertility and Endocrine Clinic, which had gained international renown during his tenure. However, in 1955, midway through the research, Rock reached Harvard's mandatory retirement age and was forced to retire from the clinic's directorship. He continued his clinical work at the new Rock Reproductive Clinic and continued to receive private funding for research on the pill. But his resources were strained, and so was his relationship with the Free Hospital. Ironically, some of the most high-impact research that came out of the Free Hospital in the mid-twentieth century was some of the most meagerly supported.[5] The pill was approved by the Food and Drug Administration (FDA) for contraceptive use in 1960, and within a few years, millions of women were taking it.

OLIVE WATKINS SMITH AND GEORGE VAN SICLEN SMITH

At the same time that Rock was examining endometrial tissue and retrieving early embryos, endocrinologist Olive Watkins Smith and gynecologist George Van Siclen Smith were investigating the hormonal causes of pregnancy loss and pregnancy-related illnesses. At the Fearing Laboratory, established at the Free Hospital in 1928, the wife-husband team worked to understand how hormones interacted to initiate and maintain pregnancy. They were searching for some way in which the newly isolated hormones might be able to save the pregnancies of women who habitually miscarried or delivered prematurely and lost their babies, and also save the health and lives of women who suffered from diabetes and eclampsia. When DES, an estrogenic compound, was synthesized in 1938, they saw its tremendous potential as a therapy for troubled pregnancies. They developed a protocol for administering it in high-risk pregnancies on the theory that it would stimulate the secretion of progesterone, which is necessary to support pregnancy. In 1946, they reported impressive results in women who had previously miscarried. Buoyed by pharmaceutical company promotion, DES as a therapy to support pregnancy spread rapidly, despite other researchers' failures to replicate Smith and Smith's results.[6]

If DES had turned out to be an effective therapy, the Smiths might now be seen as heroes of American obstetrics. If DES had turned out to be ineffective but harmless, it would be long forgotten. But instead, the story of DES has become an object lesson in medical hubris.

The postwar period was an era of tremendous optimism about modern medicine. Antibiotics, for

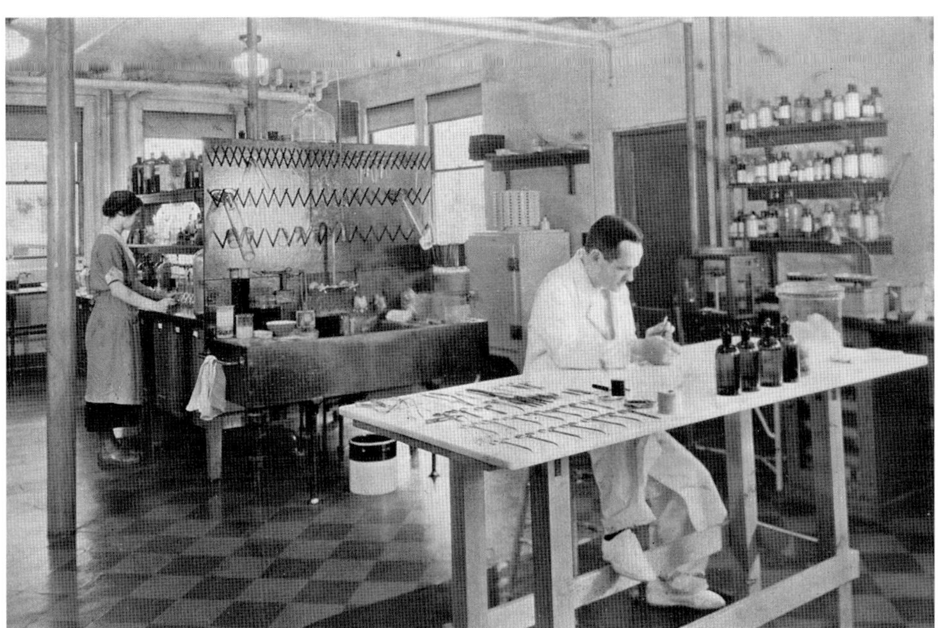

FIGURE 4-2 Olive Watkins Smith and George Van Siclen Smith in Fearing Lab, Free Hospital for Women, circa 1940s.

instance, developed for large-scale use after World War II, had effects that seemed almost miraculous. In days, even hours, they could bring someone from the brink of death back to perfect health. If that pill could save a person's life, maybe another pill could save a pregnancy. In that can-do, adventurous moment, doctors and their patients tried new drugs with abandon. The FDA's rules for drug approval were much more lenient than they would soon become, and DES had been thoroughly tested by the standards of the time.[7] Doctors were enthusiastic about DES because they had little else to offer a woman who suffered from recurrent miscarriages, and patients who had heard about the drug often demanded it. In hindsight, however, there had been warning signs: some animal studies had shown that DES was potentially carcinogenic and teratogenic, and human studies had failed to replicate the Smith's success.[8]

It is one of medicine's great mistakes that these warning signs were not heeded. In the late 1960s, one of George Smith's former students, Howard Ulfelder, saw a sudden rash of teenage girls with a rare form of vaginal cancer. One of the girls' mothers said that she had taken DES during her pregnancy. Ulfelder and Harvard colleague Arthur Herbst, another former student and friend of the Smiths, began collecting cases and created a carefully controlled retrospective study to demonstrate the link between DES and clear-cell adenocarcinoma. They published their results in 1971 in the *New England Journal of Medicine*. In that issue, Alexander D. Langmuir wrote an editorial on their work, stating: "Physicians must think more seriously before administering any drug to a pregnant woman."[9]

As it would turn out, DES use was linked to a variety of cancers and reproductive system abnormalities in the women who took the drug, as well as in their children and possibly even their grandchildren. Physicians and patients learned, in the most tragic way, about the potential impact of drugs taken by a woman on her developing fetus. This painful and powerful lesson ushered in a time of greater caution in research and was connected to widespread public critique of modern medicine and its practitioners.[10]

HISTORICAL CONTEXT OF THE NURSES' HEALTH STUDY

At the same time that Ulfelder and Herbst were starting to suspect DES's terrible side effects, another Harvard physician began to worry about a different widely prescribed estrogenic compound: the birth control pill. Frank E. Speizer's groundbreaking epidemiological work on the health effects of the pill and the genesis of the Nurses' Health Study is described by him in this chapter. However, it is also worth noting the historical context of his work.

By 1974, when Speizer had received his first grant from the National Cancer Institute to begin a study of the pill's health effects at the Channing Laboratory (then located at Boston City Hospital), the birth control pill had already been embroiled in widespread cultural and political debates about its safety for several years. The women's health movement was underway, and feminist activists were questioning the intentions and practices of doctors and drug companies alike. Journalist Barbara Seaman had published *The Doctors' Case Against the Pill* in 1969, prompting Congressional hearings about its safety in 1970.[11] Seaman and others pointed out that more than 9 million American women were now taking the pill after only relatively brief and small-scale studies of its safety and effectiveness. Like Speizer, she was alarmed that a potent drug was being casually prescribed to millions of healthy women. As a result of the highly publicized hearings, pharmaceutical companies were required to include warnings of side effects in a package insert, the first patient education insert of its kind for a prescription drug. This included warnings about the elevated (though still small) risk of potentially fatal blood clots, as well as acknowledgment of studies in animals that suggested the birth control pill might be carcinogenic.[12] (Ken Ryan, chief of staff of the Boston Hospital for Women and later chair of the Department of Obstetrics, Gynecology, and Reproductive Biology at Brigham and Women's Hospital, publicly supported the insert of health warnings into hormonal birth control packaging even as the American College of Obstetricians and Gynecologists publicly objected.) Women were only spooked enough to give up the pill briefly, but residual anxiety persisted.[13]

This feminist political activism apparently barely registered in the halls of the Channing Laboratory. As Speizer recalls, "We were pretty naïve in terms of what was going on." The political environment may have made the National Cancer Institute more disposed to fund Speizer's work, although it was not the Institute primarily responsible for research on the pill. The full-scale study finally got underway in 1976. "By going to nurses," Speizer says, "we did perhaps even better than we would have done with doctors' wives, in knowing their own bodies."

The Nurses' Health Study's questionnaire started out brief and to the point and focused on oral contraceptives and breast cancer. The choice had to do both with the interests of the people who were working on the project as well as concerns about breast cancer among the broader public. Walter Willett, who had joined Speizer's study in 1977, had long focused his work on nutrition and breast cancer. Women's health activism may have helped to focus new attention on breast cancer as a concern within the National Cancer Institute, which enthusiastically supported Speizer and Willett's work. Thus Speizer, Willett, and their collaborators shared many of the concerns of Seaman and other women's health activists but arrived at their concerns via the culture of epidemiology and public health rather than the culture of feminism.

The questionnaires have reflected concerns that span the range of health and chronic illness, including psychosocial factors and environmental factors in participants' neighborhoods. Says Willett: "We've used this to look at almost every conceivable health outcome you could imagine, including mental disease and neurodegenerative disease, right across the spectrum." The wealth of information already collected makes each new piece of data that much more valuable, because it can be compared and correlated with a huge database of existing information about the participants. Investigator Janet Rich-Edwards says, "We fight for space on these questionnaires. You should see these meetings!"

As the scope of the Nurses' Health Studies has expanded, it has required many more collaborators, working across a wide range of specialties, to pull it off. The Channing Laboratory's home at Brigham and Women's, where it had moved in 1977, was ideal. As Willett puts it: "If you're at the Brigham, you can find the world's best people within 100 yards of where you're sitting." Hundreds of researchers have contributed to the study, nurtured it over the years, and mined the data collected. "In some ways," explains Willett, "I regard what we have done as creating a platform that has allowed people from many different disciplines—clinical people, basic science people, statistical people—to come to this platform and interact, and use resources there, and contribute expertise. There are no other studies like this."

The Nurses' Health Studies have profoundly shaped our understandings of the relationships among lifestyle, diet, and health. Their conclusions have informed federal policy, popular culture, and medical practice. The richness of their resources will only grow, as they collect data over a longer time and follow participants into old age. As Willett concludes, "it has turned into something I think no one at the beginning imagined it would. It has been much more amazing than anyone had anticipated."

When Speizer initiated the Nurses' Health Study, "women's health" was not yet defined as a medical specialty or respected as a research interest. As Speizer reflected, "There was nothing called 'women's health' at that time." Yet, at a time when drug trials were mostly conducted on white men, and knowledge of the health status of women (as well as minorities, children, and the elderly) was lagging more and more behind, the study represented an enormous investment in women's health research.

Interestingly, because the Nurses' Health Study only has women participants and yet aims to inform health practices for men as well, its investigators have thought carefully about what its results mean for women's health and how they might be extended to men. For example, Willett explains: "In some ways, women are a better gender to study diet and heart disease, because in men, heart disease is accumulating from adolescence and onward, so when we start men off at age 50, we've missed the first 4 decades of atherosclerosis development. But in women, the ovarian hormones protect against the development of atherosclerosis until menopause, so we get almost a complete picture of their atherogenic experience."

Willett and other Nurses' Health Study investigators recognize differences between women and men and use that information to inform their research.

THE CONNORS CENTER

Over the last decade, this approach to women's health and the biology of sex differences in health and disease has been taken to a new level by the Mary Horrigan Connors Center for Women's Health and Gender Biology. Plans for a center began in 1995, with a gift from Jack Connors, then chair of the Brigham and Women's Board of Directors, in honor of his mother. Connors saw an opportunity for the Brigham to distinguish itself in women's health, drawing on its history and its impressive scope of existing faculty with relevant expertise.

The time was ripe for an interdisciplinary clinical and research push to tackle major issues in women's health and the biology of sex differences. The women's health movement gained strength in the 1970s, and by the 1980s had led to new National Institutes of Health (NIH) guidelines advocating equal inclusion of women in federally funded health research. When congress members Patricia Schroeder and Olympia Snowe discovered, in the early 1990s, that the guidelines were largely being ignored, and that in many important areas women's medical care was based on research performed solely on men, they were outraged. They collaborated with women's health activists and concerned scientists and administrators within the Department of Health and Human Services (DHHS) to pass legislation mandating that the NIH enforce its guidelines. In 1993 the NIH Revitalization Act put the mandate in place.[14] Also in the early 1990s, "women's health" received recognition as a field of investigation through the creation of the NIH's Office of Research on Women's Health and the DHHS' Office on Women's Health.[15] In addition, the FDA revised its guidelines, originally designed to protect children from prenatal exposures by excluding women of childbearing age from most kinds of research, to allow women using birth control to participate in clinical trials.[16] Thus the caution sparked by the DES tragedy had caused its own unintended side effects, but by the 1990s policymakers decided that the risk of involving women of childbearing age in research trials could be managed sufficiently with the modern, reliable contraception

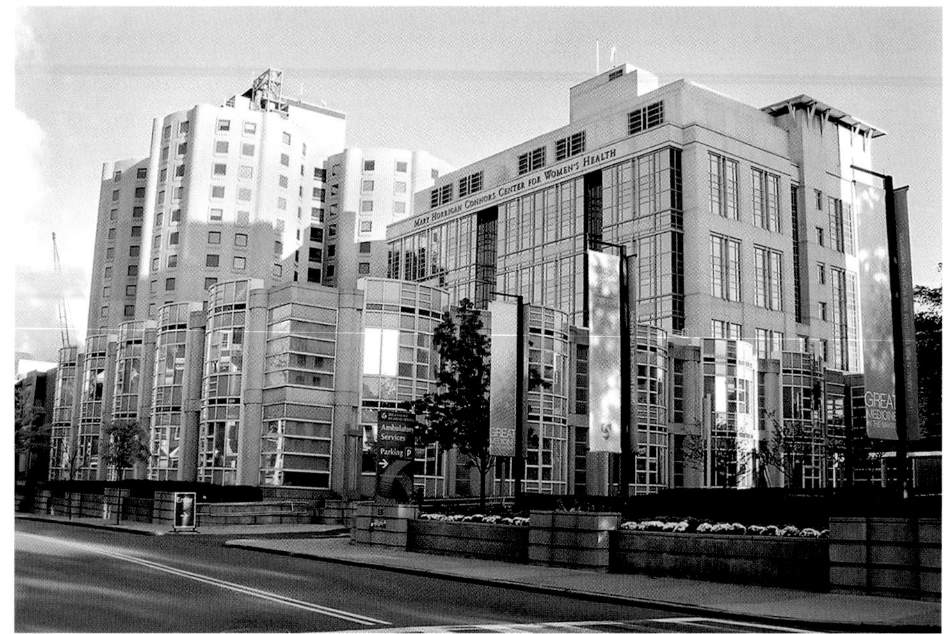

FIGURE 4-3 Connors Center for Women's Health.

of the birth control pill and the intrauterine device (IUD). Congress, the public, and the national agencies that fund the bulk of medical research had seen the need for research that includes women and is attentive to sex differences in health and disease, and had begun to build the necessary financial and administrative support.

In parallel, a consumer movement fueled the development of women's health care as a clinical specialty. Women patients were voting with their feet. As more women were admitted to medical schools, and the numbers of women internists and obstetrician-gynecologists grew dramatically, women patients began to seek them out, hoping for more respectful, thoughtful treatment than many felt they had received from their male physicians. In 1965, fewer than 7% of medical school graduates were women; by 1995, that figure had reached almost 40%, giving many more patients the option to choose female doctors.[17] Although this consumer movement relied on important changes in medical care prompted by the feminist health movement, it was not directly related. A woman did not need to be a feminist health activist to decide she felt more comfortable being examined by another woman. And although women might arrive as patients primarily because they preferred women doctors, leaders in women's health knew that they could offer not only a sensitive, respectful clinical setting, but also expertise. This was not only about reproductive health: many diseases present differently in women than in men. Cardiovascular disease and diabetes may come with different symptoms, may require different diagnostic tools, and may respond better to a somewhat different set of treatments. Many immunological diseases, such as multiple sclerosis and lupus, are not only tremendously more common in women, but have different typical courses in women and men, as do musculoskeletal issues such as arthritis and hip fracture. An academic center that offered a combination of sensitive care of women by women, plus expertise in the biology of sex differences in presentation, diagnosis, and treatment of illness, would be tremendously valued by its community.

With the Connors gift, the Brigham integrated these two powerful strands of health activism and federal funding support and began its development into a leader in women's health research and the translation of that research into clinical care. Initially, the work was carried out under the newly formed Division of Women's Health in the Department of Medicine. In its first years, with the Brigham in the lead, Harvard was named a Center for Excellence in Women's Health by the Office for Women's Health at DHSS. Organized around the problem of health disparities, programming included creating an integrated model of care for women, advancing the careers of minority women researchers, and facilitating research on women's health.

As the vision for women's health research at the Brigham developed, it became clear that a full-fledged center was necessary to fulfill the mandate of the Connors gift. Paula Johnson was named the director of the new Connors Center for Women's Health and Gender Biology and the chief of the Division of Women's Health. Johnson and her colleagues envisioned a center that would promote interdisciplinary research in women's health across Harvard, focus

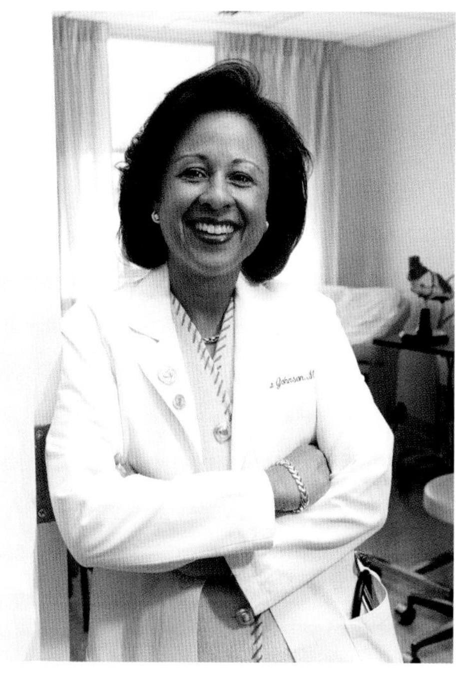

FIGURE 4-4 Paula Johnson, Executive Director of the Connors Center for Women's Health and Gender Biology; Chief, Division of Women's Health; Associate Professor, Harvard Medical School.

attention on sex and gender differences in health and illness, and tie research closely into clinical care.

Early in its existence, the Connors Center won a key training grant, indispensable for developing young investigators hoping for a career in women's health or gender biology. Because "women's health" is not the focus of any particular institute at the NIH, it takes creativity, persistence, and a robust network to launch a career. As a primary site for an Office of Research on Women's Health program called Building Interdisciplinary Research Careers in Women's Health (BIRCWH), the Connors Center can support and coach an investigator through the early, most difficult years in establishing her career. Through BIRCWH (pronounced "birch"), the Connors Center awards several-year grants to junior faculty members to help them get careers in women's health off the ground. In addition to funding, the Connors Center provides intensive, thorough mentoring from advisors selected from across the Harvard campuses and hospitals. Each BIRCWH awardee has a career mentor, a mentor in her or his primary field, and a translational mentor, who helps make the connection to clinical practice. Principal Investigator Jill Goldstein and Program Director Ursula Kaiser advise each BIRCWH scholar as well.

Past BIRCWH scholars have investigated problems as diverse as the neuroendocrine regulation of puberty, the epidemiological risk factors associated with systemic lupus erythematosus and rheumatoid arthritis in women, the role of genes and estrogen receptors in the development of aggressive forms of breast cancer and in the resistance to breast cancer drugs, and abnormal food motivation and reward processing in women with depression. Some have continued their careers at the Brigham, while others have left to build research programs in women's health at other research institutions.

Another key component of the Connors Center is the powerhouse team of nineteen senior researchers from across the hospital that comes together several times a year to shape the Connors Center research vision and brainstorm about specific research initiatives. The members of this Research Advisory Council independently perform research in women's health and gender biology in all corners of the Brigham. Some might have collaborated without the existence of the Connors Center, but never would all nineteen of them have been in the same room.

Sometimes council meetings spark new research questions for individual investigators, who then create interdisciplinary research projects, pulling together configurations of junior researchers who might otherwise never have met. Jill Goldstein, professor of psychiatry and medicine, initiated an investigation of the comorbidity of depression and heart disease in women when it became clear, in the course of a council discussion, that the pathways of the two disease processes were likely to be related. At other times, they connect colleagues with crucial resources. Epidemiologist Janet Rich-Edwards was planning a study of the relationship between vascular function and preeclampsia in Mongolia, where she could easily recruit study participants while they were planning pregnancies and measure vascular function before, during, and after pregnancy. She discussed her plans at a council meeting, and JoAnne Manson offered to connect her to the Society for Women's Health Research (SWHR), which eventually supplied pilot funding for the project. Rich-Edwards says, "This was terrific not only for the funding, but for the colleagues there, who are national experts in women's cardiovascular health. And that in turn has put me on a national stage." These new connections led to funding for a trainee to do research and present her findings to the SWHR. And every research plan discussed at a council meeting is enhanced by the tremendous extent and diversity of experience council members bring to the conversation.

Faculty with primary appointments within the Connors Center meet regularly to brainstorm and support each other as well. Faculty representing the research, clinical, policy, global health, and educational aspects of the Connors Center get together to tackle specific problems. As Rich-Edwards describes, "We take a puzzle." For instance, Rich-Edwards introduced an issue: women who have had preeclampsia are at two-fold risk of dying from heart disease, and yet in the United States we have no regular mode of educating those women and their clinicians about the risk. With an interdisciplinary group, there are "people thinking about different parts of this elephant, right here."

She says that she can now ask, "How much do primary care doctors and obstetricians currently know about this issue? What kind of actionable information would they need? How do electronic medical records work—how can we get information about who is at risk to you? Who is interested in this nationally—insurance companies, large employers, clinician organizations? I can get all of these perspectives, from clinic and from policy, and bring my own research perspective to it."

Rich-Edwards' approach of involving clinicians in the development of the research question as well as the intervention she is trying to develop is standard practice at the Connors Center. As Paula Johnson explains, this is an important innovation. "Traditionally," she says, "clinicians are just the recruiters. We're really focused on clinicians being part of the thinking process. What are the right questions, if you're doing clinical research? They are collaborators, and they are very important to the development of hypotheses." Johnson has witnessed clinicians become excited about research who have never done research before. And they are active in the translation of research back to care, as well. The Fish Center, the primary clinical aspect of the Connors Center, is truly integrated into the research effort.

A third central function of the Connors Center is to promote attention to gender difference in research across the hospital and across Harvard. Sometimes this means, as Jill Goldstein puts it, getting on her "soapbox" and reminding fellow investigators that "every tissue in the body has sex differences." Or, as Janet Rich-Edwards says, "raising the awareness so that people think, 'well, maybe we should include some female animals.'" At other times, this means coordinating seminars to bring people together, some of whom may never have researched sex differences, and thinking collaboratively about cross-disciplinary questions in the field. It can also mean providing the nitty-gritty kinds of practical support that allow an investigator to venture into uncharted territory. Rich-Edwards wanted to branch out into global health issues, working in Mongolia on how to provide vitamin D to schoolchildren, and more recently to study preeclampsia and cardiovascular health. However, it is no straightforward matter to organize and fund a local team when that team needs money up front to start the work and cannot work within the usual reimbursement process. "Simple things like that are a huge deal when you're trying to work with a developing country," she says, and impossible to execute without an experienced administrator. "It's not that sexy, but it's really important."

As work at the Connors Center embarks on its second decade, the center is in the process of creating a prospective cohort of families to be recruited from the Brigham's obstetrics department. Once it is developed, it will be a resource that, like the Nurses' Health Study, will serve as a platform for researchers across Harvard.

In its first decade, the Connors Center focused on developing networks of researchers and research projects on women's health and the biology of sex differences, drawing on the "richness of investigators that existed at Brigham and Women's," as Paula Johnson puts it, "this amazing protoplasm" that served as a foundation for the Connors Center's goals. In its next decade, as the Connors Center continues to facilitate these networks, the family cohort is expected to create a center of gravity for the center as well, to draw researchers closer and create even tighter and denser networks in the pursuit of better health care for women and a fuller understanding of the biology of sex differences.

From reproductive health research in the 1930s, 1940s, and 1950s at the Free Hospital for Women that reshaped American reproductive culture, to the preeminent prospective cohort study on women, to the comprehensive approach to women's health and the biology of sex differences that defines the Connors Center, Brigham and Women's Hospital and its affiliated hospitals have for decades been innovators in research on women's health. And over those decades, women's health research has moved from the periphery of attention to become a central focus in the Brigham's vision of its place in medical research culture and the provision of health care in Massachusetts. The vitality of current research, and the ambitious trajectory its leaders have envisioned, suggest that the Brigham will continue to be a leader in research on women's health and the biology of sex differences for decades to come.

BIOGRAPHY

JOHN ROCK (1890-1984)

Margaret Marsh

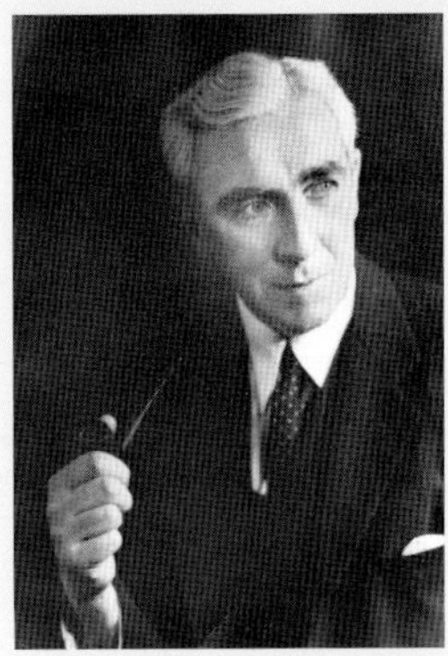

FIGURE 4-5 John Rock.

When Harvard gynecologist John Rock died in 1984 at the age of 95, *Boston Globe* columnist Ellen Goodman—referring to his work on "the pill"—called him a certified member of that small band of human beings who change the world. But to think of Rock primarily as a "father of the pill," as many still do, can obscure rather than illuminate his broader significance to the medical and cultural history of modern America.

Born into an Irish-Catholic family in 1890 in Marlborough, Massachusetts, John was the youngest son, and a twin. His father kept a saloon, dabbled in horse racing, and speculated in real estate, while his mother raised the five children. At nineteen, with his family in financial difficulties, he was shipped off to Guatemala to work for United Fruit Company as a timekeeper on a banana plantation. Fired within a year for siding with the Jamaican and indigenous workers during a wildcat strike, he knew he was not cut out to be a success in business, which had been his father's dearest ambition for him.

Instead, John decided to become a doctor, having been inspired by Neil MacPhail, the young Scots physician who befriended him in Guatemala. Entering Harvard College in 1911, he graduated from its medical school in 1918 and completed his residency training in 1921. Four years later he married Nan Thorndike. In spite of her Boston Brahmin upbringing, she brought an unconventional zest to his life as well as down-to-earth common sense. Nan and John had five children and a close, loving partnership until her death in 1961.

When he took the helm of the new "Sterility Clinic" at the Free Hospital For Women in 1926, it was one of the nation's first centers devoted to the treatment of infertility. At the time, doctors could view a woman's pelvic organs only by performing a major surgical procedure called a laparotomy. There was no way to predict accurately when a woman would ovulate, and medical researchers and practitioners barely understood the process in which a human sperm fertilized an egg. They knew even less about such things as the length of time it took a newly fertilized egg to find its way into the uterus and successfully implant. John Rock's work would change all that.

Rock's first major contribution to the new field that would become reproductive medicine appeared in the mid-1930s, when he and Marshall Bartlett developed a procedure called endometrial dating, which allowed doctors to discover, albeit after the fact, whether, and if so, when, ovulation occurred—bedrock knowledge without which there could be no reproductive technology. Then, beginning in 1938, he and pathologist/obstetrician Arthur T. Hertig began the study that would provide the first visual record of human embryonic development, research that earned both men numerous professional accolades, including the 1949 American Gynecological Society Research Prize.

In 1944, Rock had his initial brush with media celebrity when he and his research assistant Miriam Menkin achieved the first in vitro fertilization of human ova. Journalists besieged him, predicting the arrival of "test tube" babies in short order, despite Rock's insistence that such pregnancies were not on the immediate horizon. Most of the attention he and Menkin received was positive, which, given later controversies over human in vitro fertilization (IVF), might seem surprising. But this was an era that both celebrated new scientific discoveries and was strongly pronatalist. A technology to help the infertile conceive was clearly welcome.

Rock also devoted his energies to helping women who wanted to limit the size of their families. When he opened the first free birth control clinic in Massachusetts in 1936, it could legally provide women only with instruction in the rhythm method of contraception. Although his staff was careful not to overstep the law, Rock publicly spoke out against it and clandestinely subverted it in numerous ways, including teaching his Harvard medical students about the prescription and use of appropriate contraceptive devices.

By the end of the 1940s, Rock was the most visible infertility specialist in the nation. When the famous Hollywood actress Merle Oberon came to Boston in the late 1940s asking for "the fertility doctor," she was immediately sent to him. By the early 1950s, young doctors from all over the world vied for the opportunity to train with him while their more established colleagues converged on the Free Hospital in Brookline to observe his methods. He was known for his kindness and compassion toward all his patients, whether they were movie stars, African royalty, Boston society matrons, or the wives and daughters of elevator operators and laborers.

Rock was sixty-two when he began his now-famous collaboration with biologist Gregory Pincus to develop the oral contraceptive—the last act of his extraordinary career. As an infertility specialist and a practicing Catholic, he defied everyone's stereotype of a birth control advocate. His argument that the Catholic Church should allow its members to use the pill, expressed most famously in a book called *The Time Has Come: A Catholic Doctor's Proposals to End the Battle over Birth Control* (1963), made him an international celebrity.

During the backlash against the pill in the late 1960s, Rock drew the ire of feminist health activists mistrustful of medical authority and became a target of some fundamentalist Christians and others who considered his earlier embryo research to have been immoral. At his death, he was eulogized as a "true visionary," praised for his work on in vitro fertilization, and recalled as "the point man for the social medicine that initiated a sexual revolution." Today, he is remembered as one of the leading progenitors of the twentieth century's reproductive revolution, a revolution that has still not run its course.[18]

THE NURSES' HEALTH STUDY

Frank E. Speizer

In 1957, John Rock, professor of obstetrics and gynecology at Harvard Medical School and the Free Hospital for Women, reported on the use of synthetic progesterone as a regulator of menstrual cycles in fifty fertile women. As part of his study, he observed that none of the women became pregnant. Although this preparation was not initially marketed as an oral contraceptive, by 1960 approval was obtained, and within a period of five years, more than 6.5 million U.S. women were using "the pill." The pill had a similar history in Great Britain and was clearly an effective contraceptive.

In the mid-1960s I was working in the offices of the Medical Research Council of Great Britain in a unit directed by Sir Richard Doll, who, with Sir Austin Bradford Hill, conducted the British Doctors and Smoking Study linking smoking and lung cancer. We were receiving reports of rare but serious thromboembolic side effects, including death, among healthy young women who were using the pill. Moreover, I was surprised to learn in 1966 that no one from government, academic or industrial agencies had given thought to systematically assessing the potential long-term consequences of placing otherwise healthy women on such potent synthetic progesterone/estrogen preparations. We believed that a cohort of women followed prospectively in a manner similar to the British Doctors and Smoking Study could answer questions related to potential long-term consequences of the pill. Our initial problem was to determine the nature and size of the cohort of women to be included in such a study. To obtain unbiased estimates of their risk of developing disease, the subjects had to provide data on their past medical histories at the time of enrollment. We would need repeated assessments and updates to assess their behavioral and lifestyle factors that might modify or contribute to subsequent risk of disease. Once specific disease conditions were reported,

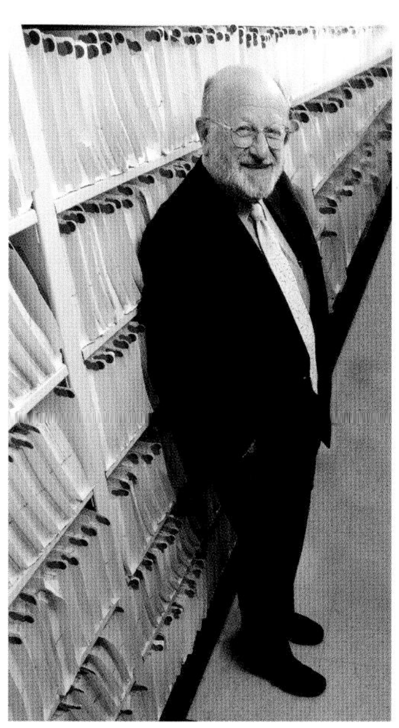

FIGURE 4-6 Frank Speizer.

we would need permission to access their medical information to verify their reports, while maintaining confidentiality and continued cooperation. Because this had to be done over a relatively long period of time, a cost-effective method was needed to make the study feasible.

We initially chose to study female physicians and physicians' wives, as members of such a cohort would understand medical terminology and might be more willing than other women to provide sensitive and private information. We conducted several pilot studies both in the United Kingdom and the United States and ultimately decided that the study could best be done in the United States using a mailed questionnaire. A most important discovery during this pilot testing phase was that in a number of cases, the male physicians had completed the questionnaires for their wives. Although we were upset with this discovery, because such an effect would invalidate much of the data, it led to a most important decision—to switch to nurses, and to conduct the Nurses' Health Study (NHS).

The target population consisted of married, female registered nurses aged thirty to fifty-five years and residing in one of the eleven states with the largest number of registrants: New York, California, Pennsylvania, Ohio, Massachusetts, New Jersey, Michigan, Texas, Florida, Connecticut, and Maryland. We limited the study population to married women due to the sensitivity of questions about contraceptive use at that time. The names and addresses of 238,026 nurses who fulfilled the eligibility criteria were obtained from a 1972 listing supplied by the American Nurses' Association, with approval from the state boards of nursing. Unique identification numbers were immediately assigned to each nurse to ensure strict confidentiality. The NHS cohort was established from this group of nurses via a series of three mailings of the baseline questionnaire. Starting in June 1976 (shortly before the Channing Laboratory became part of Brigham and Women's Hospital) and ending with the final mailing in December 1976, 122,690 nurses returned completed questionnaires (71.2% response rate of those not returned to us as unforwardable). The final number of 121,701 participants was established after removing from the original data duplicates and noneligible respondents, including males.

NHS participants have received a questionnaire every two years, commencing in 1976. A response rate of at least 90% has been achieved in each follow-up cycle. The original focus on contraceptive methods, smoking, cancers, and heart disease has been expanded to include many other lifestyle factors, behaviors, personal characteristics, nutritional measures, and diseases. Over the years, the women have contributed toenails, blood, and cheek cell specimens that are stored on site for use in a wide variety of biochemical and genetic studies. The NHS continues today as the longest running and largest prospective study of multiple risk factors for chronic disease in middle-aged and elderly women and is continuously funded by the National Institutes of Health.

The NHS has contributed in many ways to the research environment of the Brigham. Many investigators who as part of their training worked on the NHS have gone on to notable careers in population-based chronic disease research both within and outside the Brigham. The study has been not only a research and teaching base for a large number of successful leaders in the field of chronic disease, but also a model for additional cohort studies with substantial Brigham involvement. These include the Physicians' Health Study (a controlled clinical trial initially of aspirin and heart attack in about 22,000 male physicians), the Women's Health Study (a similar controlled clinical trial of aspirin, followed by observational studies in a cohort of approximately 40,000 older women nurses not in the NHS), the Health Professionals' Follow-up Study (a prospective cohort of 55,000 male nonphysician health workers carried out in a similar fashion as the NHS, with similar outcomes), Nurses' Health Study II (a prospective cohort of 116,700 younger nurses designed in part to assess the use of oral contraceptives before first pregnancy—not possible in the original NHS), and the Growing Up Today Study (a cohort of 17,000 children of NHS II mothers to assess early life diet and other risk factors for subsequent development of chronic diseases). All of these studies have taught us that the Brigham is not only is an outstanding primary, secondary, and tertiary care facility, but also a rich environment for the study of risk factors that can lead to prevention by assessing large population-based groups before they become patients.

Among the studies conducted by the NHS investigators, the findings primarily relate to the risks associated with (1) oral contraceptives, (2) postmenopausal hormones, (3) smoking, (4) physical activity, and (5) diet, including alcohol use. One of the more unique qualities of the NHS has been our ability to do repeated assessments using a semiquantitative food frequency questionnaire of dietary intake, with updates and cumulative assessments of long-term nutrient intake. The variety and quality of the data being collected in the NHS have been used by researchers to study (1) breast and other reproductive organ cancers; (2) colon, lung, and other cancers; (3) coronary heart disease, diabetes, and stroke; (4) hip fractures; and (5) eye diseases and other chronic conditions. More recently, because of the age of the population, some of the focus has shifted to assessments of cognitive function and healthy aging.

The findings of the NHS have contributed significantly to the scientific bases for public policy decision making in a number of arenas. These relate to the changing pattern of oral contraceptive and postmenopausal hormone use, the role of physical activity in the prevention and survivability of both heart disease and cancer, support of changing smoking policies resulting from findings related to both active smoking and second-hand smoke exposure, the impact of the control of weight gain, and the recommendations of dietary changes to reduce the intake of animal fats. Because we had the foresight to collect biological specimens on a large number of these women before the onset of any disease, these specimens have become a precious resource for studies of gene-environment interactions in the development of a variety of chronic diseases.

The success of the NHS in large part has resulted from the devotion of nurses who trusted us some thirty-six years ago to be involved in a grand experiment in which the only satisfaction was the promise that future generations of women might have better lives. The efforts of a large group of talented investigators, posing important questions that could be tested with the data, also contributed to our success. Harvard Medical School has acknowledged the importance of population-based medicine by promoting over the years to full professor at least a dozen individuals whose primary work has been in the NHS. Furthermore, these commitments have been supported by the Brigham through provisions of space and resources to support faculty development and foster an atmosphere of collaboration that is consistent with the mission of the hospital. The Brigham, by its continued commitments to the NHS and its progeny studies, will remain a leader in the field of population-based medicine and thus in incorporating preventive strategies into the nation's healthcare system.

BIOGRAPHY

ARTHUR T. HERTIG, 1904-1990

James E. Zuckerman

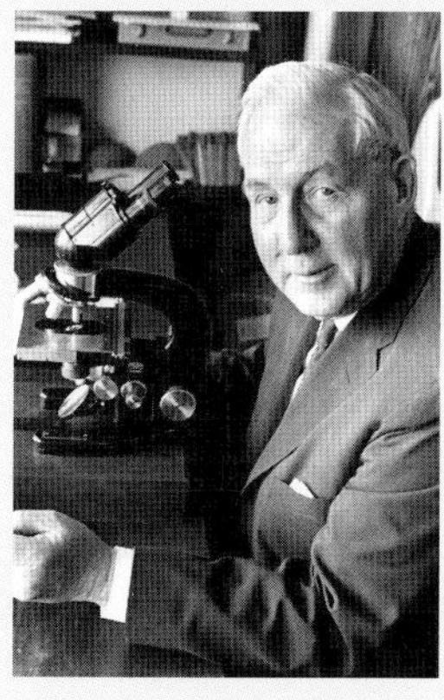

FIGURE 4-7 Arthur Hertig.

In 1852, Louis Pasteur said, "In the field of observation, chance favors only the prepared mind." Arthur Hertig's mind must have been well prepared, because chance did seem to favor him.

Born in Minneapolis in 1904, Hertig was a sophomore in high school when he decided to study medicine, prompted in large part by his fondness for his family doctor. He was also attracted to the field of entomology. His elder brother, Marshall, who was an entomologist, got Arthur a part-time job in the laboratory at the Department of Entomology at the University of Minnesota. As Hertig later wrote, the "vista of science opened for me. At 40 cents an hour the pay and intellectual climate were better than working in a bakery-ice cream establishment, good though that was."[19]

After his first year at the University of Minnesota Medical School, in 1925, Arthur worked for two years in China as an assistant to Marshall on the insect transmission of kala azar. They developed a system for artificially feeding sand flies and infecting them with *Leishmania donovani*, the causative agent of kala azar. Visited in China by David Edsall, dean of Harvard Medical School (HMS), Arthur Hertig demonstrated the technique of artificial feeding. Edsall was impressed by both the technique and the young medical student and invited him to transfer to HMS.[20] Hertig finished his second year at the University of Minnesota and transferred to HMS in 1928.

Hertig's next "chance," combining his interests in entomology and medicine, came a year later. S. Burt Wolbach, the Shattuck Professor of Pathological Anatomy and pathologist-in-chief at the Peter Bent Brigham Hospital, hired Hertig to do field research on the control of wood ticks on Martha's Vineyard. Although it was, as Hertig said, "a lovely summer job and well paid," it was cut short by an acute appendicitis. Nonetheless, his association with Wolbach led Hertig to the field of pathology.

After graduating from HMS in 1930, Hertig interned in pathology at the Brigham. On Valentine's Day in 1931, with only eight months of training, he was asked to establish the first pathology laboratory at the Boston Lying-In Hospital.[21] He accepted this position, disregarding the opinion of colleagues that there was no future in obstetric pathology because reproduction and childbirth were normal phenomena.[22] Indeed, before the laboratory opened in July 1931, fourteen maternal deaths had already been autopsied. Hertig did everything during his year in this new laboratory, including "making blood typing serum, struggling with bacteriological media, doing hospital bacteriology, performing autopsies, including sewing up bodies, learning about placentas, spontaneous abortions, etc."[23]

While planning further training in pathology, Hertig was encouraged by Frederick Irving, Richardson Professor of Obstetrics at the Boston Lying-In Hospital, to study with George L. Streeter, an eminent embryologist at the Carnegie Institution in Baltimore. Hertig found his year at the Carnegie Institution (1933-1934) "great fun and stimulating," and it sparked his lifelong interest in early human development and obstetric and gynecologic pathology. While at Carnegie, he completed important studies on the in situ origin of placental blood vessels from the trophoblast, which he described in an illustrated monograph.[24] He also studied the pathogenesis of spontaneous abortions, and, most importantly, learned both a technique of isolating early fertilized ova from primates and how to examine normal and abnormal human embryologic material.

Upon his return to Boston, Hertig completed his training both in pathology at the Children's Hospital under Sidney Farber and in clinical obstetrics at the Boston Lying-In Hospital. In 1938 Hertig became pathologist at the Free Hospital for Women. He began a fruitful, long-term collaboration in embryological studies with "Dr. John Rock (of 'pill' fame) . . . in our successful search for a series of fertilized human ova ranging in age from 1 to 17 days,"[25] using the egg-harvesting technique he had learned at the Carnegie Institution. Hertig's simple method was to scan the surgically removed uterus and fallopian tubes with a dissecting microscope to find a fertilized ovum, examine and photograph the ovum grossly, and serially section it for microscopic analysis.[26] Hertig and Rock collected thirty-four normal and abnormal human ova from uteri and fallopian tubes removed for gynecologic disease between 1938 and 1954. These ova were the substrate for the first organized studies of embryogenesis. Their findings, published in five monographs and papers between 1941 and 1956, laid the basis for modern embryologic research, fertilized egg transplantation, and the development of therapy for infertility.

Hertig's many scientific publications—numbering about 200, despite his dislike for writing—encompass the breadth of obstetric and gynecologic pathology. His monograph, *Human Trophoblast*, published in 1968, is the synthesis of his lifelong fascination with this tissue. Overall, Hertig made pioneering and significant contributions in placental pathology, precancerous lesions of the endometrium and cervix, and trophoblastic disease. But his greatest pleasure was in his studies of the early ovum.

Hertig began teaching at HMS in 1942. By 1948 he had risen to the rank of professor and pathologist at Boston Lying-In Hospital and the Free Hospital for Women. In 1952, he was appointed Shattuck Professor of Pathological Anatomy and, subsequently, chair of the HMS Department of Pathology. His skill as a teacher resulted in two awards for excellence in teaching by Harvard medical students, and he was made an honorary member of one of the graduating classes. His lectures were described as "clear and concise, scholarly and logical, and laced with a delicious sense of humor, personal anecdotes and mordant wit." An example of his concern for his students and for teaching is that for some years he endeavored to have every student in his class, in small groups, to tea in his office.[27]

Hertig retired as chair of the HMS Pathology Department in 1968 and moved to the New England Primate Research Center, where he focused on nonhuman primate reproductive pathophysiology and electron microscopy. In 1979, he was awarded the Gold Headed Cane, the highest award of the American Association of Pathologists. In accepting the award, Hertig looked back on his work, which he had described a few years earlier as "Forty years in the female pelvis—a case of prolonged dystocia."[28] He repeated maxims that he had lived by, including "Pygmies placed on the shoulders of giants see more than the giants themselves,"[29] that is, we all stand on the shoulders of our teachers and associates. He added: "One must take the job but not one's self seriously," and "We need high-powered workers using low-powered tools."[30]

Arthur Hertig died at the age of eighty-six on July 20, 1990. As noted by former trainee Ralph M. Richart:

> *Dr. Hertig was instrumental in establishing Ob-Gyn pathology . . . Because he focused attention on the pathology of the female genital tract at a time when little was known about the subject, he was able to make many significant contributions . . . He was also a compelling teacher . . . I still remember him sitting on the second floor of D Building overlooking the quadrangle with Hazel Gore, signing out consult cases with two rows of chief residents behind him hanging on his every word.*[31]

POPULATION STUDIES, RANDOMIZED PREVENTION TRIALS, AND WOMEN'S HEALTH: STUDIES OF AND BY WOMEN

JoAnn E. Manson

The Brigham has been an internationally renowned leader in population-based epidemiologic research for at least thirty-five years. Many of the studies focus on women's health and are directed by female research scientists. Moreover, the institution's large-scale prospective cohort studies and randomized prevention trials have served as a training ground for a large cadre of students, residents, fellows, and junior faculty members, helping to launch successful careers in epidemiology and translational research for several hundred investigators.

The prototype for the large population-based cohort with cost-effective mail-based follow-up was the Nurses' Health Study (NHS), a study of 121,701 U.S. female registered nurses (see essay by Frank E. Speizer in this chapter). Launched in 1976 by Frank

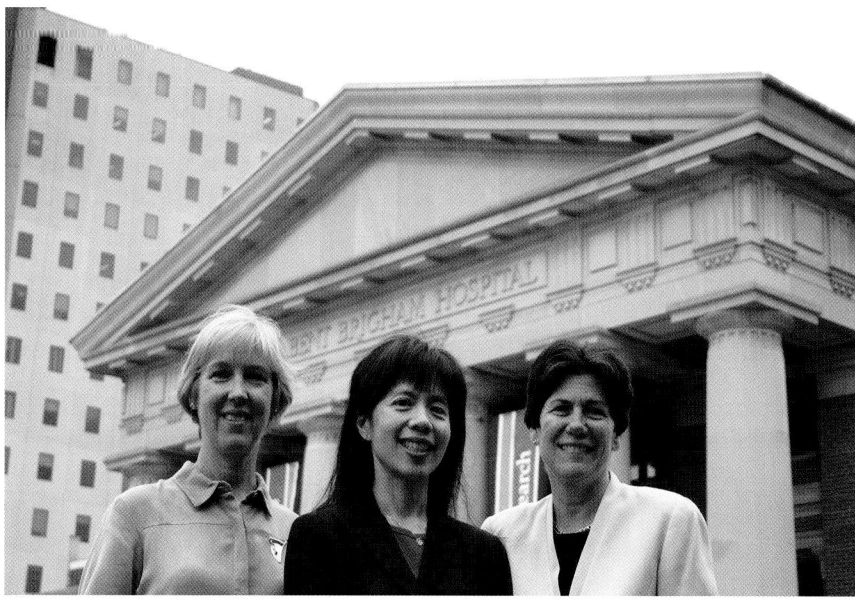

FIGURE 4-8 Left to right: Nancy Cook, Associate Biostatistician, Brigham and Women's Hospital; I-Min Lee, Associate Epidemiologist, Brigham and Women's Hospital; Julie Buring, Senior Epidemiologist, Brigham and Women's Hospital.

E. Speizer, the NHS has been directed by Susan E. Hankinson and is currently codirected by Francine D. Grodstein and Meir J. Stampfer. The NHS is widely recognized as a pivotal and pioneering study that is the "grandmother" of many subsequent women's health studies. This study and the Nurses Health Study II (NHS II), a cohort study directed by Walter C. Willett and including 116,700 women in younger age groups, have provided extraordinary opportunities to study women's health throughout adulthood.

Nearly every Brigham department and division is actively involved in women's health research. However, most of the population-based epidemiologic research and randomized prevention trials have been, or are currently being, conducted at either the Channing Laboratory or the Division of Preventive Medicine, often in collaboration with researchers in other divisions or at the Harvard School of Public Health. The Brigham has earned an international reputation for its leadership in the design and conduct of large, simple, cost-effective trials that focus on prevention. The first randomized controlled trial at the Brigham, a cost-effective study conducted primarily by mail, was the Physicians' Health Study (PHS), a trial in 22,000 U.S. male physicians of aspirin in the primary prevention of cardiovascular disease. Following the completion of the PHS, a diverse set of population-based cost-effective trials, primarily directed by female faculty members and conducted by mail, were initiated in the Division of Preventive Medicine.

The Women's Health Study (WHS), initiated in 1992, was a randomized, double-blind, placebo-controlled trial of the balance of benefits and risks of low-dose aspirin and vitamin E in the primary prevention of cardiovascular disease and cancer in 39,876 U.S. female health professionals. The randomized trial component ended in 2004 and has been converted to an observational follow-up study. Julie E. Buring, an epidemiologist and professor of medicine at Harvard Medical School, has been its principal investigator, and is currently a codirector with I-Min Lee. The WHS demonstrated that low-dose aspirin has a role in preventing ischemic and total stroke in women but, in contrast to the findings among men in the PHS aspirin trial, did not reduce the risk of myocardial infarction overall. Results appeared to be influenced by age: women sixty-five years of age and older experienced a reduction in major cardiovascular disease (CVD) events, myocardial infarction, and stroke on aspirin treatment. Women younger than sixty-five years had a reduction in stroke but not in other vascular events. Beyond its primary goals, the WHS also includes multiple ancillary studies related to cancer, cognitive function, diabetes, age-related macular degeneration and cataract, and biomarker and genetic predictors of chronic disease. The WHS is an invaluable resource for women's health research by virtue of the extensive data collection on nearly 40,000 women over twenty years of follow-up, including detailed annual medical histories, dietary assessments, and blood collections on more than 27,000 participants. A wide array of biomarkers, including lipoproteins, inflammatory markers, and thrombotic/hemostatic variables, have been measured on the stored blood samples, and genome-wide association studies have also been conducted. The processed and stored blood, including DNA, allow faculty and trainees to explore a virtually unlimited number of biomarker and genetic hypotheses.

The Women's Antioxidant and Folic Acid Cardiovascular Study (WAFACS, initiated in 1993) is a randomized, double-blind, placebo-controlled trial of the balance of benefits and risks of vitamin E, vitamin C, beta-carotene, and a combination of folic acid, vitamin B_6, and vitamin B_{12} in the prevention of cardiovascular events among 8,171 female health professionals (5,442 participated in the B-vitamin trial) with a prior history of or at high risk for cardiovascular disease. Leadership includes JoAnn Manson, principal investigator and Chief of the Brigham's Division of Preventive Medicine, and co-investigators Christine Albert and Shumin Zhang. Additional outcomes of interest in WAFACS include breast and colorectal cancer, colorectal adenomas, age-related macular degeneration, cognitive function, depression, and skeletal fractures. Although the trial confirmed the absence of cardioprotection from either antioxidant vitamins or homocysteine-lowering agents, it showed a statistically significant reduction in age-related macular degeneration with folic acid and B-vitamin supplements. Other analyses are underway, including analyses of cognition and depression by Francine Grodstein and Olivia I. Ookereke.

In 1993, the Brigham's Division of Preventive Medicine became one of the sixteen original clinical sites for the nationwide Women's Health Initiative (WHI), the largest set of randomized clinical trials ever conducted in postmenopausal women. The WHI is an National Institutes of Health–initiated, nationwide, multicenter, randomized trial to assess the benefits and risks of menopausal hormone therapy, a low-fat dietary pattern, and calcium/vitamin D supplementation in the prevention of cardiovascular disease, cancer, and osteoporosis-related fractures in postmenopausal women. JoAnn Manson, principal investigator at the Boston site since study inception, participated in the design and protocol development for the study. The clinical trial components of this project ended in the early 2000s and have subsequently been in an observational follow-up phase through 2012. The landmark WHI has clarified the balance of benefits and risks of estrogen-progestin and estrogen-alone therapy in relation to chronic disease prevention, provided conclusive evidence on the role of calcium/vitamin D supplementation for fracture prevention, and assessed cancer and cardiovascular disease outcomes associated with a low-fat dietary pattern. A large number of other women scientists have been active contributors to WHI-related science, including Meryl S. LeBoff (bone health), Kathryn M. Rexrode (stroke and CVD), Aruna Pradhan (diabetes), and Shumin Zhang and Jennifer H. Lin (cancer).

The VITamin D and OmegA-3 TriaL (VITAL) is a newly launched double-blind randomized clinical trial assessing the effects of vitamin D and two marine omega-3 fatty acids (EPA + DHA) in the primary prevention of cancer and cardiovascular disease among 20,000 U.S. men and women. Trial leadership includes JoAnn Manson, Julie Buring, and I-Min Lee. Baseline blood collections are planned for at least 80% of the cohort (~16,000) and follow-up blood collections in ~6,000. Ancillary studies are assessing the interventions' effects on additional health outcomes, including diabetes and glucose tolerance, lung function and autoimmune diseases.

BWH is a leader in population-based observational cohort studies and randomized clinical trials. Its investigators have directed landmark studies related to women's health and have trained and nurtured the careers of women scientists.

BIOGRAPHY

MERYL S. LEBOFF

Peter V. Tishler

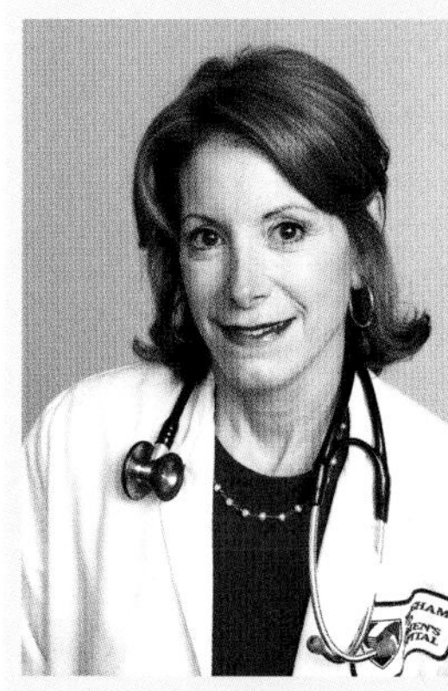

FIGURE 4-9 Merle LeBoff.

Meryl S. LeBoff is representative of the young, exceptionally achieving women physicians and scientists at the Brigham. An endocrinologist specializing in osteoporosis and metabolic bone disease, she founded the Skeletal Health and Osteoporosis Center in 1987. Under her directorship, this center has become a program of many objectives, including clinical care, education, and research. Building on her documenting the high prevalence of vitamin D deficiency in women admitted to the Brigham with hip fractures, she has championed the interdisciplinary Brigham Fracture Team, also involving members of the Department of Orthopedics, to advance the care of hip fracture patients. She contributes to educational initiatives and guides on osteoporosis and women's health policy and is an active mentor of fellows and students. Her research, an equally major commitment, focuses on the causes of primary and secondary osteoporosis and skeletal health across the life cycle, mechanisms facilitating osteoblast generation in human marrow stromal cells, the genetics of osteoporosis, and clinical approaches to facilitate fracture healing. LeBoff has received numerous honors, including inclusion on the Honor Roll of top 1% of doctors in *U. S. News and World Report*, and the Mary Horrigan Connors Award for Outstanding Leadership in Women's Health. She has served as a trustee and on the Scientific Advisory Board of the National Osteoporosis Foundation, the Advisory Board to the Massachusetts Department of Public Health Osteoporosis Program, and the National Institutes of Health's Calcium, Vitamin D and Osteoporosis Committee for the Women's Health Initiative since its inception. She contributes to national and international committees and task forces to systematically improve fracture care. As an elected Councilor to the American Society for Bone and Mineral Research, she is working on strategies to reduce the burden of fractures, including serving on the task force that is preparing a report on "Systems Approaches to Osteoporotic Fracture Secondary Prevention."

In 2009, LeBoff became the first female Harvard Professor of Medicine in the Brigham's Endocrine, Diabetes, and Hypertension Division. In the fall of 2012, she was presented with the Brigham and Women's Hospital distinguished Chair in Skeletal Health and Osteoporosis. As such a multifaceted achiever, she is an inspiration to all of us.

A BRIEF HISTORY OF THE DEPARTMENT OF OBSTETRICS AND GYNECOLOGY

Donald Peter Goldstein

The Department of Obstetrics and Gynecology began with the founding of the Boston Lying-In Hospital (BLI) in 1832 by Walter Channing, an eminent physician and dean of the Harvard Medical School (HMS) from 1826 to 1847. (More details about Channing's life can be found in Chapter 6.) The concept of in-hospital delivery was revolutionary since most respectable women delivered at home while poor women went to the House of Industry. David Humphreys Storer, succeeding Channing as the leader of Boston obstetrics, was an advocate for medical education reform and also dean of HMS from 1855 to 1864. Milestones during those early years included the introduction of anesthesia to alleviate labor pains in 1848 by Channing and the first cesarean hysterectomy by Horatio Storer (son of David Storer) in 1868.

The BLI moved from Washington Street to more a more elaborate facility on Springfield Street in 1854, but soon closed because of financial duress. It reopened in 1868 at a new location on McLean Street, directed by William L. Richardson. The first free outpatient clinic began in 1880, affording Harvard Medical students the unique opportunity to learn and deliver obstetric care. This service, which continued until the outbreak of World War II, was hugely popular with medical students. Under Richardson's leadership, Alfred Worcester, a junior member of the BLI staff, demonstrated the efficacy of antiseptic obstetrical technique in the 1880s, resulting in a marked reduction in postpartum infection. During Richardson's tenure as HMS dean from 1893 to 1907, he ensured that obstetrics became an integral part of the medical curriculum.

Coincident with these early developments in obstetrics, the nascent field of gynecology was becoming a specialty, largely because of the pioneering work of J. Marion Sims, founder of the Women's Hospital in New York City. The visionary surgeon William H. Baker trained with Sims and founded Boston's Free Hospital for Women (FHW) in 1875 for "the free treatment of poor women affected with diseases peculiar to their sex." Baker's intent was to "advance the healing art through study, experiment and invention." After overcoming public anxieties about the propriety of exposing female patients to physicians-in-training, Baker forged a close alliance with HMS, and the FHW soon became an epicenter of research and teaching. The centerpiece of the hospital was its pathology laboratory, founded in 1891 by William P. Graves, who had worked in the first gynecologic pathology laboratory in the country under the direction of William S. Cullen.

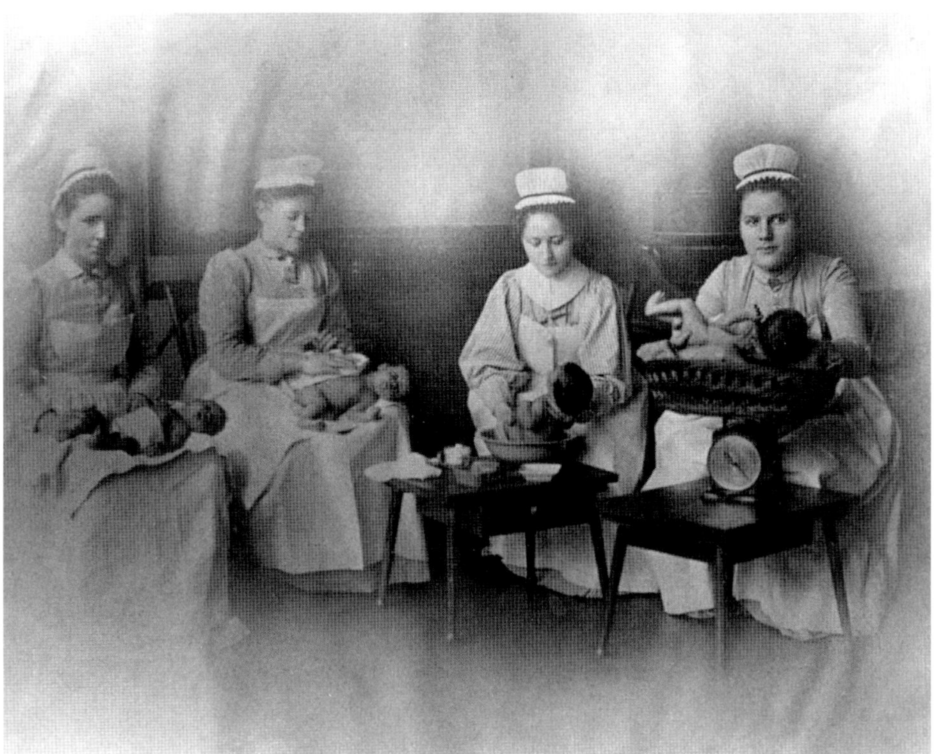

FIGURE 4-10 Nurses at the Boston Lying-In Hospital, circa 1890.

The FHW relocated from Springfield Street to Pond Avenue in Brookline in 1901. In 1908 Baker was succeeded by Graves. His tenure was notable for the development of major abdominal and vaginal procedures, the establishment of the first cancer ward, the use of radium to treat gynecologic cancer, the introduction of diagnostic imaging, and the invention of the Graves vaginal speculum, still used today. The opening of the Parkway Hospital for private patients in 1922 allowed the staff to integrate their private practices with their clinic responsibilities. Graves was succeeded by Frank A. Pemberton in 1933.

At the BLI, Charles M. Green succeeded Richardson as chief of staff in 1907. During his tenure, the American obstetrical community recognized the importance of prenatal care, and a pregnancy clinic was established for this purpose in 1913. Under the leadership of Franklin S. Newell, commencing in 1916, the relationship between the obstetrical service and HMS became solidified. Newall, an exceptional surgeon, established standards for performing cesarean sections. Spinal anesthesia for cesarean birth became widely practiced, as did labor induction. Concern about alleviating the pain of labor led to the use of "twilight sleep" with scopolamine and morphine, as well as "sacral anesthesia." Newall facilitated the establishment of the first cardiac clinic in an obstetrical hospital in 1921, led by Paul Dudley White and Burton E. Hamilton. He expanded other outpatient services to include clinics for urology, toxemia, and postpartum follow-up. In 1925 the first well-baby clinic for newborns was started in collaboration with the Children's Hospital under Kenneth Blackfan. A sixteen-person residency program in obstetrics was formally begun under the supervision of Judson Smith, the first resident physician, and a loose affiliation with the FHW was established for training in gynecology. A new BLI facility, necessitated by these multifold activities, was opened in 1923, on Longwood Avenue opposite the medical school.

In 1930, Frederick "Fritz" Irving became the first William Lambert Richardson Professor of Obstetrics and Chief of Staff at BLI. He created a full-time obstetrical pathology service, headed initially by S. Burt Wolbach, at that time also chair of pathology at the Peter Bent Brigham Hospital (PBBH). In 1942, Irving established the first full-time anesthesia service in an obstetrical hospital, headed by Burt B. Hershenson.

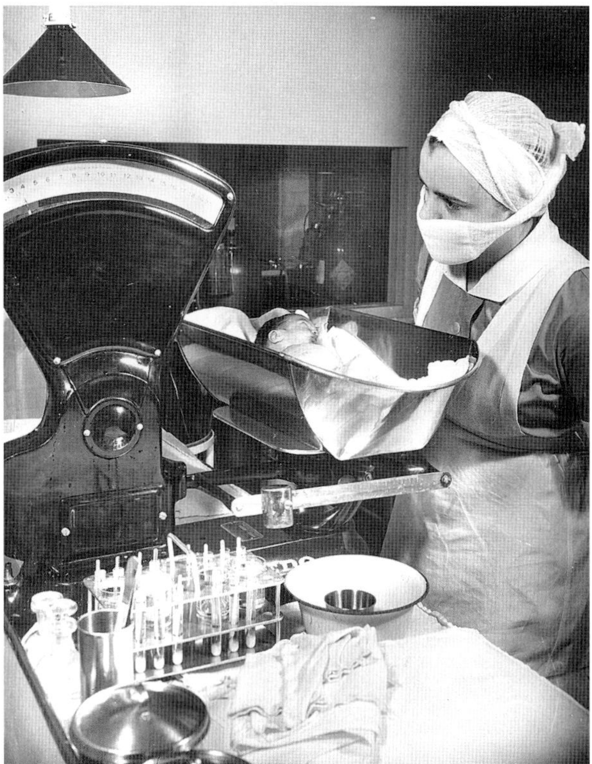

FIGURE 4-11 Boston Lying-In Hospital Premature Nursery, 1939.

During his tenure (1930-1946), he facilitated many advances in understanding and managing obstetric hemorrhage due to placenta previa, abruptio placenta, and placenta accrete, first described in 1937 by Irving and Arthur T. Hertig, then head of pathology and later the Shattuck Professor of Pathologic Anatomy at Harvard. Other major advances during Irving's tenure included early intervention and exchange transfusion of patients with erythroblastosis fetalis (with Children's Hospital pediatrician Stewart Clifford and pathologist Arthur Hertig), description of the morphology of molar disease (Hertig), and delineation of the proper role of cesarean section and pituitary extract for the management of labor. The incidence of both maternal and fetal mortality dropped precipitously during Irving's leadership.

Over the years, the FHW was also recognized for innovations in the field of infertility and reproductive endocrinology, the result of research at both the Fearing Laboratory and the Rock Reproductive Center. In 1928, the pathology laboratory became the George Fearing Research Laboratory, supervised by George and Olive Smith, who were concerned with elucidating the complex pathways of action of ovarian and placental hormones, including estrogen's role in menstruation and pregnancy. George Smith was a gynecologic surgeon who spent his entire career at the FHW, working as a telephone operator and orderly during medical school, training there in gynecology, and becoming a staff member and ultimately chief of staff and HMS professor of gynecology. Olive, a PhD biochemist, collaborated with George on numerous studies. The Rock Reproductive Center was started by John C. Rock, who had trained in obstetrics and gynecology at the BLI and FHW. In 1944, after working on human reproduction at the FHW, Rock and his associate Mirriam Menkin carried out the first fertilization of an ovum in vitro. In collaboration with Arthur Hertig, Rock also studied the human embryo, ultimately identifying a nine-day embryo known as the Hertig-Rock embryo. In 1949, nearly a decade before Food and Drug Administration approval of the first oral contraceptive, Rock coauthored a book entitled *Voluntary Parenthood* presenting a number of contraceptive methods at a time when dispensing contraceptives was illegal in Massachusetts. In the 1950s he began his research on the effects of progesterone and estrogen on ovulation, which led, in collaboration with Gregory G. Pincus of the Worcester Institute for Experimental Biology and Medicine, to the development of oral contraceptives. (Details about the accomplishments of the Smiths, Hertig, and Rock are found elsewhere in this chapter.)

In 1946 Duncan E. Reid followed Irving as Richardson Professor and BLI chief of staff. Reid and his team, expanding on Irving's work on obstetric hemorrhage, introduced fibrinogen for treatment of obstetrical disseminated intravascular coagulation (1950), successfully delivered a mother who had undergone a kidney transplant at the PBBH (1954), established the first clinic for evaluation of abnormal Pap smears in pregnancy with Lorna Jackson and Charles E. Easterday, and created a clinic for DES-exposed daughters (1971). Dedicated to developing academic leaders in the obstetrics, he received financial support from the Josiah M. Macy Foundation for the training of

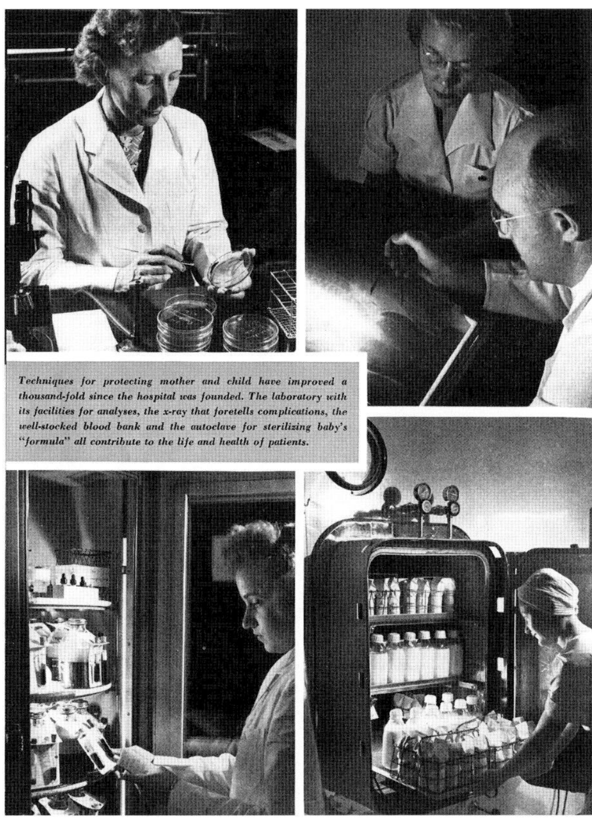

FIGURE 4-12 Boston Lying-In Hospital pamphlet, Safe Anchoring Ground: "Techniques for protecting mother and child have improved a thousand-fold since the hospital was founded," circa 1940s.

residents who were committed to an academic career. This highly successful program, in addition to producing a number of leaders in the specialty, supported John Josimovich's work on the isolation and purification of human placental lactogen. Reid also facilitated the establishment, with National Institutes of Health support, of the New England Trophoblastic Disease Center in 1965, in collaboration with pathologists Hertig, Hazel Gore, and Shirley Driscoll, and with the Gynecologic Endocrine Laboratory of the PBBH. The effectiveness of chemotherapy in patients with choriocarcinoma and related trophoblastic tumors proved to be an impetus for the field of medical oncology and was the prototype for the use of biomarkers for diagnosis, monitoring the effect of treatment, and follow-up to identify recurrences. In 1966, during Reid's tenure, the BLI and FHW merged to form the Boston Hospital for Women.

In 1973, Kenneth J. Ryan was appointed chair of the combined department, after extensive research on biochemical pathways of estrogen metabolism at the Fearing Laboratory under Olive Smith, and chairing obstetric/gynecologic departments at Case Western Reserve in Cleveland and the University of California/San Diego. Under Ryan the department continued to grow and prosper, with the establishment of subspecialty divisions with full-time faculty and fellowship training programs. In 1975 Robert C. Knapp was

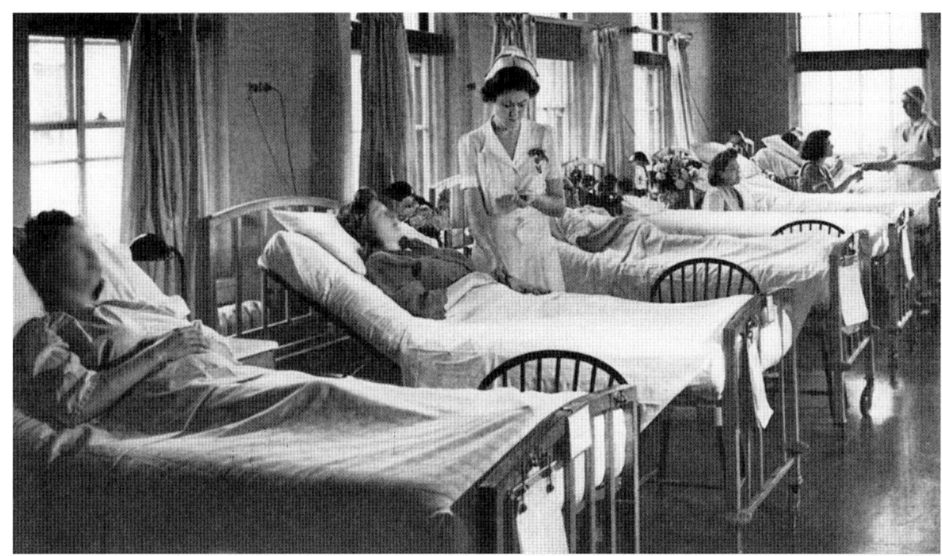

FIGURE 4-13 Boston Lying-In Hospital nurse in large ward, circa 1940s.

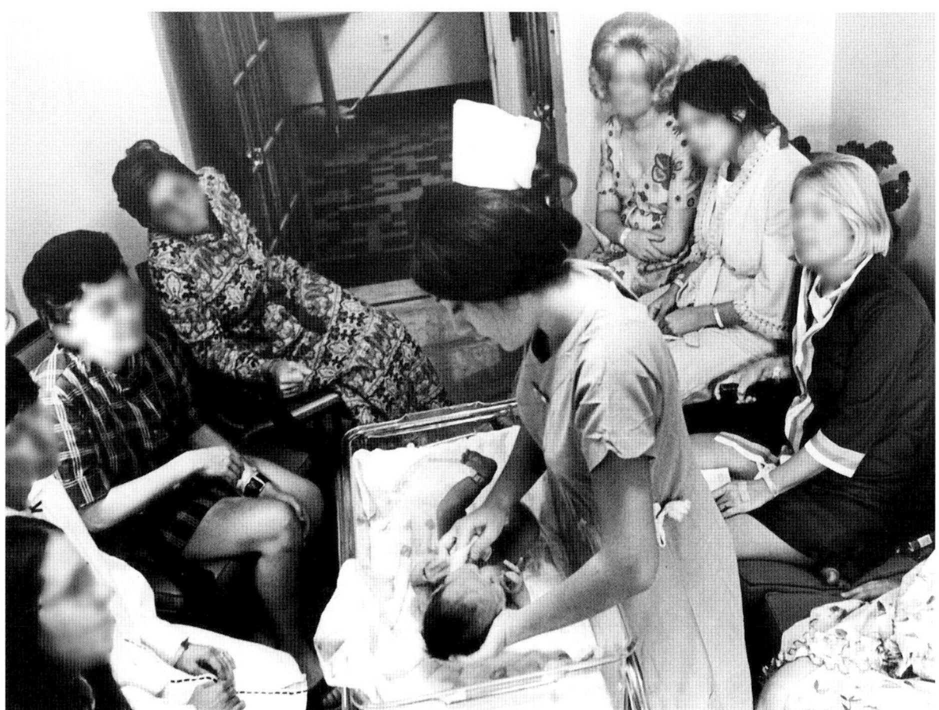

FIGURE 4-14 Boston Lying-In Hospital patient education, circa 1960s.

recruited from Cornell University Medical College to head the Division of Gynecologic Oncology at the FHW, and the Divisions of Maternal and Fetal Medicine and Reproductive Medicine were established. During this same year, the Boston Hospital for Women merged with the PBBH and Robert Breck Brigham Hospitals to form the Affiliated Hospitals Center and then the Brigham and Women's Hospital (1980), after which all facilities of the Boston Hospital for Women were moved to the current Brigham facility.

In 1993, Ryan was succeeded by Robert L. Barbieri, the current department chair and Richardson Professor, who also had trained in this department and had excelled in the field of reproductive medicine. Under Barbieri's leadership, the department and the full-time faculty have expanded to include subspecialty programs in urogynecology and reconstructive pelvic surgery, global obstetrics and gynecology, African women's health, minimally invasive surgery, fetal medicine and prenatal genetics, pediatric and adolescent gynecology (in collaboration with Children's Hospital), and family planning. The residency

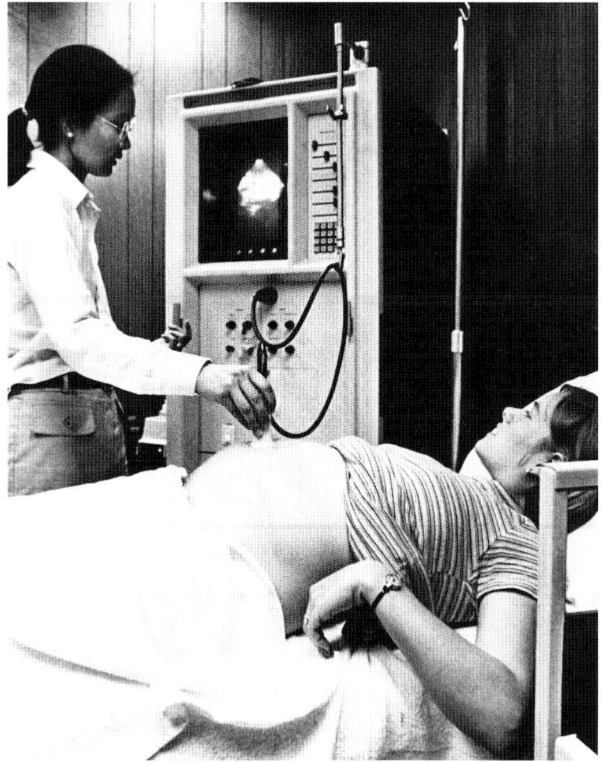

FIGURE 4-15 Brigham and Women's Hospital ultrasound, circa 1980s.

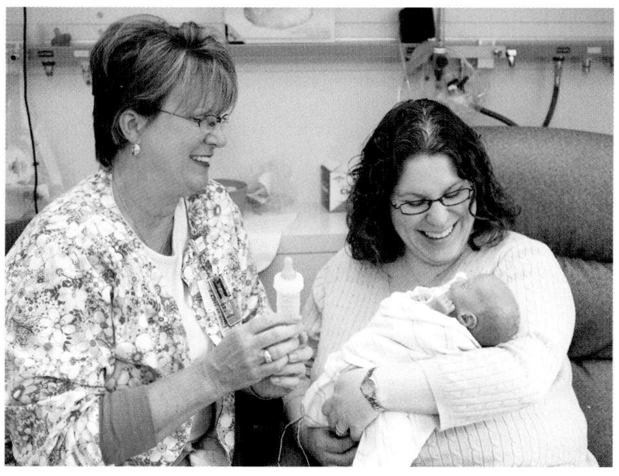
FIGURE 4-16 BWH mom with newborn and nurse Karen Green.

program expanded to four years and utilizes the facilities of multiple hospitals in addition to the Brigham. Research activities have also grown in the fields of cytogenetics, genital tract biology, gynecologic oncology, and epidemiology.

The Department of Obstetrics and Gynecology at the Brigham and Women's Hospital began in 1832 with the vision of one man who believed that all women had the right to "safe deliverance." Its mission, in addition to training the next generation of leaders and advancing knowledge through research, is dedicated to providing exceptional medical care continuously through the entirety a woman's life.[32]

BIOGRAPHY

DUNCAN EARL REID, 1905-1973

James E. Zuckerman

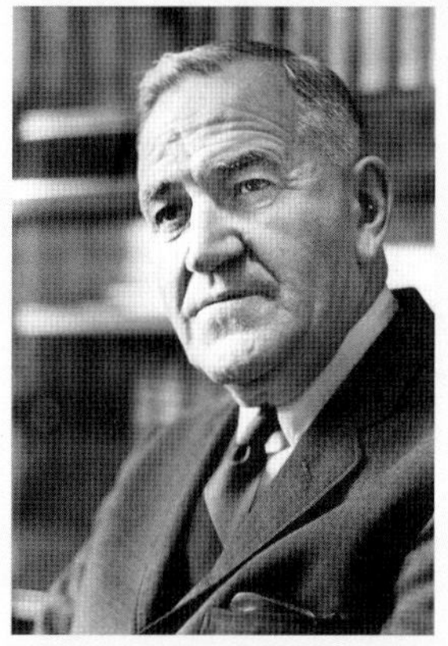
FIGURE 4-17 Duncan Reid.

A brilliant and compassionate doctor, Duncan Reid was born in Burr Oak, Iowa, on December 22, 1905. His mother died six weeks after his birth, and her death might have been one of the forces that led him to a career in obstetrics. His father died when Duncan was twelve, and he was raised by his paternal aunt and her husband, David McDougall. Reid attended Ripon College in Ripon, Wisconsin, graduating in 1927. He was a keen athlete, participating in track, football, and basketball. To help pay for college, he worked at a factory and as a medical librarian. Reid attended the Northwestern University Medical School in Chicago, graduating in 1931. He remained in Chicago during his internship in gynecology at Passavant Hospital, a residency year of general surgery at St. Luke's Hospital, and work in pathology at the Cook County Hospital.

Reid joined the Boston Lying-In Hospital in 1933, the first non-Harvard resident in obstetrics under Frederick C. Irving. He was a teaching follow at Harvard Medical School (HMS) from 1938-1939, an instructor from 1941-1947, and the William Lambert Richardson Professor of Obstetrics and Boston Lying-In Obstetrician-in-Chief commencing in 1947. He received an honorary MA from Harvard in 1947. In 1948, he aided in the amalgamation of the residencies in obstetrics at the Boston Lying-In Hospital and gynecology at the Free Hospital for Women. In 1959, as chief-of-staff at the Boston Lying-In, he was instrumental in fusing Harvard's Departments of Obstetrics and Gynecology, and he was named head of the combined department. In 1966, when he spearheaded the merger of the two hospitals, forming the Boston Hospital for Women, he was appointed chief-of-staff.

In 1954, Reid implemented a Josiah Macy, Jr., Foundation Fellowship for the recruitment and training of talented persons for academic careers in obstetrics and gynecology. The Macy Foundation also endowed the Kate Macy Ladd Chair in Obstetrics and Gynecology at HMS in 1963, and Reid became the first incumbent of this chair in 1964.

As a teacher, clinician, and researcher, Duncan Reid made valuable contributions to the care of women in pregnancy and childbirth and wrote more than 140 scientific papers on a wide range of topics. His focus on medical complications in pregnancy and on the biology of reproduction improved obstetrical care by taking it far beyond the principles of midwifery. In his early years, he was concerned with precisely defining the types of hypertension that complicated pregnancy. He published early, definitive papers on the causal relationship of severe pregnancy toxemia to cardiovascular or renal disease—a medical controversy of the day. In 1944-1946, he introduced posterior pituitary extract for the treatment of prolonged labor. In later years he dealt with such diverse topics as defects in coagulation due to fibrinogen deficiency, estrogen production in normal and abnormal pregnancies, and the anatomy and physiology of the pregnant uterus. Distilling twenty-five years of experience into a book, in 1962 he published *A Textbook of Obstetrics.*

In 1952, Reid performed the first therapeutic abortion in Boston on a patient who had been exposed to rubella. He was among the earliest to urge that elective abortions be performed after consideration of the relevant factors in the woman's home environment, present and future, as well as mental or physical characteristics. With foresight, and perceiving the need long before its acceptance, he established a contraception clinic. He played a large part in easing Massachusetts' laws against birth control and in 1970 urged that federal funds be used to establish special centers for abortions as part of a national policy of population control. In 1964, in collaboration with Howard N. Jacobson, he proposed that maternal care be given in large part by family nurse practitioners—individuals who would provide most of the medical supervision in the prenatal and postnatal periods at a community-centered clinic. At the time, this represented a significant change from the traditional pattern of American maternal care.

Reid was a compassionate man with unmatched devotion to patients. During World War II, he worked constantly to care for the patients of doctors who were in the service. To the frustration of his efficient office nurse, he would often see a sick ward patient in consultation with the resident staff if his private patients did not need his attention. Rubie M. Smith, who served at Boston Lying-In for decades, said of him:

> *Dr. Reid never hurried—always kept his cool when things were flying right and left around him. In the Out-Patient [Clinic] he gave the individual patient a feeling of warmth and sincerity. He felt something should be done to help the poor woman to regulate the size of her family and worked for the cause. ... Dr. Reid radiated his quiet warmth and sincerity to all who worked with him.*

Reid was equally devoted to education. His efforts were described by at a farewell dinner on June 9, 1971, by Gerald W. Mungerson, then director of the hospital: "For twenty years, beginning in 1945, [Duncan] and I spent unnumbered hours working on ways to improve teaching, to select doctors for appointments, both Harvard staff and research, and on hospital interrelationships."

Duncan Reid retired from Harvard and the Boston Hospital for Women in 1972 and joined the faculty of the University of Arizona Medical School. He was responsible for house staff and student teaching. He also participated in public health work among local Mexican-Americans and Native Americans a joint effort of the American College of Obstetricians and Gynecologists, the University of Arizona, U.S. Indian Health Services, and the University of New Mexico. In a 1971 interview, Reid said, "The problems of the Indians are those common to people living in poverty everywhere. The sickness and death rate for mothers and babies is higher than for the general population. While the Indians often live in wide open spaces, they can be as deprived as people in the ghettoes."

Unfortunately, Duncan Reid died in Tucson on November 6, 1973, of complications of a patient-transmitted viral hepatitis. Shortly before his death, his revised obstetrical textbook, *Principles and Management of Human Reproduction*, was published under joint authorship. Fitting Duncan's lifelong appreciation for and dedication to humanity, they dedicated the book to "those who work toward achievement of the initial right of man to be born without handicap and the privilege for women to bear without injury."[33]

THE HISTORY OF NURSE-MIDWIFERY AT BRIGHAM AND WOMEN'S HOSPITAL

Christine Wenc

With the merging of the Peter Bent Brigham with the Boston Hospital for Women, itself a merger between the Boston Lying-In Hospital and the Free Hospital For Women, babies began to be born in what had been the Peter Bent Brigham Hospital complex on Francis Street. Today, Brigham and Women's Hospital (BWH) is among the top hospitals in the country for gynecology and women's health, and nearly 8,000 babies are born at BWH every year. Nurse-midwifery has had a presence since the start of Brigham and Women's Hospital, and the practice is one of the oldest in the United States.

Midwives have always attended births, but the nurse-midwife did not exist until the 1920s in the United States, when the Children's Bureau, the first national research and advocacy group focused on women and children, created a plan to address serious problems with infant mortality and the absence of prenatal care. According to the American College of Nurse Midwifery, during the same period, a group of nurses, mothers, and physicians formed the Maternity Center Association in New York to address these problems as well. They found that the countries with the best maternal-child health records used a nurse-midwife model of care, and they thought that such a model could improve care in the United States. Unfortunately, at the time there were lay and traditional midwives but no nurse-midwives here. Lay midwives were routinely excoriated by the medical profession. To address this problem, Mary Breckenridge, who had founded the Frontier Nursing Service in eastern Kentucky, brought British nurse-midwives to the United States. Eventually, schools of nurse-midwifery were formed, and by the 1950s, there were seven American training programs. The American College of Nurse-Midwifery was created in 1955 to set standards for nurse-midwifery practice. In 1969, the name changed to the American College of Nurse-Midwives (ACNM) and today is still the professional organization for certified nurse-midwives in the United States. It also sets the standards for practice and accredits educational programs.

The ACNM provides the following definition: "Certified nurse-midwives (CNMs) are licensed healthcare practitioners educated in the two disciplines of nursing and midwifery and are certified by the American Midwifery Certification Board. They provide primary healthcare to women of childbearing age including: prenatal care, labor and delivery care, care after birth, gynecological exams, newborn care, assistance with family planning decisions, preconception care, menopausal management and counseling in health maintenance and disease prevention. CNMs attend almost 8 percent of the births in the United States. 96 percent of these births are in hospitals."[34] According to the history of nurse-midwifery on the ACNM website,

> *The popularity and acceptance of nurse-midwifery increased dramatically in the 1970s and 1980s. The number of CNMs in practice jumped from 275 in 1963 to 1,723 in 1976, to 2,550 in 1982, to over 4,000 in 1995. Certified nurse-midwives (a title adapted after the implementation of formal certification measures) were no longer only caring for indigent women and children. More affluent consumers discovered the benefits of the personalized, holistic healthcare that the modern-day nurse-midwives had to offer. Birthing centers began opening around the country offering prenatal counseling, extensive personal care during birth and close collaboration with physicians-all characteristics of the nurse-midwifery profession.*
>
> *Today, over 7000 certified nurse-midwives practice in all 50 states and many developing countries... In 2005, CNMs attended over 306,000 deliveries, mostly in hospitals. This number accounts for almost 8 percent of all U.S. births. Furthermore, certified nurse-midwives continue to be highly regarded in the health care community. Two reports by the Institute of Medicine and the National Commission to Prevent Infant Mortality praise their contributions in reducing the incidence of low birthweight infants and call for their increased utilization.*[35]

In 1977, Massachusetts, known for its conservative obstetrics community, became the 49th state to legalize this modern form of nurse-midwifery. (Worth noting, however, is that hospital birth did not become the most common form of birth in the United States until after the 1940s. Before that time, the Boston Lying-In Hospital had an established home birth practice, and educational materials produced for Lying-In clients from the period give detailed instructions for both hospital and home birth preparation. See Figure 4-18.[36]) When nurse-midwifery became legal in Massachusetts, there were already three midwives working as nurses at the Affiliated Hospitals Center (later renamed Brigham and Women's Hospital), who had not trained in the United States but rather in Australia and England, where midwives had long delivered a sizeable percentage of babies. With legalization, they began to provide prenatal care, assist women in labor, and "catch" babies in the hospital. In 1978, three more midwives were added to the staff.

In 2012 there were twenty BWH-based certified nurse midwives, who, combined with the midwifery practice at the Harvard Vanguard Medical Group, which delivered at BWH until 2013, delivered around a quarter of the approximately 8,000 babies born at BWH that year. Their mission is: "to provide culturally sensitive full-scope midwifery care to an ethnically and socioeconomically diverse population of women. We support each person's right to active participation in health-care decision-making. We are an integral part of the health care system of The Mary Horrigan Connors Center for Women's Health. Our practice is actively committed to the education of students in the disciplines of midwifery, medicine and nursing."[37]

In early 2012, state legislation was passed to allow certified nurse-midwives (the only type of midwife licensed in the state) to operate without the direct supervision of a physician. Most states are moving away from requiring a supervising doctor for nurse-midwives, and with this new ruling, only five states will still require routine physician supervision of certified nurse-midwifery.[38] Midwives are still required to work within a healthcare system and have a clinical relationship with a physician. One commentator wrote: "At a practical level, the law means that nurse-midwives, who long have been able to write prescriptions and order tests, won't need a doctor to oversee their decisions."[39] Advocates say that the changes will make it easier for women to access health care. For example, "in a rural area with few health care providers, nurse-midwives no longer will have to find supervising physicians, who may be reluctant to assume liability for them."[40] Critics say that the law leaves too much ambiguity and that midwives may make errors without direct physician oversight. However, nurse-midwives will continue to work under the same standards of care as before, which require them to consult with physicians when appropriate. The Massachusetts Medical Society opposed the law. It remains to be seen what changes, if any, the ruling will bring to the labor and birth experience at BWH.

Midwifery is often thought to take a less interventionist and technological approach to birth than that used by many obstetricians. In 1979, Nancy Haley, senior nurse-midwife at BWH, said, "We tend to be less operative, and to let nature take its course...knowing when to intervene when the birth is not progressing normally, but not interfering when things are okay." In 1978, the Affiliated Hospitals Center (later BWH) began to offer "alternate birth rooms" where couples could experience labor, birth, and recovery in the same room rather be switched from one to another at different stages of the birth process, "a further extension of the family-centered care philosophy."[41]

Notable about the BWH midwifery practice is its long tradition of connection to the community. Midwifery in the 1970s began playing a very important role in the Brookside and Jamaica Plain community health centers and continues to do so. As BWH nurse-midwife Kathleen Sullivan, who has been a midwife at BWH since the 1970s and has worked in the community health centers for decades, puts it, midwifery became "the face of the Brigham" in the community because so many women received their regular gynecologic health care from nurse-midwives as well as their prenatal, birth, and postpartum care. By 1990 the community center and the BWH practices had merged into one large group practice, and

YOUR HEALTH DURING PREGNANCY

For nine months your baby depends entirely upon you. For nine months your body is under the additional strain of pregnancy. For the sake of your baby's life and future health and for the protection of your own health:

See your doctor As soon as you know you are pregnant go to your doctor. Do exactly what he tells you. Ask questions of him and the nurses at any time, but do not take advice from others.

On your first visit the doctor will inquire about your past health and pregnancies and will give you a complete general physical examination. In addition, he will measure your pelvis (the passage-way for the baby), observe the condition of your womb and of the baby, take your weight and blood pressure, and test your blood and urine. Because changes take place all through pregnancy, you must be seen at least once a month for the first six months, every two weeks for the next two months, and then every week until the baby is born. At these visits the doctor will ask about any changes in your health and the condition of your baby. He will take your weight and blood pressure, and test your urine, and at certain times will examine you for the baby's position and heart beat. If anything unusual happens between visits, call the doctor or hospital immediately.

The nurses in the clinic and the Community Health nurses will help you to follow the doctor's instructions.

See your dentist Have your teeth examined. Brush them after each meal.

Eat properly Follow the instructions in the separate diet folder.

Rest Work Exercise Sleep at least eight hours at night with the windows open according to the weather. In addition, plan one or two rest periods during the day. Take a nap or relax with a book or magazine. Do not allow yourself to become over-tired.

You may carry on ordinary occupations, if they do not involve heavy work, until the doctor tells you to stop. Be sure that you have your extra rest periods. You may do light housework but not heavy work, such as scrubbing, heavy washing, beating rugs, moving furniture, and the like. Sit down at your work whenever possible.

You need a certain amount of exercise daily. Walking out of doors is one of the best forms. Ask the doctor about sports. Do not exercise to the point of becoming over-tired.

Bathe daily The water should be neither very hot nor very cold. A sponge bath or a shower may be taken. Because of the danger of infection, do not take a tub bath in the last two months.

Be regular You should have a daily bowel movement. This depends upon regular habits, proper diet, and exercise. If you become constipated, ask the doctor for instructions.

Wear proper clothing Clothing should be loose, comfortable, and attractive. *Tight* girdles, *tight* brassières, and *round* garters should never be worn.

Maternity dresses allow for increase in size, are more comfortable, and make you less conspicuous than ordinary dresses. The nurses will give you patterns for them and for smocks, skirts, slips, and garter belts.

Shoes should be comfortable, with a low or medium heel broad enough to give you adequate support as your weight increases.

Ask the doctor if you need a maternity corset or binder for abdominal support. The nurses can show you a pattern for one that can be made easily at home.

Keep a calendar Mark off the days on which you would be having your monthly periods if you were not pregnant. At these times avoid any unusual activity. Do not have relations with your husband at these periods, and not at all during the last two months. Avoid traveling at these period times. At any time avoid long tiring automobile trips.

Do not worry If anything bothers you, consult the doctor or the nurses. Plan ahead so that preparations do not have to be made in a rush at the end. Follow a regular daily routine. Remember that anything that bothers you is important. Ask about it.

Be Sure to Report

Swelling of your ankles, hands, or face	Bleeding	Illness
Headache	Cramps	
Vomiting		
Eye trouble		

SIGNS OF LABOR

False labor pains may occur at any time during the last two months. They come in the lower back or abdomen, as do real labor pains, but are usually short, irregular, and not too severe.

Real labor may begin with one or more of the following signs:

1. Lower back or abdominal pains or cramps. These come and go but gradually become harder, more frequent, and last longer.
2. A showing of blood or bloody mucus.
3. A gush or leakage of the "waters."

If any of these should occur at any time, call the doctor immediately or go to the hospital.

PREPARATIONS FOR HOME DELIVERY

Be sure to have all of your supplies ready by the seventh month. Keep them in a separate drawer or box, well protected from dust.

You will need for yourself:

- 3 large and several small newspaper pads and plenty of extra clean newspapers
- 1 rubber sheet or oilcloth
- 2 large basins
- 1 pail (may be used later for diaper pail)
- 2 lbs. absorbent cotton
- clean towels
- light blanket
- bedpan
- sanitary pads (to be sterilized before use)
- extra change of bed linen

When labor begins:

1. Call the doctor, nurse, and your helper.
2. Boil two kettles of water and cover them. Let one cool off.
3. Clear a table or bureau.
4. Have your baby's clothing, crib, and a small blanket or flannel square ready and warmed (but do not leave hot water bottles or hot covered irons in bed with your baby).

PREPARATIONS FOR HOSPITAL DELIVERY

Pack your bag ahead of time with kimono, slippers, and toilet articles.

Have ready for bringing home your baby:

- 1 shirt
- 2 diapers with safety pins
- 1 nightgown (or dress and slip)
- 1 sweater (or coat and bonnet)
- 2 blankets
- 1 pr. stockings or bootees
- 1 pr. knitted (or rubber) pants

FIGURE 4-18 "Health During Pregnancy," a pamphlet produced by the Boston Lying-In Hospital and the Harvard School of Public Health, 1941.

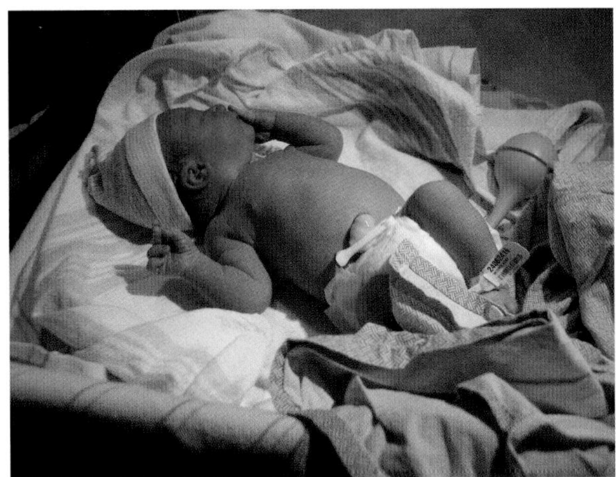

FIGURE 4-19 Cecelia P. Michael, shortly after being born on September 22, 2009 at BWH with the help of nurse-midwife Helen Dajer of the Harvard Vanguard Medical Group.

today BWH midwives have an important presence at ten different community centers in six Boston neighborhoods. Along with pregnancy-related care, midwives are also "experts in family planning, decision making, menopausal management and counseling in health maintenance and disease prevention." Miriam Mahler, former director of the midwifery program at BWH, has said, "Midwives support the spiritual, mental and emotional health of the whole family." The nurse-midwifery program at BWH and the community health centers has "a profound impact on the health and well-being of the communities they serve."[42]

Kathleen Sullivan says, "I came from a feminist perspective in the 1970s. There was a huge response to a lack of control over aspects of care and the mechanization of care and high levels of intervention. Many women who came to midwifery at that time came specifically so that they would feel that their birth process would not be interfered with." Changes came to medical obstetrics at this time as well. In a 1978 *Boston Globe* article, reporter Herbert Black noted, "a profound change in the attitude of doctors and nurses toward childbirth—a shift from the "doctor-knows-best" and "do-as-you're-told" atmosphere to one in which parents are accepted as people with feelings, emotions, and a right to have some say in a very personal experience. Frigoletto, chief of obstetrics at the Boston Hospital for Women at the time, said that more and more doctors "are trying to tailor-make delivery. This is comforting and rewarding to mothers. We hope it will continue."[43]

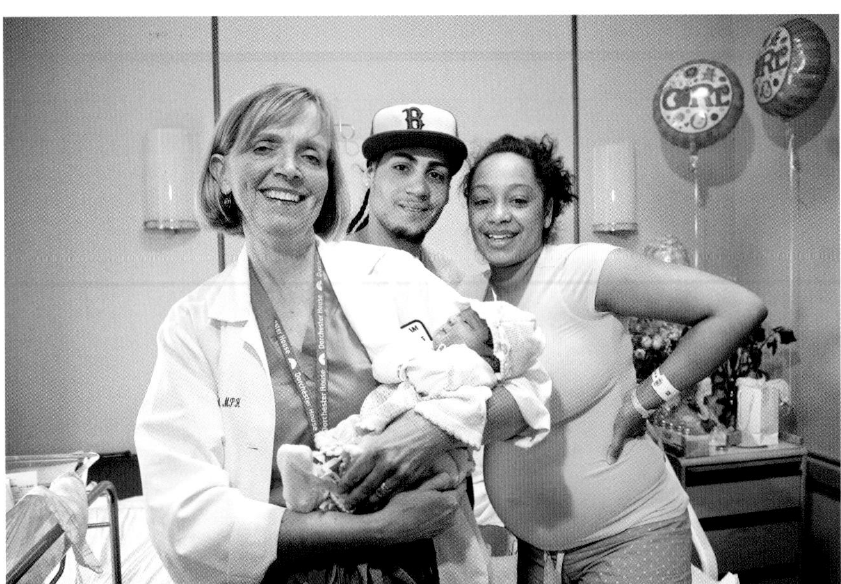

FIGURE 4-20 Certified nurse-midwife Miriam Mahler with new family.

BIOGRAPHY

KENNETH RYAN

Christine Wenc

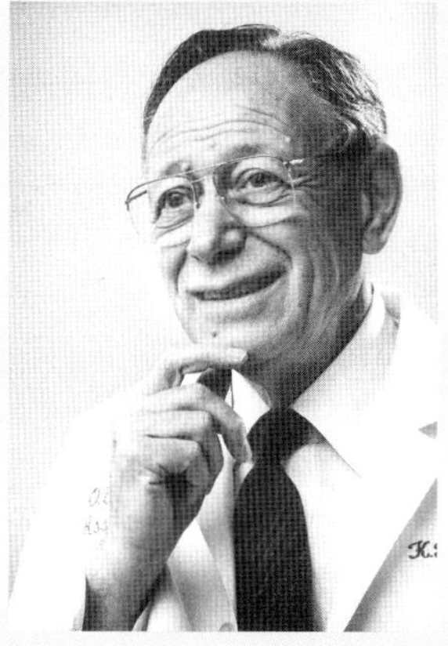

FIGURE 4-21 Kenneth Ryan.

Kenneth Ryan, chair of the Department of Obstetrics and Gynecology at Brigham and Women's Hospital from 1980 to 1993, was known nationally for research into sex steroid biosynthesis and his leadership role in the development of the field of medical ethics. He inspired many with his teaching and his commitment to women's reproductive rights.

Ryan was born and raised in New York City, the son of a wealthy father who lost everything in the Great Depression. His mother died when he was ten years old, and he went into foster care, graduating from high school at seventeen. He served in the Navy in World War II, obtained his bachelor's degree from Northwestern University while working full time, and graduated from Harvard Medical School in 1952.[44] Ryan started his training in internal medicine at the Massachusetts General Hospital and completed it at Columbia Presbyterian Hospital in New York. He then returned to Harvard, where he completed a residency in obstetrics and gynecology at the Boston Lying-In Hospital and the Free Hospital for Women.

Ryan studied the pathways of sex steroid biosynthesis with Nobel Laureate Fritz Lipman and Olive W. Smith at the Fearing Laboratories, where they characterized the ovarian enzyme system that synthesizes estrogens. In 1961 he moved to Cleveland to become the chair of obstetrics and gynecology at Western Reserve University, where he expanded the department with National Institutes of Health support, played a major teaching role, and continued his laboratory investigations. He then went to California to become the first professor and chair at the new medical school of the University of California at San Diego. He moved back to Boston in 1973 to become the Kate Macy Ladd and William Lambert Richardson Professor of Obstetrics, Gynecology and Reproductive Medicine at Harvard Medical School and chief of staff of the Boston Hospital for Women, where a few years later he played a major role in the merger with the Peter Bent Brigham Hospital and the Robert Breck Brigham Hospital.

At the new Brigham and Women's Hospital, Ryan then became chair of the Department of Obstetrics, Gynecology, and Reproductive Biology. He retired as department chair in 1993. Current chair Robert Barbieri has said: "Dr. Ryan was instrumental in developing specialty training programs for obstetrics and gynecology as well as broadening basic research in the field...Today's ob/gyn physicians owe much to Ryan for elevating and expanding their medical field."[45]

His most important research discoveries include the following: (1) the identification of the aromatase enzyme system that converts androgens to estrogens; (2) the development of the "two-cell" theory of steroidogenesis; (3) demonstration of metabolism of sex steroids by neuroendocrine tissues; (4) the discovery that 21-hydroxylase is a cytochrome-dependent enzyme; and (5) the demonstration that estradiol and estrone are interconverted. In addition, "through his leadership he inspired many obstetrician-gynecologists to pursue basic research careers."[46] He was an author on more than 300 scientific publications, some of which are considered classics.[47] The biochemistry of steroidogenesis plays an important role in fertility treatments and in the treatment of endocrine dependent cancers such as breast and prostate cancer.

Ryan was also nationally known for his work in bioethics. He chaired several federal panels in the 1970s examining ethical issues, including the National Commission for the Protection of Human Subjects of Biomedical and Behavioral Research, which met from 1974 to 1978. The committee was formed partly as a response to research scandals like the Tuskegee syphilis study in which black patients with syphilis were left untreated from 1932 to 1972, even after penicillin had been discovered to be an effective cure in the 1940s. Ryan's commission's recommendations became the basis for the informed consent rules that now govern human subjects research in the United States. Later, in 1988, Ryan also was cochair of a panel that recommended lifting the ban on fetal tissue research.

Ryan was a "firm if soft-spoken supporter of abortion rights"[48] and created the first abortion service in a university hospital along with a resident training program at the Boston Hospital for Women soon after the Roe v Wade decision in 1973. Ryan also was a founding fellow of the Ethics Center at Harvard and played a major role in the creation of the Division of Medical Ethics at Harvard Medical School and in starting the bioethics service at Brigham and Women's Hospital. He was also a Hastings Center fellow.

Ryan was not afraid to be controversial. As one writer put it:

> *His belief in "broad disclosure to patients" occasionally placed him at odds with organized members of his own profession. When the FDA required an informational package insert for the patient to accompany oral contraceptives, IUDs, and estrogens, the American College of Obstetricians and Gynecologists sued on the grounds that this was an unwarranted and unnecessary infringement on the doctor-patient relationship. Ryan chided them in the pages of the New England Journal of Medicine: "At a time when the credibility of organized medicine's interest in the public good is being challenged, our parry to each governmental initiative should not be reflexively negative."*[49,50]

Ryan served as chair of the Ethics Committee of the American College of Obstetricians and Gynecologists from 1984 to 1988, the chair of the Department of Health and Human Services Scientific Issues in Human Transplantation Research Panel from 1988-1989, and chair of the American Fertility Society Ethics Committee from 1993-2001. He also served as the chair of the Department of Health and Human Services Commission on Research Integrity. He was the president of the Society for Gynecological Investigation and the American Gynecological and Obstetrical Society and was a member of the American Academy of Arts and Sciences and the Institute of Medicine. Today, his legacy is still felt at BWH as well as across the United States.

THE AFRICAN WOMEN'S HEALTH CENTER: CULTURAL SENSITIVITY AND COMPASSION

Nawal Nour

In 1994, Nawal Nour began her residency at Brigham and Women's Hospital. A Harvard-trained gynecologist who grew up in Sudan, Egypt, and Great Britain, her work began attracting patients from the Boston area's African refugee and immigrant community. In July 1999, the practice that had grown up around Nour's compassionate interest and expertise became formally recognized as the African Women's Health Center (AWHC).

The mission of the AWHC is to provide culturally and linguistically appropriate obstetric, gynecologic, and reproductive health care. Its patients are women from Somalia, Sudan, Ethiopia, and Nigeria, the vast majority of whom have undergone the practice variously referred to as female circumcision, genital mutilation, or simply female genital cutting (FGC). The center is the first and only African health practice in the United States focused on this issue, providing access, understanding, and community to women who have long-term complications from FGC and who seek reproductive health care.

The World Health Organization defines FGC as "procedures that involve partial or total removal of the external female genitalia, or other injury to the female genital organs for non-medical reasons." The most severe form of the practice can result in problematic scarring, chronic urinary tract infections, menstrual and sexual complications, and difficulty in delivering a baby if the woman does become pregnant. Among other services, the AWHC offers these women surgical procedures that help restore both the natural appearance and normal function of the

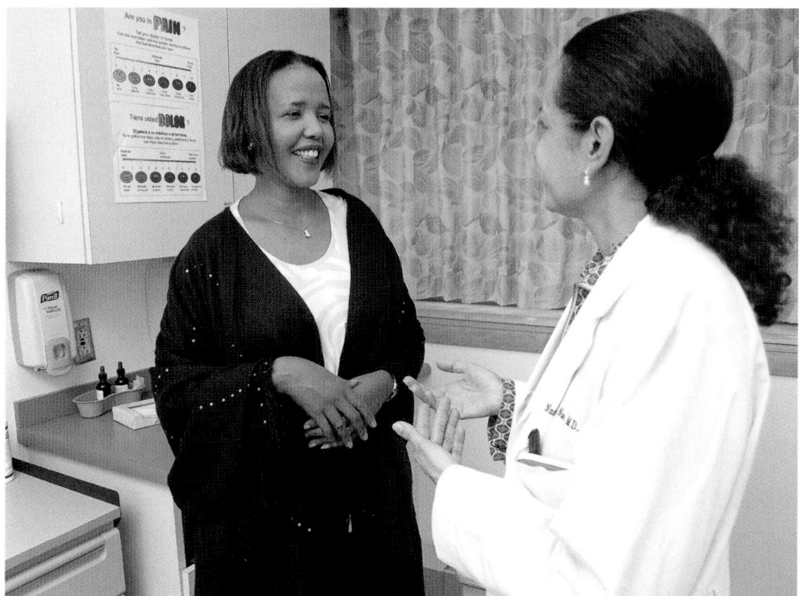

FIGURE 4-22 Somali interpreter Layla Guled (left) and Nawal Nour.

external genitalia, easing urination and menses and alleviating pain.

Although her main goal in founding the center was to relieve the suffering of these women, Nour also sought to establish a platform for organizing doctors, other professionals, and patients themselves against the practice of FGC. They work to prevent the practice from being perpetuated in the United States and discourage their patients from sending their daughters back to Africa to undergo the procedure.

Another central goal for Nour and her colleagues is to educate other healthcare providers about caring for women who have undergone FGC. Although a thorough understanding of the physical/medical aspects of the practice is of course necessary, a holistic approach requires also that caregivers understand the suffering these women have lived through and continue to live with. Fulfilling its mission and its founder's intent, the AWHC offers expert medical care—delivered with both compassion and cultural sensitivity.

REFERENCES

1. Margaret Marsh and Wanda Ronner, *The Fertility Doctor: John Rock and the Reproductive Revolution* (Baltimore: Johns Hopkins University Press, 2008), p. 51.
2. Ibid., p. 71.
3. Ibid., pp. 92-104.
4. Ibid., pp. 104-110.
5. Ibid., pp. 139-211.
6. Robert Meyers, *D.E.S.: The Bitter Pill* (New York: Seaview/Putnam, 1983), pp. 56-73; Roberta J. Apfel and Susan M. Fisher, *To Do No Harm: DES and the Dilemmas of Modern Medicine* (New Haven, CT: Yale University Press 1984), p. 20; Elmer Osgood Cappers, *History of the Free Hospital for Women 1875-1975* (Boston: Boston Hospital for Women, 1975), pp. 66, 76; Olive W. Smith, George V. Smith, and D. Hurwitz, "Increased Excretion of Pregnanediol in Pregnancy from Diethylstilbestrol with Special Reference to the Prevention of Late Pregnancy Accidents," American Journal of Obstetrics and Gynecology 51 (1946), pp. 411-415.
7. Apfel and Fisher, *To Do No Harm: Des and the Dilemmas of Modern Medicine*, pp. 15-20.
8. Meyers, pp. 61-73.
9. Alexander D. Langmuir, "New Environmental Factor in Congenital Disease," New England Journal of Medicine 284 (1971), pp. 912-913.
10. Ibid., pp. 93-110; Arthur L. Herbst, Howard Ulfelder, and D.C. Poskanzer, "Adenocarcinoma of the Vagina: Association of Maternal Stilbestrol Therapy with Tumor Appearance in Young Women," New England

Journal of Medicine 284 (1971), pp. 878-81; Alexander D. Langmuir, "New Environmental Factor in Congenital Disease."

11. "Medicine: The Pill on Trial," *Time*, January 26, 1970.

12. "Text of the Proposed Leaflet on Birth Control Pills," *New York Times*, March 5, 1970.

13. Elizabeth Siegel Watkins, *On the Pill: A Social History of Oral Contraceptives, 1950-1970* (Baltimore: Johns Hopkins University Press, 1998), p. 4.

14. Steven Epstein, *Inclusion: The Politics of Difference in Medical Research* (Chicago: University of Chicago Press, 2007), pp. 76-82.

15. Ibid., p. 126.

16. Ibid., p. 86.

17. Jennifer Leadley and Rae Anne Sloane, *Women in U.S. Academic Medicine and Science: Statistics and Benchmarking Report 2009-2010* (Association of American Medical Colleges, 2011), figure 1.

18. This essay is drawn from Margaret Marsh and Wanda Ronner, *The Fertility Doctor: John Rock and the Reproductive Revolution* (Baltimore: Johns Hopkins University Press, 2008).

19. Arthur T. Hertig, "Forty Years in the Female Pelvis. An Unusual Case of Prolonged Dystocia," Obstetrics and Gynecology 42 (1973): 907-909.

20. Arthur T. Hertig, "Acceptance of the Gold Headed Cane Award," *American Journal of Pathology* 96 (1979): 368-371.

21. J.G. Gruhn, H. Gore, and L.M. Roth, "History of gynecological pathology. IV. Dr. Arthur T. Hertig," *International Journal of Gynecological Pathology* 17 (1998): 183-189.

22. Hertig, "Acceptance of the Gold Headed Cane Award."

23. Arthur T. Hertig, Quoted in the *Harvard Medical Area Focus*, October 30, 1980, p. 6.

24. Arthur T. Hertig, "Angiogenesis in the Early Human Chorion and the Primary Placenta of the Macaque Monkey," *Contrib Embryol* 25 (1935): 38-82.

25. Arthur T. Hertig, "Acceptance of the Gold Headed Cane Award."

26. G. Majno and K. Benirschke, "Presentation of the Gold-Headed Cane to Arthur T. Hertig," *American Journal of Pathology* 96 (1979): 365-368.

27. Gruhn et al., "History of Gynecological Pathology. IV. Dr. Arthur T. Hertig."

28. Hertig, "Forty Years in the Female Pelvis."

29. Hertig, "Acceptance of the Gold Headed Cane Award."

30. Majno and Benirschke, "Presentation of the Gold-Headed Cane to Arthur T. Hertig."

31. R.M. Richart, personal communication, October 15, 2011.

32. J.F. Jewett, "Sesquicentennium of the Boston Lying-In Hospital—150 Trailblazing years," *Contemporary Ob/Gyn* (1983): 198-206; Department of Obstetrics and Gynecology, Brigham, and Women's Hospital, Annual Reports 1997-2011; The Free Hospital for Women: A brief history (Boston: Brigham and Women's Archives, Countway Library of Medicine, Harvard Medical School).

33. George V. Smith, "Duncan Earl Reid, 1905-1973," *Harvard Medical Alumni Bulletin* (January/February 1974): 41-42; C.L. Easterday, J.F. Enders, J.F. Jewett, K.J. Ryan, G.V. Smith, H. Ulfelder, and A.T. Hertig "Duncan Earl Reid," Memorial Minute Adopted by the Faculty of Medicine of Harvard University, February 22, 1974, *Harvard University Gazette* 1974; LXIX: #29; D.E. Reid, K.J. Ryan, and K. Benirschke, *Principles and Management of Human Reproduction* (Philadelphia: Saunders, 1972).

34. American College of Nurse Midwives, "Differences between Nurse-Midwives, Other Midwives, and Doulas," http://www.mymidwife.org/Differences-Between-Nurse-Midwives-Other-Midwives-and-Doulas . Accessed December 13, 2012.

35. American College of Nurse Midwives, "A brief history of nurse midwifery in the U.S." http://www.mymidwife.org/A-Brief-History-of-Nurse-Midwifery-in-the-U-S. Accessed December 13, 2012

36. Samuel B. Kirkwood, M.D. and Madelen Pollock, RN, "Health During Pregnancy," Department of Child Hygiene, Harvard School of Public Health and Boston Lying-In Hospital, 1941

37. http://www.brighamandwomens.org/Departments_and_Services/obgyn/Services/midwifery/mission.aspx?sub=0. Accessed December 13, 2012.

38. Sarah Barr, "Mass. Nurse-Midwives No Longer Need Physician OK to practice." Capsules: The Kaiser Health News blog, February 9, 2012. http://capsules.kaiserhealthnews.org/index.php/2012/02/mass-nurse-midwives-no-longer-need-physician-ok-to-practice/. Accessed December 14, 2012.

39. Ibid.

40. Ibid.

41. *Inside AHC*, News, June 1978, p. 11.

42. "Partners Healthcare Brigham and Women's Hospital: Promoting Healthy Families," *Bay State Banner*, March 24, 2011, Vol 46, No. 33.

43. *Inside AHC*, News, June 1978, p. 11.

44. Fredric D. Frigoletto, Jr., Leon Eisenberg, Steven Gabbe, Michael F. Greene, Rudolph Kass, Brian Little, Kenneth J. Ryan, Jr., Isaac Schiff, Dennis Thompson, "Kenneth John Ryan. Faculty of Medicine—Memorial Minute," *Harvard Gazette*, October 28, 2004. http://www.news.harvard.edu/gazette/2004/10.28/27-mm.html. Accessed September 4, 2012.

45. "Obituary: Kenneth John Ryan, MD, 75." BWH Bulletin, January 11, 2002. http://www.brighamandwomens.org/about_bwh/publicaffairs/news/publications/DisplayBulletin.aspx?articleid=1633. Accessed September 4, 2012.

46. "Kenneth J. Ryan, MD." Physicians for Reproductive Health, http://prh.org/provider-voices/kenneth-j-ryan-md-memorial-program/programs-kenneth-j-ryan-md/. Accessed September 4, 2012.
47. Frigoletto et al., "Kenneth John Ryan."
48. Eric Nagourney, "Kenneth Ryan, 75, Obstetrician and Leader in Medical Ethics," *New York Times*, January 28, 2002. http://www.nytimes.com/2002/01/28/us/kenneth-ryan-75-obstetrician-and-leader-in-medical-ethics.html. Accessed September 4, 2012.
49. Frigoletto et al., "Kenneth John Ryan."
50. "Obituary: Kenneth John Ryan, MD, 75." *BWH Bulletin*, January 11, 2002, http://www.brighamandwomens.org/about_bwh/publicaffairs/news/publications/DisplayBulletin.aspx?articleid=1633, accessed September 4, 2012.

CHAPTER 5

HISTORY OF PATIENT-CENTERED CARE

INTRODUCTION: PATIENT-CENTERED CARE AND THE HISTORY OF BRIGHAM AND WOMEN'S HOSPITAL

Christine Wenc

Care of "the whole patient" as a concept has existed at the Peter Bent Brigham Hospital since its founding. The idea has also been an important part of the history of the Boston Hospital for Women and the Robert Breck Brigham Hospital. In 1954, Dorothy Vernstrom, director of the School of Nursing at the Peter Bent Brigham, wrote in the *Brigham Bulletin:* "We speak often these days of taking care of the whole patient, recognizing his physical, psychological, social and spiritual needs. Unless, however we have a definite plan for implementing and meeting these spiritual needs of the patients, we are not carrying out our ideals."

In this section of the book, we present a number of essays relating the history of services at the hospital primarily over the past decade that are intended to "carry out the ideals" of patient care that extend beyond medical diagnoses and treatment, such as the chaplaincy, social work, palliative care, medical interpretation, Schwartz Rounds, and patient and family services. In addition, we relate the history of intensive care unit (ICU) nursing, a major aspect of profound changes to the hospital and the patient/family experience that happened after World War II, as well as some stories told by nurses themselves.

Together, all of these hospital services work to create what is often called "patient-centered care," a major shift in the way hospitals and patients interact since the paternalist days of only a generation or two ago, when doctors gave orders and patients were expected to obey. (No one was bringing a folder full of internet printouts about their condition to medical appointments in 1965, and, compared with today, few were doing so even in 1995.) Today, the patient-centered experience is not merely a pleasant turn of phrase; it is now a stated part of the hospital's long-term strategy, one that requires concrete and specific actions to become possible.

It is perhaps not going too far out on a limb to suggest that twenty-first century patient- and family-centered care could be something akin to the way care was provided in most households before the modern hospital came into being at the beginning of the twentieth century. Prior to this time, sickness, infirmity, and injury were almost always tended to at home. Only the most destitute and friendless ended up in hospitals, which were often little more than almshouses. In many important ways, patients in this pre–twentieth-century period were actually not "patients" at all, in the way entering a hospital and putting on an ill-fitting gown removes people from their social context. Instead,

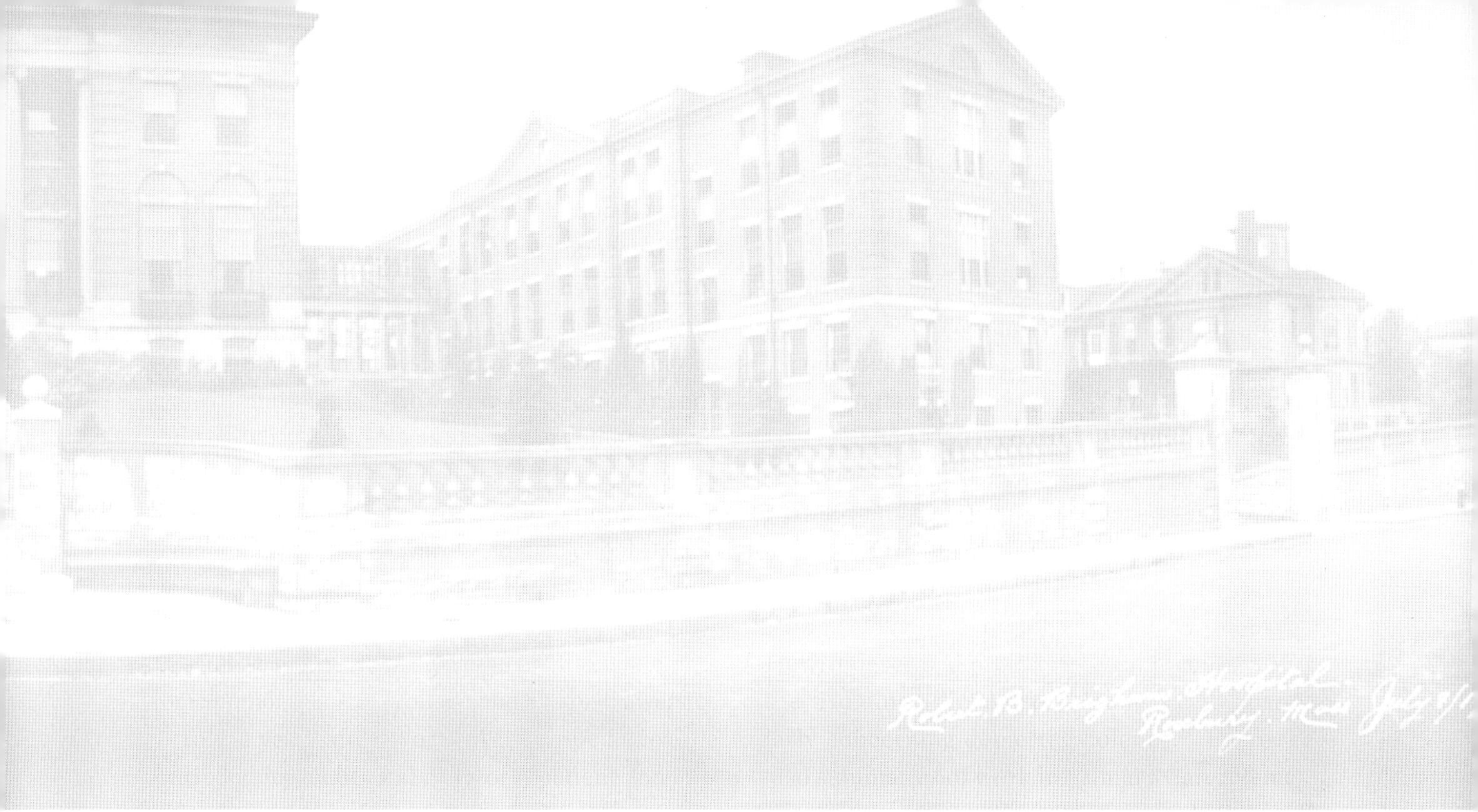

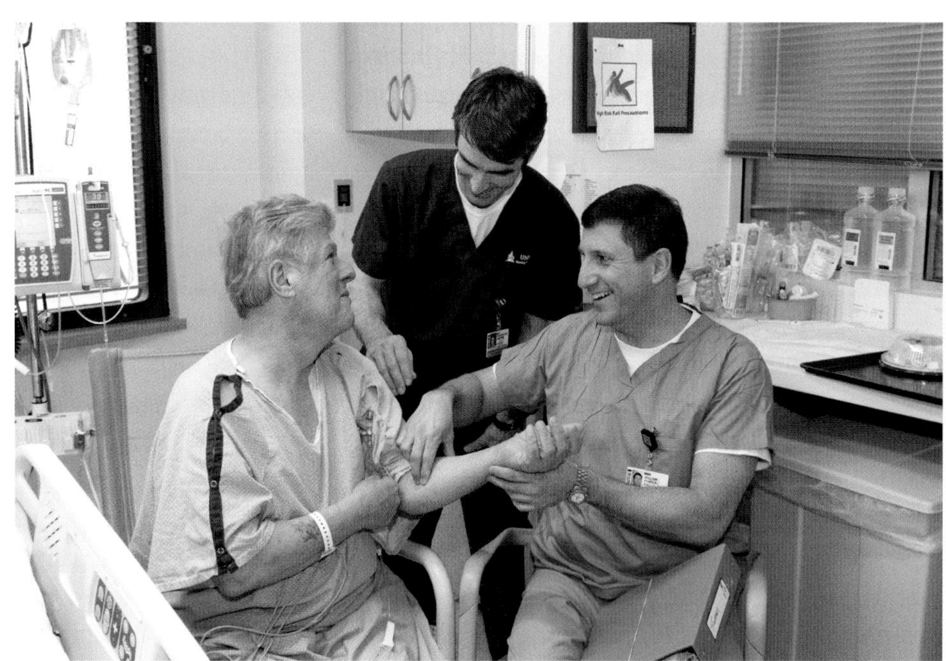

FIGURE 5-1 Patient Charles P. Truman (left), student Jason Gabaree (center), and nurse Bill Poirier.

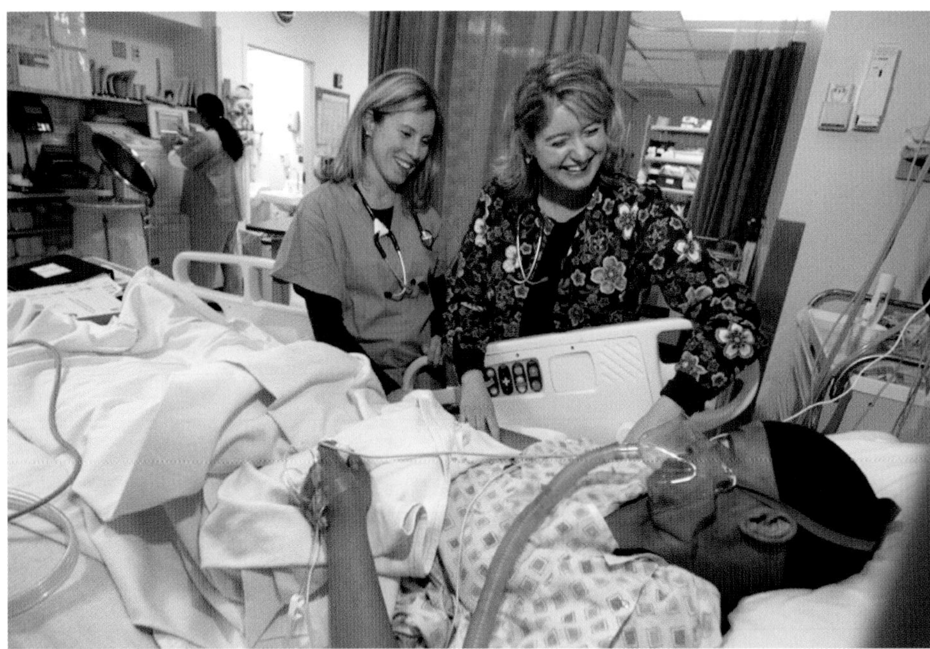

FIGURE 5-2 BWH nurses with a patient.

they remained in their positions as members of a family and a community, even though they might not have been able to fulfill their usual duties while sick or injured. Women provided most of the care at this time, in their domestic roles as mothers and keepers of the home, although doctors and midwives were also involved if they were available and trusted and families could afford their services. (In any case, the care provided by doctors prior to the twentieth century was not often much different from, or even preferable to, what the lay public could provide for themselves.) Surgeons were typically used only as a desperate and very last resort—understandable in an age before anesthesia or an awareness of antisepsis and asepsis. Most babies were born at home until the 1940s in many parts of the United States, and when things went well, the experience was likely much more intimate than a hospital birth. Death also took place at home, where the majority of us still say we would like to conclude our lives.

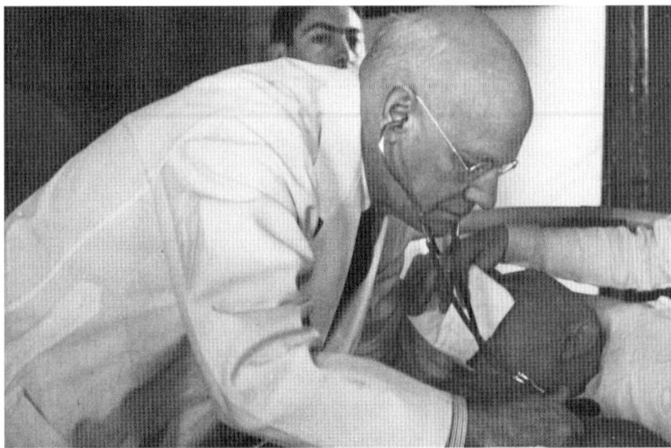

FIGURE 5-3 Henry Christian with a patient.

The downside of this comfortable and familiar home environment, of course, is that many conditions that are easily treated today caused significant morbidity and mortality, and aside from the use of morphine and other opiates, pain relief was not available in the way it has been used in the hospital. The possibility of cure and the hope that engenders has been the primary reason why people have been willing to enter a space that historically has stripped them of their social and community role and to consent to painful, frightening, and sometimes humiliating procedures carried out by strangers.[1] No one likes going into the hospital. As the current Brigham and Women's Hospital head of chaplaincy services, Kathleen Gallivan, told me, "Everyone who enters here is in crisis."

Today, however, concrete efforts are being made at BWH to help patients retain some of their "social

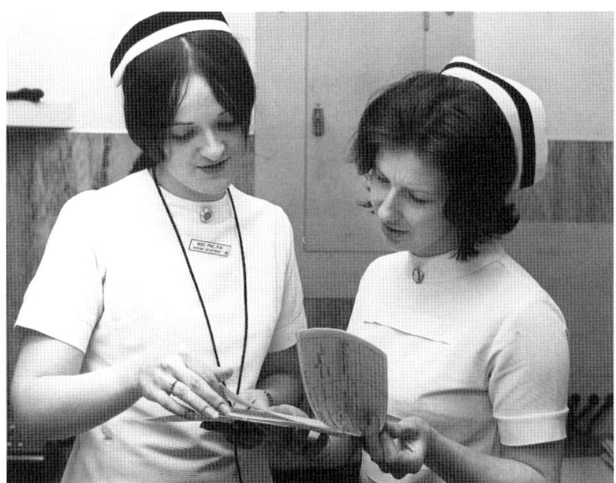

FIGURE 5-4 Two Boston Hospital for Women nurses, circa 1970.

context" while receiving care and to have medical and surgical experiences that take into account the patient as a whole person as well as their families. Patients, if they choose, can now be at the center of their care and play a full role in the decision-making process.

In the history of twentieth and twenty-first century medicine, this is a shift that is probably just as profound as the development of heart surgery or organ transplantation. It was only a few decades ago, after all, that fathers were first allowed into the delivery or operating room when their children were born. Until recent decades, new mothers who gave birth in a hospital did not have the option of rooming in with their infants; babies were separated from their mothers after birth and taken to the hospital nursery. Newborns in neonatal critical care units were not allowed to be touched by their parents. Today, "kangaroo care," long periods of skin-to-skin contact between parent and baby, is common and has been shown to improve outcomes by many measures.

Family visiting periods in the adult ICU were limited to a few minutes per hour, and limiting or ending futile care was difficult or carried out surreptitiously. Patients with terminal cancer were not given their diagnoses. Married women had to get their husbands' consent for a breast biopsy. Questioning your doctor was not something that happened very often during the "golden age" of American medicine between World War II and the 1960s, when so many surgeries, drugs, and technologies in common use today were first developed. Formal attention to patients' psychological or spiritual needs was considered irrelevant or soft. As Renee Fox writes in her introduction to *Experiment Perilous*, her pioneering work of medical sociology based on her observations of a metabolic research ward at the Peter Bent Brigham in the early 1950s, at the time no one had ever studied the psychosocial dynamics of serious illness before. She writes:

> *If anything, the academic medical and social scientific climate of the 1950s ran counter to it. A strong commitment to "being scientific" prevailed, with a heavy emphasis on achieving the highest possible standards of rationality, objectivity, and rigor. Even in medical settings conducive to it, for example, serious, outright discussion about death, dying, or terminal illness were generally considered too philosophical and too emotional to conform to this image of science.*[2]

Even for patients who were not dying, the patient's emotional response to illness and accommodations for

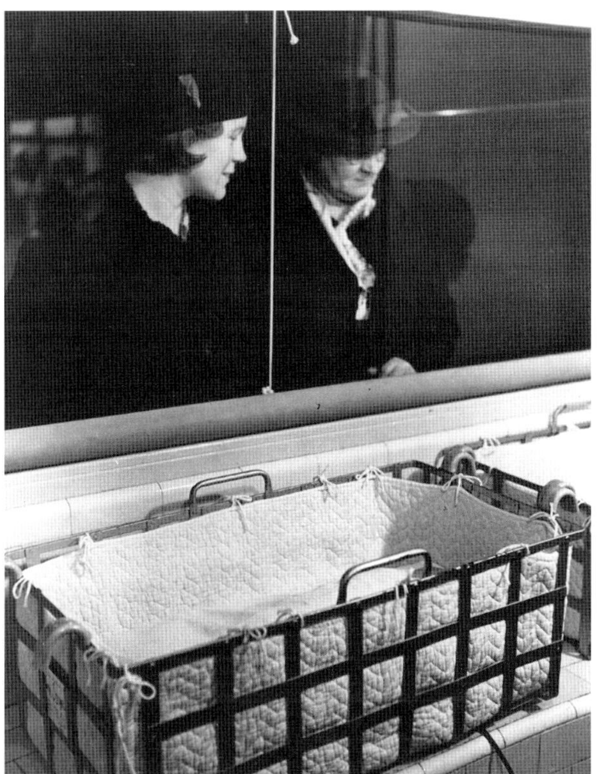

FIGURE 5-5 Women gazing at newborns through nursery window, Boston Lying-In Hospital, 1930s.

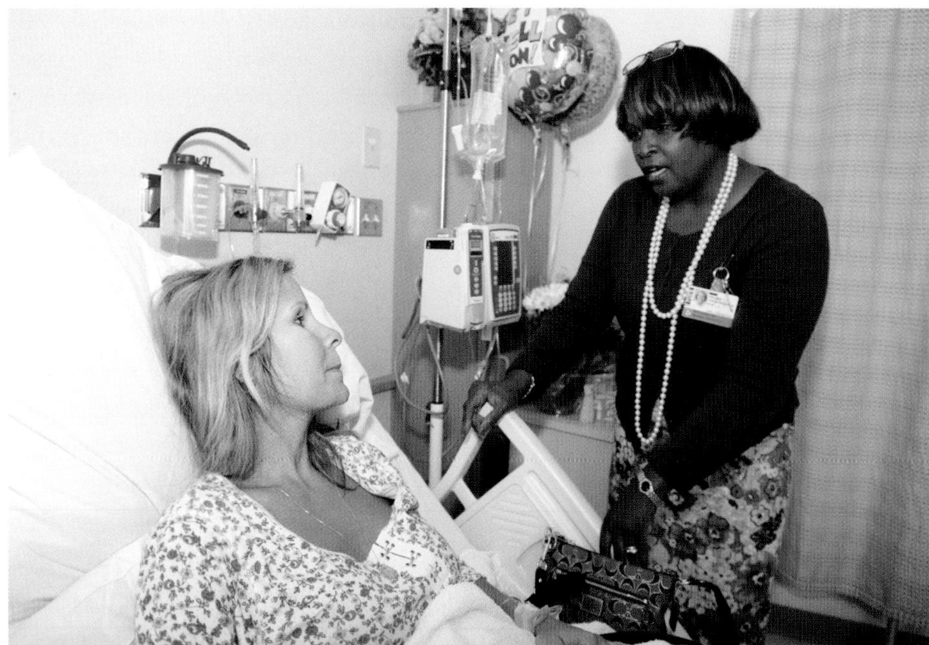

FIGURE 5-6 Wilma Frieson-Gaskin, Care Coordination, with a patient.

family were not a priority in most hospitals. However, in the last few decades, this has changed profoundly, even within the memories and careers of some physicians and nurses still working at the hospital today. The Joint Commission now requires attention to patients' spiritual well-being as a condition of hospital accreditation. Patient/consumer activism has also been of major importance in bringing the patient into a more active role in health care. Important stages of this have been the women's health movement in the 1970s, AIDS activism in the 1980s, and breast cancer activism in the 1990s.

The social structure within hospitals has undergone significant changes too. Today, nurses hold some of the highest administrative ranks in the hospital, and some of them have PhDs. About half of medical students today are women, and some predict that women will make up a majority of clinicians in the

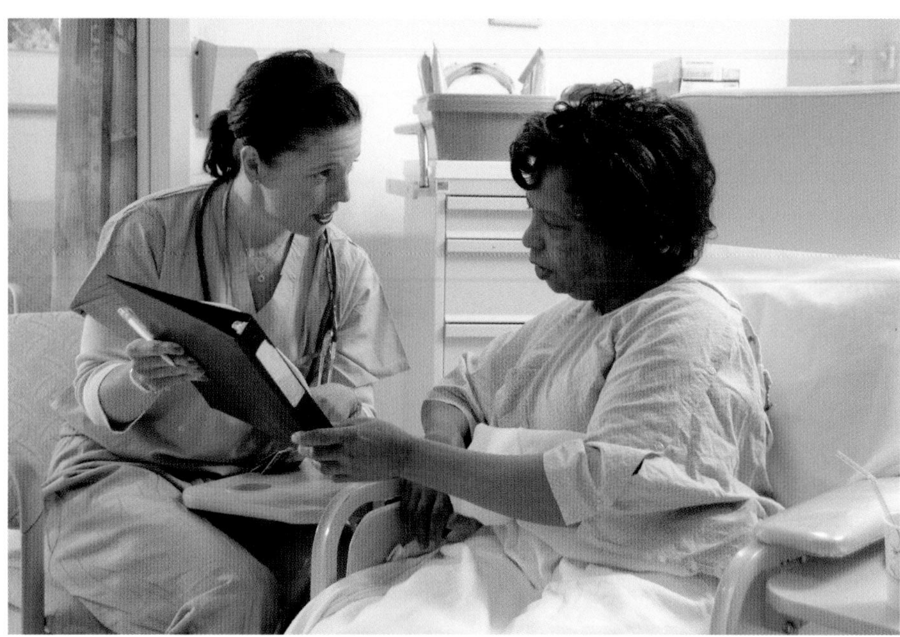

FIGURE 5-7 A BWH staff member talks with a patient.

not-so-distant future. (Already most OB/GYNs are female, and pediatricians and primary care doctors probably come in a close second.) Physicians and staff are more diverse in race, nationality, and ethnicity; today, it would not be unusual to see a surgical team at BWH that included a female surgeon, a resident from India, a Chinese American anesthesiologist, and a nurse from Australia. The picture would have been very different only thirty or forty years ago. Black Americans, after being barred from many medical schools as well as the American Medical Association until the 1960s, still only make up about 3% of physicians and medical students. In future years one hopes this figure will improve.

Also of importance is the move in recent years toward a team approach to care, which involves not only physician and nurse but a suite of other services including nutrition, pharmacology, and social work. Patients have recently even been invited to give rounds as part of the work of the Bretholtz Center and the BWH Patient and Family Advisory Council. All of this is still evolving, but in many ways the patient- and family-centered care movement could become something that brings together the best of two worlds: the patient's family/community context and effective scientific medicine.

CHANGES IN PRACTICE AND QUALITY IMPROVEMENT

The efforts being carried out by BWH to achieve the goals of patient- and family-centered medicine extend into the past decade. Leadership that focuses on patient and family centeredness is now a priority, as are improvements in care protocols and facility design. Other long-term goals involve creating a "distributed campus," where sister hospitals (including the Brigham and Women's Faulkner Hospital, the VA Boston Healthcare System, and Dana-Farber Cancer Institute), community health centers, rehab facilities, and clinics can deliver the best and most appropriate care "in the right setting at the right time," whether that care is preventive, acute, episodic, or chronic. Through a new referral and access system, "seamless" care is also a goal, surmounting the common modern problem of fragmented medical care and repetitive testing, which is not only inconvenient (and unpleasant) for both patients and providers but also costly. More care is also likely to be delivered at home in the future with the help of innovations in technology, communications, and nursing. Translational research integrated with clinical care is also an important focus and an area in which BWH is likely to continue being an innovative leader. Medical education is a deeply important historic component of the hospital's mission and will continue to be a top priority. Health equity and addressing health disparities is also part of BWH's historic focus and will remain such. Workforce development and cultivating diversity is also essential to the further success of the hospital, which exists in a diverse world and serves a diverse array of patients.[3]

Another important change taking place since the 1990s is the application of new quality management and quality improvement techniques to the hospital setting. Much of this can be traced back to former BWH President H. Richard Nesson, who also played a major role in orchestrating the creation of Partners HealthCare with Massachusetts General Hospital. (Nesson was also supportive of expanding services like the BWH chaplaincy, which, although it had been a presence at BWH for decades, has recently taken on a much more active role; now chaplains go on regular rounds with the rest of the caregiving team and visits are recorded in patient charts. Virgina Hermani, a Brigham chaplain for many years, says, "The need for chaplaincy was becoming more apparent across the board. Any admission to the hospital is stressful if not traumatic. Even if it's going to turn out OK it's still stressful. In order for people to do well and heal well, heal faster, you have to think about not just the body but the mind and the spirit.")

Tom Lee, who worked with Troy Brennan, Sheridan Kassirer, and Mairead Hickey to create the first quality improvement programs in the hospital, recalls his experiences:

> *Troy and I started working formally with the Hospital in 1992, when Dick Nesson invited us to spend part of our time performing research on improvement of quality and efficiency within the institution. At that time, Troy and I were both fairly prolific*

young researchers—Troy had done major research on medical malpractice, and I had worked with Lee Goldman on risk stratification of patients with common cardiovascular syndromes such as acute chest pain. We of course had ideas of implications of our research for clinical practice, and it was not lost upon us that not everyone was consistently following our well-considered recommendations.

One day in the winter of 1990-1991, Dick Nesson said to me (in the Pike, right where Phyllis Jen's portrait hangs today), "You guys are always writing things saying what people should do—how would you like to spend part of your time seeing if you can get people to do it?" He had a similar conversation with Troy, and we agreed to spend 20% of our time doing "improvement research" for the Brigham.

Sheridan Kassirer very much held our hands and taught us how the hospital worked—she was already deeply interested in what was a relatively new body of work at the time—Total Quality Management, or TQM. In 1992, we formed the Clinical Initiatives Development Program for the Hospital. We developed measurement frameworks, organized teams to figure out what interventions should be made systematic, worked to implement those interventions, and evaluated their impact.

It was very much the same basic approach that we are using today at a Partners level and at the Brigham—measure, plan, do, evaluate. Dick Nesson was visionary in being willing to invest in us, giving us resources to hire people like Mairead [Hickey], who helped us figure out what we really ought to measure, and how we ought to try to act. Mairead taught us about concepts like "self-efficacy"—patients' confidence that they could do what they were supposed to do to. We worked on implementing "critical pathways" and wrote some of the first articles about what they could and couldn't do. The work was really early manifestations of what people call "Patient Centered Care" and Atul Gawande's "checklist manifesto" approach today.[4]

Dorothy Goulart, director of performance improvement, says: "It's really about building a workforce of improvers, a workforce of problem solvers." She says that today the belief is that being in the 90th percentile isn't good enough—when it comes to quality, "we need to be closer to the 99th percentile." To carry this out, she and her team work not just to manage quality but to directly improve it, by communicating with staff to find out what a particular part of the hospital might want to see improved and then work directly with them to make it happen. Efficiency and removing redundancy and waste are of prime importance. Often, small changes can make a significant impact. The need for customizing care for the individual patient, of course, will always remain and is one reason why healthcare delivery can get complicated; however, Goulart and her team are always looking for whatever processes can be streamlined and improved, from pharmacy compounding to ICU protocols. They are also finding ways to make individual patients have a better stay. One seemingly innocuous change that has undoubtedly improved many patient experiences is the new availability of meals on demand rather than at set mealtimes. The emergency department has also undergone a very significant change in operations, resulting in a shift from being in the 40th percentile for patient satisfaction to the 90th in just two years.

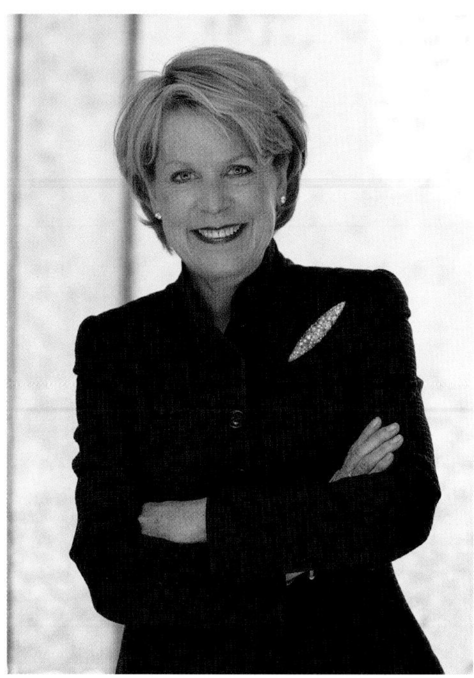

FIGURE 5-8 Mairead Hickey, executive vice president and chief operating officer at Brigham and Women's Hospital.

Nursing has also been a focal point for change in recent years. Along with her pioneering work with Tom Lee and Troy Brennan, Mairead Hickey, now BWH executive vice president and chief operating officer, was previously chief nurse and senior vice president of Patient Care Services. As chief nurse, appointed in 2005, she led the hospital in developing a philosophy and model for patient- and family-centered care. She also developed a strategic vision for the Department of Nursing that advanced the practice of nursing and compassionate care for patients and families and supported clinical development and research efforts. A book detailing the process by which she led major changes in nursing culture and practice at the hospital, *Change Leadership in Nursing: How Change Occurs in a Complex Hospital System*, edited by Hickey and Phyllis Kritek, was published in 2012. Hickey writes that in the fifteen years prior, the department of nursing had "weathered significant challenges" arising from organizational restructuring. However, the "energy and pride" she witnessed among BWH nurses was motivating, and she focused on her "most critical challenge"—to move from a state of high variability in nursing practice to a state of "sustained high reliability, where every BWH patient and family was assured of receiving excellent nursing care throughout their care experience, and every nurse consistently demonstrated excellent practice." Her vision statement for the Department of Nursing was "to provide excellent care to patients and families, with the very best staff, in the safest environment." Hickey also emphasized the cultivation of nursing research and a restructuring of nursing leadership, with the creation of several new roles at the executive level. She also launched the Center for Nursing Excellence, "an engine of innovation and a hub that would integrate nursing education, research, professional development, and innovation in support of clinical practice." By 2007, "change had been set in motion."[5] These changes are not yet complete, but progress is ongoing, now being carried out by Chief Nursing Officer Jackie Somerville, Executive Director of Nursing Practice Development Mary Lou Etheredge, and other nursing leaders.

Making sure all BWH nurses are following the new goals of the department is of prime importance, and new education techniques developed in the past thirty years focus on moving nursing practice beyond mere technical competence and finding ways for nurses to learn from each other. Evidence shows that nurses can be divided into categories depending on where they are in their professional development: novice, competent nurse, and expert nurse. Ideally nurses will move through all these phases until they become expert. In some cases, though, this does not happen. Etheredge says:

> *There are supports and conditions in an environment that can either facilitate that development or can prohibit that development such that it becomes each individual nurse's responsibility to develop themselves as opposed to a mutual responsibility. How do we ensure that every patient and family is cared for by a nurse who is developing in his or her practice, wherever that may be, as opposed to somebody who may be stuck in a certain stage of development? We want to provide that patient with that kind of nursing. We want to provide the nurse with the opportunity to keep developing in their practice.*

One of the ways BWH nurses educate each other and develop clinical wisdom is through the use of a particular kind of storytelling. Nursing narratives, such as the example written by ICU nurse Roger Blanza presented at the end of this chapter, are more than just catalogs of events. At their best, nursing narratives reveal the hidden knowledge and intuition created by years of experience in a way that can be accessed and used by other nurses. Important to note, Somerville says, is that such narratives do not have to be about "heroic" situations. "They can be about an average day, what they did, how they touched a patient, how they touched a family," she says. "What they learned in that process. The cues the family or the patient gave them that made them think about driving the care in a specific direction." In this way, she says, "the knowledge that oftentimes is invisible becomes more public to other nurses and the general public," and can then be shared in ways that help nurses move from competence to expertise.

The quality improvement movement is important for patient care, but what might not be obvious is its importance for hospital finances. With twenty-first century healthcare reform, many changes are taking place in how healthcare organization will be reimbursed; what this will eventually look like is still unknown. Some changes related to quality have already taken place. Medicare payment rates, a significant source of hospital revenue, are now partly determined by patient satisfaction scores. The Health Maintenance Organization (HMO) movement of the 1980s and 1990s, which brought a business model to medicine in ways that had not taken place before, has also had an effect. Tom Lee says: "I think Dick [Nesson] was ahead of his time—but only a bit, as pressures for efficiency were beginning to build in ways that are obvious in retrospect." These pressures were created by HMOs that, among other things, pushed for shorter length of stay, which required major rethinking of how care is delivered.

TRANSFORMATIONS

In the end, though, the patient experience is what matters the most. The hospital is a place where profound emotional and spiritual as well as physical transformations take place among patients and families every day. In the early twenty-first century, almost all births take place in the hospital; women become mothers and men become fathers here for the first time every day. The hospital is also a place where patients become free of illness and heal from injury, where they leave the hospital different in soul as well as body from who they were when they entered. Even an outpatient surgery that is commonplace for a seasoned physician can be life changing for the patient. Some patients experience severe illness and recovery as a kind of rebirth. In her 1997 book *The Patient's Voice: Experiences of Illness*, Jeanne Young-Mason presents the words of a number of patients going through different serious maladies. A writer living in Boston related:

> *The medical term for hauling someone back from the brink of death is "resuscitation," the act of restoring consciousness, vigor, or life. This term is perhaps too arrogant in its attribution: both the mechanism by which one is revived and the factors that determine who lives and who dies are far from understood. A better term might be "resurrection," the act of rising from the dead, which leaves the causal agent unstated –God, medicine, the will to live, and luck*

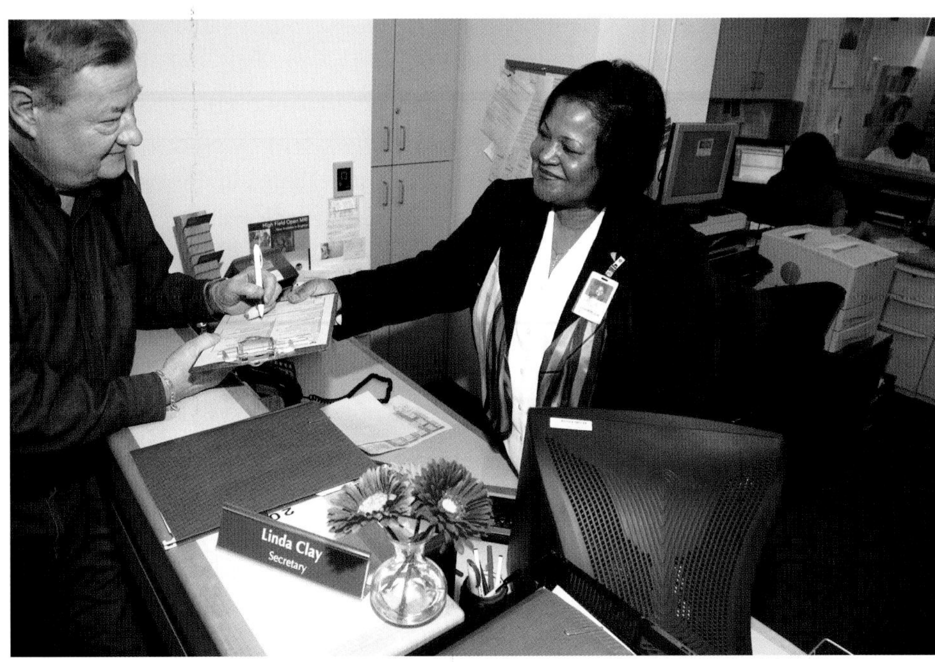

FIGURE 5-9 Linda Clay talks with a patient at Brigham Internal Medicine Associates (now the Phyllis Jen Center at Brigham and Women's Hospital).

are equal contenders. To one who has been there and back, however, neither term feels quite right. Coming back from a near-death experience feels less like resuscitation or resurrection, both of which imply a return to what was, than it does like rebirth, a second or new birth, a reincarnation.[6]

Most deaths also take place today in an institutional environment. Families and friends have said goodbye to someone they love at BWH thousands of times, making it a place where the deepest human emotions are experienced on an everyday basis.

Esther Lucile Brown, a social anthropologist known for her influential study of nursing education published in 1948 called *Nursing For the Future*, has noted that personal transformations can also take place among the caregiving staff as well as among patients. This is an important idea to keep in mind as we contemplate the history of care at the hospital, the movement toward patient-centered care, and what this means for the future. How do these new modes of care affect the caregivers? And how might this change transform the hospital as a whole?

Those who provide patient care might well be considered fortunate: they do not even have to search for an environment where human nature stands revealed, for it is ever present. Nor do they have to try to find a place, as do so many others, where they are urgently needed, and where every increment of growth in knowledge, perceptiveness, and sympathy can be at once translated into greater everyday effectiveness. To them is given the opportunity for the development of those qualities both of knowing and feeling that permits the caring for patients of which Dr. Peabody wrote. And from such caring comes the kind of care of the patient that is not only a comfort to him but an act of creativity capable of giving deep satisfaction to those who perform it.[7]

Over the years the hospital has recognized caregiving staff with various honors, including the Dennis Thompson Leadership and Compassionate Care

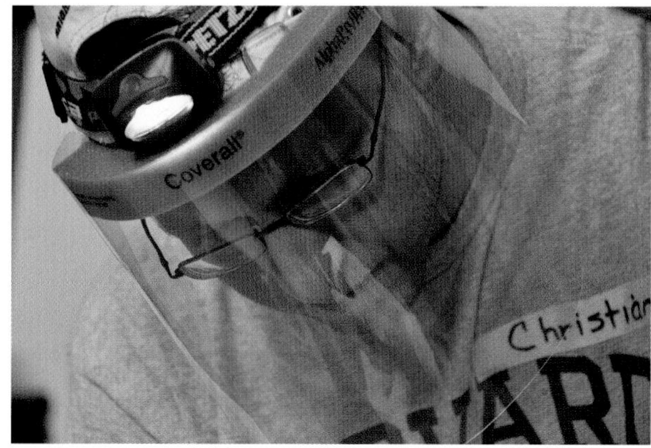

FIGURE 5-10 Christian Arbelaez, winner of the 2007 Thompson Compassionate Care Award, suturing in the field in Haiti.

Scholar Awards, which "recognize employees or teams of employees from any discipline who embody the principles of compassion in their daily work and exemplify it most at the bedside of patients,"[8] and the Starfish Award. Ray Reilly, a BWH gynecologist from Ireland who trained at Johns Hopkins, started his Boston career at the Lying-In Hospital in the early 1960s, and has been here ever since, explains the Starfish Award this way:

This hospital, as I see it, is all about the patient. It is built around the patient. The Starfish Award is an award given by this hospital that is based on the starfish story, where millions of starfish are washed up ashore one day and there is an individual guy on the shore picking up starfish and throwing them back into the water. And there is a guy up the road watching this and doesn't know what is happening and comes down and says, "What are you doing?" The guy picks up a starfish and throws it back in the water. So the guy looks around the whole millions of these starfish and says: "That's not going to make any difference." And the guy picks up a starfish and throws it back in and says: "Well, it will to that one."

This is about the individual person. You take care of the individual person. This hospital has that attitude. It is a wonderfully run, beautifully executed hospital. I've lived all over the world, England, Ireland, Germany—and this one by far beats them all.

THE PATIENT/FAMILY RELATIONS DEPARTMENT AND THE BRETHOLTZ CENTER

Maureen Fagan

The Brigham and Women's Hospital Patient/Family Relations Department seeks to provide a supportive environment for patients and families who wish to share feedback about the quality of care and service they receive at BWH. Patient/Family Relations was the strategic vision of Mairead Hickey and former Chair of the Board of Directors Rob Bretholtz and was first conceptualized in the 1990s as American health care began a national movement toward a patient- and family-centered care environment. Their vision was to create a comprehensive resource center that was dedicated to the needs of patients and families and to support them with comfort and information while they received care at the hospital. The vision was realized with the creation of the Bretholtz Center, located at 75 Francis Street, just behind the information desk in the main lobby. The center opened in 2000 and provides a wide range of services to patients and families seeking respite from the high demands of being a patient, or the loved one of a patient, during a complex hospital stay.

In addition to Patient/Family Relations, the Bretholtz Center is home to Family Liaison and the Kessler Library. Family Liaison is a reception area for the loved ones of surgical patients with a staff dedicated to keeping families informed of patients' progress throughout their operation and immediate recovery. The area includes private rooms so that families may speak with their loved ones' surgeon postoperatively or take a moment of pause during the day. Additionally, light refreshment, computers with internet access, and reading materials are available. The Kessler Library, made possible through the generosity of the Kessler Family Foundation, opened in December 2000 and is a welcoming, peaceful place where patients and families find resources and patient- and family-centered assistance to understand the medical diagnoses of loved ones, to explore paths to lifelong wellness, and to formulate questions about their medical conditions for their providers. Patients and families also spend time at the library simply to enjoy some personal time for rest and reflection or to catch up on work and email.

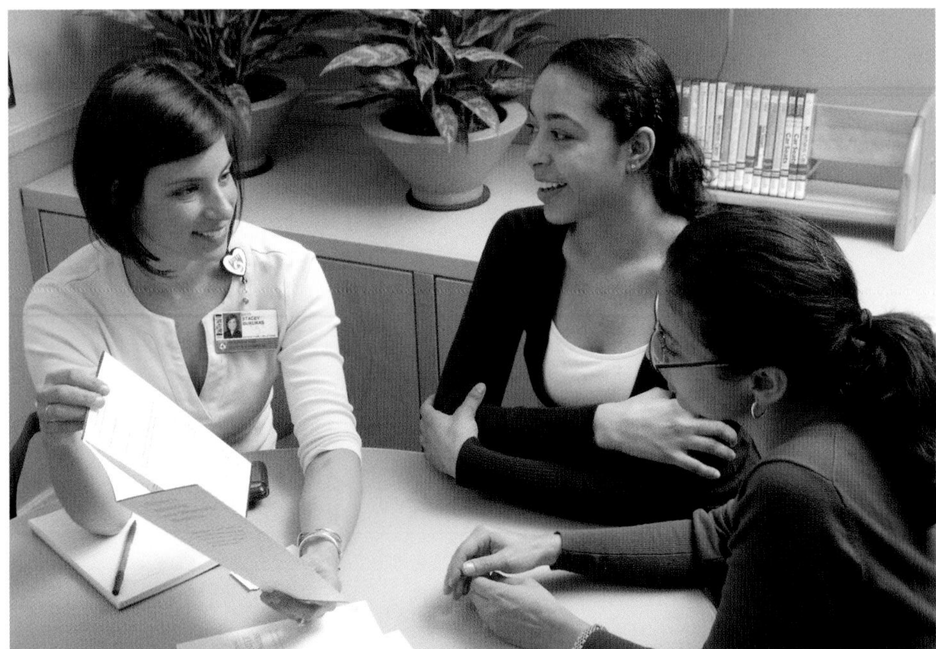

FIGURE 5-11 Stacey Bukuras, Patient/Family Relations Representative at Brigham and Women's Hospital, discusses the Welcome to Brigham and Women's Hospital pamphlet.

Over the years, the Kessler Library has also become a place where patients, providers, and staff share their areas of expertise at special events or other ongoing initiatives and groups. By participating in experiences that encourage personal control of one's health and independence, patients and families can build on their strengths and aim to improve their health outcomes. Bridging the gap between the language of the biomedical disciplines and the need to communicate effectively to diverse populations of patients and families is the heart of the mission of the Kessler Library.

In January 2001, Kathleen Gordon became director of Patient/Family Relations. She was tasked with building an infrastructure and resources to assure that in addition to amenities, there was a formal process for patient feedback to be reviewed and responded to. With the popularity of the internet, Gordon observed that patients and families were more informed and wanted to be part of healthcare decision making.

In 2005, the concept of patient- *and family*-centered care came to the forefront of the healthcare agenda at Brigham and Women's Hospital. It is an approach to the planning, delivery, and evaluation of health care that is grounded in mutually beneficial partnerships among healthcare providers, patients, and families. Gordon worked closely with Mairead Hickey, then chief nursing officer, to outline the core concepts of patient- and family-centered care, which were identified as Dignity and Respect, Information Sharing, Participation in Care and Decision Making, and Collaboration with Patients and Families as Advisors.

Patient/Family Relations played a major role in brainstorming efforts for the design of the Shapiro Cardiovascular Building in 2006, by leading twenty focus groups within the hospital to identify the ideal design of a patient- and family-centered space. From selecting furniture to contributing ideas about the physical layout of the units, Patient/Family Relations made a robust contribution to the Shapiro Center's design, which supports family presence at the bedside of their loved one.

Today, the Bretholtz Center and Patient/Family Relations are staffed by two service coordinators, a project manager, and six representatives, who are overseen by a practice manager and an executive director. All aim to give voice to the patient experience. Patients and families often arrive to us weary, frustrated, and seeking a soft place to fall. Our service coordinators are present at the Bretholtz Center to receive in-person

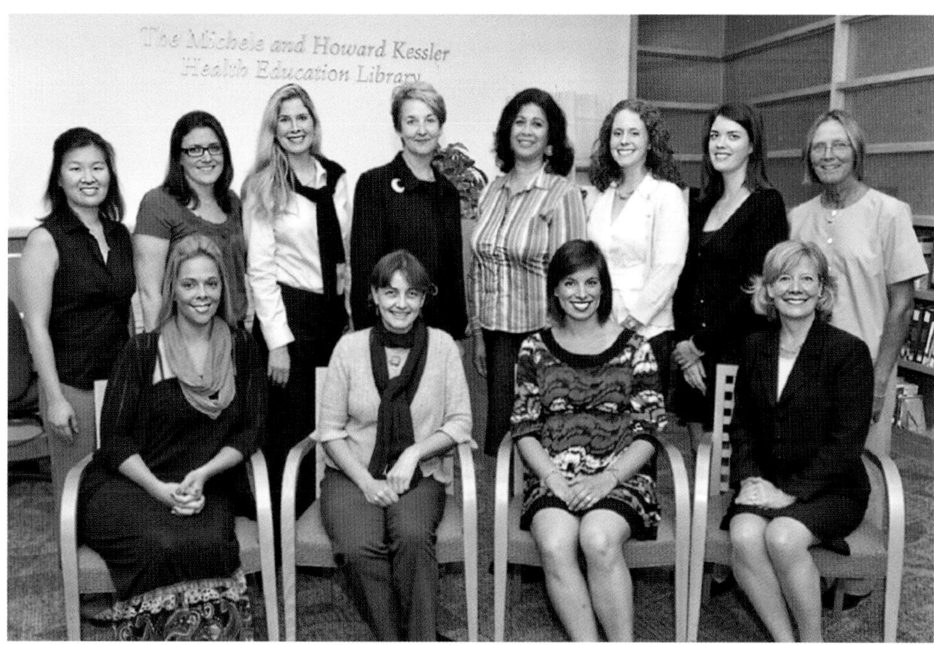

FIGURE 5-12 The staff of the Patient/Family Relations Department at BWH. From left to right, seated: Cherie Drew, Laura Zanini, Stacey Bukuras, Lynne Blech. Standing: Celene Wong, Kristen Koch, Maggie Hewit, Maureen Fagan, Adis Benitez, Erica Zaken, Kaileigh Reeves, DeeDee Mariano.

visits or telephone calls from 7:00 am to 6:00 pm, Monday through Friday. Our service coordinators triage the case to one of our representatives, who are delegated by line of service. The nature of these initial interactions is often fraught with raw emotion as patients and families often come to us because they are displeased with aspects of their experience or confused about their plan of care. When sadness manifests itself in the form of anger or frustration, our service coordinators create a safe haven by offering empathy and compassion and restoring a sense of calm. We also provide notary services to patients, accommodation information, and a host of other amenities, ranging from the provision of creature comforts to DVDs and mobile phone chargers on loan.

Our service coordinators are the first and often sole point of contact in a patient or family member's experience with Patient/Family Relations. However, when patients and families express concern with regard to the quality of care or service they receive, a representative is assigned to help facilitate a resolution. The representative's role is unique in that they are not "advocates" but neutral liaisons between patient and provider, serving as facilitators, mediators, and negotiators.

Patients and families most often seek our help because they perceive that there has been a breakdown in communication, or that their needs, fears, and concerns are not being heard. Patients often have a profound reverence for their physicians and are not always able to advocate for themselves, as they do not wish to appear ungrateful. The representative begins by serving as a supportive listener, allowing patients and families simply to "vent" about their experience. Being able to tell their story is cathartic in itself, and patients and families will often express appreciation that "someone listened." The representative will next summarize the feedback, employing reflective listening tactics, to help identify the crux of the concern, which often reveals itself through the "venting" process. In this way, Patient/Family Relations representatives help to focus and deescalate patients and families when they are feeling frustrated and overwhelmed.

Our representatives are skilled in the art of written and verbal communication and recognize that so often, the content of a message is not as important as the way in which it is delivered. To that end, the representative's next step is to share the patient and family's concern with the clinical provider(s) and propose suggestions on how to alleviate their distress. The intervention of Patient/Family Relations is typically viewed positively by staff; representatives are strategically assigned by service line so that they may cultivate relationships with physicians, nursing staff, social work, and other members of the care team. In time, our representatives become familiar with individual style preferences with regard to communication and conflict resolution so that they may craft an often unpleasant message from patients and families in a way that is well received. This mediation allows for healthy dialogue to take place between patient, family, and provider, so that information can be communicated and heard in the way that it was intended. Depending on patient and provider preferences, the representative might participate in this conversation to help moderate and restore trust that may have been impaired.

Likewise, our representatives are called on by administrative and clinical staff to intervene with patients whose behavior is challenging to manage so that the provider may resume focus on the provision of care. One of the representative's roles is to "hold a mirror up to the patient's behavior" or to help patients understand how their words and actions are being perceived by staff. This often involves setting limits and redefining expectations of what a therapeutic relationship looks like.

In 2010, Maureen Fagan assumed the role of executive director of the Center for Patients and Families. Her work is focused on building on the patient- and family-centered care foundation that Hickey and Gordon initially established. Fagan is also creating many patient advisory councils that portray the distinct voices of patients and families who have or are currently receiving care by Brigham and Women's Hospital's interprofessional teams.

In 2011, Jackie Somerville joined Brigham and Women's Hospital as chief nursing officer. Somerville brings extensive knowledge of patient- and family-centered care, having established and cochaired the first patient and family advisory council at Massachusetts General Hospital. Somerville and Fagan are partnering to implement an extensive infrastructure of patient and family advisory councils that will enable the diverse voices of our patients' and families' care experiences to be heard.

Brigham and Women's Hospital established their first Patient and Family Advisory Council in 2007 with the goal of creating mutually beneficial partnerships with our patient and family members. Since the inception of this council, our patient and family advisors have advised us in multiple areas and have sat on various hospital committees. Bringing the perspective of patients and families directly into the planning, delivery, and evaluation of care improves the quality and safety of the care that we provide to our patients. In 2010 and 2011, several of our clinical service lines have either launched their own patient and family advisory council or have included a patient or family member on their care improvement council. We currently have fourteen councils and more than forty patient and family advisors and are consistently working to build additional councils and recruit new advisors. Each council is unique, but the goal is the same: to provide excellent care to our patients and families.

TWO INTERNISTS' VIEW OF SURGICAL CARE IN 2012: UP CLOSE AND PERSONAL!

Peter V. Tishler and Sigrid L. Tishler

"Dr. Tishler, you have a mass in your right lung."

The radiologist called me in the late afternoon of February 1 with this terse, unexpected message, as I was shopping in Harvard Square. A serendipitous finding; a total shock! What brought this to light? I had seen orthopedist Scott D. Martin a few days earlier for nagging shoulder pain. My claustrophobia precluded the usual magnetic resonance imaging study, so I had a diagnostic computed tomography scan instead. The scan visualized the lung adjacent my aging shoulder and highlighted the mass. Was it for real? Why was it there? For how long? Was this a death-knell? I am an active older adult, totally healthy except for the shoulder problem. I had not smoked in forty-five years. Could this chance discovery be fortunate, identifying the mass before it disseminated? Images from my early days as a medical student and doctor haunted me: patients dealing with painful thoracic surgery, struggling to breathe and ultimately losing to lung cancer.

My anxiety receded the next day, when Steven J. Mentzer, a well-known thoracic surgeon at the Brigham, and his associate Syed O. Ali, calmly took charge of my care. A plan was presented, including a host of corroborative studies. The mass was there, but spread was not. A positron emission tomography scan showed modest metabolic activity, most likely, according to Mentzer, the activity of an indolent form of lung cancer. I hoped, irrationally, that it was something else (infection?). He described the procedure, video-assisted thoracic surgery, that he would perform early next week. There would be two small incisions, nothing like the larger operations of the past. The postoperative pain for the first few days would be controlled by an epidural anesthetic, and with the comfort I could take deep breaths, walk soon after surgery, and avoid complications. This was not like the thoracic surgery of yesteryear.

With my family in tow, I entered the Brigham for a right upper lobectomy on the morning of Valentine's Day. The admitting office had all my information and whisked me to the preoperative area. My family members waited in the comfortably furnished Bretholtz Center, where staff members kept them updated on my progress and knitting projects were available to help nervous relatives pass the time. The surgery went smoothly, and I was awake by mid-afternoon. Mentzer told me that the frozen section obtained at surgery did identify the mass as a cancer, but more specific information must await the detailed pathologic study. My remaining hospital stay on unit 12B was shepherded by the nursing staff, the house staff, Mentzer, and Ali, and my very concerned wife and children. Care was wonderful. The nurses were concerned for my well-being, attentive to my problems of convalescence, and accessible to us as we needed them. Even my grouchiness, one of my "birth defects," did not discourage them! The room was super clean. My doctors were optimistic concerning my recovery and prognosis. There was no problem that escaped the staff. When I developed an irregular heartbeat (atrial fibrillation), the physicians and nurses responded competently and were reassuring. When my wife felt she had to stay overnight, a compassionate nurse covered her with a warm blanket as she tried to sleep in a lounge chair.

Since discharge, my recovery has progressed as anticipated. I am back at work, writing for this book. On detailed pathological examination, the mass was indeed a lung cancer, the relatively favorable type predicted by Mentzer ("adenocarcinoma, predominantly lepidic"). This cancer grows and spreads very slowly if at all. Because all studies demonstrated no spread of the cancer, my surgeon suggested that the prognosis is very favorable—but with frequent follow-up to substantiate this.

Like every patient, I need a long time to deal with the psychiatric aspects of this terrible mess and mass. Why did I, a paragon of good preventative health, develop lung cancer? This defies all logic. I had planned to live forever. Is that still likely? Rationally, no. How do I remain healthy for as long as possible? Maybe whatever I do will have little or no relevance. How do I exploit what time I have left? Maybe I should modify my "workaholism," or perhaps not. How do I show my family members that I am intact, devoted to them, and willing and able to help out as they grow and develop? These are all essential life questions with which I must grapple.

Psychic uncertainties aside, thoracic surgery has provided me with life-prolonging therapy, with the best possible attention to my medical care and recovery. I am so grateful to be the recipient of a century of medical excellence at the Brigham. What aspect of a hospital and its care could be better?

SCHWARTZ CENTER ROUNDS: CARING FOR THE CAREGIVERS

Christine Wenc

Patients are not the only ones who can become stressed by the hospital experience. Caregivers—physicians, nurses, and others—also feel the impact of playing central roles in the life-altering events that take place daily in the hospital. In the early twenty-first century, medicine is making a conscious and evidence-based effort to alter older styles of medical work that tended to deny or repress caregivers' emotional reactions. Important to note is that the goal is not merely to make caregivers feel better but to improve care in measurable ways.

The "Schwartz Rounds" are one way that Brigham and Women's Hospital (BWH) caregivers are participating in this effort. The Brigham is one of more than 200 sites across the country and fourteen in the United Kingdom,[9] including academic hospitals, community hospitals, nursing homes, and community health centers, to host "Schwartz Center Rounds," which offer caregivers a safe place where they can "share their experiences, dilemmas, joys, concerns, and fears (both for their patients and for themselves)." The goals of the Rounds are "to improve relationships and communication with patients and among providers and to enhance providers' sense of personal support."[10] Rounds are attended by physicians, nurses, social workers, the chaplaincy, bioethics staff, and others involved in care.

The Schwartz Center for Compassionate Healthcare, an entity outside of BWH, was created in 1997 by Kenneth B. Schwartz, a Boston lawyer who died of lung cancer in his early forties. The center's rounds were piloted at Massachusetts General Hospital (MGH). Beth Lown is now the medical director of the Schwartz Center and has been a member of the board since 2005.

> *The Rounds are one-hour, case-based, interactive discussions held monthly or bimonthly and led by a physician and/or a professional facilitator. Each session begins with a brief presentation of a patient (or family) case by members of the health care team who cared for the patient. This presentation introduces multiple perspectives on selected psychosocial topics. Audience members and the presentation team participate in the facilitated group discussion that follows.*
>
> *The Rounds address a wide range of important topics rarely discussed elsewhere. These topics include the management of team conflict, stories of hope and miracles, instances when providers become patients, the impaired professional, the impact of patient violence toward providers, instances when cultural or religious beliefs impair providers' ability to communicate, the impact on providers of making a mistake, humor and healing, and many others.*[11]

The Rounds are

> *one of several approaches that have emerged in recent years to help health care workers unload the stresses of their jobs, both to help them avoid burnout and to regain the empathy that is central to patient care...Most meetings center on a single case or incident, such as the death of a longtime patient, an outburst by a combative patient, or a medical error ending in a lawsuit. Hospitals have traditionally held clinical rounds at which physicians discuss the medical care of a difficult or interesting patient. In contrast, Schwartz Center Rounds highlight feelings—guilt, fear, anger, or sadness—that might lead caregivers to withdraw emotionally from their work.*[12]

Thomas Lynch, formerly an oncologist at MGH, Kenneth Schwartz's physician when he died, and chair of the Schwartz Center Board, put it this way: "One thing that the Schwartz Center has learned and has taught others is that for so long we always felt that compassion was innate. And the ability to connect with a patient was something you had or didn't have. And that's wrong. Just like any other skill in medicine, communication and connection absolutely can be taught and it can be role modeled."[13]

The Rounds "challenge the traditional medical culture that discouraged emotional attachment between physicians and their patients."[14]

Beth Lown and Colleen Manning have written of this work:

> *High-quality interpersonal relationships, communication, and "whole-person" knowledge of patients have been correlated with improvements in clinical and functional status, adherence, patient trust, reduced malpractice suits, and the satisfaction of both physicians and patients with their encounters. As the medical profession has shifted from "physician-centered" care to "patient-centered" or "relationship-centered" care, patients' experiences of care are now valued and measured. In addition, empirical studies have shown the correlation between close integration of care teams and improved patient health outcomes, reduced mortality, shortened length of stay, and better organizational outcomes, including enhanced workforce morale and reduced burnout and staff turnover.*[15]

The issue of provider behavior and its connection with patient satisfaction also matters to hospitals both financially and for accreditation and certification. Since October 2012, for instance, Medicare is basing 1% of its payments on providers' "patient experience" scores.[16] Since 2008, the Joint Commission's standards for patient care have included the assessment of patients' spiritual well-being.

Still, because there have been many efforts over the years to humanize high-tech medical care, with varying degrees of success, some skepticism among medical personnel about this latest venture is perhaps understandable. The culture of academic medicine has also perhaps tended to discourage emotional or philosophical reflection, if for no other reason than there is little time to do so. Lown's work shows that attending Schwartz Rounds may result in enhanced communication, teamwork, and provider support. The more Rounds attended, the more likely an impact. Thus "the Rounds represent an effective strategy for providing support to health care professionals and for enhancing relationships among them and with their patients."[17]

THE HISTORY OF SOCIAL WORK AT THE PETER BENT BRIGHAM HOSPITAL AND BRIGHAM AND WOMEN'S HOSPITAL

Ann Conway

Professional social work at the Peter Bent Brigham Hospital (PBBH) originally came out of the same progressive impetus that established the institution—the idea that illness came not from personal immorality but from scientifically identifiable causes and that its course was often connected to social and environmental factors. The PBBH model reflected the emerging ideas of Richard Cabot, a senior physician at Massachusetts General Hospital (MGH), who with Ida Cannon is considered the founder of the medical social work profession. Cannon, who had been a visiting nurse, was hired at MGH and formed the Social Work Department there in 1914. In an unusual arrangement, as chief of social work, Cannon was placed on a par with the chief of medicine and chief of surgery.[18]

Social Service also had a long history at the Boston Hospital for Women, the Robert Breck Brigham Hospital, and in Boston in general. The late nineteenth and early twentieth century embrace of progressive ideas was not limited to men; the "bright and beautiful sisterhood" of charitable women in Boston were also involved in education, temperance, prison reform, charity to women and children, the abolitionist movement, and eventually, women's suffrage. Nevertheless, the development of medical social work was a new frontier.

At the PBBH, Alice Cheney, who was also a nurse, was hired as the first head of Social Work in 1914. Although there was significant interest at the hospital in the relation of the hospital to community problems, Cheney did not have the same status as Cannon. Like Carrie Hall and others, and unlike the powerful chiefs, she reported to the superintendent, not the trustees. In many ways, her first decade of work was a process of carving out her role. Cheney found herself caught in the debate about the function of the teaching hospital as a provider of community service with a larger educational and research mission, all in the context of limited resources. As she wrote in the Second Annual Report:

> *To give a patient who enters the hospital the most thorough and scientific treatment possible would seem to be the logical course for the good of the patient and of society. However, if the funds of the hospital are diverted largely into a department so that the social conditions of the patient and his family may be improved...the regular work of the hospital suffers and less efficient diagnosis and treatment result, and herein lies the danger of extending the work of a social service department too far beyond the immediate needs of a thorough cooperation with the medical world of the institution.*[19]

Eventually, Cheney and her successors became greatly involved in the work of the Outdoor Department, particularly in health education connected with the existing clinics, as well as an extensive resource and referral for inpatients and outpatients. In this, they were frequently assisted by the Social Service Ladies Committee (which eventually became Friends of the Brigham), as well as a corps of volunteers. In addition, Social Service had teaching responsibilities—the Annual Report for 1940 mentioned participation in Friday Harvard Medical School (HMS) Medical Rounds for students, and the department was accepted as a teaching site for Simmons College in the same year. The report for 1945 mentions students from Simmons, Boston College, and Boston University.

In the years after World War II, Social Service continued its traditional roles of inpatient and outpatient case work and referral, teaching, participation in the integrated care provided in the Geriatric Clinic, the Alcoholic Clinic, the Gynecological Clinic, and other new endeavors, including the Medical-Social Rounds. The 1958 Annual Report also notes the complexities of the new era of transplantation and the social worker's role in providing services to patients and affected families. By this time, social workers were not only involved in nursing education; they provided orientation for fourth-year HMS students in general and on the clinics to which they were assigned.

By the Fiftieth Annual Report, in keeping with the enhanced attention to community evidenced on every front, Social Service referred to itself as a "community agency." It noted: "An organized program of visiting nursing homes by a designated worker has been in operation since September 1956, with the growing recognition that the medical-nursing discipline should be an integral part of such a venture."[20] Social Work subsequently was very involved in the nursing home visitation/quality rating program started by Andrew Jessiman, as well as many of the community health efforts increasingly undertaken by the hospital.

In 1979, just before the physical merger of the three hospitals (the Social Work departments, like others, engaged in years of planning), the PBBH Social Work Division[21] of what was temporarily called the Affiliated Hospitals Center, or AHC, reflected on its history and changes in its mission:

> *Patients' problems have increased in complexity under the influence of regulations on utilization of hospital beds; the problems involved in obtaining adequate resources (such as finances for services in the home or other care facilities); and the very serious shortage of nursing-home beds. We share these problems with many departments, especially the Continuing Care Service.*[22]

Then PBBH Director of Social Work Barbara Hewitt described programs in Emergency Service, the "Holding Unit," and the "Walk-in Unit," particularly concerning domestic violence.[23] There were also summaries of work in Primary Care, Hematology, and Inpatient Services; the employment of a Spanish-speaking social worker was mentioned, as was the presence of students from Simmons School of Social Work and much in-house interdisciplinary training.

Today, the BWH Social Work Department, directed by Martha Byron Burke, is part of the Department of Care Coordination. Approximately fifty licensed social workers provide multifaceted services to patients, focusing on improvement of quality of life, ameliorating psychosocial barriers, care coordination, and providing education for patients, staff, students, and families. The scope of care includes identification, assessment, clinical intervention, short-term therapy, and follow-up, including discharge planning and addressing needs related to the impact of illness, hospitalization, and discharge.

Social Work works closely with other health care providers, particularly the Care Coordination nursing services directed by Joanne Hogan. The team covers fourteen services, including medicine, transplant, surgery, neurology, cardiovascular, infectious disease, oncology, and psychiatry.[24] It is also involved in a number of initiatives centering on quality and performance improvement, as well as discussions of the legal and ethical issues attendant on twenty-first century health care. The service offers a multifaceted suite of support groups for patients and families, including a

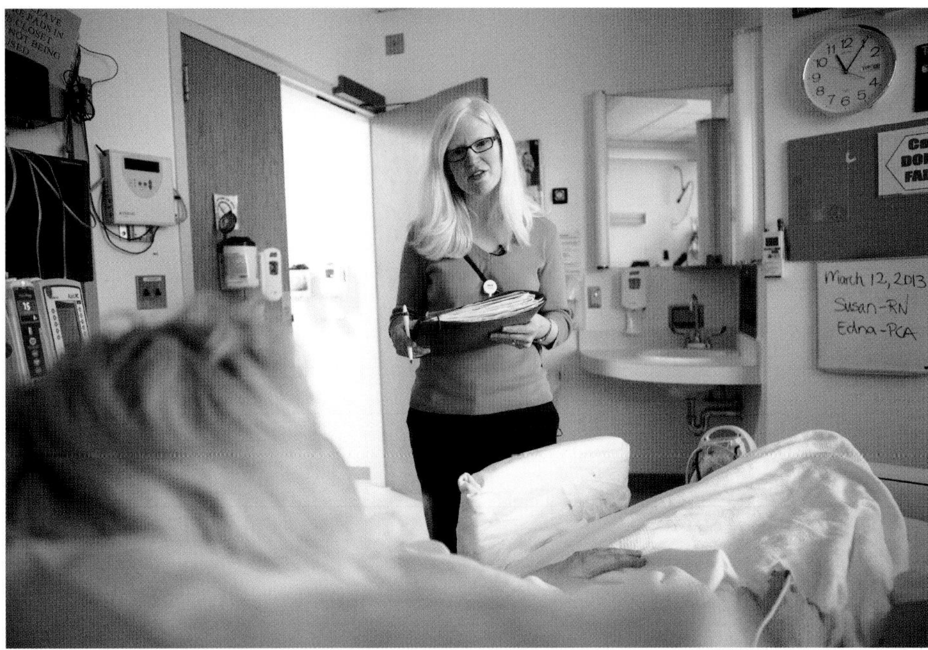

FIGURE 5-13 BWH social worker Ellen Golden in action, March 2013.

Bereavement Support Group, Diabetes Group for Spanish Speakers, MS Partners in Care Support Group, Parent Support Group Following the Loss of an Infant, and many more.

Medical social workers have always been faced with a number of challenges. In the twenty-first century, these include the rise in domestic and societal violence in Boston, the infant mortality crisis, immigration-related issues, homelessness and economic disempowerment, and advanced care planning and end-of-life issues in an aging population—all complicated by budget cuts on the state and federal levels. Nevertheless, BWH social workers exhibit the same ability to adapt to the challenges of a rapidly transforming health care and community environment as did their predecessors.[25]

INTERPRETER SERVICES AT BRIGHAM AND WOMEN'S HOSPITAL

Yilu Ma

Interpreter Services has grown from a one-person show more than thirty-three years ago to what is now one of the largest hospital-based interpreter services in Boston. In the late 1970s, there was only one Spanish interpreter in the whole hospital: Pedro Sanchez, presently of the Jen Center. A medical student at that time, he was hired by a "coordinator," Eileen Amy, a nurse who is still with the hospital at the Obstetrics Clinic. Interpreting service was sporadic at best, available only during the day, and certainly was not sufficient, considering this small staff's limited availabilities and other responsibilities.

In the years that followed, the needs crept up as the patient population became more diverse. The service expanded, adding another four to five Spanish interpreters. It really began to formalize into a department in 1995, when my predecessor, Ileana Jimenez-Garcia, came on board. From then on, more interpreters were hired. Languages were added, resources secured and allocated, and office spaces sprawled in different buildings and locations.

Today, the department has twenty-five part- and full-time staff interpreters and seventy per diems, providing interpretation and translation service in more than forty languages, twenty-four hours per day, seven days per week. In addition to face-to-face interpreting, which accounts for more than 75% of the total requests, telephonic interpreting has been added into the mix and has seen an upsurge. This latter modality, mostly via a vendor, Pacific Interpreters, increased to more than 1,000 calls a month and is capable of providing interpretation in more than 200 languages. In 2011, the department provided nearly 48,000 interpretations, and it anticipates a 20-25% increase this year. Compared with the ad hoc interpreters in the early days of the interpreter services, interpreters now are all professionals. As members of the International Medical Interpreters Association, they are certified by the National Board for Medical Interpreters.

To be more effective and expand language coverage to the increasingly distributed institution, Interpreter Services is also working diligently to leverage technology to provide remote interpreting via video conferencing. As of late 2012, more than ten service areas have installed video devices; they are fully tested and ready to use. This innovative interpreting modality will eliminate interpreters' travel time and patient/caregiver wait time, allowing Brigham interpreters to provide immediate remote interpretation from their office booths. In addition, Interpreter Services has teamed up with the information technology service to develop a daily operation management system that enables us to develop quality benchmarks on patient wait time, interpretation time, and statistics updating and compilation and to effectively deploy our resources in a timely fashion. Technology is transforming the service into a customer service–orientated and rapid response program. We are very confident that with the firm support of the leadership and the collective wisdom of the interpreters, we will bring the service to an even higher level.

Despite the incredible expansion of resources and manpower, the core of the service has never changed: interpreters are deeply committed to providing professional, competent, and timely responsive interpretation services to patients with limited English proficiency and/or hearing impairment. As part of the care team, interpreters proudly play the crucial role of language conduit, bridging the linguistic gap between the patients and the providers. They also offer intercultural advice, clarify information, facilitate communication, and advocate for patients. They work closely with doctors, physician assistants, nurses, social workers, occupational/physical therapists, and dieticians/nutritionists, to name a few. One can see them in ambulatory clinics, inpatient bedsides, family meetings, consults, emergency rooms, operational rooms, at discharges, and at registrations. Their contribution to patient care is omnipresent throughout the gamut of care provision, from diagnosis to treatment delivery, from establishing physician–patient rapport to facilitating conflict resolution. Our interpreters are invaluable. As they put it: "We are the mouth of the patients and their families."

THE NUTRITION DEPARTMENT: A HISTORIC BRIGHAM PROGRAM WITH MULTIFACETED ROLES IN PATIENT AND COMMUNITY CARE

Christine Wenc

Dietetics may be the oldest branch of medicine. Written works for both practitioners and for the public on the connections between diet and health, as well as the use of diet as a form of medical treatment, go back hundreds of years. Since the later nineteenth and early twentieth century, when vitamins and other diet-related concepts began to be researched in the laboratory in earnest, nutrition has been a science and clinical hospital nutrition a specialty that has evolved to encompass many aspects of care inside and outside the hospital. The Peter Bent Brigham Hospital and later Brigham and Women's Hospital (BWH) have been noted twentieth and twenty-first century innovators and proponents in this field.

The original Peter Bent Brigham Hospital was a "pioneer in providing nutrition services as an integral part of medical care."[26] The Brigham nutrition program has long been integrated into patient care at the hospital, and Brigham dieticians have been involved in community outreach, research, and leadership in the field for generations. The Brigham nutrition program is also important historically for its dietetic internship program, one of the oldest nutrition training programs in the United States. From the program's inception in 1913, students (uniformly female until the 1970s) had college degrees and came from all over the country to attend; students attended the one-year internship program from many different states, including Hawaii. In the first half of the twentieth century, classes averaged around ten students per year. The program also had a relatively diverse and international student body for the time, and some young women came far from home for their training in Boston. Archival documents show that interns came to the program from Canada, China, Ireland, the Philippines, Columbia, Puerto Rico, and Haiti between the 1920s and 1960s. Starting in the 1950s, small numbers of African American students were admitted as well from different parts of the United States.

The work of BWH dieticians has gone far beyond mere meal planning. A 1976 *Brigham Bulletin* article described the dietetic internship program as training students at the graduate level in "Food Administration, Nutritional Care, Teaching, Ambulatory Services, Research and Nutrition Services in the Community." Some of the Nutrition Department's accomplishments include the following: In 1969, Mary Ellen Collins, at the time associate director of the Department of Dietetics (the earlier name for the Department of Nutrition) assisted Harvard Professor

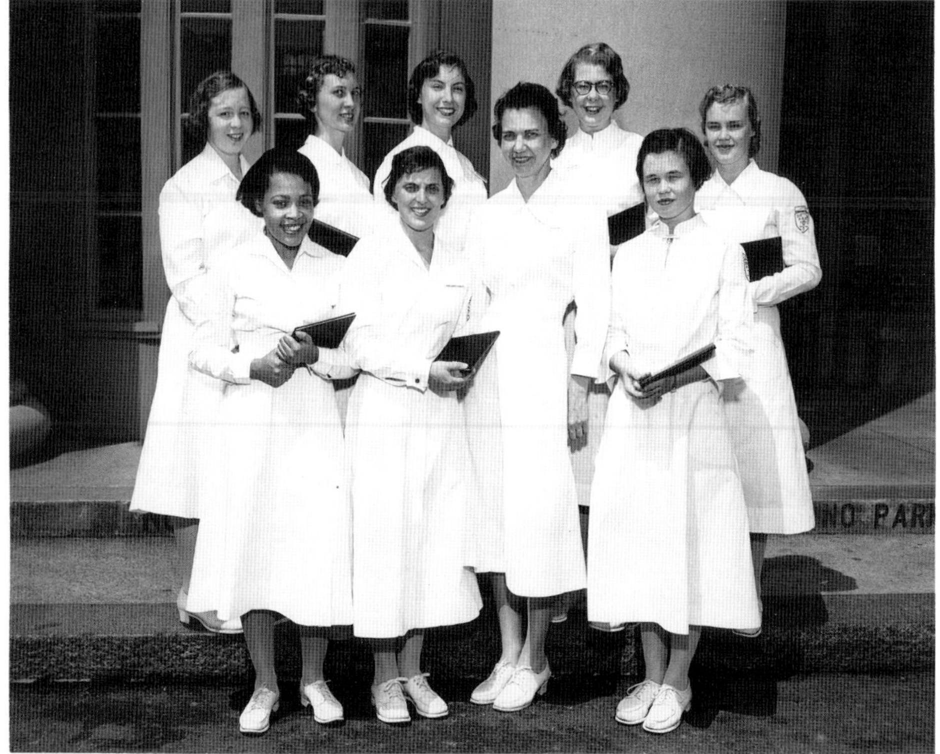

FIGURE 5-14 1954 Dietetic Internship class graduation photo, Peter Bent Brigham Hospital. Pictured are (order unknown): Nancy Keirans, Katherine Ellis, Bernette Neun, Dorothy Risley, Janet Cawley, Gertrude Nicholson, Gloria Flowers, Chieko Abe, and Margaret Mack.

of Nutrition Jean Mayer in organizing President Richard Nixon's White House Conference on Food, Nutrition, and Health, which Nixon stated was to be "the beginning of a national commitment to end hunger and malnutrition among the poor, to make better use of our agricultural bounty and nutritional knowledge, and to make it possible for all Americans to have a healthful diet."[27] Collins later became director of the department and was involved in other community-related projects; she also made numerous media appearances as an expert. Doug Wilmore, who with Stanley Dudrick was a pioneer in the development of lifesaving total parenteral nutrition, became the director of the hospital's nutrition support service in 1978 and was a faculty member in the Department of Surgery for many years. In the 1970s, the Brigham offered nutrition instruction in Spanish at the Spanish-speaking clinic at the hospital, cooperated with nursing homes in Jamaica Plain, and worked with the Roxbury Federation of Neighborhood Health Centers to provide home-delivered meals to the elderly.[28] The department also participates in nutrition-related outreach programs to the community via the BWH-affiliated community health clinics and has done so since the clinics' creation in the 1970s. The Peter Bent Brigham Hospital offered classes for diabetics and other patients from the very first years of the hospital's existence; such classes still exist today.

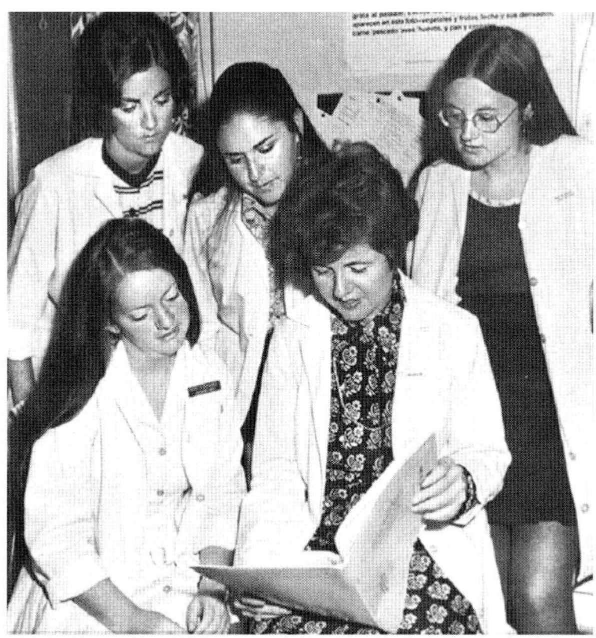

FIGURE 5-15 1974 Peter Bent Brigham nutrition staff. Pictured are: (top row) Julie S. Daly, Fanny Guterman, and Wendy Midgley; (bottom row) Peggy L. Kloster and Mary Ellen Collins.

Kathy McManus currently directs the Nutrition Department at BWH. The department reports to the senior vice president of Patient Care Services and Chief Nursing Officer Jackie Somerville. Dieticians are responsible for looking after the nutritional needs of medical, surgical, oncology, obstetrical, and neonatal intensive care unit patients. All transplant patients must be evaluated by a dietician before and after surgery. Several members of the staff also do ambulatory care at Dana-Farber Cancer Institute. Brigham nutritionists also participate in interdisciplinary rounds along with nursing, pharmacy, social work, the chaplaincy, and others. The department also participates in translating nutritional data from many of the large epidemiologic trials conducted at the Harvard School of Public Health into recommendations for the public (and for the Brigham cafeteria!). The department has also recently been centrally involved in research on obesity reported in the *New England Journal of Medicine* and in creating a pregnancy food guide that is used throughout the country.

Given the role of diet in coping with common American health conditions such as diabetes, the changing dietary needs of an aging population, and the need for attention to dietetics in many other conditions both acute and chronic, the BWH Nutrition Department will undoubtedly continue to play an important role both inside and outside the hospital.

KEEPING THE HEART IN MEDICINE: THE HISTORY AND EVOLUTION OF THE BRIGHAM AND WOMEN'S HOSPITAL CHAPLAINCY SERVICES DEPARTMENT

Kathleen Gallivan

The history of the Brigham and Women's Chaplaincy Services Department reflects the evolution of healthcare chaplaincy in the United States. There has been a broader culture shift from expecting that religious needs of patients will be met by local clergy to a realization that the religious and spiritual needs of patients and families are an important dimension of patient- and family-centered care, and that board-certified chaplains are an integral part of the health care team. In 2012, the chaplaincy estimated that about 60% of Brigham and Women's patients have contact with a chaplain. Many of these visits are referrals, but Brigham chaplains also try to visit as many patients as possible preoperatively to help relieve their anxiety. They also make regular rounds through the hospital.

Prior to 1980 there was very little chaplaincy presence in the hospitals that merged to form Brigham and Women's Hospital (BWH). The Peter Bent Brigham Hospital (PBBH) had the strongest chaplaincy presence. Beginning in 1955, Protestant, Catholic, and Jewish chaplains, who were probably area clergy, donated some of their time or were supported financially by the Archdiocese, the Jewish Chaplaincy Council or local congregations. Before that time, local clergy would simply come to visit people from their congregations in the hospital.

BWH CHAPLAINCY SERVICES DIRECTOR: WILLIAM LEACH (1965-1982)

In 1965, William Leach, an Episcopal priest, was hired as the first full-time chaplain, paid for by the Episcopal Diocese of Massachusetts. A 1971 document, likely written by Leach, outlined a model for a Chaplaincy

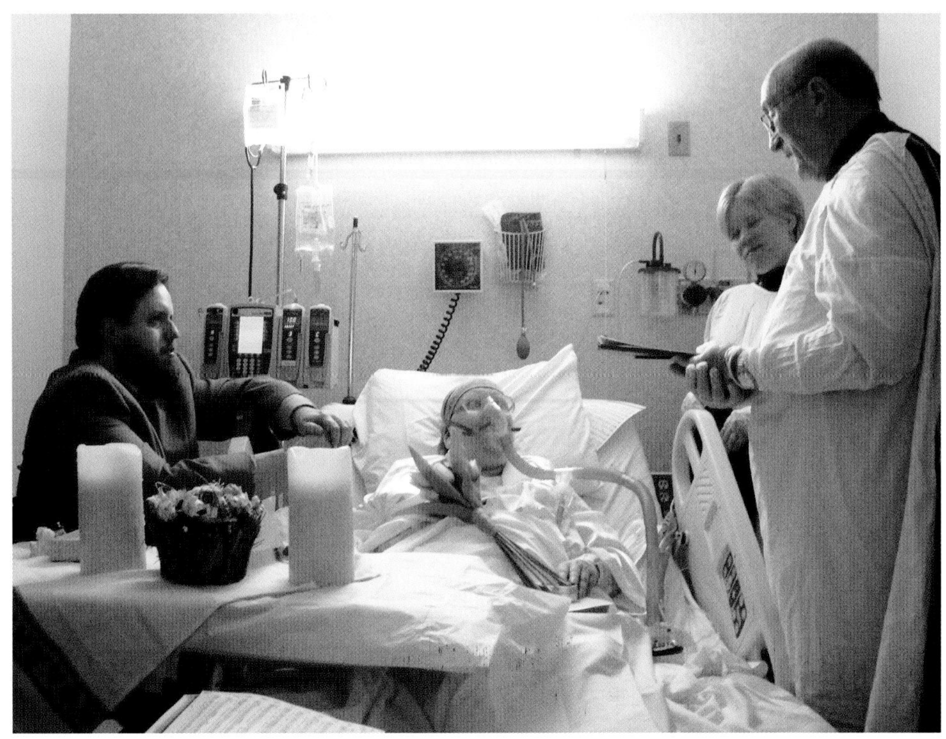

FIGURE 5-16 Patient wedding, performed by BWH chaplain Ron Hindelang.

Service for the hospital. There would be "one chaplaincy service, directed by a Resident or House Chaplain, who would have a position similar to the 'Chaplain in Chief' in the armed forces. This particular chaplain should function on a nondenominational basis" and should be an "employee of the Affiliate."

In 1976 a Chaplaincy Service Department was officially created when the PBBH took over some financial responsibility for the chaplains, and Leach became an employee of the hospital. The 1976 Brigham Annual Report indicated that twelve student chaplains were also involved in the department, from Harvard Divinity School and Episcopal Divinity School, and that the department also hosted services at the Children's Hospital Medical Center. Leach also joined the newly formed Patient Care Committee at the hospital. In the next several years, Leach worked to expand and develop the Chaplaincy Department, which likely worked on a traditional model in which chaplains in each of the three main religious traditions represented visited with patients in their traditions. Leach and Thomas Putnam, an Episcopal deacon who was the hospital's first full-time chaplain intern, also developed and implemented a Pastoral Visitors Program for Protestant (probably mostly Episcopal) laypeople. Started in the late 1970s, preparation for this program included a yearlong course through which participants became "senior pastoral volunteers." The Pastoral Volunteers Program has continued to the present, and two of the staff chaplains, Virginia Hemani and Katherine Mitchell, first came to BWH through this program.

Leach's personal annual reports from the late 1970s indicate that he provided counseling services, officiated at weddings and funerals, had numerous speaking engagements including at other hospitals, and was involved with many local professional associations. Leach also started a weekly discussion group, open to all hospital staff, under the title "Human Aspects of Medical Care" that met regularly for at least four years. Leach planned for the new Chaplaincy Department at Brigham and Women's Hospital and became its first director. Space was granted for a new chapel, which opened in 1981 as the Elizabeth Louise Dieterich Cutler Memorial Chapel, and weekly services took place.

Leach continued to develop the Pastoral Visitors Program, advertising for volunteers through Episcopal publications. At the graduation ceremony for a group of pastoral volunteers in February 1982, Leach described his approach to chaplaincy, explaining that chaplains and pastoral volunteers offer "presence." "Attention is the presence," he explained. "Everyone that passes through the doors of a hospital is made in the image and likeliness of God." What makes a chaplain different from other visitors "is in the effort to reflect the wholeness of the patient...to help a person strike a balance of acceptance between what he can manage in his life and what he cannot control." Chaplains "help [patients] recognize the hallowedness of their lives, to help them celebrate what has been joyful, to help them work through the pain, and to bring them with wholeness to the point where they may depart in peace."

BWH CHAPLAINCY SERVICES DIRECTOR: DIANA PHILLIPS (1983-1989)

Following Leach's departure in 1982, Pastoral Visitors provided much of the chaplaincy support. In 1983 Diana Phillips, an ordained minister in the United Church of Christ, was hired as the new director. The department grew, and a Catholic sister was hired, the first time a Catholic staff chaplain was paid directly by the hospital. Volunteer and educational programs continued in the 1980s. A relationship also developed between BWH and the Dana-Farber Cancer Institute (DFCI) through which a BWH chaplain visited with DFCI inpatients. Phillips was a member of the hospital's Ethics Committee from its inception and served on other committees.

Phillips outlined her approach to chaplaincy in a 1984 BWH magazine, emphasizing that chaplains are there to listen and have broader conversations with patients, which are not always about religion:

We try to bring that other dimension—what I call God and others might call something else—into that room. We say to the patient, "You're loved, you're important." But that message might come across while we're talking about the Red Sox, the weather, or the patient's favorite place on earth. It doesn't have to be in a specifically religious context.

It is important to note that religion is rarely discussed in the normal course of pastoral visiting. In Phillips' words, "I believe we are called upon to be representatives of the love of God...how we express that love depends on the needs of the particular patient."

Often there were not enough chaplains to meet all the requests in these years. Phillips dreamed of more staff and having specific chaplains responsible for particular units. Her annual reports describe a desire to find ways to keep the "heart in medicine" even as technology develops.

BWH CHAPLAINCY SERVICES DIRECTOR: MAUREEN MANNS (1990-2002)

Phillips left BWH at the end of the 1980s, and Maureen Manns was hired as the director. Manns had completed an MDiv at Andover Newton Theological School and a PhD at Boston University. She was also certified as a Clinical Pastoral Education (CPE) supervisor, the nationally recognized training program for professional chaplaincy.

Manns took steps to make the department more multifaith. She hired two clinically trained Catholic priests and a Muslim imam. An interfaith model was developed in which chaplains were assigned to particular units and were responsible for the patients on their units. The wishes of patients who wanted to see a chaplain from their own tradition were respected. The department moved from faith-specific services in the chapel to interfaith services. Faith-specific services continued to be offered on important religious holy days.

Manns said:

We see a patient or family whether or not they have a religious affiliation and work with them to access the resources which help them to cope with the crisis. For some, this means traditional resources of prayer and ritual. For others, it means supportive conversation. For others, it may mean teaching guided relaxation or exploring options about their medical treatment.

Chaplaincy also changed in the 1990s to reflect changes in hospital medicine: As hospital stays continued to shorten, chaplains were called to see more patients coming into the hospital for same-day surgeries. Chaplains were also called to support patients making complex ethical decisions in light of increasingly sophisticated medical technology.

Like her predecessors, Manns served on various hospital committees, including the Ethics Committee, Medical Intensive Care Unit Ethics Committee, Uncompensated Care Committee, and Cancer Committee. Individual chaplains were involved with committees including Bereavement, Cancer, Domestic Violence, Emotional Support, Ethics, Human Research, and Reward and Recognition. Chaplains also assisted with ethics consultations, the training of cardiac liaison volunteers, educational sessions, and support groups. The hospital's Palliative Care Service first included a staff chaplain as a member of their interdisciplinary team in the early 2000s.[29]

One of Manns' most significant contributions was the introduction of chaplains recording their visits in patients' charts, documenting their presence as members of the healthcare team. A chaplaincy system was developed that captured statistics, allowing the department to analyze and identify best practice. Manns also founded the Brigham's Clinical Pastoral Education program and hired an additional CPE supervisor.

BWH CHAPLAINCY SERVICES DIRECTOR: KATHLEEN GALLIVAN (2002-PRESENT)

After Manns retired in 2002, Kathleen Gallivan became the next director. A Catholic sister with the

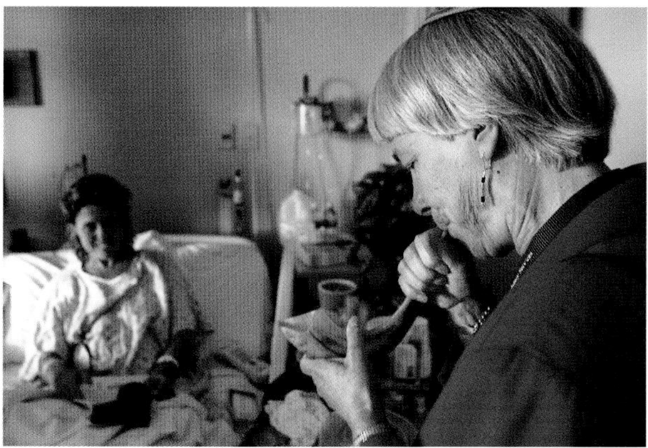

FIGURE 5-17 Rabbi Katy Allen blowing the shofar.

Sisters of Notre Dame de Namur, Gallivan was trained at Emmanuel College and Andover Newton Theological School. She also has a PhD in pastoral psychology from Boston University and is certified as a CPE supervisor.

Gallivan envisioned a multifaith, diverse Chaplaincy Department that was fully integrated into the hospital. The staff developed a mission, vision, and values statement that charged chaplains to "take a leadership role in fully integrating spiritual care into the healthcare system." Chaplains broadened their involvement in hospital committees, interdisciplinary rounds, and attending to staff support. The hospital's Palliative Care Service and the Mesothelioma Program included staff chaplains as members of their interdisciplinary teams.

Gallivan hired several more chaplains, including the first rabbi to be salaried by the hospital, an African American bishop, a Nigerian Catholic priest, and a Hispanic chaplain. All chaplains were required to be nationally board certified. The Eucharistic Ministry, Field Education, and Pastoral Visitors programs grew. As the relationship between BWH and Faulkner Hospital strengthened, Gallivan also took over responsibility for the spiritual care at Faulkner.

Extensive renovations were undertaken in the chapel to make it a more welcoming multifaith space to be used by patients, families, and staff. The current chapel includes very few explicitly religious symbols and is used for noontime interfaith services, memorial services, family meetings, and other activities as needed. It is open twenty-four hours a day, seven days a week.

CLINICAL PASTORAL EDUCATION

As a way of contributing to the hospital's mission to educate next-generation healthcare professionals, Gallivan focused on expanding the Clinical Pastoral Education Program. A CPE residency began in 2003 to prepare students for professional chaplaincy and for national board certification. An additional internship program began in 2008, and the CPE program became accredited to train future CPE supervisors. A third CPE supervisor was hired. This program is also offered for local clergy and for women and men preparing for other professional careers in ministry. BWH's CPE program is accredited by The Association for Clinical Pastoral Education, a national multicultural, multifaith organization.

Chaplaincy students represent a variety of faith traditions including Catholic, Protestant, Jewish, Buddhist, and Muslim, and they learn to function as interfaith chaplains while they are at BWH. Their program consists of a combination of clinical work, didactic instruction, and individual and group supervision. The core philosophy of clinical pastoral education is that patients and families are our teachers and that learning takes places through engaging in the relationship and then reflecting on and learning from that encounter. Students develop specific learning goals in the areas of Pastoral Formation, Pastoral Competence, and Pastoral Reflection, and they are evaluated in relation to meeting their goals. Acceptance into the BWH CPE program is highly competitive, and applications far outnumber available spaces. Graduates of the BWH CPE Internship and Residency are now serving in hospitals, hospices, prisons, community services agencies, parishes, and synagogues throughout the country and internationally.

A HISTORY OF INTENSIVE CARE UNIT NURSING AT THE PETER BENT BRIGHAM HOSPITAL AND BRIGHAM AND WOMEN'S HOSPITAL

Christine Wenc

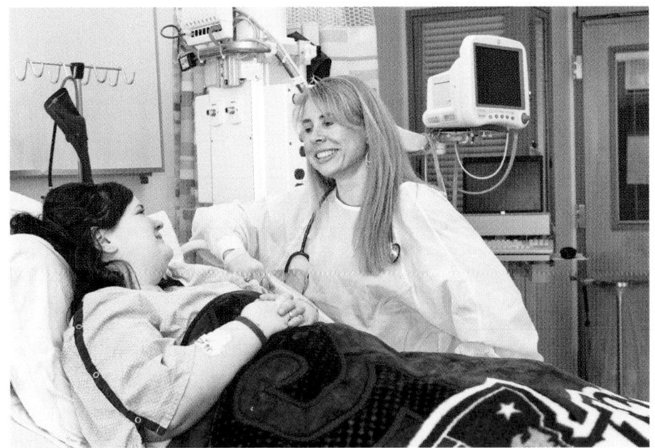

FIGURE 5-18 Nurse Karen Politano and patient.

The Intensive Care Unit (ICU), also called the Critical Care Unit, developed in the 1950s and 1960s at the Peter Bent Brigham Hospital (as well as around the United States and the world) and brought many changes to nursing. Intensive care came into being after World War II as a response to major changes in medicine, surgery, government support, and investment in hospitals, technology, and society at large, and its growing importance in the postwar American hospital is a significant part of the story of twentieth century American medicine. The ICU has also been a site of particular importance in the broad national movement in the past few decades toward patient- and family-centered care and away from paternalism, as decision making surrounding end-of-life care, medical "futility," and other related issues connected to ICU and other technology-intensive care in the hospital have moved toward a much more family-centered approach than was the case in the early days. The number of inpatients requiring intensive care has also come to represent a significant proportion of hospital patients and will likely stay that way or increase in coming years as more nonacute care moves out of the hospital. Today, about 18% of Brigham and Women's Hospital (BWH) inpatients are in a critical care unit, including premature babies and other newborns with medical problems in the neonatal intensive care unit (NICU).[30]

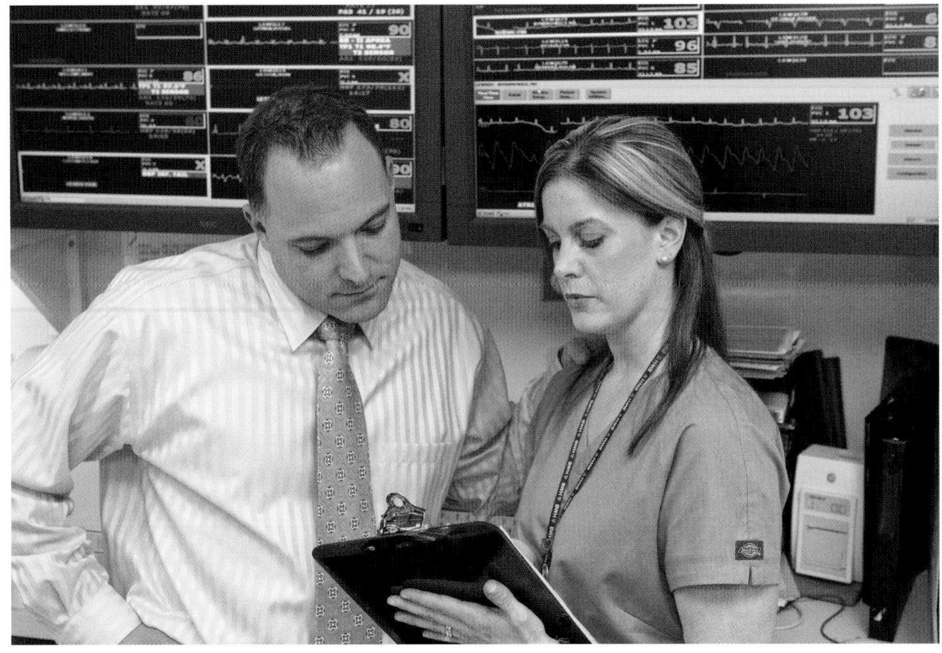

FIGURE 5-19 Matt Quin, nursing director, and Leslie Sabatino, Cardiac Surgery ICU.

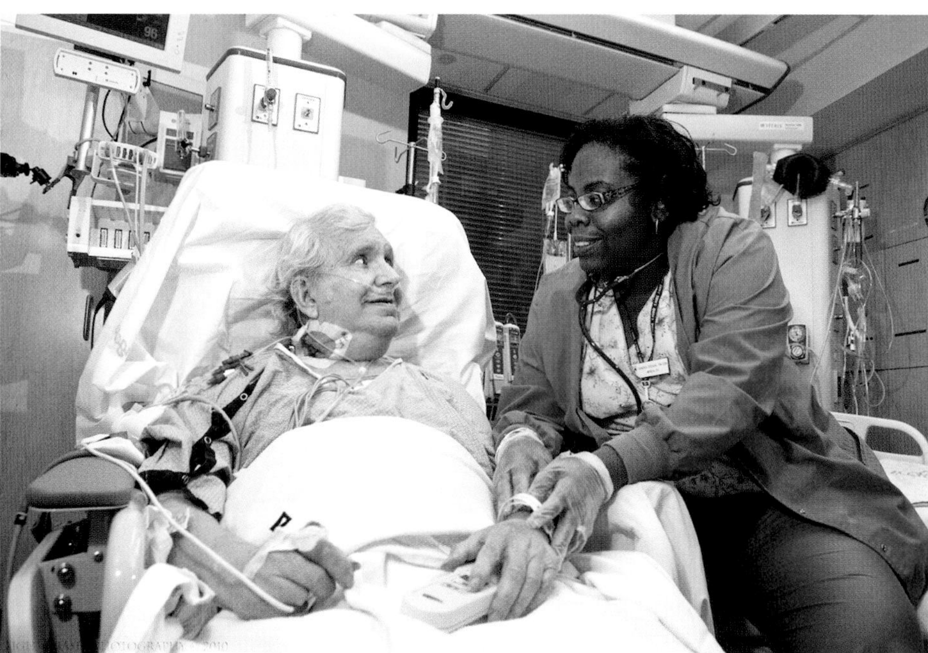

FIGURE 5-20 Sandra Dougal, of the BWH Medical Intensive Care Unit, with a patient.

The changes to nursing engendered by the development of the ICU centered on the need to develop much more advanced levels of knowledge and technical skill among ICU nurses. This accompanied a changing relationship with physicians, in which nurses came to be partners in patient care rather than only subordinates. (Providing nurses with advanced training and the pressing need for more highly skilled nurses during a period of shortage is a continual theme in the Peter Bent Brigham Annual Reports as the ICU developed during the 1960s and 1970s.) In the ICU, nurses also developed more clinical autonomy than had been the case in previous hospital nursing; the need for constant, round-the-clock care of the critically ill and unstable patients found in the ICU, combined with rapid technological advances, necessitated that nurses be able to make a higher level of clinical decisions on their own. Finally, as advocates for those they care for, ICU nurses have played a special role in the hospital for many years, one in which they often have the closest relationship and the most frequent contact with the fear, anxiety, and pain experienced by their patients and their families. And for patients who will not leave the hospital, nurses have also played a role in initiating and participating in the many ethical discussions and advancements surrounding end-of-life care in the ICU that have transpired in past decades in critical care. As constant advocates for their patients, they continue to be on the front lines of these complex problems, which in many ways are still evolving.

According to the American Association of Critical-Care Nurses (AACN), critical care nursing is:

> *that specialty within nursing that deals specifically with human responses to life-threatening problems. A critical care nurse is a licensed professional nurse who is responsible for ensuring that acutely and critically ill patients and their families receive optimal care...Critically ill patients are defined as those patients who are at high risk for actual or potential life-threatening health problems. The more critically ill the patient is, the more likely he or she is to be highly vulnerable, unstable and complex, thereby requiring intense and vigilant nursing care.*

Although there had always been a population of very ill hospital patients, prior to the 1950s not much could be done for someone having a heart attack, an especially poor recovery from surgery, or a respiratory crisis. Most hospital patients were there for routine operations such as tonsillectomies and appendectomies or to convalesce a "stable hospital population" who sometimes stayed in their beds for weeks and did not require much specialized nursing care.[31] The existing model of hospital nursing before World War II, which relied on free or cheap student labor provided by the hospital nursing schools and would seem low-tech today, seemed to be adequate for this patient population. (At the Peter Bent Brigham, of course, the development of brain surgery under Cushing and heart surgery under Dwight Harken likely led to expertise in nursing such patients. Nurses at the Free Hospital for Women likewise probably became adept at nursing gynecologic patients, and nurses at the Boston Lying-In Hospital skilled with laboring mothers and newborns.)

However, during and especially after World War II, the United States experienced a burst of scientific and technological development and innovation. In the United States, this was enabled both by new sources of federal funding for research as well as industry. The creation of Medicare and Medicaid in the 1960s, which paid for health care for seniors and destitute families, also sent impressive amounts of money into the health-care system as people who could not have afforded care previously began to receive it at the same time that many new effective procedures and treatments became available. This included surgical and technological improvements in specialties such as cardiology and oncology, the evolution of organ transplant, the availability of antibiotics and other new drugs, new physiological monitoring devices and life-support technology (some of which had origins in the space program), and new research into the body's response to the shock of surgery and effective treatments for this shock, important aspects of which were conducted by Francis Moore in the 1950s at the Peter Bent Brigham. Also of major importance during this time was the willingness of physicians and their patients to attempt new and sometimes radical treatments, especially with surgery. Many of the men and women who would create and develop the new critical care units had military experience in World War II and the Korean War, and their experiences in these extreme conditions influenced their activities back home in the hospital. Current institutional review board (IRB) restrictions on human subjects research did not exist, nor did many present state and federal regulations affecting practice, and in this bold "cowboy" atmosphere (as one senior BWH physician characterized it to me), experiments, surgeries, and procedures took place at hospitals, and in other contexts that would likely never be allowed today. Some of these activities eventually contributed to the perceived need to create IRB protocols and bioethics review panels. Much activity in this field was led by the Brigham's Chief of Obstetrics and Gynecology Kenneth Ken Ryan in the 1970s and 1980s, who served on some of the first national-level bioethics committees.

The 1950s and 1960s was a time for the medical miracles long promised by scientific medicine to finally be delivered in a significant way: Antibiotics brought children, parents, relatives, and friends back from the brink of death to perfect health (grandparents and great-grandparents today can tell you stories of such incidents); the defibrillator stopped life-threatening rapid heart rates; life support allowed people to recover from what would have been fatal conditions only a few years earlier; new vaccines seemed to create the possibility of eliminating certain diseases; and many others.

However, the aftermath of some of these new treatments and procedures created a new class of patients who needed a far higher level of nursing care than hospitals were accustomed to providing—something that was often left out of the medical miracle stories. As nursing historians Julie Fairman and Joan Lynaugh put it:

> *Patients undergoing chest surgery, the then-novel heart-valve commissurotomy and replacement procedures, and vascular and large-scale abdominal surgeries experienced postoperative complications ranging from respiratory failure and shock to wound infections or wound drainage problems. These gravely ill people overwhelmed the postoperative recovery room or private nursing systems then in place. Ultimately, these surgical and cardiac patients, later joined by patients whose lives were prolonged by kidney dialysis, began to constitute a larger subpopulation of hospital patients whose*

demanding and time-consuming care requirements created a growing hospital nursing crisis. At the same time, these gravely ill patients were coming to be evaluated by the public as "saveable."... Patients and their families, as well as their doctors and nurses, thus began to share a different and much more expansive idea of routine treatment in the face of life-threatening, devastating illness.[32]

Despite all these changes, the hospital system in most places in the 1950s and 1960s was still very much a top-down hierarchy, and nurses were not typically a major part of senior hospital administration. On the floor, nurses were almost uniformly female, and physicians usually addressed them by their first names. They still wore the iconic white uniform dresses and caps. Many were still students in the hospital nursing schools—sometimes only a year or two out of high school—and so were young and inexperienced. Physicians were almost entirely male, were to be called "Doctor," and their orders were not to be questioned—only carried out. Nurses were expected to stand when doctors entered the room and give up their chairs to them if none was available. Independent thought and independent action had been explicitly discouraged in hospital nursing for generations. Wages were low (or in the case of hospital nursing school students, nonexistent), and turnover was high. The popular perception that nursing involved more sentiment than skill and was the quintessential "woman's work," with all that implies about status, authority, and autonomy, also undoubtedly had an impact. Educational standards for nurse hires and training programs varied widely in quality. In the 1950s, 80% of American nurses had graduated from a hospital diploma program such as the one at the Peter Bent Brigham, the Free Hospital for Women, and many of the other Boston hospitals. In many cases, however, "hospital-based training often was functional and task-oriented. Education in physiology, pathophysiology, and pharmacology was usually rudimentary; nurses were expected to rely somehow on physicians' knowledge rather than their own to solve complex clinical problems."[33]

But on many general medical or surgical wards, a wide variety of patients were now present, with some needing far more care than others. During this period, team nursing was often the model of care used at the Brigham and elsewhere, which typically consisted of a mix of a few graduate nurses with a larger group of students and licensed practical nurses (LPNs) or assistants who divided up tasks among themselves, so that each patient saw a multitude of nursing staff and assistants over the course of a day, performing different tasks. (Today, primary nursing, relationship-based care, or patient/family-centered care are preferred models of care, because they are based on nurses entering caring relationships with patients and their families, a much more holistic approach then that compartmentalized task-driven role of the past. This allows the individual nurse to develop a far more detailed and nuanced awareness of how the patient is doing.) Fairman and Lynaugh write: "On any single unit, patient conditions varied widely and changed rapidly. Often, inexperienced nurses faced new emergency situations with little assistance or appropriate knowledge." One physician commented: "Many nurses in their training and immediately afterward have been in contact with so few cases requiring intensive therapy...that they know relatively little about their management."[34] Complicating the matter was the high rate of turnover among all levels of nursing staff. This all resulted in a "diluted" nursing skill pool at the precise moment that hospitals required the opposite.[35]

Many nurses were aware that in this situation they could not provide the individualized care necessary for critically ill patients nor keep pace with rapid changes in patient condition:

All over the country, in erratically staffed but expanding hospitals, nurses found themselves responsible for desperately ill and dying patients whose medical and nursing needs exceeded the nurses' availability, knowledge, and authority. Left on their own to cope with these difficult and frustrating situations, some physicians and nurses were powerfully motivated to find a better way.[36]

What would this way be? Systems that gave nurses and physicians ideas included the postoperative recovery room (also a new idea in the 1950s) and the iron lung polio wards of the 1940s and 1950s. Wartime experience in both World War I and World War II, with special field hospital unit care for patients suffering from emergency life-threatening conditions like gas poisoning or chest wounds, also informed domestic hospital ideas about how to care for the critically ill, as did a new system of hospital nursing care called progressive patient care, developed in the 1950s by the U.S. Army to classify patients according to illnes. Four levels of care were called for in this system, including "intensive care" or "critical care"—and although the other three levels did not catch on, physicians reportedly embraced the idea of critical care right away.[37]

At the Peter Bent Brigham Hospital, Francis Moore established the Bartlett Critical Care Unit in 1954 with a gift from E.B. Bartlett. The focus was on respiratory care. As the *Brigham Bulletin* put it in an article commemorating the first twenty years of the Bartlett unit in 1973, "This became a special area where sick patients were cared for, seemingly hopeless patients got well, and a place where we had our first decade of experience with prolonged endotracheal intubation and respiratory assistance in patients with recoverable pulmonary failure."[38] Following "the visitation of the King of Arabia," another gift was given to Moore and the Department of Surgery and was matched by a government grant for a "Study and Care Unit" in intensive care; Bartlett also made another gift. With these funds, a new unit with eleven beds was built with "a metabolic diet kitchen and an adequate nurses station." Carol Paduano was named head nurse, nursing supervisors included Helen Kordis and Eleanor Toochey, and the nursing staff included Lois Toothaker. The Bartlett Unit was the site of all the Peter Bent Brigham's "intensive respiratory management." In 1964 a three-bed ICU for postoperative patients was also added one floor below, adjacent to the eight-bed Recovery Room, which relieved overcrowding after surgeries.[39] The Bartlett Unit was "the scene for the care of virtually all our burns, many patients with drug toxicity and central respiratory failure from the medical service, patients with multiple severe injuries, patients with disabling gastrointestinal fistulae, and many patients after open-heart surgery."

> *Any such group of very sick patients will naturally have a very high and prolonged morbidity and a considerable mortality. But from the beginning it has been the conviction of Dr. Moore, Dr. Morgan, Dr. Collins, Dr. O'Connor and the others concerned with the management of these patients, that this precious social resource of intensive care should not be wasted on hopelessly ill patients such as those with terminal cancer. They should be kept as comfortable as possible, given every comfort and assurance, but there should be a conscious avoidance of modern Intensive Care techniques merely to prolong the end stages of a ravaging disease...*
>
> *Although any Intensive Care Unit sees many tragedies each year as patients...succumb to their injuries or illnesses, the Unit also has a remarkable record of returning to their home and to society, completely well and recovered, hundreds of patients who otherwise would have been lost. There are hundreds of patients who owe their lives to the Bartlett Unit.*[40]

Nursing was essential to the success of the Bartlett Unit, as was continuing education of nurses and the expanding nursing role. As the 1963-1964 annual report stated:

> *With the rapid increase of new clinical programs in medicine and surgery, we see the generalized staff nurse at this hospital evolving into a clinical nursing specialist, having to assume new and greater responsibilities. With the establishment of Intensive Care and Cardiac Monitoring Units and the expansion of organ transplant and thoracic surgical programs, it is essential that the nurse practitioner have a broad scientific background, specialized knowledge, increased technical skill and the ability to participate in medical and nursing research.*[41]

At BWH, several early critical care nurses have gone on to major leadership roles at the hospital.

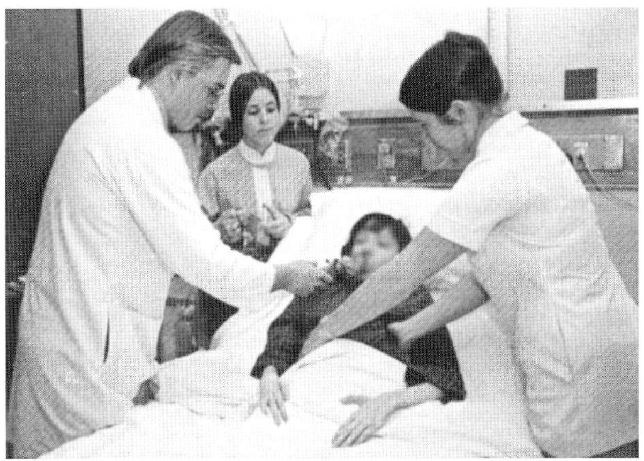

FIGURE 5-21 The Bartlett Unit, February 1973. A patient recovering from respiratory failure is given treatment by James Berryman, Technical Director of Respiratory Care; Carolyn Rogers, Bartlett Unit staff nurse; and Kathryn Melhado, Supervisor of Chest Physiotherapy.

Mairead Hickey, now executive vice-president and chief operating officer at BWH, was a critical care nurse at the Peter Bent Brigham in the 1970s and worked in the Bartlett Unit. She recalls that this was an exciting time to be part of a clinical team that was at the forefront of new technologies and innovations to advance care and treatments for patients. "It was a time in which cardiac surgery was relatively new and the volume was rapidly increasing. I still remember the drama and sounds of the Bartlett Unit doors flying open as the surgery and anesthesia teams rushed their postoperative cardiac surgery patient from the operating room to a bed where they were greeted by nurses and respiratory therapists who would join the clinical team. This was the beginning of what we now refer to as a 'hand off.'"

By 1972 Brigham surgeons were performing six to eight open heart operations per week.[42] Hickey says that this was a period when much of what is taken for granted in the ICU today was first being developed. New technologies such as the membrane oxygenator (an early prototype of extracorporeal membrane oxygenation), advancements in mechanical ventilation, and long-term hyperalimentation were examples of early translational research at the bedside. She recalls bed to bedside research as being "the norm." Hickey remembers working with critically wounded patients as well. "We cared for patients with huge burns. There was a crash at Logan Airport in the 70s. I remember taking care of a patient who was burned over 80% of his body and we tested different ways to graft skin... the beginning of what we now do every day." Much of Francis Moore's research in the 1950s had to do finding ways to remedy the shock and extreme metabolic changes that burn and other trauma patients' experience.

Dorothy Goulart, a nurse who is now director of Performance Improvement at BWH, worked as a cardiac surgical clinical nurse specialist in the 1980s; she also remembers the beginnings of many technologies and practices that are now everyday events, such as the precise administration of pharmaceuticals via "smart pumps" that regulate how much medication a patient should receive through their IV. She says: "The degree to which these pumps can monitor and track and calculate doses given is just amazing as compared to what I did as a nurse on a general surgical floor in the 70s, where I literally would use my watch and count the drops to make sure that I was giving the intravenous medication at the right rate." The vastly expanded range of drugs available today for critical care alone is of great significance and is also due to intense research and development efforts both at the hospital and by industry in the past fifty years. Although Goulart remembers being impressed by what was available back then, "it pales to the armamentarium of devices and medications that we have now." The Bartlett was also the site of important research and innovation in the area of total parenteral nutrition (TPN), which was called hyperalimentation in the 1970s. Kathy McManus, presently head of the Department of Nutrition, says: "This was huge. Before that people would die if they couldn't be fed or their GI tract couldn't absorb the nutrients that we were giving them." TPN is now standard care all over the world.

In 1965, Bernard Lown organized and opened one of the first specialized ICUs in the United States at the Peter Bent Brigham, a coronary care unit (see essay in Chapter 3) called the Samuel A. Levine Coronary Care Unit, or the LCU. Like other early ICUs in American hospitals, which were installed in underutilized spaces like closets and croup treatment steam rooms,[43] Lown's coronary care unit used makeshift hospital space. He also understood that the level of nursing required for this unit would be different from that utilized by the hospital previously and that nurses who cared for patients there would require further training. He writes: "The 14 young Brigham nurses whom we recruited were given a three-week course in electrocardiography, arrhythmia recognition, emergency cardiovascular medicine, and cardiopulmonary resuscitation . . . I have never since encountered a brighter, more committed, and more enthusiastic group of nurses."

In addition: "Nurses assumed a major role in patient management. They participated in morning rounds and invariably had much to contribute. They alerted physicians to significant heart rhythm changes, and instituted prompt lidocaine prophylaxis. They were the first responders to cardiac arrest. To combat depersonalization that might be brought on by cutting-edge technology, nurses related interpersonally to the patients. In addition, nurse-led weekly family rounds explored the social dimensions of a patient's illness."

As a 1965 guide to coronary care stated, the success of these new units was "predicated almost wholly on the ability of nurses to assume a new and different role."[44] George Thorn's report on the Department of Medicine in the 1966-1967 Peter Bent Brigham Hospital Annual Report noted: "Even more important than the outstanding technical devices built especially for this unit are the effectively trained group of nurses responsible for the minute-to-minute supervision of these dangerously ill patients."[45]

In his report on the LCU in the same year, Lown noted that the mortality rate continued to be "remarkably low" and that a primary element in the success of the unit was "the devotion and hard work of the nurses," including three "pioneering members" of the original staff: B.J. (Betty Jane) Bonneville, head nurse; Yvonne Schmidt, director of nursing education; and Patricia Parente.[46]

Margaret (Peggy) Bernazzani, a Peter Bent Brigham School of Nursing graduate and currently a nurse in the BWH Surgical ICU as well as a nominee for the 2012 Essence of Nursing Award, started working at the Peter Bent Brigham right out of school in 1976 and moved to the Bartlett Unit in 1977. She says: "The relationship between nurses and doctors changed when I moved from floor to ICU. There was a degree of respect from the doctors that I didn't appreciate when I worked on the floor. It was as though there was recognition that the nursing care is not routine, but rather that the nurse is putting in more thought, making a larger contribution to the patient's plan of care and its execution. Through the years this sliver of respect has evolved into a collaborative relationship which is tremendously rewarding as an active contributing member of the healthcare team."

Although the ICU could be a site where nurses could demonstrate their significant technical skills and scientific knowledge, the new ICUs could also be difficult for caregivers emotionally, as the *Brigham Bulletin* had implied about the Bartlett Unit. ICU nurses all over the country were now being confronted "with an unrelenting stream of physiologically fragile, disfigured, often comatose patients and the daily occurrence of death." By 1978, the Affiliated Hospitals Center chaplain, William Leach, was holding meetings with a nursing group on "stresses associated with intensive care." The chaplaincy also offered a weekly open-ended discussion group for hospital staff on Human Aspects of Medical Care, where there was "a particular and prolonged emphasis on subjects that had to do with involvement of patients and staff in treatments that demonstrate the effect and power of modern technology. We dealt with many ethical issues, the meaning and power of money in medicine, and several unusual 'case histories' that affected the discussants in some profound way."[47]

Ongoing courses in ICU nursing associated with both the Bartlett Unit and the LCU were available at the Peter Bent Brigham Hospital all through the 1960s and in subsequent decades, and ICU-related courses and rounds continue at BWH into the

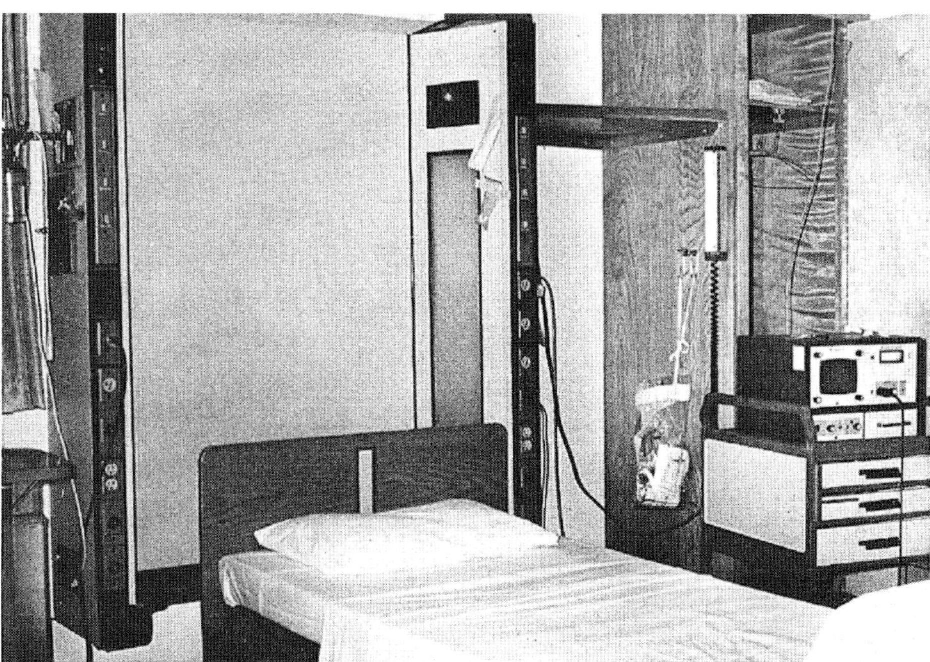

FIGURE 5-22 Photo from the Brigham Bulletin, October 1974, from an article about the renovation of the Levine Cardiac Unit.

present. At the same time, "nurses taught the physicians how the patients responded to treatment and what patient behavior to expect during the course of illness."[48] The increase in responsibility accorded to ICU nurses could be dramatic.

> *Thus, in a matter of months, nurses who previously had been forbidden to give aspirin for headaches found themselves restarting stopped hearts. Nurses reached an accommodation with physicians, a way to collaborate, by articulating a clear conception of critical care nursing, that is, intervening to stabilize the condition of unstable patients. Most important, nurses and physicians learned to trust each other as each practiced his or her own area of expertise.*[49]

In 1978, the head of nursing wrote: "The past year has also been noteworthy from the standpoint of experiencing an increasing number of more acutely ill patients. Review of types of surgical procedures and of admissions by primary and secondary diagnostic category provides the basis for this conclusion. Nursing care in the intensive care units (ICU) has reached a level where it is routine to provide a single nurse for a single patient for 22 out of 24 hours."

The number of patients needing high levels of care continued to develop, and the hospital also established "secondary care units" where: "the nursing coverage, although not as intense as in the ICU, far exceeds that of a standard medical-surgical unit. This trend toward treating increasing numbers of intensively ill patients has been gradual but continuous."[50]

Peggy Bernazzani says: "ICU nursing is very different from nursing in other parts of the hospital. It is an opportunity to practice true primary nursing, allowing the nurse the ability to care for all the patient's needs . . . The ICU patient, as the most vulnerable with their multisystem insults, provides the healthcare team with the ultimate challenge of care. In my mind, the ICU nurse becomes the truest, purest advocate for her patient."

As part of the 1980 BWH merger, the Peter Bent Brigham Bartlett Unit was divided into three separate ICUs: a cardiac surgical unit, a burn-trauma unit, and a general surgical ICU. In 1981 the Special Care Nursery from the Boston Hospital for Women was moved to BWH and renamed the neonatal intensive care unit (NICU), with space for forty newborns.[51] (The Robert Breck Brigham hospital had no ICU.) The additional beds were welcome; the previous year, Marion Metcalf, vice-president for nursing, had remarked: "The absolute need for additional intensive-care beds becomes more pressing each year, as the Bartlett and intensive care units run at 98-100% capacity."[52]

ETHICS

Concern with end-of-life nursing care at the Peter Bent Brigham goes back at least to 1968, when the philosophy of the Peter Bent Brigham School of Nursing was revised. Along with the opening statement, "We, the Faculty of the Peter Bent Brigham Hospital School of Nursing, believe in the essential dignity and worth of the human being and his potential for personal fulfillment and service to society," the new philosophy stated: "We believe that nursing is an art and a science which renders personal service to the patient as an individual, a member of the family, and of the community. It is concerned with the promotion and maintenance of health and preventive and rehabilitative aspects of disease including the palliative and supportive needs of the dying patient."[53] Most ICU nurses today have been through complicated experiences with families, patients, and the healthcare team surrounding the question of whether or not to continue certain kinds of care. Chris Day, ICU float nurse and also a 2012 Essence of Nursing nominee, says: "I am a stat nurse throughout the hospital and have seen so many codes and end of life struggles with families dealing with patients trying to die with dignity." One way to prevent such struggles, he suggests, is to get the family involved from the beginning of the dying process. Another way is to let the family be present during a code, which in real life can be very different from what happens on a TV show—typically a family's only previous exposure to the process. He says: "Letting them see us doing CPR, shocking, hanging drugs, poking their loved ones with needles, brings reality into the mix, and usually the family member does not want their loved one to go through all that." Bernazzani says that many of her experiences with end-of-life care in the ICU have been "very frustrating situations with wishes that the whole experience had been conducted differently." She has seen many family members insist that "everything" be done, even when doing so goes against the patient's wishes. "Unfortunately, it is rarely seen that the brakes of care are applied, and when they are, it is typically the doctors and nurses helping and encouraging the family to open their eyes to see the consequence of this futile care which was not the wishes of their loved one in the first place. It is a struggle, to say the least." There are, however, she says, situations where "sensibility and humanity prevail, and living wills and DNR orders are respected. After a valiant attempt the healthcare team and family come together and provide for this patient a peaceful death. The differences in deaths are indescribable." She states: "This particular issue with medical care has affected me and many of my colleagues tremendously." Susan McDonald , an oncology ICU nurse who has been at BWH since 1986, says that in her experience, end-of-life care "has changed for the good." Frequent conferences on end-of-life issues are available for all caregivers. The hospital also has developed the Intensive Pain Care Unit for palliative care. "They are consulted all the time now on patients at end of life."

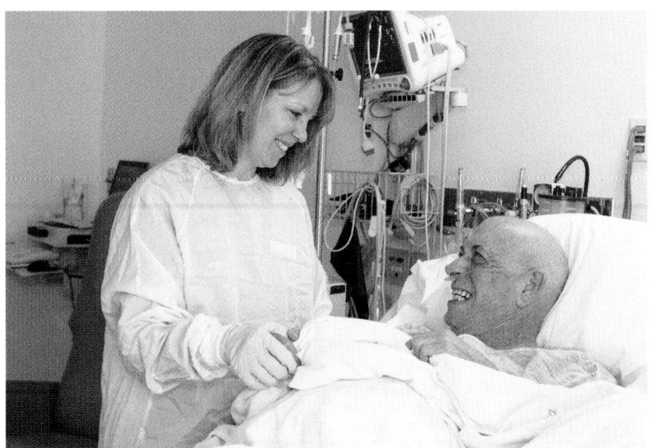

FIGURE 5-23 Bone marrow transplant nurse Susan McDonald.

CLINICAL WISDOM

Of course, the point of ICU care is not about death or dying at all, but, rather, to support patients through a crisis long enough for them to recover enough to leave the ICU and leave the hospital. Thankfully this is frequently successful, and a substantial body of research has built up since the 1950s on how best to care for ICU patients and help them to recover enough to go home. Early publications were often focused on technical and scientific issues, as of course many do now, but an important development is that the nursing research that has come out of the ICU focuses on the nontechnical aspects of caring for patients. Many experienced nurses develop not just very high-level technical skills—the ICU technological environment has been compared to the cockpit of a jet—but also refined intuition and clinical knowledge based on their years of experience. Beginning in about 1992, the AACN sought to encourage the idea of "patient-centered care." "The AACN leadership urged greater emphasis on the principles of coordination of care, patient and family education about clinical status, physical comfort, pain control, emotional support, involvement of family and friends, and problems of transition to other settings."[54] Today we recognize that the expert critical care nurse uses a particular kind of knowledge and intuition, called "clinical wisdom" in a recent 2011 clinical care nursing textbook, that extends into many areas, including problem solving, anticipating and preventing clinical and technological problems, managing crises, providing comfort measures, caring for patient families, end-of-life care and decision making, teamwork, patient safety, education, and moral leadership.[55]

As length of stay decreases and hospitals increasingly become the site of primarily acute care rather than convalescent care, this knowledge necessarily also spills over in other kinds of patient care at the contemporary acute care hospital. Since about 2000:

> *The boundaries between the acute and critical care health systems have blurred, and many hospitals are offering multiple layers of critical care from stable critical to intensively critical. They require skilled and wise nurses to deal with high levels of uncertainty, ambiguity, unpredictable clinical situations, rapidly unfolding clinical trajectories, and complex patient situations...Within this context, the nurse's role is to keep the patients at the center of care—getting to know them as a person, recognizing their unique ways of responding to insults, and advocating for them to provide care that is grounded in understanding, knowledge, and wisdom.*

The idea of "wisdom" is important because the state of clinical and scientific knowledge is constantly changing. But clinical wisdom "is at the heart of nurses' ethical and moral comportment that ultimately defines nursing excellence."[56]

Jackie Somerville, chief nursing officer at BWH and senior vice-president of Patient Care Services, puts it this way: "With advances in medicine, the number of ICU beds have increased over the years. What ICU nurses do brilliantly is preserve the personhood of our patients in the midst of overwhelming amounts of equipment and technology. They are the eyes and ears of the team at the bedside 24/7. They integrate and synthesize the massive amounts of data and alarms coming at them every minute, titrating the care based upon the unique patient response."

She also says, "I think as nurses our role is to always remember that there is a human being in the middle of all this." The nurse is there "to be on the journey with the patient wherever that takes us," whether that is to health and home or to the end of life. The goal "is to make sure that our practice isn't driven by the technology" but rather that the technology supports the highest quality patient care.

The physical design of new hospital space also can make a fundamental difference for patients and families. Anyone who has spent the night trying to get a few hours' rest under a coat in a hospital reclining chair while worrying about a loved one will be delighted by the spaces and options available to families in the new Shapiro building, which include, among other things, couches that open into beds for family members to get some rest. Visiting is also more open. Goulart says, "In

1980 in the ICU, family members could come in for 10 minutes every hour between the hours of 1 pm and 8 pm. Now we have an open Cardiac Surgery ICU in the Shapiro Center. Now a family member can stay in the hospital with the patient. The Shapiro is designed to support that comfortably."

The best ICU outcome is a story that ends well. Chris Day, the ICU float nurse, tells a story about a new mother and her baby. He had been called one night to the Center for Women and Newborns because a new mom had been admitted to a surgical ICU for bleeding, blood pressure, and heart rate issues. She had also been intubated—not a very pleasant introduction to motherhood. "I was asked to stay with her the whole time and help. Those patients can go critical very quickly," he says. Her doctors were able to stop the bleeding and the patient received a transfusion. However, she remained intubated. "When we got her to the ICU, I remember being so busy—hanging blood, giving her fluids and blood pressure meds," he says, painting a picture of the speed and competence experienced nurses exhibit. By the end of his night shift, though, things had calmed down. Her vital signs became more stable, and the staff started to wean her from the ventilator. Eventually, the tube was removed.

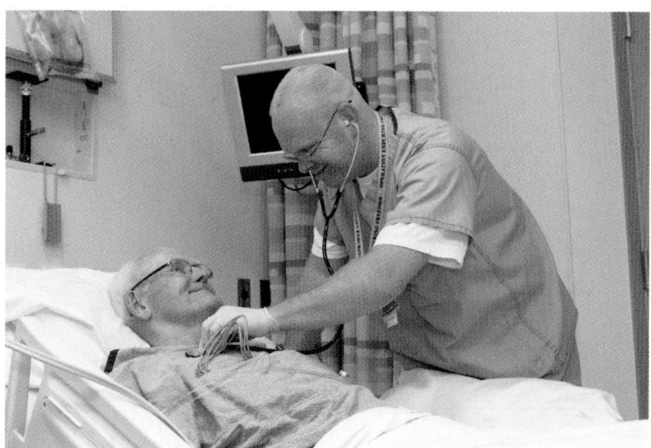

FIGURE 5-24 ICU float nurse Chris Day, with a patient.

The next night Day came to see how she was doing. "She was awake and nursing her baby," he said. "That was definitely a happy ending."

PALLIATIVE CARE AT BRIGHAM AND WOMEN'S HOSPITAL

Janet L. Abrahm

Although hospice care has been available in the United States since the mid-1960s, the subspecialty of hospice and palliative medicine was first recognized by the American Board of Medical Specialties only in 2006. Hospice programs care for patients with six months or less to live, if the disease takes its expected course. Palliative care practitioners, however, treat patients from the onset of a life-limiting illness until their death, which can be for periods of one to two years for adults; pediatric palliative care practitioners can follow patients for much longer periods of time.

What do palliative care practitioners do for patients with advanced, life-limiting illnesses? According to the palliative care professional organization for physicians, the American Academy of Hospice and Palliative Medicine:

> *The goal of palliative care is to prevent and relieve suffering, and to support the best possible quality of life for patients and their families, regardless of their stage of disease or the need for other therapies, in accordance with their values and preferences. Palliative care is both a philosophy of care and an organized, highly structured system for delivering care. Palliative care expands traditional disease-model medical treatments to include the goals of enhancing quality of life for patient and family, optimizing function, helping with decision-making and providing opportunities for personal growth. As such, it can be delivered concurrently with life-prolonging care or as the main focus of care.*[57]

Until the new specialty was recognized, and experts joined medical school faculties and teaching hospitals, physicians, nurse practitioners, and even social workers were not trained in the expert assessment and management of symptoms that accompany advanced illnesses and their treatments (e.g., pain, nausea and vomiting, delirium, dyspnea, anxiety, or depression), in the communication skills needed to break bad news skillfully or to help patients identify and modify their goals when the burdens of therapy outweighed the benefits, in the set of skills needed to help patients and their families as patients die, or in the needs of the grieving bereaved families and of the doctors and nurses who cared for those patients. Clinicians were not trained in how to respond to patient requests for hastened death; they did not know how to prevent or recognize compassion fatigue in themselves or colleagues.

My own story began in oncology in 1980 when I completed my fellowship in hematology and oncology and joined the faculty at the Hospital of the University of Pennsylvania. Then, we were taught to "use" complaints of pain to determine what was wrong with the patient—for example, the characteristics of the pain appendicitis caused were an important component in its diagnosis—and then reverse the problem. We were not taught to treat the patients' pain while we were making the diagnosis. Neither were we taught how to respond to patients' complaints of pain when the underlying pathology could not be reversed, as was the case for patients with advanced, refractory cancer. When no more effective therapies to reverse a condition remained, patients were told, "There is nothing more I can do for you."

My communication skills were so poor that the first time I told a patient she had leukemia, she responded, "I'm all right, dear, are you?" We had very few drugs with which to treat pain in a sustained way because the preparations we had lasted only about three to four hours. Patients set their clocks to awaken them to take these medications and prevent the pain from recurring. We also had little to prevent the nausea and vomiting induced by chemotherapy, and patients started to equate the efficacy of the therapy with the severity of the side effects they were having. In those days, the sight of me was enough to start my patients vomiting, even in a grocery store or at an airport. Some of my younger patients could not tolerate the side effects of treatments that could cure them and instead turned to unproven, unconventional therapies and died.

We did not routinely establish health proxies, discuss resuscitation pros and cons with patients, or let patients and their families know that when time was short, they should use their energy to tie up any loose ends and spend good time with their loved ones. Instead of explaining why we weren't offering treatment, we would say we were waiting..."until you get stronger." In 2003, I published an article about this lack of transparency, entitled "Waiting for the Platelet Count to Rise."[58] We rarely told patients what their prognosis was, even when asked to do so, as Christakis discusses in his book *Death Foretold*.[59]

Losing patients because they could not tolerate the side effects of therapy and having patients with uncontrolled pain asking me to hasten their deaths led me to what we would now call palliative care. In my oncology clinic, I used the most aggressive antiemetic protocols I could find and was able to control the symptoms well enough that patients could endure the lifesaving therapies. I learned to use hypnosis in a variety of ways with my cancer patients and helped my hospital add the new longer acting pain medications to the formulary. To learn more about pain management, I took a sabbatical in 1992 with the pioneers in the field, led by Kathy Foley at Memorial Sloan-Kettering Cancer Center. During that sabbatical I was introduced to what was to become the field of palliative care and found my passion in it.

When I returned to my faculty position, I started a palliative care team while continuing to practice hematology and oncology and began to learn about suffering in all its dimensions, which was quite different from pain. Before my sabbatical, if a patient with lung cancer asked me, "Why did this happen to me?" I responded, "Because you smoked." After the sabbatical, working with my nursing, social work, and chaplaincy colleagues on the palliative care team, I learned that this was a spiritual question that required quite a different answer and approach.

I moved to Dana-Farber Cancer Institute (DFCI) and Brigham and Women's Hospital (BWH) in 2001

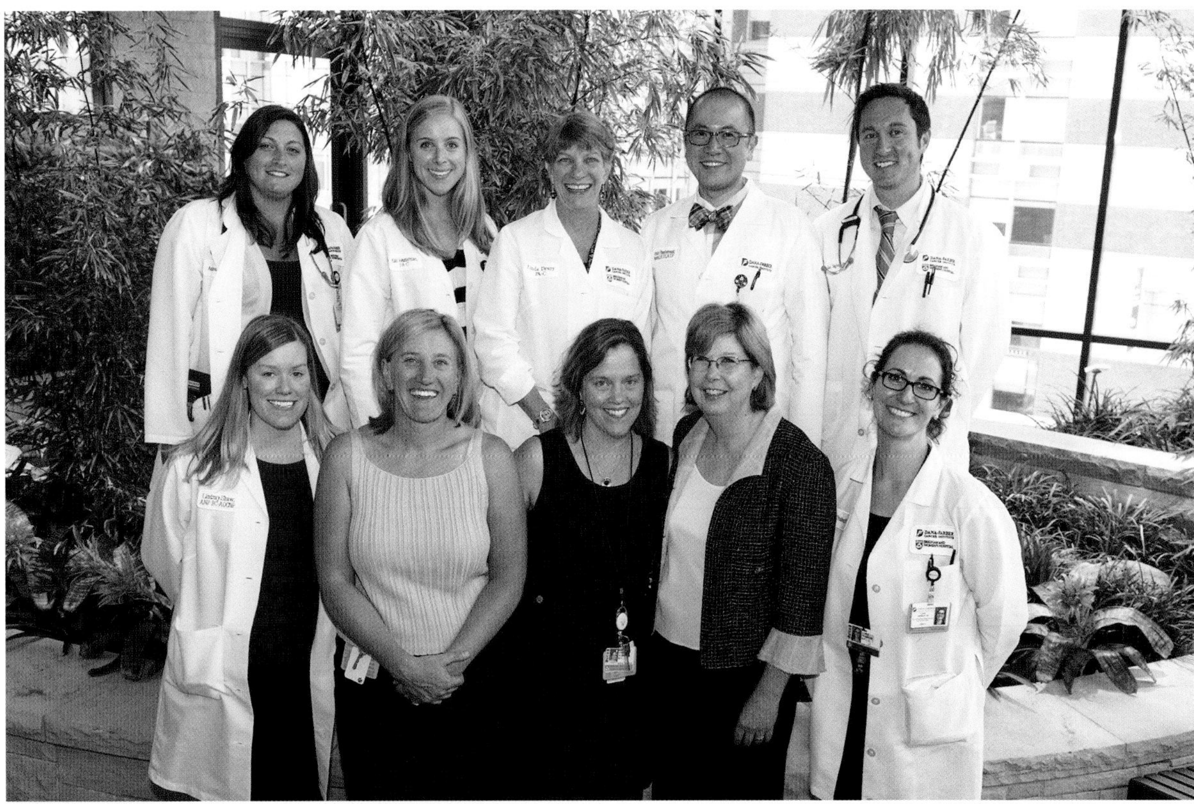

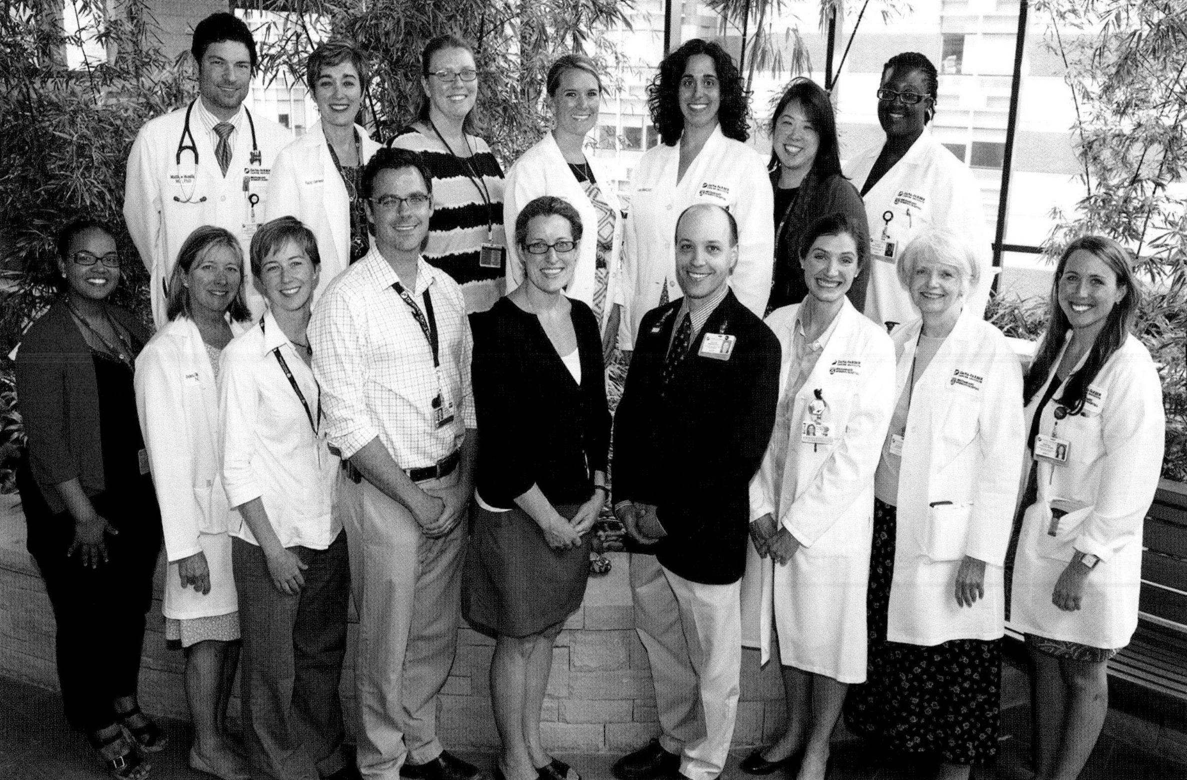

FIGURE 5-25 The BWH Palliative Care Team. Top photo: Left to right, front row: Lindsay Shaw, Rachelle Bernacki, Kristen Schaefer, Janet Abrahm, Lorie Trainor. Back row: Andrea Rines, Kate Baccari, Linda Drury, Victor Phantumvanit, Ian Nagus. Lower photo, front row: Ashley Lewis, Debra Skoniecki, Arden O'Donnell, Phil Higgins, Jane deLima Thomas, Douglas Brandoff, Elizabeth Rickerson, Maureen Lynch, Deborah Whalen. Back: Matthew Mendlik, Kathy Selvaggi, Bridget Fowler Scullion, Katie Fitzgerald Jones, Lida Nabati, Irene Yeh, Patrice Richardson.

because the leadership was enthusiastic about growing palliative care within Partners HealthCare and specifically at BWH and DFCI. George Thibault, who was then vice-president of Clinical Affairs at Partners HealthCare; Andy Whittemore, then chief medical officer of the Brigham; Gary Gottlieb, who became president of the Brigham in 2002 and is now president and chief executive officer of Partners HealthCare; and Edward Benz, president of DFCI, all had the vision to support and nurture our palliative care programs. They all told me it was the right thing to do, and they offered to Susan Block (now our department chair) and me whatever support we needed to make it work.

I was excited by this opportunity to begin a full-time practice of palliative care, to build a program, and to work with a multidisciplinary team of experts. I knew it was also the best way for me to acquire the skills I needed to offer the highest quality of palliative care to our patients and their families and to the oncology and other medical teams who have the primary responsibility for caring for these very ill patients. I continue my growth and my journey, which is a fascinating and fulfilling one, and one I know will continue as palliative care integrates itself among the other medical subspecialties at BWH.

GROWTH OF PALLIATIVE CARE IN THE UNITED STATES

Just as I was drawn from oncology to palliative care, many other physicians felt called to work in this new field. By the time palliative care was officially recognized in 2006, therefore, palliative care teams were already widespread throughout the United States. The 2006 American Hospital Association survey reported that more than 70% of hospitals with more than 200 beds had a palliative care team.[60] Though it is not a requirement for the designation, all National Cancer Institute (NCI)–designated comprehensive cancer centers have palliative care teams, as do 78% of non–NCI-designated facilities caring for cancer patients, including the vast majority of those housing oncology fellowship programs.[61,62] The Accreditation Council for Graduate Medical Education began accrediting fellowship programs in 2007, and the American Board of Internal Medicine began certifying medical practitioners in 2008, with the unique cosponsorship of nine additional boards (anesthesiology, emergency medicine, family practice, obstetrics and gynecology, pediatrics, surgery, radiology, psychiatry and neurology, and physical medicine and rehabilitation). Palliative care physicians now have National Provider Identifiers from the Centers for Medicare and Medicaid Services, validating their expertise in hospice and palliative care.

Palliative care is a multidisciplinary specialty; palliative care teams include physicians, nurse practitioners, nurses, social workers, chaplains, psychologists, pharmacists, and physician assistants. In addition to caring for patients, palliative care clinicians also support the families who care for these patients and the professional caregivers who often struggle with very difficult decisions as they weigh the burdens, benefits, and risks of the multitude of treatments they can offer. Palliative care clinicians can facilitate better communication among patients, families, and the healthcare team and prevent compassion fatigue in clinicians by helping them understand medicine's limitations, what patients truly expect from them, and how to grieve for the patients they have cared for who have died.

The development of palliative care clinical programs throughout the United States is due in large part to the efforts of the national Center to Advance Palliative Care (CAPC). As of 2008, CAPC had trained thousands of administrators and clinicians in more than 1,200 hospitals throughout the country in its six Palliative Care Leadership Centers and through national seminars, media-awareness activities, and online resources (http://www.capc.org). CAPC's practical online tools enable the collection and analysis of the financial, operational, clinical, and customer data needed to convince hospital administrators that palliative care for adults and children is not only the right thing to do but also cost-effective.[63] In 2008, CAPC's founder, Diane Meier, received a MacArthur Award for her pioneering work in palliative medicine.

PALLIATIVE CARE AT BWH AND DFCI

BWH and DFCI have been at the forefront in embracing palliative care. In 2001, the Pain and Palliative Care Team began its work at DFCI and BWH as a part of the Division of Psychosocial Oncology and Palliative Care within Medical Oncology at DFCI and the Department of Medicine at BWH. The first team included a physician, nurse practitioner, and pharmacist, who consulted only on DFCI outpatients and cancer patients at BWH.

As of 2012, the division has grown into the Department of Psychosocial Oncology and Palliative Care, and the team is now the Adult Palliative Care Division of that department. It includes nine physicians (two of whom spend 80% of their time in research), five inpatient and one outpatient nurse practitioners, a program nurse, two pharmacists, three social workers, five physician assistants, and a chief physician assistant, along with a close affiliation with departmental psychiatry colleagues and BWH chaplains and its anesthesia pain service. The physicians and nurse practitioners are all board-certified in hospice and palliative medicine, and they and their social work colleagues are among the national leaders in the field.

HEALTHCARE REDESIGN

Palliative care has a key role in the healthcare redesign at BWH and DFCI and at Partners. Our Department Chair, Susan Block, and members of the Adult Palliative Care Division participate in the strategic planning processes that enhance the continuum of care for BWH and DFCI patients. They advise and implement mechanisms by which BWH clinicians help patients express their wishes for care at the end of life through their health proxies and advance directives, and they work continually to improve the quality of care we deliver by participation in directed projects related to innovative healthcare delivery. We have mentored clinicians growing palliative care programs at Newton Wellesley and Faulkner Hospitals and DFCI community affiliate practices. We also participate in research projects designed to improve symptom management and design and lead innovative research projects to improve the quality of conversations and documentation about goals of care and advance care plans.

CLINICAL SERVICES

The clinical services we offer at BWH and DFCI include both an inpatient and an outpatient service. The inpatient Adult Palliative Care service includes a consult team that in 2012 averaged about thirty patients a day. The patients have a wide range of life-limiting illnesses, including cancer; heart, renal, or respiratory failure; strokes; or overwhelming infections. The team consults on patients seven days a week and is available by phone twenty-four hours a day. We are consulted for patients in the intensive care units, the emergency department, and on hospital wards.

In addition, the Intensive Palliative Care Unit (IPCU) team is responsible for the daily care of an average of twelve hospitalized cancer patients admitted for control of intractable symptoms or delirium. They can be receiving curative or palliative therapies and can be early or late in the course of their illness. We are the attending physicians, and the team includes an expert palliative care social worker, physician assistants, pharmacist, and care coordinator for the crucial discharge planning process. Our IPCU team has made gains in decreasing costs and length of stay, enhancing patient comfort, and training a significant proportion of the oncology physician assistants in principles and practice of palliative care. Our physician assistant leadership offers education and supportive conferences open to all the BWH physician assistants on the topics of grief, self-reliance, and other aspects of self-care to sustain them in the very difficult work they do. The outpatient team at DFCI sees twenty to twenty-five cancer patients a day referred by their oncologists for consultation for either symptom management or other forms of supportive care, including discussions about goals of care and advance directives.

EDUCATION IN PALLIATIVE CARE

We have an extensive educational mission nationally and internationally and within BWH, DFCI, and Harvard Medical School. One of our goals is to train clinicians to join the palliative care workforce. In 2010 it was calculated that the United States needed 10,810 palliative care and 4,487 hospice physicians, but there were only 4,400 board-certified members of the American Academy of Hospice and Palliative Medicine.[64] This is a palliative care workforce crisis.

Our division has offered a palliative care fellowship since 2001 at DFCI and BWH, one of the first in the nation. In 2006, DFCI and BWH joined Massachusetts General Hospital and Children's Hospital in offering the Harvard Palliative Medicine Fellowship, through which we train six to seven physicians in adult palliative care and one to two physicians, a social worker, and a nurse practitioner in pediatric palliative care each year. This fellowship was also among the first to be nationally certified.

At BWH and DFCI, we have offered internal sabbaticals in palliative care to BWH medical staff in surgery, anesthesia pain, and radiation oncology. We provide communication training as well as other basic clinical palliative care skills for the BWH medical and primary care residents as well as for the fellows in medical, surgical, and gynecologic oncology and anesthesia pain. We have been asked to train clinicians in other fields at BWH in basic palliative care skills and in how to recognize patients who would benefit from a conversation about goals of care and will be doing this training in the coming years.

Block leads international courses for faculty and program developers in palliative care, including a course offered by the Harvard Medical School Center for Palliative Care that has trained more than 800 graduate clinicians in the past twelve years. Members of our division are faculty of that course and are invited speakers on palliative care topics at internal medicine, cardiology, oncology, and geriatric meetings, and faculty in graduate level palliative care courses nationally and internationally. They contribute original articles, journal reviews, and chapters on palliative care topics to the major internal medicine, palliative care, oncology, and hematology online and print texts; serve as editors for Up-to-Date in palliative care; and write qualifying board examinations for nurses, nurse practitioners, and physicians in palliative care.

Palliative care clinicians address physical, psychological, social, emotional, and existential causes of distress; help patients have the best possible quality of life throughout the course of a life-limiting illness; and help them make decisions that can enable them to maintain their dignity and retain a voice in what happens to them as they approach the end of life. Since palliative care began at BWH and DFCI in 2001, members of the Department of Psychosocial Oncology and Palliative Care and of the Division of Adult Palliative Care at BWH and DFCI have made a major difference both in the care of patients and their families and in the professional satisfaction and proficiency in symptom management and communication skills of members of the clinical staffs of both institutions and throughout the world. We look forward to more collaboration and growth in the years ahead.

REFLECTIONS ON THE MISSION HILL HOSPICE, THE 1980S AIDS CRISIS, AND HOSPITAL COMMUNITY CONNECTIONS

Paul Thayer

The number of AIDS cases continued to rise in the mid- to late 1980s despite all attempts to find a cure. Tertiary care centers such as Brigham and Women's Hospital (BWH) focused their efforts on providing the best care, but despite the best efforts of all caregivers, the numbers of individuals to die from the disease continued to rise. In response, community groups began to think about alternatives to

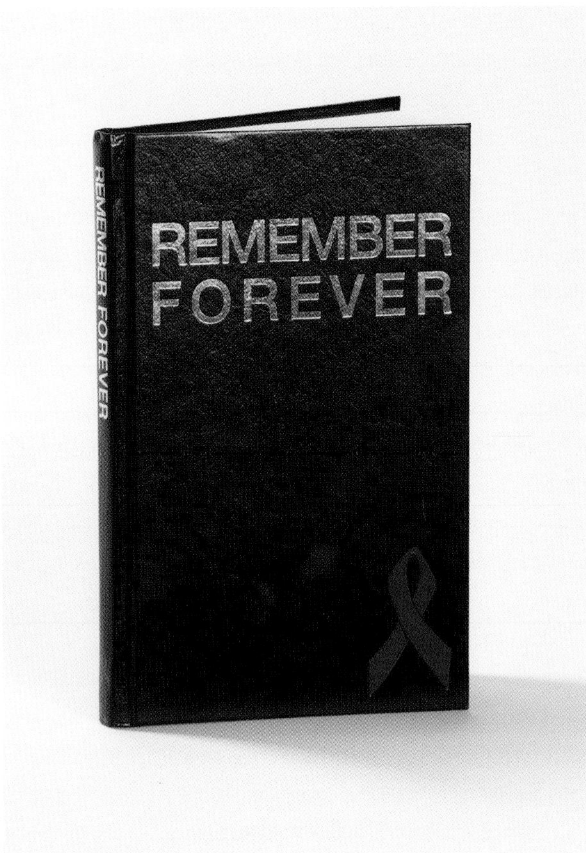

FIGURE 5-26 Memorial book given to the AIDS team at BWH in 1995 from social worker Jessica Aguilera-Steinert, now Director of Training and Technical Assistance with PACT at Partners In Health. The dedication to the book reads: "Dear AIDS Team (Anne, Susan, Paul, Scott, Joel, and all from the past and future): This book is to be used to celebrate the lives of those sisters and brothers we have lost but will never forget. It is my hope that this book will remind you of the gifts our patients have given us and that influence our lives both professionally and personally."

hospital-based care for those in the final stages of the disease. Through the efforts of many in Boston health care, community agencies, and advocacy groups, the Hospice at Mission Hill opened on Parker Hill Avenue in 1989. Brigham and Women's physicians and social workers remained in touch with patients who moved to the hospice.

Richard was one of the first to arrive from his South End apartment. He had been referred by his BWH physician who felt that the hospice focus on comfort measures and quality of life would best meet Richard's wishes. Physical pain was not the only pain that would be addressed by the hospice staff. Richard had long been alienated from his family, who had disowned him after he introduced them to his partner. Eventually with the help of his social worker, reconciliation would occur within the hospice walls, and he died peacefully with his family and his partner together at his side.

Ralph came a few weeks later, referred by the clinic where he went for methadone treatment. Ralph's mother had always faithfully stuck by her son's side through many years of addiction and periods of homelessness. Ralph entered the hospice directly from the streets, but died peacefully having experienced not just being cared for, but also being cared about.

The Boston interior design community took responsibility for designing the individual rooms. Each designer's choice of color, fabric, furniture, and design elements reflected a unique and very personal contribution to the patients who would call the room "home." Nine rooms on each of the two floors all faced the central, light-filled atrium that was the center of community life, along with gardens and an outdoor balcony. Daily meals were sometimes fancy but often just comfort food, cooked by a chef who was in every way a part of the caregiving team. Small and large group gatherings, volunteer musicians, and many visitors filled the common space with much laughter that spilled out into the rooms of those too sick to actively join in.

Ralph and Richard could not have had more different histories, but here they sat side by side sharing stories and encouragement with each other. They would have likely just passed each other on the streets of Boston, but in the spaces of the hospice they discovered a mutual respect and admiration.

Advances in medical care of AIDS have been so significant that we no longer view AIDS as a terminal illness. Because of a decreased need for end-of-life AIDS care, the hospice ultimately closed in 1996, and that is a good thing. In its short life span, it provided care for 1,200 patients. In addition to the wonderful patient care, the hospice also contributed to two hallmarks of our current understanding of outstanding care—the greater recognition of holistic healthcare needs and the greater recognition of the need to collaborate across healthcare systems.

AIDS raised emotional, social, spiritual, and political issues that were not just about a virus and a body. The medical community recognized that such a holistic disease required holistic treatment provided by a wider circle of care. Volunteers, social workers, community activists, spiritual leaders, artists and musicians, nurses and nurse's aides, family members, and friends have a broader presence in health care since the collaborative efforts to provide care for individuals coping with AIDS.

As our healthcare system has become increasingly specialized, we have learned to coordinate care across systems. The hospice was able to provide outstanding care because it recognized it was part of a much larger network of care. The hospice model allowed the hospice patients to keep their primary physician as an active part of care. Ralph and Richard were both fortunate that their Brigham and Women's physicians were more than happy to cross Brigham Circle and up the hill to continue to see "their patients." Maintaining those vital patient–doctor relationships provided security and trust. The collaborative spirit is a good reminder of the importance of relationships, coordination, and communication in an increasing diverse system of healthcare delivery.

GABE THE BARBER

(Reprinted from the November 1951 edition of the Brigham Bulletin)

Gabe the Barber was one of several well-known characters working at the Peter Bent Brigham Hospital in the middle of the twentieth century. He represents the dedication and compassion of staff members, who are often as important to the patient experience as doctors and nurses. Read his story alongside twenty-first-century nurse Roger Blanza's narrative at the end of this chapter to discover how the meaning of a certain kind of patient care remains the same even as medicine advances.

BRIGHAM PEOPLE: GABRIEL SPAGNUOLO

"Hospital barbering has been a family affair for generations to Gabriel Spagnuolo, 37, who succeeded his uncle six years ago as barber at Peter Bent Brigham Hospital.

"No doubt more than one patient coming out of anesthesia following surgery has thought that he has arrived at the pearly gates when the loud speaker system chants, 'Calling Gabriel, Calling Gabriel.' Sometimes the operator thinks to add, 'Calling Gabriel, the Barber,' but in general Gabriel is such a well-established part of the Peter Bent Brigham Hospital life that the association of his name with his angelic counterpart is overlooked by those familiar with the hospital. Only the newcomers ponder the meaning of this strange coincidence.

"But to get to the beginning of the story of Gabriel, his natural fondness for people has raised the importance of his profession to more than a mechanical chore. In fact, he represents a daily carrying out of the more subtle arts of good public relations, for Gabriel has made many friends throughout the hospital during his professional association.

"It was back in 1928 when Gabriel, then fourteen, used to visit his grandfather who was a surgical patient at this hospital, and watch with envy the activities of his uncle, Albert Terminello, who was then the hospital barber. Gabriel resolved at that early age to be a barber at Peter Bent Brigham Hospital.

"After completing school in Roxbury where the Spagnuolo family then lived, Gabriel set up his own barber shop in Dorchester. He had gained his experience by working at his father's barber shop. Similarly,

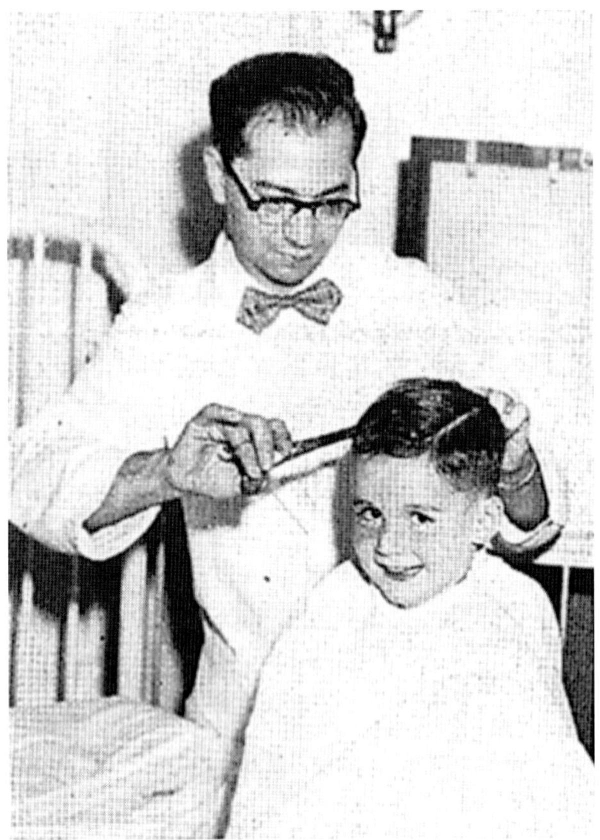

FIGURE 5-27 Gabriel the Barber—shown with a customer—little John Moynihan of Roxbury.

his Uncle Al had gained his knowledge of the tonsorial art by working for his father who was a wigmaker as well as a barber. Albert became the first hospital barber at Peter Bent Brigham beginning his work there when the hospital was completed in 1913.

"Several years before Al's death he was failing in health and so Gabriel used to take over for him at Peter Bent on the days that his uncle was unable to work, leaving his assistant to run his own shop in Dorchester. It was natural therefore, that Gabriel should 'inherit' the job when his uncle passed away.

"Two of Gabriel's cousins, sons of his uncle Al, became barbers. One of them, Anthony Terminello, went to night school, to study law, successfully passed the bar, and is now a practicing lawyer in Revere.

"Gabriel runs his schedule with as much professional system as a doctor. He makes 'rounds' three times a week on the surgical and medical wards and in the afternoon he keeps 'office hours' from 1.30 to 4.30 when he takes care of the hospital staff and their children. He also spends one day a week at the Children's Hospital doing haircuts and on the side taking magazines and other items to his child patrons.

"Gabriel has given a close shave to such celebrities as Vaughan Monroe, Louis B. Meyer, and Spencer Tracy, and has found them exceedingly friendly in the usual 'barbershop' chatter.

"There are times, says Gabriel, when very sick patients present peculiar problems in getting the job done when they can't be moved. In fact, he admits jovially, 'I almost have to crawl in bed with them.' But it's very important, both for their own comfort and for the satisfaction of the doctors, relatives, and friends, that even the very ill be kept shaved and freshened up with the delightful 'morning after' lotion which Gabriel uses. He says it is a great feeling of satisfaction to see the change in appearance and the bolstered spirit of the patient when the work is completed—and that is one of the many reasons why he loves his work. Proof that he knows his people is shown by the fact that Gabriel has a very understanding attitude towards any patient who may be 'out of sorts' and seem uncooperative. 'These are sick people who are not to blame for how they feel or responsible for what they may say,' says Gabriel, 'and I never am tempted to be touchy myself or argue with them if they give me a bit of a rough time.'

"Gabriel is more than a barber—he is a personal friend to many distinguished members of the medical profession. Among these he values highly his relationship with the late Dr. Elliott C. Cutler, for many years surgeon-in-chief at the hospital. When Dr. Cutler returned from overseas following his World War II service, one of the first things he did was to send his chauffeur after Gabriel and have both a visit and a shave on the front lawn of his home. Gabriel continued to attend Dr. Cutler several days a week right up to the time of his passing. Among his treasures is an autographed picture of Dr. Cutler, with an expression of appreciation for his service, presented to Gabriel just two weeks before Dr. Cutler's death."[65]

NURSING STORIES FROM BRIGHAM AND WOMEN'S HOSPITAL

Peggy Bernazzani, Sasha Dubois, and Roger Blanza
Introduced/interviewed by Christine Wenc

The history of American nursing is complex and multifaceted. With its connections to labor history, women's history, immigration history, African American history, and the history of technology, as well as the history of medicine, nursing is about far more than the stereotype of white uniforms and routine hygienic tasks.[66]

In 2011, Brigham and Women's Hospital (BWH) employed 3,072 registered nurses. Ninety-three percent were female, and their average age was 44.8 years. BWH nurses were recipients of numerous awards from regional and national organizations, including the Boston Business Journal, New England Regional Black Nurses Association, Nursing Spectrum, New England Nursing Informatics Consortium, the American Association of Critical Care Nurses, the Robert Wood Johnson Executive Nurse Fellow Program, the American Academy of Nursing, and the Case Management Society of America. Shapiro 6 West received the AACN Gold Status Beacon Award for Excellence. Inpatient Satisfaction nursing scores were in the 98th percentile. In 2011, BWH nurses completed the first Clinical Ethics Residency for Nurses, a collaborative effort between BWH, Massachusetts General Hospital, and Boston College funded by a grant from the U.S. Department of Health and Human Services. 2011 also saw the continuation of the Haley Nurse-Scientist Program.

The stories these accomplished BWH nurses have to tell are fascinating and illuminate the history of nursing. A book could (and should) be written featuring their stories alone. Here, however, we will give just three examples: an autobiographical reflection by a veteran nurse, thoughts from a nurse just starting her career, and a "nursing narrative" focused on a patient care experience by another veteran nurse.

AUTOBIOGRAPHICAL NURSING REFLECTION

Peggy Bernazzani

Margaret (Peggy) Bernazzani has been a nurse for more than thirty years and was a graduate of the Peter Bent Brigham Hospital School of Nursing. She is a staff nurse in the Surgical Intensive Care Unit (SICU), where "she is known to advocate for her patients and their family members with kindness and confidence" and "preserves the humanness of the care experience for each patient."[67] She was a nominee for the BWH Essence of Nursing Award in 2012. Interview by Christine Wenc.

Career choices didn't seem as plentiful back in 1972-1973 when deciding in which direction to move after high school. According to my mother, my sisters and I were advised to become teachers, nurses, or nuns. With her power of persuasion, four of the five girls in my family became nurses. My mother was the greatest influence on my decision to become a nurse, to care for others. She encouraged me to work as a nurse's aide when I was sixteen to expose me to the world of nursing and to see if I would like the "work." As a nurse's aide herself, she actually was the one to orient me, the one who taught me how to nurse, and, more importantly, how to "care" for each of the patients. She encouraged ownership, always referring to the patients as "her" patients. I was moved and impressed by the impact this actual caring made.

I started nursing school at Peter Bent Brigham School of Nursing (PBBHSON) in 1973. The nursing students were assigned to live in the high-rise apartments on Tremont Street across the street from Mission Church. The apartments were furnished and quite modern. All our classes for the first two years were conducted in the amphitheater at Carrie M. Hall. Our entire day was spent in that far wing of Peter Bent Brigham Hospital (PBBH) between the lounge area and the amphitheater, venturing only to the cafeteria for meals. My class of fifty-one was all Caucasian girls, such as myself, who had just graduated from high school and were approximately eighteen years old. There was one man. The majority of us lived in the apartments by Mission Hill, which were the SON's dorms; however, there were commuters. Students in my class were from Massachusetts, Maine, New York, New Jersey, Rhode Island, Connecticut, Pennsylvania, Vermont, and Virginia. My classmates were from middle-class to upper-class families.

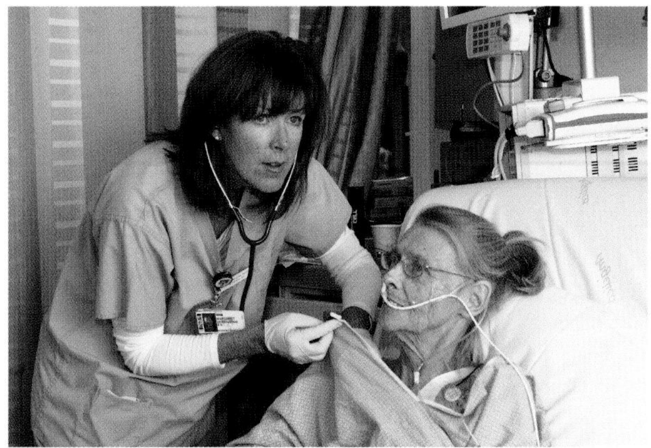

FIGURE 5-28 Margaret (Peggy) Bernazzani and patient in the ICU.

For the last semester of nursing school, a few of our classes were conducted in Emmanuel College classrooms. It was during this year that the PBBHSON was formulating a liaison with Emmanuel College. I believe it was the initiative to encourage the hospital-based nursing students to continue on with their education toward their Bachelor of Science in Nursing (BSN). College credits were given for classes held at Emmanuel.

During my years at PBBHSON, I was always haunted about whether I had made the right decision to attend a diploma nursing school or if I should have pursued a college program.

The atmosphere was ripe for promoting college nursing programs as the best program for the professional nurse, yet controversy swirled regarding whether or not the graduates of these programs were as capable in the field as the hospital-based graduates who had far more actual time on the floors in clinical, more hands-on experience. The Beth Israel Hospital created more uncertainty about my decision, when, around the time of my graduation, they were only hiring newly licensed nurses from college programs, seeking the more professional nurse for their patients.

Our clinical training began in our second semester of our first year, and we were petrified. The instructors were tough, to say the least. I think it is fair to say that "complete preparation for perfection" was the rule of the day. It was embedded in our minds how vulnerable our patients were, with "do no harm" of paramount importance. With our hair tied back, modest make-up, pristinely pressed uniforms, starched caps, run-free panty hose, and pure white clinic shoes, we were introduced to the clinical experience. This was truly the best part of the program, providing challenging and varied patient diagnoses and needs. Two days a week provided us with the time and exposure we required to help with our comfort level and our competency.

There were private floors of PBBH, but the majority of the hospital's beds were ward beds. The large wards consisted of eighteen beds in the round, with a curtain separating each bed. The sinks were in the center of the ward. The small ward was more upscale, with wooden partitions separating the beds providing more privacy. The wards were male or female, medical or surgical. Team nursing was in vogue throughout my nursing school experience. However, as students we essentially were taught primary nursing, the dawning patient care model of the future.

Our clinical experience rotated through Med/Surg, Children's Hospital, McLean's for psychiatry, the Lying-In for obstetrics, and public health with the Cambridge VNA. We were afforded a rotation through the operating rooms, intensive care units (ICUs), and recovery room, providing us a glimpse and exposure to all different areas of nursing which we could join once graduated.

Nursing school was a solid commitment. At times we were frustrated to realize that our friends at colleges were having the time of their lives, while we were so submerged in our studies with very little time to "party."

THE MERGER

To the best of my recollection, there was little impact directly on nursing at the hospital during the merger in the late 1970s. Most of the nurses conceived of the merger as exactly what it was—three hospitals coming together under one roof but maintaining their own identity. Still, many of us missed the small-town feel of the PBBH, walking the Pike, the main street of the PBBH, and seeing practically everyone who worked there. Now there were elevators taking us up to our floor with very little exposure to the other floors, the other nurses, and other patients, generating a claustrophobic feel. We became departmentalized/specialized with our one ICU now divided up into Medicine, Surgery, Cardiac, and Cardiac Surgery. Before the merger, cardiac medicine, better known as the Levine Unit on A-second, was always separate from the general ICU, but shortly before the move to the Tower, Cardiac Surgery established its own territory as a specialty, branching off from the Bartlett Unit and opening up a new separate ICU on one of the main floor wards. The ICU nurses had to decide which area they desired to pursue with the move.

The majority of us missed the variety of patients and the various specialties—there was a sense of accomplishment knowing that you had the knowledge and ability to care for an open heart patient one day and a burn patient the next. The camaraderie amongst the nurses was tremendously affected as nurses separated out and went to their floors of employment. Though friendships survived, a lot of the "fun" in working with each other was gone, at least for a little while, until the newness would wear off and everyone would adjust.

WORKING IN THE ICU

My first job was at the PBBH, in May 1976, after nursing school, and I was assigned to the male surgical ward on C-second. There was an extension to C-second called the Bridge, which was essentially the neuro/neurosurgical floor of the hospital. Upon graduation, the care model was team nursing, which quickly transitioned to primary nursing the first year out of school.

I had truly enjoyed the challenge of the ICU when I had clinical time there as a student, so that my career plan was to secure a year of general surgical experience and then apply for the ICU. In 1977 I moved to the Bartlett Unit, and I have been in the ICU ever since. It was the only ICU at the hospital, so the patient population was medical, surgical, burns, and trauma. I was paired with a couple of nurses over the course of the month of orientation, and they taught me everything on the job with no classroom time. Baptism through fire!

Once off orientation, the charge nurse was your backup. The charge nurses at that time didn't have a patient assignment. A large percentage of their day was checking up on the nursing staff to be certain that all the needs of the patients were being addressed. My experience was incredible, learning from excellent nurses who, similar to my nursing school instructors, expected excellent care with little room or tolerance for anything else. I continue to be challenged and to learn something new every day, reaffirming to me that I made the right decision years ago to pursue ICU nursing.

The biggest difference in nursing today is the vast amount of knowledge the nurse is expected to have and share with the patient, family, physician, and other nurses.

The family is very involved in patient care. It is fair to say that the nurse does not just take care of the patient, rather she/he takes care of the entire family. There is much merit in this philosophy. However, patient care can sometimes become defocused, with more attention to the family, a difficult family, detracting from the actual caring process of the patient. Patients and family members are far more informed about their illnesses thanks to the internet. However, information without complete understanding can create misinformation, which fosters an environment of distrust—again, a distraction to the caring process.

Thank goodness for multidisciplinary involvement, which is another difference in nursing care today. Social workers, care coordinators, nutritionists, and pharmacists bring their own specialized care to the patients as a collaborative effort, with the doctor and nurse providing the most complete, best care—truly a team effort.

Both my mother and my brother at different times were trauma patients in the BWH trauma unit. Both of their stories ended positively. My brother lost both his legs when he was twenty years old after being struck by a car. As a family we were and are convinced that his nurse, Ellie, who cared for him, was a vital component of his successful recovery. We as a family are forever indebted to her for her unwavering support and care, with always a positive attitude and outlook. She won the Nursing Essence Award years later.

THE START OF A NURSING AND MENTORING CAREER

Sasha Dubois

Sasha Dubois joined BWH in 2008. According to Nursing Director Ellen Clemence and Nurse Educator Erin Kelleher, "Sasha has an engaging way of 'knowing' her patients. She strives to individualize her care plan to their specific needs and effectively communicates to the multidisciplinary team, as well as her colleagues, about her patients' status and concerns. Her patients have expressed that she is a true advocate for them." DuBois has been a member of the New England Regional Black Nurses Association since 2007 and "is passionate about promoting and making health care available to African Americans, as well as other underserved communities."[68] Interview by Christine Wenc.

I was always the kind of person you got advice from even before I became a nurse, and I always wanted to take care of people. I was always interested when people became sick. So when I was choosing between nursing and medicine, I really just liked the fact that the nurse was the first and last person that you see when you are being cared for as a patient. And that really stuck to me. I loved how nurses were able to be there all the time with the patient and really make an impact in that way.

I started at the Brigham through the Student Success Jobs Program. I was hired in high school, and I would shadow nurses, physicians, and support staff. This was where I wanted to be. I went to Simmons College, where I got my Bachelor of Science in Nursing and also minored in Africana Studies and

Biology; I really wanted to focus on health disparities and barriers to achievement in health care. I also started to work at Simmons College as a mentor in a program specifically designed for students of color. Most students were not necessarily all doing poorly academically, but research showed that students fare better and actually have a better college experience and a better academic experience when they are paired with a mentor who is actually doing the things that they wish to do. When I was a student I joined the New England Regional Black Nurses Association, and I now serve as the secretary of the organization. I've also been involved in other organizations around the city, including the Young Black Women's Society. I was also on a young professional's board for Healthworks Community Fitness. I still do some things with them from time to time if my work schedule doesn't conflict. I'm a YMCA Achiever as well and the recipient of the 2012 Simmons College recent alumni award for community service.

In 2011, I won the New England Regional Black Nurses Excellence in Nursing Practice Award. For this award, you are nominated by one of your peers or someone from the administrative staff. The award recognizes people who go above and beyond the call of duty based on your work category, which may be Practice, Education, Research, or Administration; I was nominated for Practice. In my work, I bring students into the clinical setting. I make sure that they are prepared when they go into the clinical settings or if they plan to work at Simmons. I do informal mentoring and I am involved in the various community organizations.

At the Brigham I see a little bit of everything. The unit on which I practice houses medical patients, but we see surgical and oncology patients as well. We are known as the Integrated Teaching Unit. It's all about collaborative interdisciplinary work—making sure that everyone is included from the attending to the social workers and that everybody is on the same page. Nursing is also about prevention and helping people to achieve their greatest potential with whatever condition they may have. I also really work diligently on encouraging people to get preventative screening, which I think is a key factor in keeping anyone well. I also encourage people to be active and have those conversations that many people are not willing to initiate regarding illness and well-being. With a really strong backbone at the Brigham, nursing keeps patients first and also makes sure that we can advocate for ourselves.

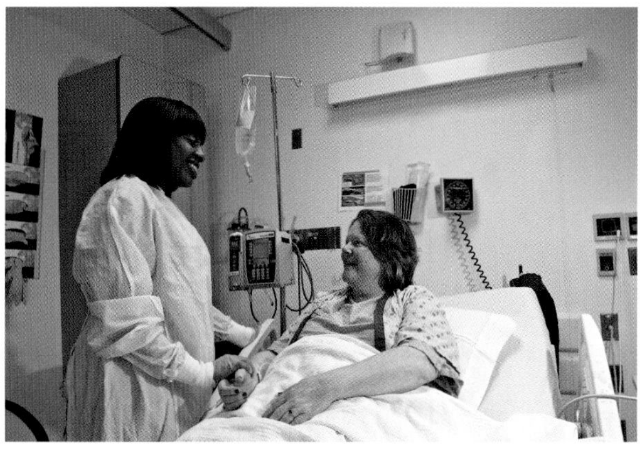

FIGURE 5-29 Sasha Dubois with a patient.

What makes it worthwhile is how the patients trust you and how they say thank you, just thank you for being here. I sometimes hear that at the end of my shift when I am going to say "have a good day" or "have a good night" to my patients. That's what makes it for me. It's those little things that really make me want to be a nurse: that I made somebody's day better, knowing that I helped them get through something that they probably didn't think they could get through by themselves.

THE PATIENT CARE EXPERIENCE: A NURSING NARRATIVE

Roger Blanza

Recent nursing research has shown the value of nursing narratives—stories about nursing experiences written by nurses—both for transmitting techniques and knowledge among nurses as well as to help others see and understand better what nurses do in the course of their daily work. Much of what nurses do takes place in private, with only patients, families, and the nurses themselves as witnesses; not even physicians see what nurses do much of the time. In addition, much of an experienced nurse's knowledge is what is sometimes called "tacit knowledge," meaning the kind of knowing that is embodied in a person's experience, expressed through actions, and is not easily explained or transmitted through writing or scholarly exchange. Because of this, the actual work of hospital nursing can sometimes be invisible or misunderstood.

Brigham nurses have participated in the recording of nursing narratives for a number of years and they are published in BWH Nurse, the nursing department newsletter, periodically "for the purpose of stimulating ongoing discussion and advancing our learning as a professional community." What follows is the narrative of Brigham and Women's cardiac ICU nurse Roger Blanza (Fig. 5-30), who won the 2012 Essence of Nursing Award at BWH. His story shows that nurses do far more than simply take pulses, monitor machines, and administer drugs; they are at the center of the patient and family experience. Blanza's clinical skills "are firmly rooted in evidence-based practice, and he possesses an intimate understanding of the needs of his patients, as well as their family members."[69]

I came to the Brigham and Women's Hospital more than a decade ago after having the experience of working in cardiac ICU settings. The experience I have gained throughout the years sustained my belief that there are miracles in life and that maybe somehow I might have been a part of some of them.

Mr. A's journey to a successful ventricular assist device implantation is one of those stories I considered a miracle. Mr. A was a sixty-three-year-old man with a complicated and sad cardiac history. His school-age granddaughter who was visiting him with her parents found him unresponsive at his home. Her parents initiated cardiopulmonary resuscitation (CPR). He was brought to the BWH emergency department in full cardiac arrest and was eventually resuscitated and transferred to the coronary care unit (CCU). He woke up in the CCU and was told that he suffered from end-stage heart failure and that his only chance of survival at that time was to have an implanted left ventricular assist (LVAD) device. He was also told that if he survived the complicated LVAD operation, he would need to have a complete recovery before he could be listed for a heart transplant. He was told that his journey to his new heart would be long and sometimes could be bumpy. After discussing his options with his family, Mr. A decided to begin his long journey to a new heart.

No one was more nervous and anxious than Mrs. A. She had been through a rollercoaster ride since she saw her husband's lifeless body that night. She just wanted her husband to have a new lease on life and spend another ten years or so with him. Mr. A went to the operating room and underwent a ten-hour LVAD implantation. This device would support his failing

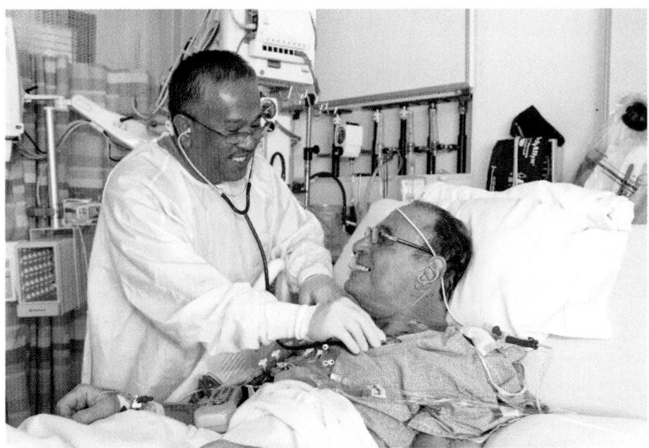

FIGURE 5-30 Roger Blanza, and patient.

heart until a new heart was found for him. This was the longest day for Mrs. A and her family.

Mr. A left the operating room (OR) bleeding, with an open chest and multiple vasopressors to support his low blood pressure. He was very sick. Mrs. A was very shocked to see Mr. A in this condition. No amount of preoperative teaching could prepare her for this scene. She was devastated and extremely frightened. All the nurses caring for her husband were very busy stabilizing Mr. A. She was told that her husband had a complicated OR course and would stay in the ICU for a while.

Mrs. A already knew the nurses who cared for her husband and wanted to keep the same nurses. She became her husband's strongest advocate. She would stay 24/7 in the room and not leave her husband's side. She did everything to make sure that her husband recovered.

One day, Mr. A's primary nurses were not on his schedule, and I was assigned to his care. I could tell immediately upon entering Mr. A's room that Mrs. A did not like me there because she did not know me. I introduced myself to Mr. and Mrs. A. I explained to them that I would be Mr. A's nurse for twelve hours. As I was going through my assessment of Mr. A, I could sense that Mrs. A was sizing me up, paying attention to every move I made, and questioning what I was doing. I had the feeling that she was trying to gauge my capabilities to determine if I was competent enough to take care of her husband. I knew this feeling, having experienced this with other patients before.

My Filipino accent can sometimes signal something "foreign" to some patients and their families. I don't take this personally, since I have noticed it can be a learning experience for some people. I patiently explained to her all the details of my actions in a slow and clear voice, for if I talk very fast my accent can be difficult to understand. I encouraged her to ask questions and to tell me if I was talking too fast. I promised her that I would not take it personally if she did not understand me. This statement made her smile. I also told her that I had been a nurse for more than twenty-five years and that I had been caring for patients like Mr. A for eleven years.

Our conversations were interrupted occasionally by nurses asking me for help and troubleshooting advice and doctors asking me how Mr. A was progressing. As the hours went by, our conversations became longer, and Mrs. A started telling me about her family, her grandchildren, and how much she dreaded losing her husband. I listened to her and encouraged her to also take care of herself by making sure that that she slept and ate. She finally agreed to leave her husband's room and have breakfast in the cafeteria.

While she was in the cafeteria, I continued my assessment of Mr. A, who was very weak. He was extubated already and still on oxygen, but the stress of surgery and long ICU stay made him a little depressed and confused. All he wanted to do was sleep. I told him that he should only sleep during the night so he would be ready for his physical therapy and other activities during the day. I bathed and shaved him.

I then asked him if I could cut his hair. He said no at first. I then told him that I was going to sit him up in the chair. It would be his first time to sit in the chair. He said he was too weak. I explained to him that it would be hard at first but it would be good for him. He agreed to sit up in the chair. I asked him again if I could cut his hair. He asked me why I insisted in cutting his hair. I asked him if he would leave his house looking like this—pointing to his long hair. Mr. A said no, he would usually go to his barber before it could grow that long. I told him that I would be his barber now and that I also cut other patients' hair. Sensing that I was the type of nurse who did not take no for an answer, he agreed, so I started cutting his hair carefully.

When the haircut was done, I gave him a mirror to look at himself. He must have thought he looked so good because even with a nasogastric tube (NGT) in his nose, he gave me a big smile and said: "Thanks, Roger, I look good." Then Mrs. A arrived. She almost dropped her cup of coffee when she saw him sitting in the chair, clean cut and smiling. Mrs. A was so overjoyed she hugged her husband and started crying and said: "You look so good, honey!" She turned to me and hugged me and said "Thank you!" Mrs. A took pictures of her husband on her cell phone and sent them to her kids. That was the beginning of my relationship with Mr. and Mrs. A.

The next day, I took care of him again. He was still confused and had pulled out his NGT. I felt frustrated because I knew this situation could turn ugly. Mr. A was malnourished and had failed the speech and swallow study two days ago. He would give us a fight if we put the NGT back. As Mr. A gave me the NGT, I calmly told him that the tube was giving him food so he could get better and go home. He said he was sorry but the tube was very uncomfortable. Mrs. A was afraid that if we forced the NGT on him, he would get more confused and we would have to restrain him, and this could tip him over the edge. After much discussion with the ICU team, I suggested that we do another speech and swallow study and if he passed, we would feed him. However, the team said that it would not be enough nutrition to meet his caloric needs and that we needed to insert the NGT again.

I argued that we might lose the little gain we had if he became combative and more confused. I explained that Mr. A could aspirate from trying to pull out his NGT again. They finally agreed with me. Mr. A passed the speech and swallow and we started feeding him. I encouraged Mr. A to eat even if he did not have an appetite. I explained the importance of good nourishment; otherwise the NGT might be inserted again. He forced himself to eat and in time became less confused and more participatory with his care.

The next day, Mr. A was able to take a few steps with much encouragement from his family. Every milestone was celebrated by picture taking and sharing with the rest of the family. Mr. A transferred to the step-down unit at the end of his third week in the ICU. When I transferred him to the intermediate floor, I reminded him to always walk and eat even if he did not feel good. I also reminded Mrs. A to rest and try to get out of the hospital from time to time so she could "recharge" and so continue to be Mr. A's greatest cheerleader. While in the step-down unit, I would come and visit Mr. and Mrs. A. As things were heading in the right direction for Mr. A, Mrs. A was now relaxed and happy.

But on the day before he was to be discharged, Mr. A's LVAD began to alarm. Further tests revealed that he developed a clot in his pump. He needed to go back to the OR to have the clot removed. I was working the day Mr. A was rushed back to the ICU, but I was caring for another patient. When Mrs. A saw me she rushed over to hug me. She was shaking and in tears and did not know what to do. She was afraid her husband would not make it.

I reassured her that things would turn out well. I told her that he was lucky that this happened while he was still in the hospital and not at home. She asked me if I could take care of her husband again. I assured her that any nurse in the unit was capable of caring for her husband and that I would care for him as well.

The second ICU stay was unbearable for Mrs. A. She was in near breakdown, as she refused to leave her husband's side. She was not getting any rest and became very critical of other nurses caring for her husband. Unfortunately, when Mr. A woke up from anesthesia and was extubated, he was a different patient this time. He was very withdrawn and became depressed. He refused to talk and participate with his care. It was back to square one and he was tired of it!

I could see that both Mr. and Mrs. A were getting impatient and stressed out with this setback. I sat down with both of them and listened to their frustrations. Although Mr. A was quiet, I knew something was bothering him. I asked Mrs. A to take a break and get herself something to eat. As I continued to explore Mr. A's feelings, he said he did not think he would make it and he was tired of fighting. I listened to him and gave him every word of encouragement I knew.

I told him that I would give him a shave and cut his hair again so he would feel better. Mr. A refused and did not want to be bothered. I told him that it would "stain" my reputation as a barber if the staff saw him with long hair and an unshaved face! He smiled and agreed.

It was like déjà vu as Mr. A looked in the mirror and smiled. Mrs. A walked in the room and again almost dropped her coffee in amazement. She could not believe that her husband was smiling again. Mrs. A hugged and kissed him then took pictures to share with their family. After much encouragement, Mr. A. eventually got better. With peace of mind, Mrs. A was able to leave him and occasionally go home to rest.

The big day had arrived when Mr. A was finally going home! He would be placed on the heart transplant list while waiting at home. Before they were discharged, Mr. and Mrs. A returned to the ICU and thanked the staff and his primary nurses. They gave me a personally made "Thank You" card, for which I was deeply touched. With tears in their eyes, they told me: "We will never forget you, Roger. You advocated for us and you will always be our friend."

REFERENCES

1. See, for instance, the 1951 address by Leo Simmons, "The 'Culture of Illness' in the Home Versus the Hospital," reprinted in Esther Lucile Brown, *Newer Dimensions of Patient Care, Part 1: The Use of the Hospital and Social Environment of the General Hospital for Therapeutic Purposes* (New York: Russell Sage Foundation, 1961), pp. 121-5.
2. Renee Fox, "Introduction," *Experiment Perilous: Physicians and Patients Facing the Unknown* (New Brunswick and London: Transaction Publishers, 1998; Free Press, 1959; University of Pennsylvania, 1974), p. 10.
3. Elizabeth Nabel, Erin McDonogh, Diana Vaprin, and Gillian Buckley, *Discovery and Innovation: Working Together to Provide Superior Healthcare* (Boston, MA: Office of Communication and Public Affairs, Brigham and Women's Hospital, 2012).
4. Author's email interview with Tom Lee, October 13, 2012.
5. Mairead Hickey and Phyllis Kritek, *Change Leadership in Nursing: How Change Occurs in a Complex Hospital System* (New York: Springer, 2012), pp. 11-18.
6. David Gordon, "Reconceptions," in Jeanne Young-Mason, *The Patient's Voice: Experience of Illness* (Philadelphia, PA: F.A. Davis, 1997), p. 82.
7. Esther Lucile Brown, *Newer Dimensions of Patient Care, Part 3: Patients as People* (New York: Russell Sage Foundation, 1964), pp. 162-3.
8. "Calling for Thompson Compassionate Leadership Award Nominations," *BWH Bulletin*, January 15, 2010. http://www.brighamandwomens.org/about_bwh/publicaffairs/news/publications/DisplayBulletin.aspx?articleid=4739. Accessed January 4, 2013.
9. Helen Shen, "Finding Healing for the Healers," *Boston Globe G Magazine*, July 15, 2012.
10. Ibid.
11. Ibid.
12. Shen, p. 1.
13. "15 YearVideo Retrospective," The Schwartz Center for Compassionate Healthcare, Brightcove.com video, 6:48, posted by The Schwartz Center for Compassionate Healthcare, 2013. http://link.brightcove.com/services/player/bcpid674388874001?bckey=AQ~~,AAAAGtzO86E~,9HXkYcv7D_n_TuMjh6EB5xkmbITH-vRy&bclid=673461974001&bctid=1968570317001.
14. Shen, p. 2.
15. Beth A. Lown and Colleen F. Manning, "The Schwartz Center Rounds: Evaluation of an Interdisciplinary Approach to Enhancing Patient-Centered Communication, Teamwork, and Provider Support," *Academic Medicine* 85 (June 2010), p. 1073.
16. Liz Kowalczyk, "Nurses Balk at Bid to Guide Dealings with Patients." *Boston Globe*, March 21, 2012. http://www.boston.com/news/local/massachusetts/articles/2012/03/21/nurses_balk_at_bid_to_guide_dealings_with_patients/. Accessed January 4, 2013.
17. Lown and Manning, p. 1073.
18. "History," MGH Social Service. Accessed June 11, 2012.
19. Alice M. Cheney, "Social Service," *Second Annual Report of the Peter Bent Brigham Hospital for the Year 1915* (Cambridge, MA: The University Press, 1916), pp. 38-9.
20. *Peter Bent Brigham Hospital Fiftieth Annual Report, 1962-1963,* p. 153.
21. At this time, PBBH, RBBH, and BHW still presented separate division (including departmental) reports in the Affiliated Hospitals Center Annual Report.
22. Barbara W. Hewitt, "Report of the Department of Social Work," *Affiliated Hospitals Center 1979 Annual Report* (1979), p. 106.
23. Hewitt was director of social work in the "PBBH Division" of the Affiliated Hospitals Center; 1979 was its last year of existence.

24. "BWH Celebrates Social Work Month," *BWH Bulletin*, March 13, 2009. http://www.brighamandwomens.org/about_bwh/publicaffairs/news/publications/DisplayBulletin.aspx?articleid=4439. Accessed June 11, 2012.
25. Information on programs and environmental challenges from "BWH Social Work," PowerPoint presentation provided by Martha Byron Burke, personal communication, August 2012.
26. "The Brigham's Nutrition Clinic," *Brigham Bulletin* XIX (June 1974), p. 1.
27. "White House Conference on Food, Nutrition, and Health," *Brigham Bulletin* 14 (March 1970), p. 7.
28. "The Brigham's Nutrition Clinic," pp. 1-3.
29. Chaplains have been involved in end-of-life care since they began at the PBBH in 1965. In 1992, a family who had lost an infant at the hospital in 1965 donated a blank book to the department to be used as a remembrance book. The dedication reads: "This Book of Remembrance is presented in loving memory of our baby son who was born in this hospital [in 1965], but lived for only a few short hours. Time is a great healer of sorrow but memories should be cherished." Since that time, parents who have an infant or child die in the hospital are invited to write in this book and many do. They also include photos, cards, letters, and other memories.
30. This history will focus on the adult ICU. The NICU has its own parallel history, and much of that story still needs to be researched and written; the Boston Lying-In Hospital and the Boston Hospital for Women have no doubt played a major role. For a history of nineteenth and early twentieth century treatment of premature infants and other newborns requiring a high level of care, see Jeffrey P. Baker, *The Machine in the Nursery: Incubator Technology and the Origins of Newborn Intensive Care* (Baltimore, MD: Johns Hopkins University Press, 1996).
31. Julie Fairman and Joan Lynaugh, *Critical Care Nursing: A History* (Philadelphia: University of Pennsylvania Press, 1998), p. 6.
32. Ibid., p. 6.
33. Ibid., p. 8.
34. Ibid., p. 10.
35. Ibid., p. 8.
36. Ibid., p. 10.
37. Ibid., p. 13.
38. "The Bartlett Unit, 1954-1973," 1973 Brigham Bulletin, p. 6.
39. Margarita M. Farrington, "Annual Report, Nursing Service and School of Nursing," *Fifty-First Annual Report, Peter Bent Brigham Hospital, 1963-1964* (1964), p. 163.
40. "The Bartlett Unit, 1954-1973," p. 7.
41. Farrington, 1963-1964, p. 161.
42. "New Techniques in Open Heart Surgery," *Brigham Bulletin* 16 (May 1972): 5.
43. Fairman and Lynaugh, p. 13.
44. Ibid., p. 17.
45. George W. Thorn, "Divisional Activities, Department of Medicine," *Fifty-Fourth Annual Report, Peter Bent Brigham Hospital, 1966-1967* (1967), p. 8.
46. Farrington, p. 193.
47. William G. Leach, "Report of the Chaplain," *Affiliated Hospitals Center 1978 Annual Report* (1979), p. 115.
48. Fairman and Lynaugh, p. 18.
49. Ibid.
50. W. Vickery Stoughton, director, 1978 Annual Report, p. 105.
51. H. William Taeusch, "Report of the Joint Program in Neonatology," *1980 Brigham and Women's Hospital Annual Report, October 1, 1979-September 30 1980*, (1980), p. 144.
52. Marion L. Metcalf, "Report of the Vice President for Nursing," *Affiliated Hospitals Center 1979 Annual Report* (1980), p. 16.
53. Marion L. Metcalf, "Report of the Director if the Nursing Service and School of Nursing 1968-1969," *Fifty-Sixth Annual Report, Peter Bent Brigham Hospital, 1968-1969* (1969), p. 22.
54. Fairman and Lynaugh, p. 115.
55. Patricia Benner, Patricia Hooper Kyriakidis, and Daphne Stannard, "Table of Contents," *Clinical Wisdom and Interventions in Acute and Clinical Care: A Thinking-in-Action Approach* (New York: Springer Publishing Company, 2011).
56. Patricia Benner et al., *Clinical Wisdom*, Foreword, p. ix-x.
57. American Academy of Hospice and Palliative Medicine, *Statement on Clinical Practice Guidelines for Quality Palliative Care*, 2006. http:www.aahpm.org/positionsquality.html. Accessed July 11, 2013.
58. Janet L. Abrahm, "Waiting for the Platelet Count to Rise: Negotiating Care at the End of Life," *Cancer Investigation* 21 (2003), pp. 772-81.
59. Nicholas Christakis, *Death Foretold: Prophecy and Prognosis in Medical Care* (Chicago: University of Chicago Press, 1999).
60. David E. Weissman, Diane E. Meier, and Lynn Hill Spragens, "Center to Advance Palliative Care Palliative Care Consultation Service Metrics: Consensus Recommendations," Journal of Palliative Medicine 11 (2008), pp. 1294-98.
61. David J. Debono, "Integration of Palliative Medicine Into Routine Oncologic Care: What Does the Evidence Show Us? Journal of Oncology Practice 7 (2011), pp. 350-4.
62. David Hui, Ahmed Elsayem, Maxine De la Cruz, et al., "Availability and Integration of Palliative Care at US Cancer Centers," Journal of the American Medical Association 303 (2010), pp. 1054-61.
63. David E. Weissman et al., "Center to Advance Palliative Care," pp. 1294-98.

64. Dale Lupu, "American Academy of Hospice and Palliative Medicine Workforce Task Force. Estimate of Current Hospice and Palliative Medicine Physician Workforce Shortage," Journal of Pain and Symptom Management 40 (2010), pp. 899-911.
65. "Brigham People: Gabriel Spagnoulo," *Brigham Bulletin* II (November 1951), p. 2.
66. Recommended books in the history of nursing and related topics include (but are not limited to): Patricia D'Antonio, *American Nursing: A History of Knowledge, Authority, and the Meaning of Work* (Baltimore, MD: Johns Hopkins University Press, 2010); Karen Buhler-Wilkerson, *No Place Like Home: A History of Nursing and Home Care in the United States* (Baltimore, MD: Johns Hopkins University Press, 2001); Darlene Clark Hine, *Black Women in White: Racial Conflict and Cooperation in the Nursing Profession, 1890-1950* (Bloomington, IN: Indiana University Press, 1989); Julie Fairman and Joan Lynaugh, *Critical Care Nursing: A History* (Philadelphia: University of Pennsylvania Press, 1998; Julie Fairman, *Making Room at the Clinic: Nurse Practitioners and the Evolution of Modern Health Care* (New Brunswick, NJ: Rutgers University Press, 2008); Susanne Gordon, *Life Support: Three Nurses on the Front Lines* (New York: Little, Brown, 1997); Susanne Gordon and Bernice Buresh, *From Silence to Voice: What Nurses Know and Must Communicate to the Public* (Ithaca, NY: ILR Press, 2006); Joan Lynaugh and Barbara L. Brush, *American Nursing: From Hospitals to Health Systems* (Cambridge, MA: Blackwell, 1996); Susan GelfandMalka, *Daring to Care: American Nursing and Second-Wave Feminism* (Chicago: University of Illinois Press, 2007); Barbara Melosh, *"The Physician's Hand": Work Culture and Conflict in American Nursing* (Philadelphia, PA: Temple University Press, 1982); Susan Reverby, *Ordered To Care: The Dilemma of American Nursing, 1850-1945* (New York: Cambridge University Press, 1987); and Margarete Sandelowski, *Devices and Desires: Gender, Technology, and American Nursing* (Chapel Hill: University of North Carolina Press, 2000).
67. "The Essence of Nursing," *BWH Nurse*, March/April/May 2011, p. 6.
68. "Three BWH Nurses Honored by NERBNA," *BWH Nurse*, March 28, 2011. http://www.brighamandwomens.org/about_bwh/publicaffairs/news/publications/DisplayNurse.aspx?articleid=1298. Accessed November 12, 2012.
69. "Blanza Honored with Essence of Nursing Award," *BWH Nurse*, March/April/May 2012, p. 1.

CHAPTER 6

THE BRIGHAM AND ITS COMMUNITIES

THE BRIGHAM AND ITS COMMUNITIES

Ann C. Conway

INTRODUCTION

"Our first patient entered the Brigham hospital on January 27 of 1913...It is the month of Janus, the god of the beginning and origin of all things...usually represented with two faces looking in opposite directions...likened to a gate which opens either way and is never locked."[1]

—Harvey Cushing, November 12, 1914, "Founder's Day"

"By such an affiliation...the humane intentions of the founder are more perfectly realized."

—William Welch, on the relationship between the Peter Bent Brigham Hospital and Harvard Medical School

On Founder's Day and the years to follow, the Peter Bent Brigham Hospital (PBBH) would continue to redefine the hospital and its communities. This would occur not only in medicine and surgery, but also in nursing, hospital administration, social work, and other important services once seen as ancillary. History shows that while the Brigham has served as a sanctuary for staff as well as patients, its boundaries have never been entirely rigid. This permeable character has deepened over the past fifty years. Today, Brigham and Women's Hospital (BWH) serves its community by engagement—whether it is with Brigham Circle, the city, the nation, or the world

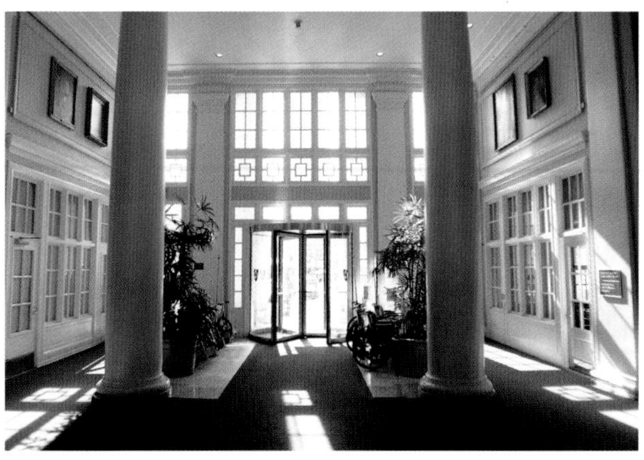

FIGURE 6-1 Interior of the original Peter Bent Brigham hospital building at 15 Francis Street.

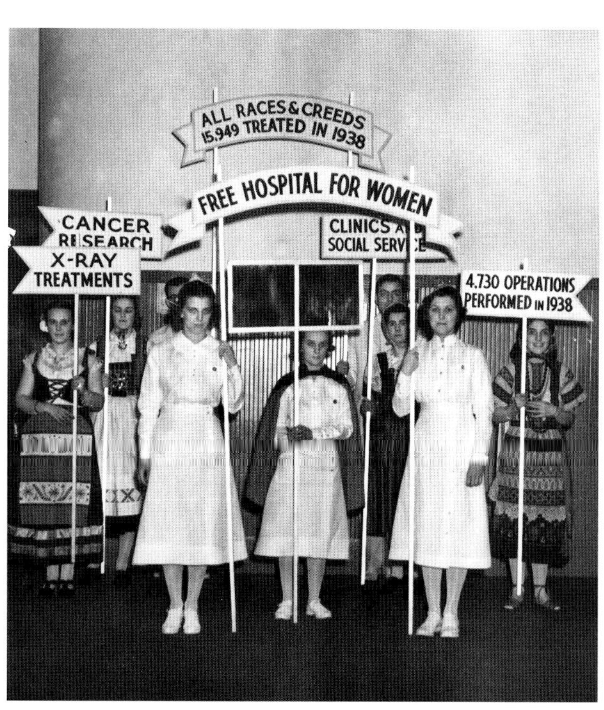

FIGURE 6-2 Nurses hold community service signs at the Free Hospital for Women, circa 1940.

that has passed in and out of its doors. It has also continually reinvented itself.

The community that the hospital serves exists both inside and outside the hospital. Underlying the vibrancy of BWH is a questioning inward and outward gaze. Harvey Cushing expressed this idea when he discussed the PBBH's close relationship with Harvard Medical School (HMS), noting that the hospital would incorporate a "centripetal" focus. This is the "inward vision" to which historian Charles Rosenberg has referred: in the twentieth century, doctors and other healthcare providers developed professional communities based on shared training and experience.[2] However, even as it created an internal community, the hospital would not neglect its traditional "centrifugal" role of service and outreach outside its doors. Both perspectives are foundational to the Brigham.

ANTECEDENT HOSPITALS: THE LYING-IN, THE FREE HOSPITAL FOR WOMEN, AND THE ROBERT BRECK BRIGHAM IN HISTORIC CONTEXT

The BWH community is based on that of a number of elite institutions, the oldest of which is the Boston Lying-In Hospital (BLI). Its story begins in 1832, when the Lying-In opened its doors on Washington Street in Back Bay.

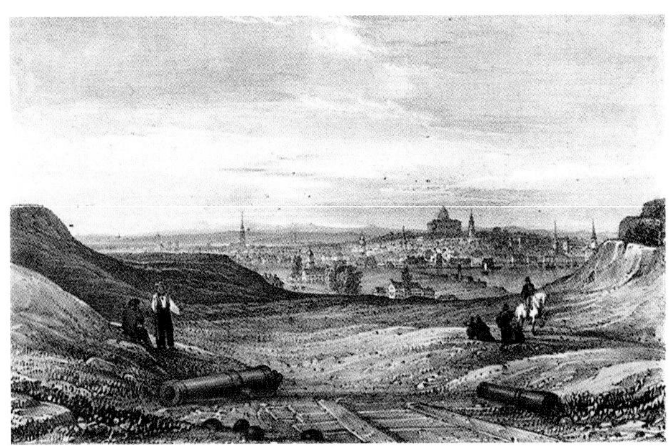

FIGURE 6-3 Boston from Dorchester Heights in the 1830s.

The Lying-In (founded 1832)

The founding of the Boston Lying-In Hospital reflects the particular physical and cultural landscape of Boston. In the 1830s, Boston was a culturally homogenous community, proud of its revolutionary heritage and reputation as a great seaport. Although prosperous as the result of far-flung trading concerns, expansion was limited by the city's tidal geography. For much of the century, Back Bay was a marshy flat, and Parker (later Mission) Hill, overlooking what would become the Longwood Medical Area, was a peninsula bordered by the Muddy River, Back Bay, and Stony Brook.[3] Cambridge and Roxbury were rural suburbs.

Though within this pastoral landscape, social problems such as poverty, drunkenness, and prostitution existed, Boston at this time was primarily "a well-to-do city in which people managed to lead comfortable and healthy lives."[4] Affluent Bostonians were sophisticated—one account notes that by 1848, 100 periodicals flourished in Boston, with circulation of half a million.[5] Its optimistic and rational ethos was that of Emerson: "Nature is thoroughly mediating... It offers its entire kingdom to man as the raw material into which he may mould all that is useful."[6] Many Bostonians were well traveled and influenced by revolutionary European notions of the possibilities of man and of reform. Its culture was broad and humanist, "defined by the pulpit, the lectern and the arts" as much as by industry.[7] Charitable reform had a religious, specifically Protestant cast, but recognized the possibilities of science to heal and serve others. The life of the Lying-In's founder, Walter Channing, exemplifies these Boston tendencies.

BIOGRAPHY

WALTER CHANNING (1786-1876) AND THE FOUNDING OF THE BOSTON LYING-IN HOSPITAL

Amalie M. Kass

When Mary Connor entered the Boston Lying-In Hospital as its first patient on October 24, 1832, she could hardly have known what to expect. Although New York and Philadelphia had provided maternity facilities for decades, only the Almshouse in Boston offered a refuge in which a homeless or indigent woman might deliver her child.[8] Since 1821, the Massachusetts General Hospital (MGH) had provided medical care to the "worthy poor" who could not be adequately cared for at home, as was the custom for most Bostonians, but it did not admit obstetric cases. Women without either a person to assist them in labor or a clean, safe place in which to deliver risked grave harm to themselves and their babies. Ordered to exercise as usual and eat plain, nutritious food, Mary Connor was the only occupant of the Lying-In until December 1. She delivered a healthy seven-pound daughter on December 8 and was discharged eleven days later.

The founding of the Boston Lying-In Hospital came about through the compassion and civic responsibility of Boston philanthropists and the leadership of several of its most respected physicians. Initiating the endeavor

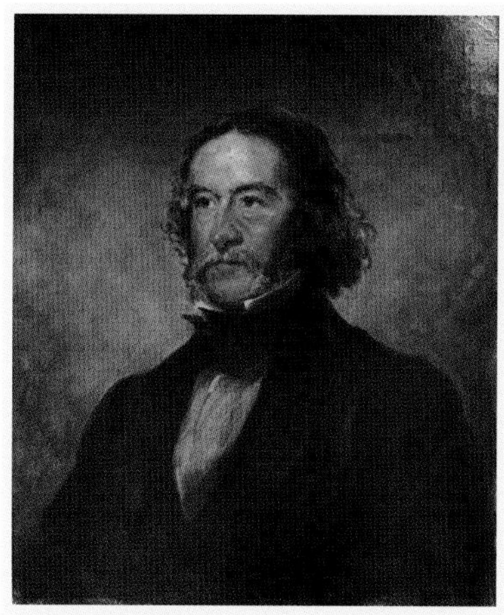

FIGURE 6-4 Portrait of Walter Channing.

was the Humane Society, founded in 1796 to resuscitate drowning victims and others in danger of asphyxiation. Over the years, the society's assets grew faster than its expenditures, and the officers sought additional causes. In 1830, a committee appointed to recommend other charities reported that it knew of "no object more deserving or more needed in the present condition of the community, than an establishment for lying-in women." The society offered to contribute $5,000 for such an undertaking if an equal sum were pledged by another organization.

When invited to collaborate in the proposed enterprise, the MGH trustees agreed that a lying-in ward was "highly desirable" but declined to participate, citing "the present state of the funds at their disposal." Unstated were assumptions that parturient women who sought obstetric care in a hospital were prostitutes or unmarried women who had sinned and that their admission would drive away the virtuous women for whom the hospital was intended. The trustees also feared that the physicians who used the hospital for clinical instruction might expect their students to witness childbirth, risking an additional affront to the sensibilities of the other patients.

Fortunately, another Boston charity, the Massachusetts Charitable Fire Society, was looking for worthy organizations to support. Organized in 1792 to assist people whose homes had been damaged or destroyed by fire, this society had also amassed assets in excess of its expenditures. Its leaders readily agreed to join the Humane Society in the creation of the Lying-In Hospital and to contribute $5,000. Individual contributions ultimately brought the total amount to more than $12,000. Legislation by the Commonwealth permitted both charities to use their funds for this purpose, which was different from their original charter. Each was empowered to designate two men to the new hospital's board of trustees. From the inception, the sponsors and trustees insisted that the Lying-In Hospital would admit married women only, thus avoiding any taint of immorality. With the legal and financial arrangements complete, a house was purchased at the end of Washington Street, close to the Roxbury Neck and discretely remote from neighbors.

The trustees appointed two attending physicians, Walter Channing, professor of midwifery and medical jurisprudence and dean of the faculty at Harvard Medical College as well as assistant physician at the MGH, and Enoch Hale, a colleague and good friend of Channing. They then named three consulting physicians: John Collins Warren, professor of anatomy and surgery at Harvard and chief of surgery at the MGH; Jacob Bigelow, Harvard professor of materia medica and botany; and George Hayward, junior surgeon at the MGH, member of the Humane Society and an early advocate for a lying-in hospital. These appointees were members of Boston's elite, professionally and socially. Edward Hook, a recent graduate of the medical school, was named resident physician. Hook, who was required to live at the hospital, admitted patients, kept case records, and provided daily patient care. Twenty-four directresses were also selected from Boston's upper class to visit weekly and "add delicacy to the benevolent objects of the institution." The trustees were all men.

Behind the activities leading to the opening of the Lying-In Hospital was Walter Channing. Although his name did not appear in the official correspondence, act of incorporation, or list of officers, he is considered the founder. He came from a family whose members fit the mold of leading Boston citizens. His brother, William Ellery Channing, was Unitarianism's most renowned minister. Another brother, Edward Tyrrel Channing, was Harvard's Boylston Professor of Rhetoric and Oratory. His wife's family, the Higginsons and Perkins, were wealthy merchants. Samuel Perkins, his father-in-law and a long-time member of the Charitable Fire Society, was one of the initial trustees of the Lying-In Hospital.

Channing received his medical degree in 1809 from the University of Pennsylvania and continued his studies in London and Edinburgh, focusing on obstetrics. When he returned to Boston in 1811, he had skills few physicians could claim, especially with obstetrical instruments. His patients had confidence in him, and his colleagues frequently asked him to consult on difficult cases. He instructed generations of young men in the "art of midwifery." He is known as the first American to approve and promote the use of anesthesia in labor, thereby relieving women of unnecessary pain. Channing was Boston's most eminent obstetrician, although he also practiced general medicine. A genial, often witty man, he was sometimes depressed, which is understandable considering the tragedies he endured: the death of two wives and his youngest daughter and a complicated relationship with his son.[9]

Channing was an active participant in major antebellum reform movements, including abolitionism, pacifism, and temperance. He was also engaged in less well-known causes such as prevention of poverty, better housing for the poor, employment for ex-prisoners, and educational opportunities for young men lacking the skills that would move them ahead in life. He organized support and proposed programs, often rather impractical, to benefit the men and women he wanted to assist. "I do not remember a day in my varied life when I was not able to minister to the wants of the poor," he once wrote, "and that . . . has been the source of the best and most enduring happiness of my long life."

In the early years of his career, Channing had attended parturient women at the Almshouse, where he saw firsthand how difficult their lives were. Six babies out of seventeen he delivered were stillborn or died shortly after birth. One woman died of convulsions after a self-inflicted abortion. As his practice expanded to include middle- and upper-class women, Channing continued to care for lower-class women, some of whom were unable to pay for his services, with the same compassionate attention. He knew the fears and risks of poor women who faced childbirth alone and understood the need for a lying-in hospital. He thus had ample experience with which to convince the leaders of the Humane Society and the Charitable Fire Society, with whom he was well acquainted, of the need for establishing and perpetuating the Lying-In Hospital.

Contrary to expectations, the Lying-In Hospital was never full. From 1832, when Mary Connor was admitted, until 1854, when it was relocated in a more elegant building on Springfield Street, the hospital accepted only 650 patients. The requirement that patients be married or recently widowed was not enforced, perhaps because it was difficult to verify stories of widowhood or desertion. Like Mary Connor, many arrived well before the onset of labor and stayed after delivery. If physically able, they were expected to contribute by helping with house chores and working in the garden. Despite some complaints, most patients appreciated the decent shelter, nourishing food, sympathetic attendants before delivery, encouragement received during labor, and advice and medical care postpartum. Case notes describe the difficulties and privations patients had experienced: desperate poverty, too many children, previous abortions, abusive husbands, and excessively strenuous work. Obstetrical procedures did not vary from private practice, although instruments were used less frequently. Puerperal fever was a frequent threat, but the hospital did not have epidemics as devastating as did many large maternity hospitals in other cities.

Channing resigned as attending physician in 1838 but remained a consultant for many more years.[10] Few people associated him with the beginning of the Lying-In Hospital until October 23, 1940, when Frederick C. Irving, William Lambert Richardson Professor of Obstetrics at Harvard Medical School and visiting obstetrician at the hospital, proclaimed "Walter Channing Day," marking the 108th anniversary of Mary Connor's admission. By then the hospital and its staff were world-renowned for their contributions to obstetrics and gynecology. Papers were read by notable doctors; tours of the hospital, then located on Longwood Avenue, were offered; and a gala dinner was held at The Country Club in Brookline. There have been occasional repeats of Walter Channing Day, but his most long-lasting memorial may well be his portrait, which hangs in the rotunda of Brigham and Women's Hospital.[11]

During the era when the Lying-In was founded and developed, Boston was transformed. Until the 1840s, immigration had been limited and manageable, in part because many immigrants chose to spend only a short time in the city, stopping briefly before moving westward for better opportunities. However, with the famine-driven Irish arrival came a tidal wave of change. Before 1845, Boston was a city "where the lifespan was long and disease rare."[12] From 1845 to 1855, however, 230,000 immigrants arrived in Boston, overcrowding the city and forever changing the social, political, and economic landscape in which charitable institutions like hospitals operated.[13]

Morbidity and mortality grew rapidly among the new immigrants. Smallpox, once virtually eradicated, became widespread among the Irish in their miserable

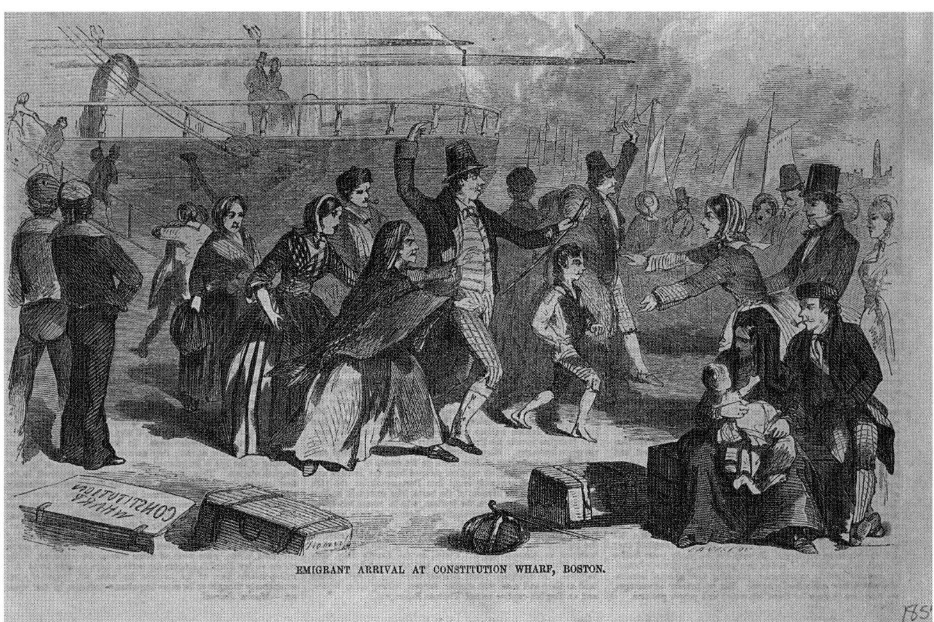

FIGURE 6-5 Nineteenth century Irish immigrants arriving in Boston, as portrayed by Winslow Homer.

living conditions, along with other infectious diseases, particularly tuberculosis. By 1855, infant mortality had risen to a level of 4.57 deaths per thousand. One estimate posited that the Irish lived an average of only fourteen years after reaching Boston.[14]

Penniless, uneducated, and ill, these new Bostonians lived at a remove from the reformers who had established hospitals, although many Irish women—more likely than men to be employed—filled menial positions in them.[15] The existing economic, physical, and intellectual community accentuated divisions between the Irish and the rest of the population and engendered fear of a "foreign group whose appalling slums had destroyed the beauty of a fine city and whose appalling ideas threatened the finest ideas of universal progress, grand reform and a regenerated mankind."[16]

BIOGRAPHY

THE BOSTON LYING-IN HOSPITAL'S ELIZA HIGGINS, 1846-1918

Ann C. Conway

Brigham and Women's Hospital's history is full of individuals who devoted their lives to their institution, but the commitment of Eliza Higgins to her work and patients is difficult to surpass. She took on her role as "Matron" of the Boston Lying-In Hospital in 1873, later becoming superintendent as the hospitals became modernized during her forty-one-year tenure.

A midwife by training, Higgins was efficient and organized. However, in many ways, the hospital during her time was still a domestic rather than a scientific institution. She kept a daily diary filled with notes about house staff, attending physicians, nurses, other staff, and patients. The terse entries mention problems in retaining staff, kindness toward patients, and the heartbreak of puerperal sepsis. Before the 1880s, when a fuller understanding of both asepsis under the leadership of Alfred Worcester and the responsibility of physicians for spreading this frequently fatal condition among hospitalized laboring women, epidemics devastated the Lying-In. In 1879, not long after four women died of "childbed fever" within the space of sixteen days, Higgins wrote of "the dreadful state of things

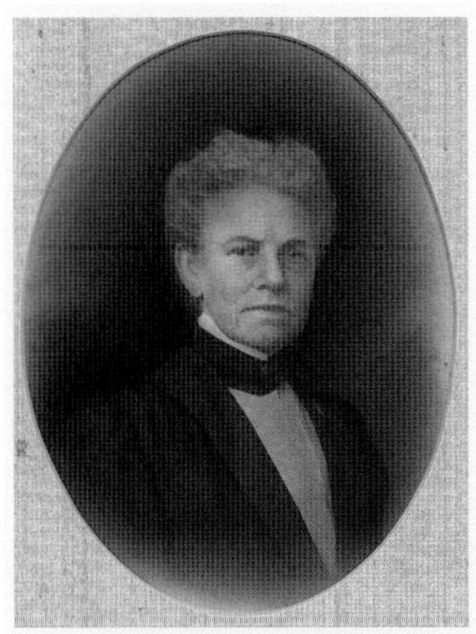

FIGURE 6-6 Eliza Higgins, matron of the Boston Lying-In Hospital.

prevailing as to the patients....speaking personally I do not care if I live or not."[17]

By this time, moralistic attitudes directed toward patients had lessened; half the patients were unmarried women, often immigrants. One of the most interesting aspects of Higgins's tenure was her attempts to find wet nurse employment for her patients, particularly the unmarried, who were desperately poor. Wet nursing (breast-feeding another woman's baby) for more affluent women was one of the few opportunities available to them and was a common practice in Boston, eventually leading to the establishment of the Wet Nurse Directory (1910) and, later, The Directory for Mothers' Milk (1930).[18]

After her despairing 1879 diary entry, Higgins stayed at the Lying-In for another thirty-five years, first bringing in nurses from the Boston Training School for Nurses and later establishing the Lying-In's own school in 1888, headed by Emily Rogers, who had trained at Boston City Hospital.[19] Higgins witnessed the advancement of nursing and understanding of bacteriology, making hospital-based childbirth an entirely different experience. She would retire in 1914, as a new era was dawning in the flatlands around Harvard Medical School, near which the Lying-In would soon relocate.

The Free Hospital for Women (founded 1875)

The Free Hospital for Women (FHW) was founded in 1875. Located in rented rooms on Boston's East Springfield Street, it expanded rapidly over the next twenty years. William Baker, its founder, had served as a surgical resident under Marion Sims of the New York Hospital for Women, an early explorer of better treatment for the diseases of women. By 1882, the FHW had expanded to twenty beds and established one of the first cancer wards. It began to offer free medical care for poor women and it also affiliated with Harvard. Planning and funding efforts for a newer, larger facility in the "wilderness" of Brookline commenced in the 1880s and resulted in the opening of a new building in January 1895.

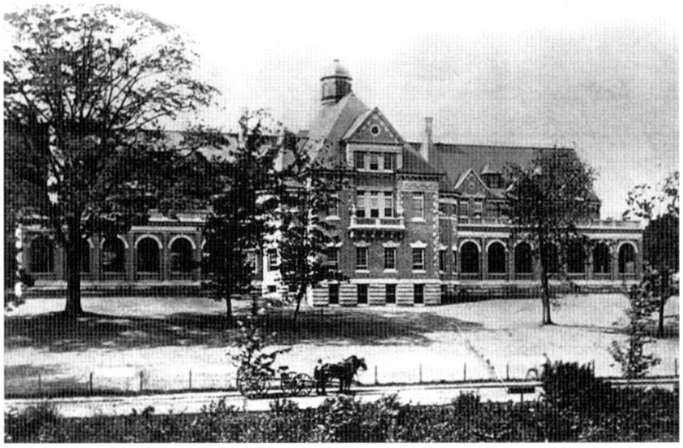

FIGURE 6-7 Free Hospital for Women, Pond Avenue, Brookline location.

Like the BLI, an ethos of service permeated the early development of the hospital. Baker was a Congregationalist minister. Edward Everett Hale, a well-known Unitarian clergyman noted for his support of education, abolition, and "liberal practical theology," headed the committee to obtain the support of several churches.[20] Seven out of nine of early trustees were clergymen, and the first nurses were from "The Episcopal Sisterhood," an order of nuns.[21]

Early FHW history foreshadows the critical role of women in funding, supporting, and staffing the hospitals that would one day comprise BWH. Long before the modern feminist movement brought women in great numbers into work roles outside the home, generations of Boston women supported the hospital as philanthropists, "directresses," committee members, social workers, and nurses. As at the BLI (and later at the Peter Bent Brigham and Robert Breck Brigham Hospitals), the FHW's "Lady Visitors" would be significant benefactors of the hospital—not only in endowments, but in practical relief, such as the "Donation Days" held for decades. They even took

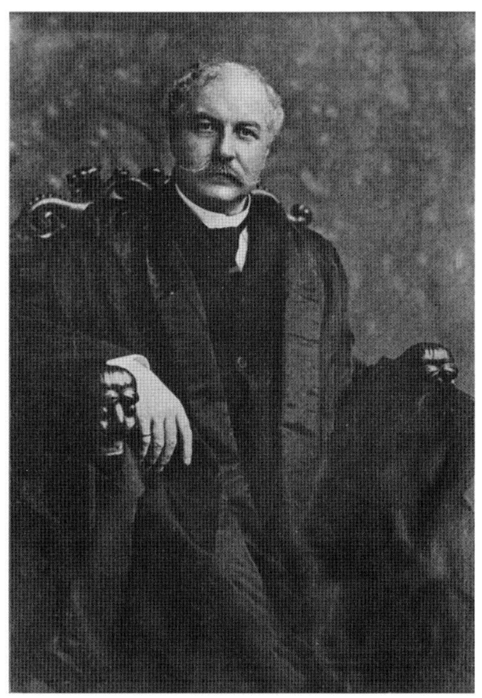

FIGURE 6-8 William Baker, founder of the Free Hospital for Women in 1875.

on housekeeping tasks during staff shortages, which were especially frequent during wartime.

The FHW broke new ground in medical education, surgery, and, particularly, outpatient services.[22] In contrast to inpatient admissions, which grew slowly, outpatient demand was high. In 1879 alone, almost 3,000 women received outpatient services, even though the hospital was closed in summer.[23] In 1900, it was estimated that more than 100,000 outpatient visits had taken place during the twenty-five years of the hospital's existence.[24]

The Board of Lady Visitors' philanthropy was essential, providing funding for outpatient clinics to be open in summer. They also took on leading roles in funding the new hospital when it moved to Brookline and helped "put the rooms in order." Later, they provided funding for electricity and other services, including free care.[25] As the acceptability of inpatient hospital care for all classes increased, so did demand; by 1910, 200 were on the waiting list for 300 yearly admissions. [26]

BIOGRAPHY

THE FREE HOSPITAL FOR WOMEN'S HANNAH EWIN, 1861-1937

Ann C. Conway

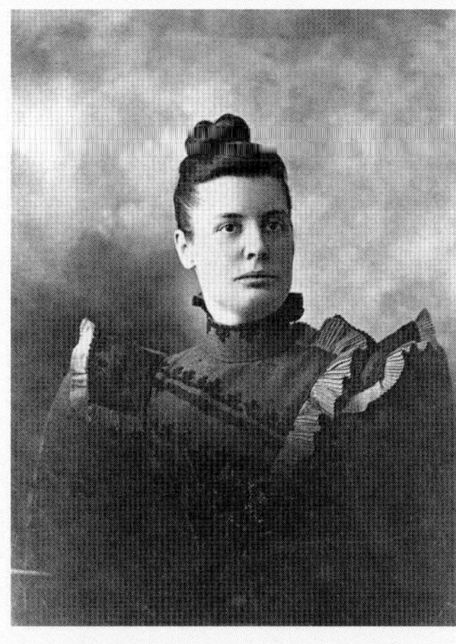

FIGURE 6-9 Hanna Ewin, head nurse at the Free Hospital for Women.

Hannah Ewin arrived at the Free Hospital for Women (FHW) as superintendent of nurses in 1895 and started a nursing school there almost immediately. Like Carrie Hall, Ewin represented the new world of professionalized nursing. She had trained at Newburyport's Anna Jacques Hospital and done postgraduate work at General Memorial Hospital in New York, the city that would become an epicenter of professional nursing education.[27]

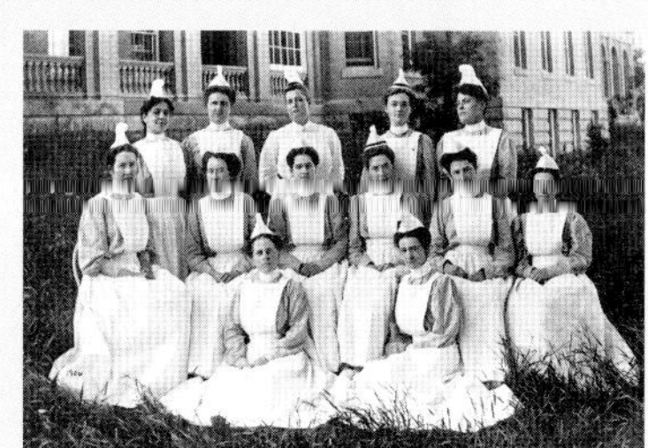

FIGURE 6-10 Free Hospital for Women nurses, 1916.

The FHW nursing school placed an emphasis on prior education and qualifications. Ewin first called for a nine-month course of study for those with no prior training, but quickly altered it to a four-and-a-half month course that required prior formal nursing experience. Students did stints in the operating room and the busy outpatient department.[28] Later, members of the Ladies' Board, with whom she worked closely, helped her build a Nurses' Home, which opened in 1909.[29]

Ewin worked closely with William Graves, chief surgeon at the FWH, who praised her "energy, resourcefulness, honesty of purpose, humor and sympathy."[30]

By the early twentieth century, the connection with Harvard Medical School had deepened: "Harvard was expecting more from the Free Hospital for Women than from any other hospital in respect to the development of the science of surgery and gynecology."[31]

Ewin stayed at the hospital for more than twenty-five years, during a period when the FHW served thousands of women—mostly poor and working class—who crowded the outpatient department and wards. The FHW was exactly that—free—until the increasing cost of care necessitated more private patients. It would not be until the 1920s that the middle class accepted hospitals as an appropriate place to go for medical care. Ewin witnessed this shift, along with nursing's professionalization. She also saw FHW's building expansion and, a few miles away, the opening of the Peter Bent Brigham Hospital in 1913, with its show place School of Nursing.

Ewin died in 1937 at age seventy-seven. In what was seen as an innovative move, diagnostic X-rays had been introduced at the FHW years before. Ewin's death released her from suffering engendered by "deep incurable radium burns on her hands caused by handling the silver-colored capsules without instruments."[32]

The Robert Breck Brigham Hospital (founded 1914)

The Robert Breck Brigham Hospital (RBBH) was the first American hospital devoted exclusively to the care of arthritis and rheumatic disease. Like his uncle, the founder of the Peter Bent Brigham Hospital, Robert Breck Brigham would make his mark as a restaurateur and landowner, live penuriously with a female relative, and earmark a sizeable estate for the "indigent poor" of Suffolk County."[33] Brigham died in 1900, followed by his sister Elizabeth in 1909, who would leave the $1.5 million vital for the hospital's building atop Mission Hill.[34]

Both Alfred Worcester and Richard Cabot were members of the RBBH's initial advisory board and helped select initial hires and the hospital's systems of care—Worcester representing the new world of scientific discovery through his pioneering use of antiseptic technique at the BLI and Cabot through his pioneering establishment of the first hospital social work

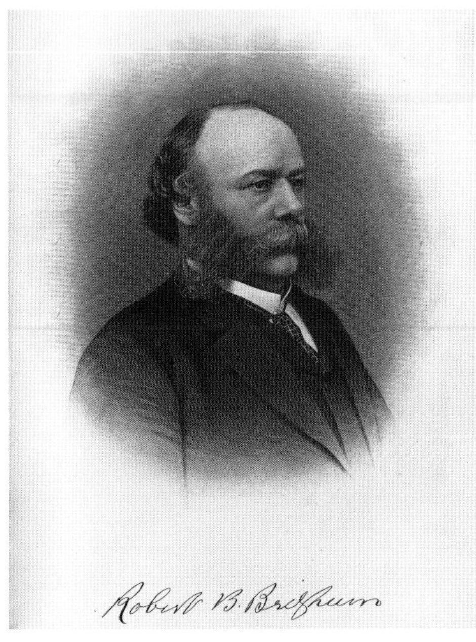

FIGURE 6-11 Portrait of Robert Breck Brigham.

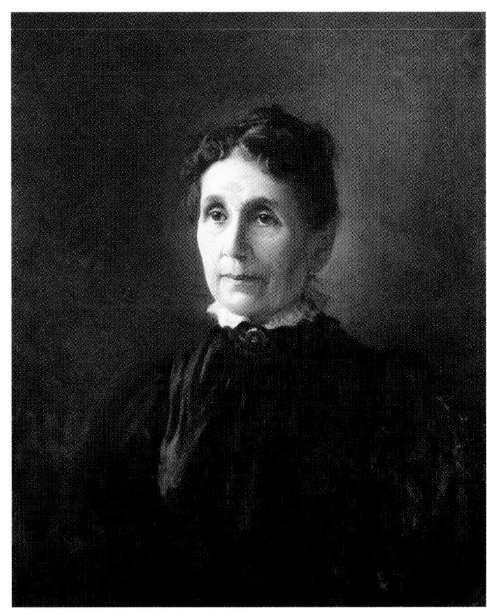

FIGURE 6-12 Portrait of Elizabeth Fay Brigham.

department in the country at MGH and his emphasis on the holistic nature of patient care. As Cabot wrote: "Beyond the special disease of a special child or adult who comes to us in the dispensary stands a family problem, ultimately a community problem, poverty, bad housing, and food, bad habits, and associations, ignorance of the ways and means of making a clean and healthy life on scanty means."[35]

Like the PBBH, the RBBH was established on the cusp of the modern hospital era; thus its history elucidates a conflict between the nineteenth-century concept of the hospital as a solely charitable institution for the indigent and its modern form as an institution devoted to research and teaching. Although the RBBH gave a considerable amount of free care, its endowment was never large, and care for the indigent became more and more expensive with each technological advance. In 1925, the hospital was taken to court by one trustee who charged that, by admitting curable patients and paying patients, the RBBH was not adhering to the founder's will. The remainder of trustees disagreed, and in 1926 the court ruled in their favor.[36]

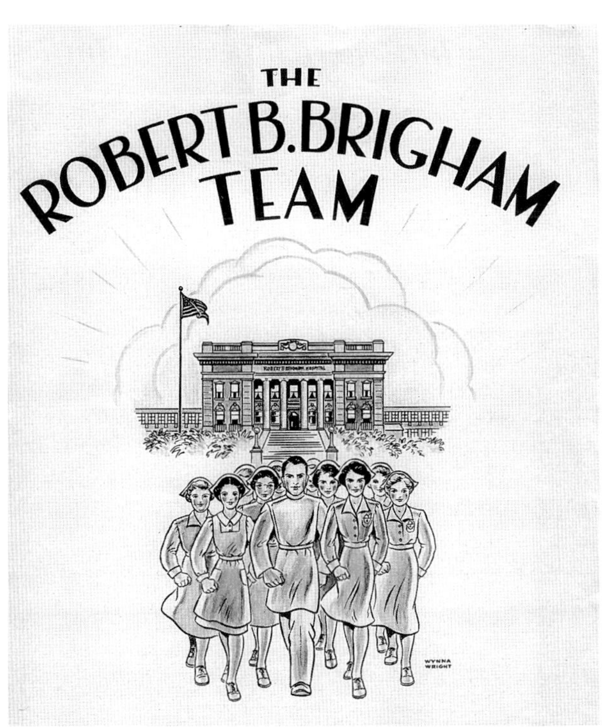

FIGURE 6-13 Robert Breck Brigham "Team" sheet music.

The foundational belief that the hospital's mission was for those people who were suffering from chronic diseases, not for the diseases themselves,[37] came from orthopedic surgeon Joel Goldthwaite, a remarkable figure in the history of orthopedic surgery and an original trustee of the RBBH hospital corporation. A specialist in rheumatic fever, Goldthwaite was concerned about the lack of facilities for "adult cripples." By 1899, he had established MGH's original outpatient department and first orthopedic ward. He had also created Boston's first clinic for adults with disabilities, located at Dorchester's Carney hospital.

Goldthwaite was instrumental in choosing the initial staff for the RBBH and establishing the social service and occupational therapy departments. Later, he was to be involved in the development of physical therapy as a profession. One of the hallmarks of RBBH's care was its "consultation" model for patients—that not simply one physician would be responsible for patients, but a team.

The RBBH also was responsible for the first hospital-based occupational therapy (OT) department in the country as well as the eventual separation of physical therapy and OT. In keeping with the rapid development of professionalized nursing education, the hospital also established a school for practical nurses, which focused on orthopedic nursing and was extant from 1924-1951.[38]

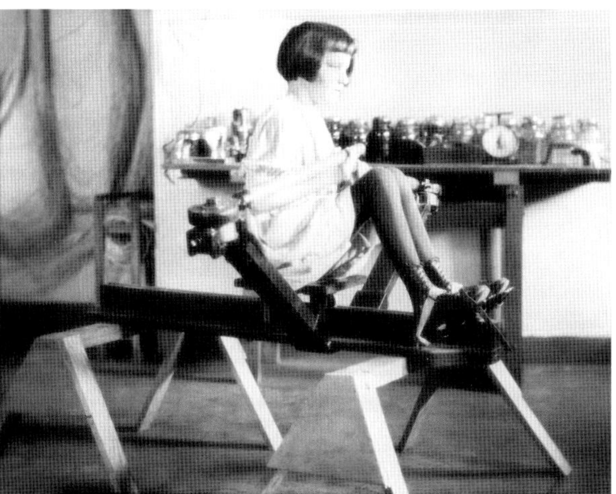

FIGURE 6-14 Robert Breck Brigham Hospital physical therapy, 1920s.

In future years, RBBH would contribute to many areas, including a vast expansion of research through a Clinical Research Center. But its culture would remain distinctive because of its location, its small size, and the nature of its patient care. Prior to World War II, some patients stayed for months or even years. Even after hospital stays shortened, staff at every level established particularly long and close relationships with patients.

SPOTLIGHT

HISTORY OF FAULKNER HOSPITAL

Cara Marcus

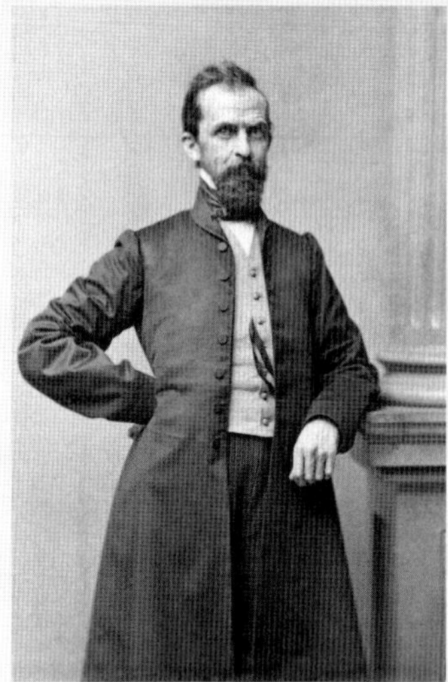

FIGURE 6-15 George Faulkner, founder of Faulkner Hospital.

On December 5, 1900, Faulkner Hospital was incorporated with funds received from George Faulkner and his late wife Abby's estate in memory of their beloved daughter Mary.[39] Hospital founder George Faulkner (1819-1911) was born in Billerica, Massachusetts, and received his MD from Harvard Medical School in 1847. He was a familiar and venerated figure in Jamaica Plain. "Comfort, support and cheer your patient" was his maxim, and he endowed the hospital with its own creed: "The patient is at the hub of the wheel."[40,41]

Faulkner Hospital, a twenty-six-bed "free" hospital given to the old town of Old West Roxbury, opened for its first two patients on March 9, 1903. The three-story hospital afforded sanitary and hygienic advantages, stood on a high, southerly slope of seven acres, and received abundant sunshine and fresh air.[42] The French Renaissance style building was made of red brick laid in white mortar with elaborate cream terracotta and granite and copper trimmings.[43] Wards were separated into male and female units. The operating room boasted a glass roof and side wall, which afforded an abundance of light.[44]

During the first twenty months, physicians at the hospital treated 514 patients, provided 3,043 hours of free treatment, performed 277 operations, and welcomed twenty-three newborns. Early patients included a blacksmith, icemen, lamplighter, charwoman, and "maker of mathematical instruments."[45] The hospital was originally purported for all medical and surgical cases that were not contagious, although the latter intent was not realized. The hospital's first patients included those with typhoid fever, bronchitis, and malaria.[46]

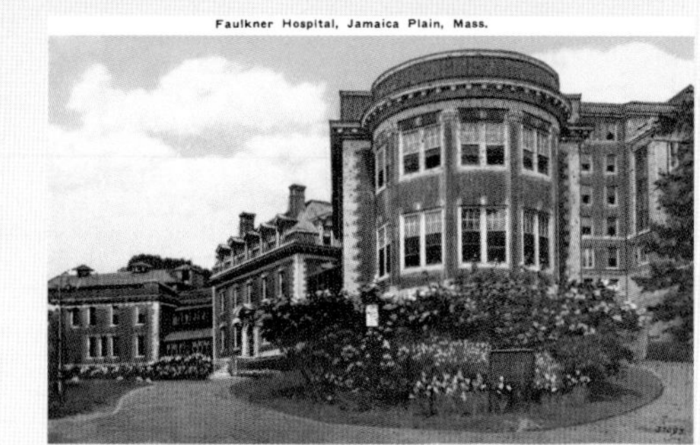

FIGURE 6-16 Faulkner Hospital, 1905.

The original medical staff consisted of an advisory physician, an advisory surgeon, and four additional physicians. Papers by Faulkner Hospital staff were published as early as 1906. Some of the first cases described a tumor removed with "marked benefit to the patient," stomach-ache following a hearty meal of clams, girdle pains, and the successful passage of a flower corsage pin from the stomach of a fifteen-year-old boy.[47] An official Medical Department was opened in 1930 and a doctor with the title of Physician to the Faulkner Hospital was hired in 1932. Faulkner Hospital became fully accredited by the Joint Commission on Accreditation of Healthcare Organizations in 1954.

Faulkner Hospital has served as a major teaching hospital to Harvard and Tufts Medical Schools as well as many other academic institutions. Throughout the years, Faulkner has affiliated with academic programs that included Boston College, Boston University, Bunker Hill Community College, Emmanuel College, Harvard University, Labouré College, Massachusetts College of Pharmacy, Northeastern University, Roxbury Community College, Simmons College, and Tufts University. With these affiliations, the hospital sponsored an array of medical, nursing, laboratory, and pharmacy student programs, residency programs, fellowships, internships, and postgraduate training. The educational focus extended into patient education, extensive community education, and comprehensive staff training programs as well.

Faulkner Hospital opened its own Training School for Nurses in March 1903, on the same day the hospital opened, with nine pupils under the direction of the superintendent. Applicants in the early years of the Training School (which was limited to twenty-one- to thirty-five-year-old unmarried women) had to pass an examination in English and practical arithmetic.[48] The school updated its policy in 1962 to allow students to marry, and in 1970 the first two male students entered the school.[49] The School of Nursing continued for seventy-five years to graduate hundreds of nurses who worked all around the world.

The 1930s heralded the hospital's first major enlargement of medical services, with the introduction of Physiotherapy and Tumor Clinics and Departments of Neurology, Bronchoscopy, Anesthesia, and Occupational Therapy, as well as a laboratory technical course and the employment of a dietician.[50] Unique services at Faulkner Hospital have included nuclear medicine, stoma therapy, diversional therapy, an incontinence clinic, an alcohol detoxification unit, eye surgery, a lung sounds research program, a vein center, a foot and ankle center, and a pacemaker clinic. A walk-in clinic called "Faulkner Express Care" began in the 1980s, serving about 500 patients each month.[51]

Some of Faulkner Hospital's services have become world-renowned, such as its Graham Headache Center, started in 1961, Psychiatry and Addiction services, and the Faulkner-Sagoff Breast Center.[52] The Faulkner Hospital Psychiatric Service began in 1966, which soon merged with the Adams Nervine Psychiatric Hospital.

Faulkner Hospital soon outgrew its original facilities, and planning for a new building to meet the hospital's growing demands began as early as 1950. In 1968, the trustees requested architects Perry, Dean, and Stewart to undertake a master development plan.[53] On the official Moving Day, May 22, 1976, the twenty-sixth Yankee Infantry Division's 114th Medical Battalion of the National Guard was in place to help staff move patients from the old to the new hospital. The sixteen-acre new hospital was seven stories high and 300,000 square feet, with 259 beds and an emergency room ten times larger than the old one.[54]

The new building spurred a number of original ideas, based on the "Friesen Design" that focused on reengineering for patient-centered care.[55] Plans called for Nurses' Stations to be eliminated and replaced by Administrative Control Centers and Team Conference Centers. Each patient room had a Nurserver (locked supply cabinet) with special airflow mechanisms to prevent infection, containing medications, linens, dressings, and IV supplies. Another futuristic idea was an Automatic Cart Transportation System to deliver supplies and patient meals throughout the hospital via a monorail conveyer. Pneumatic tubes transported messages, such as doctor's prescriptions, by a "whoosh" air mechanism at a rate of thirty to thirty-five feet per second.[56] Although these ideas worked better conceptually than in practice, they were bold and fascinating experiments for the "modern" hospital.

Faulkner Hospital and Brigham and Women's Hospital (BWH) have had a longstanding relationship. In 1974, when the Boston Hospital for Women, the Robert Breck Brigham Hospital, and the Peter Bent Brigham Hospital were consolidated, some Harvard Surgical Services were transferred to Faulkner Hospital.[57] In 1997, Faulkner Hospital and BWH began to explore ways to collaborate.

On April 8, 1998, Faulkner's leadership met with several of Brigham and Women's key leaders to discuss creation of a new corporation, Brigham and Women's/Faulkner HealthCare, Inc. through a merger of Brigham Medical Center and the Faulkner Hospital Corporation. Faulkner Hospital's Strategic Initiative Group felt that this model would make good sense for many reasons, including greatly enhancing Faulkner Hospital to continue its mission in the communities that it served. Faulkner Hospital had already developed relationships with the Brigham in several areas. On September 22, 1998, trustees voted that Faulkner Hospital would affiliate with Partners HealthCare System, Inc., The Brigham Medical Center, Inc., and The Brigham and Women's

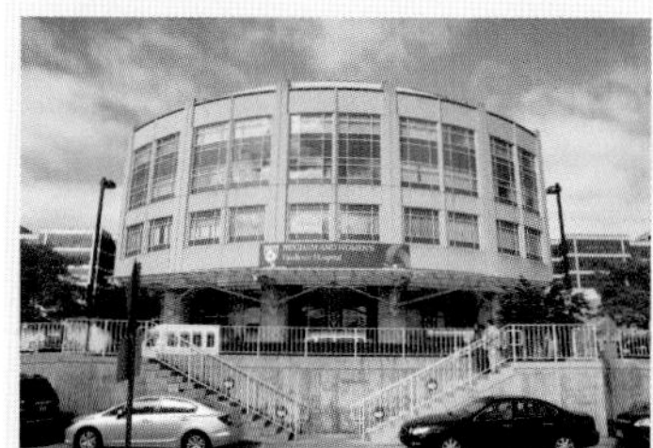

FIGURE 6-17 Faulkner Hospital today.

Hospital, Inc., to become Brigham and Women's/Faulkner Hospital, a member of Partners HealthCare System, Inc. This new relationship allowed for development of complementary services, such as psychiatric inpatient care and orthopedics, to be directed to the most appropriate hospital. A number of joint programs were developed, such as cardiology and neurology. Brigham and Women's surgery and medicine residents began rotations at Faulkner, and Faulkner chiefs were integrated to serve as vice-chairs of the corresponding Brigham and Women's Hospital departments.[58]

On March 6, 2012, the Faulkner Hospital Board voted to move to common membership on the boards of Faulkner Hospital, Brigham and Women's Hospital, and Brigham and Women's/Faulkner Hospital while retaining separate corporate entities and separate hospital licenses. On October 1, 2012, Faulkner Hospital was renamed Brigham and Women's Faulkner Hospital. The new name better reflects Faulkner Hospital's level of integration, common mission, and shared goals with Brigham and Women's Hospital.

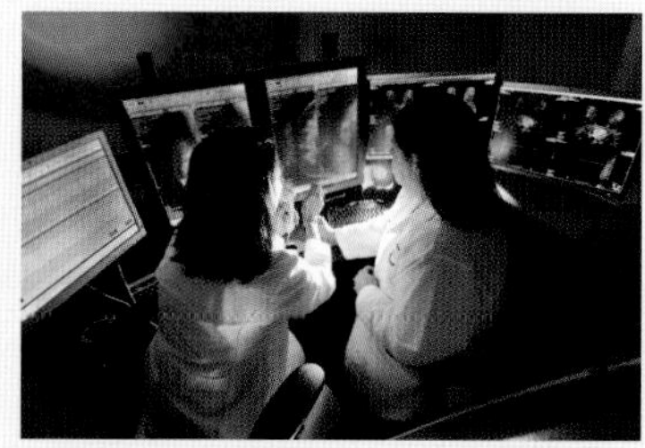

FIGURE 6-18 Breast imaging at Faulkner Hospital.

The Community Outside: Mission Hill

By the time the Peter Bent Brigham Hospital opened in 1913, Boston, the contingent neighborhood of Parker Hill, later called Mission Hill, had changed substantially. Waves of Irish and later Southern and Eastern European immigrants had altered the physical landscape and socioeconomic character of the city. Back Bay and its environs—including what would become the Longwood Medical Area—were filled in to provide housing for Boston's expanding population. Ever larger populations moved into the once-rural villages of Roxbury, Dorchester, and Jamaica Plain. Parker Hill had become a target of this expansion in the 1860s, when German families began to settle at the base of the Hill and to build the first of many breweries there.

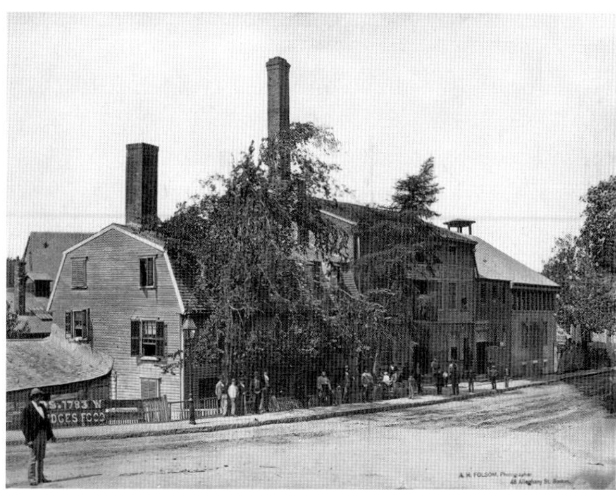

FIGURE 6-19 Old Roessle Brewery, Roxbury Crossing, late nineteenth century.

Colonial estates still dotted the Hill's slopes, giving it a rural flavor. By 1869, "Boston (had) extended street railway service and sewage systems to Roxbury (which had annexed itself to Boston in 1867) and the Irish working class poured into undeveloped suburban areas like Parker Hill."[59] The center of the Irish community was the shrine of Our Lady of Perpetual Help (popularly known as Mission Church), which had been built two years after the Catholic Redemptorist Fathers acquired the former Brinley Farm in 1869. A huge stone church, accommodating 4,000 parishioners, replaced the original in 1878 and still stands today; patients being treated at Longwood Area hospitals and their families can sometimes be found there seeking solace.

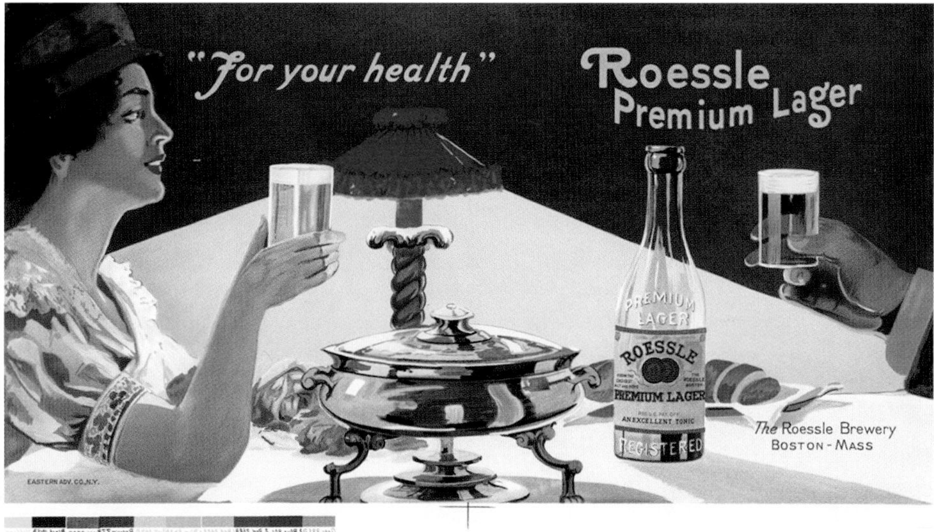

FIGURE 6-20 Old Roessele Brewery advertisement, "For Your Health."

One account gives a sense of what the area was like in the two decades before the PBBH was built:

In 1898...triple-decker houses had been built about three-quarters of the way up Parker Hill of Hillside Street, and as far west as Wait Street. Above Hillside Street were a cow farm and pasture, a reservoir, and a small building which since 1893 had housed the New England Baptist Hospital. There were some houses on Wait Street and a few more on the far end of the Hill near Parker Hill Avenue but in between was Gray's Field, an orchard filled with pear trees and apple trees, which ran all the way from Hillside Street to Huntington Avenue...Across Huntington Avenue were open fields where the circus kept its horses when it came to Boston each year. Most of the streets throughout the neighborhood were unpaved. Sidewalks, when they existed, were made of two-by-ten foot wooden planks which protected pedestrians from mud and manure.[60]

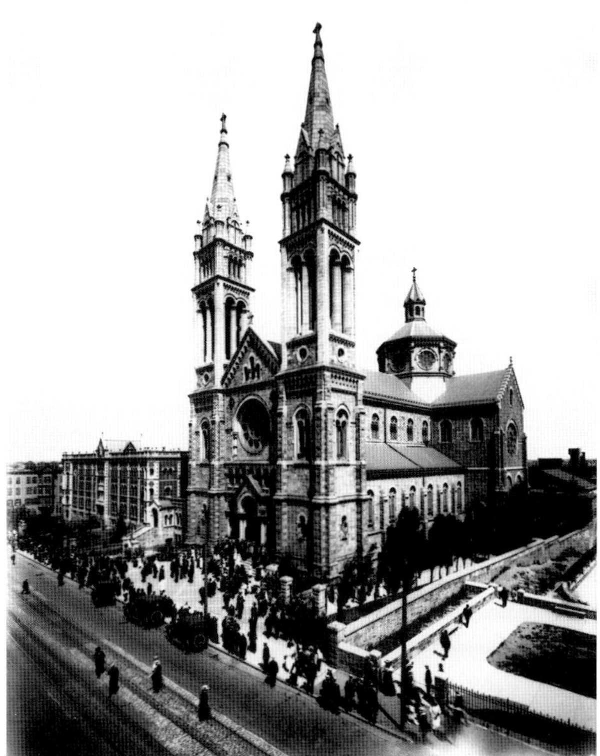

FIGURE 6-21 Mission Church, circa 1919.

Connecting Inside and Out: Community Outreach and the Out-Door Department

In its first decade, the PBBH's Out-Door Department (OD) was set up to deliver services to the community. For the first few years, there were no appointments; patients simply showed up and waited until they could be seen by a doctor or nurse. In a style reminiscent of today's efforts to engage consumers, the OD attempted to make its hours consumer friendly: it was open in the afternoons when other similar services in Boston were only open in the morning. Care was provided by house officers who were spending the final part of their training in the department. However, a more

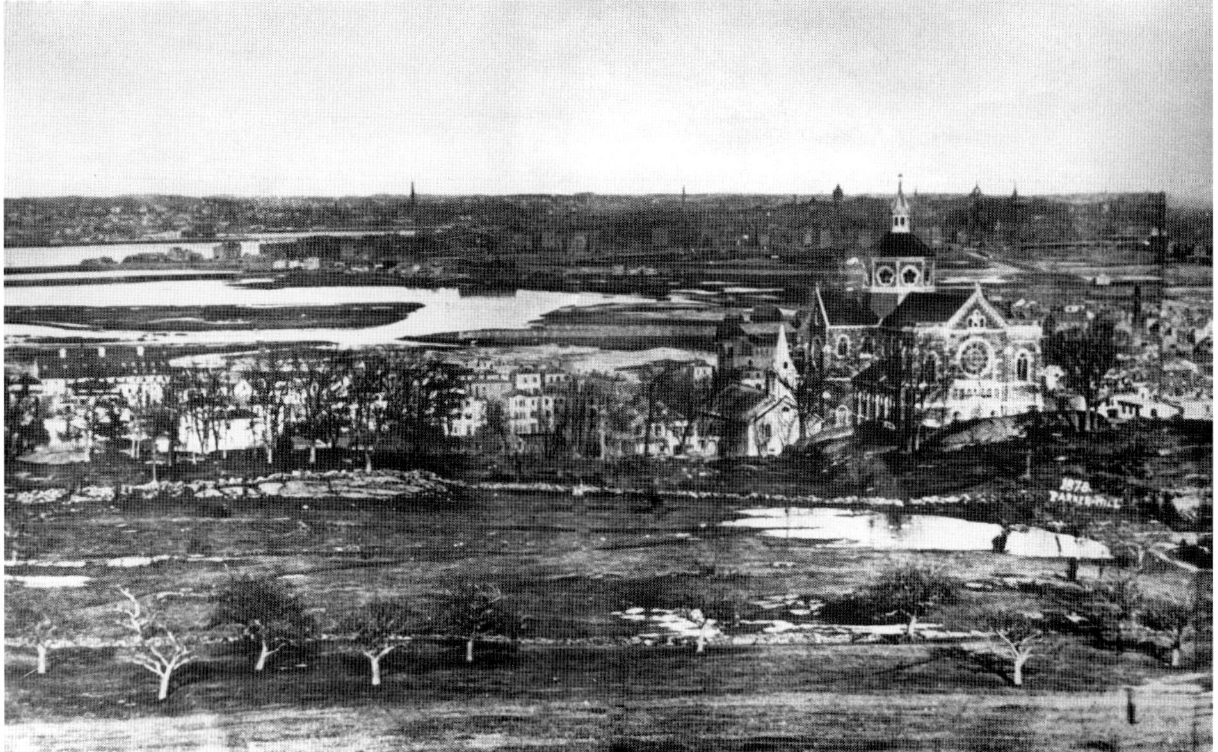

FIGURE 6-22 A view of Parker Hill, circa 1878.

advanced resident physician consulted on difficult cases, and both Christian and other physicians not only spent regular hours in the OD, but also provided consultation. The annual reports note that the "specialized laboratories" and "more complicated apparatus" available to ward patients were available to OD patients as well. Patients were also referred from the Boston Dispensary to the PBBH in a collaboration between the two entities. By its second year of operation, 8,500 visits were recorded.

An integrative approach to community-based services came early to the Brigham. The Medical Service worked closely with the Social Service Department, which initially consisted of one paid worker, Alice Cheney, and volunteers. Social work was a new profession in the early twentieth century, and the social worker's role in the hospital was still in the process of definition. Community-oriented social work efforts, however, were intensive from the start. In the two months after the Outdoor Department's opening, "100 patients [were] referred to Social Service, 84 homes were visited, and 78 visits were made to ward patients and 73 to outdoor patients."[61] Eventually Social Service became involved in the OD's "class system" of health education for first tuberculosis patients and later diabetics.[62] These educational efforts focused on environmental concerns and aftercare in the first case and collaborating with the dietitian in the second. Shortly thereafter, regular classes for patients were also implemented in cardiac and renal care. Another early collaborator in outpatient services was the occupational therapy department, which was, like social work, an emerging profession.

Coordinated patient follow-up also began early, with discharge planning systems for both in- and outpatients initiated by 1915. Social Service coordinated with the Outdoor Department and other hospital entities to refer and collaborate with dozens of outside entities, including the Robert Breck Brigham Hospital, the Boston Lying-In Hospital, Associated Charities, Federated Jewish Charities, the Women's Educational and Industrial Union, and many others. Given the newness of the hospital, concerns about patient demand and staff capacity quickly appeared. Many health issues with which patients—often recent immigrants—struggled were a result of poverty, family problems, unhealthy physical environments, isolation, adjustment to an alien culture, and other factors, as demonstrated in this snippet from an early case study:

> *Patient: A girl fourteen years of age in hospital ward.*
>
> *Diagnosis: Severe case of chorea; chronic; middle ears.*
>
> *Reason Referred: District nurse telephones that patient should not come home from hospital—mother works out all day—rooms hot and stuffy (time of year, July), food poorly prepared.*
>
> *Action taken: Patient sent to country (Farrington Memorial) for three weeks. Returns much improved. Mother in the interim has moved to Revere (seashore) for summer. Mother is shown how to take proper care of ears.*[63]

The use of scientific management techniques to provide quality care began in the Brigham's first decade, when demand for outpatient services escalated so rapidly that it threatened to overwhelm PBBH staff. After noting that MGH had more staff devoted to their own "OD," Christian examined department staffing and the amount of time spent with new and "old" patients, finding that an average of twenty-four minutes was spent with "new" patients and eight and a half minutes with returning patients. As a result of his study, measures were taken to improve patient flow.[64] Staff shortages later become so pressing that an appointment system was begun. By the eighth annual report, 52,000 visits to the OD were recorded, and medical social integration was more firmly a part of daily practice.[65]

By the hospital's fifteenth anniversary in 1928, the work of the OD was in full swing, with arthritis and dental clinics added to the existing efforts. Social Service and dietitians aided in much of the follow-up and family-visitation activities. Alice Cheney recommended one medical record integrating all information about a patient so doctors and social workers could collaborate more effectively, although she noted, "there are great difficulties in fusing Out-Door Department and house records into a system with everything about each patient contained in a single continuous clinical record."[66] Other problems included patients who could be seen by private practitioners coming to the clinic—so much volume meant less personalized care—and other patients not keeping appointments.

The Depression Years at the PBBH

> *"The past year has presented an unusual number of serious social problems occasioned by the continued hardship of unemployment. In several instances families previously well above the dependency group have this year required financial assistance."*[67]
>
> —From the Eighteenth Annual Report

Community-related efforts in the 1930s attempted to address patient issues resulting from the poor economy. Unsurprisingly, service demand was heavy during the Depression. By 1934, the OD reported more than 83,000 annual patient visits.[68] A number of new services, such as blood and tumor clinics, were instituted. The gastrointestinal clinic experienced a surge in cases, in part because of the "continual mental and emotional upsets" patients were experiencing.[69]

By 1934, due to this increased patient demand as well as rising prices in virtually every area, the PBBH was dipping deep into its capital. Christian reported with alarm: "If some way is not found to bring about a change, then we will become bankrupt."[70] Noting that the hospital had established an excellent reputation, he was heartened that scientific investigation had continued unabated. However, he was forced to reflect on the balance between clinical care, research, and teaching. If the PBBH were to reduce its emphasis on research to save money, it would not attract the best faculty candidates.

By 1938, when the PBBH's twenty-fifth reunion was celebrated, usage of the OD was still very high. Community-based referral, wrote Social Service, fell mainly into "convalescent, nursing, institutional, and terminal care; orthopedic appliances, housekeepers, transportation, interpretation to agencies, and miscellaneous requests."[71] While aided by students

Table III

Birthplaces

	1915	1914
Alabama	6	5
Arkansas	2	1
California	17	11
Colorado	3	..
Connecticut	37	27
Delaware	2	1
District of Columbia	4	6
Florida	4	3
Georgia	8	4
Idaho	1	3
Illinois	14	16
Indiana	7	2
Iowa	5	13
Kansas	3	6
Kentucky	7	5
Louisiana	2	4
Maine	140	98
Maryland	16	8
Massachusetts (except Boston)	757	876
Boston	463	165
Michigan	7	4
Minnesota	7	4
Missouri	6	3
Nebraska	3	4
New Hampshire	78	56
New Jersey	16	12
New Mexico	3	..
New York	125	94
North Carolina	12	17
North Dakota	1	..
Ohio	21	21
Oklahoma	2	2
Carried forward	1,779	1,471

REPORT OF THE SUPERINTENDENT

	1915	1914
Brought forward	1,779	1,471
Oregon	..	1
Pennsylvania	33	15
Rhode Island	41	13
South Carolina	5	10
Tennessee	2	6
Texas	6	6
Utah	3	1
Vermont	32	41
Virginia	35	24
West Virginia	3	3
Wisconsin	8	13
Wyoming	..	1
Total Americans	1,947	1,605
Africa	..	1
Argentina	1	..
Australia	..	2
Austria	20	26
Belgium	1	6
Bulgaria	1	1
Canada	325	226
China	2	1
Denmark	6	6
East Indies	..	1
England	141	113
France	4	4
Germany	61	52
Greece	42	24
Holland	5	3
Hungary	4	..
Ireland	273	281
Italy	85	100
Norway	23	6
Panama	1	1
Poland	..	4
Portugal	8	..
Roumania	4	3
Carried forward	1,007	861

PETER BENT BRIGHAM HOSPITAL

	1915	1914
Brought forward	1,007	861
Russia	333	274
Scotland	28	27
Spain	7	1
Sweden	40	29
Switzerland	..	3
Tasmania	..	1
Turkey	52	33
Venezuela	..	1
Wales	2	1
West Indies	1	7
Total foreigners	1,470	1,238

FIGURE 6-23 Peter Bent Brigham Hospital patient birthplaces listed in the 1915 Annual Report.

from Simmons College School of Social Work and by volunteers, especially those from the "Social Service Ladies Committee," which would become the Friends of the Peter Bent Brigham Hospital in 1940, providing adequate community services would continue to be challenging, even though new Works Progress Administration programs—such as housekeeper services for patients returning to the community—assisted the hospital.

Looking back on the period in 1945, hospital Director Norbert Wilhelm noted that although the OD had been very busy during much of the 1930s, the hospital had been operating well under its inpatient capacity. Wilhelm attributed this to a lack of middle-income patients—the wealthy and very poor were provided for. He thought that for such patients, group or Blue Cross insurance could be a solution. Another problem was that the PBBH had outgrown its original facility endowment. Somehow these problems required resolution, either through greatly increased philanthropy or through federal grants. As Wilhelm noted:

> *As one looks ahead, it becomes increasingly apparent that the future of American medicine, in urban areas at least, is group practice, and as this is essentially what medical care in an Out-Door Department consists of, we must prepare for a steady increase of patients in this department.*[72]

THE FRIENDS OF THE BRIGHAM

As was the case in the other parent hospitals, the Peter Bent Brigham Hospital's Ladies Social Service Committee, precursor of the Friends of the Brigham, had a prominent role at the institution. This consisted of not only the provision of funds, a practice initiated by the sisters of both Peter Bent and Robert Breck Brigham, but in working closely with the Social Service staff, the School of Nursing, dietetics, and other parts of the hospital. For many years, Ladies Committee members provided and solicited the bulk of contributions to the Social Service Fund; of the dozens of contributions noted in the Tenth Annual Report in 1924, almost all were from women.[73]

Often, in a time when few middle-and upper-class white women worked outside the home, Ladies Committee members were wives of or otherwise related to physicians. But they fulfilled central roles at the hospital. Long before the establishment of a formal PBBH Volunteer Department under their aegis, the committee members spent long hours volunteering in Social Service and the Out-Door Department. As early as the Second Annual Report, Mrs. Kenneth Mark and Miss Katherine Homans were respectively honored for their work in the diabetic and heart clinics.[74] The work of the committee that would eventually become Friends of the Brigham was particularly central during wartime, when the membership took on vital volunteer roles in the face of shortages.

The hospital was always pressed for funds, and the committee and auxiliary had an important role in addressing this—not only generally, but for specific projects, often concerning the nursing school. In addition, and not unimportantly, the committee was able to provide many of the touches that made the Brigham a "home." They held teas for staff and nurses, decorated the hospital, helped to maintain the grounds, honored key employees, and held dozens of fundraising events. They were early public relations and development professionals at a time when the hospital did not structure these as formalized roles.

All of these contributions helped develop the esprit de corps of the hospital over years that were never easy—as the PBBH created its identity while experiencing war, epidemics, Depression, and war again. Beyond the work inside the hospital, the Ladies Committee helped with resources and referral processes for Social Service, which worked extensively with Boston charities—entities with which committee members were often familiar through their own charitable work. The help was usually very pragmatic; for instance, during the Depression, at a time when the hospital was challenged on all fronts, the Junior League was brought in to do volunteer work in the overloaded clinics.[75]

In 1940, the committee was reorganized into the Friends of the Brigham and then took on an ever more integral role in the PBBH's operations. In that year, the Social Work Department reported that "37 individuals served as volunteers in the Out-Door and Social Service Departments. Two thousand five hundred and forty-seven (2,547) hours or 318 working days were rendered by this conscientious group of workers," led by Mrs. Dorothea (Roger) Merriman.[76]

The volunteer service became so busy and complex that, also in 1940, the director of Social Service called for a paid volunteer coordinator. She also noted that there were 1,662 calls for "motor and ambulance service" at a time when the Red Cross Motor Service was cut back and eventually shut down during August. In response, a volunteer group, led by Mrs. Stanley Hoerr, provided "motor transport throughout the year to make up for the reduced service."[77]

The mission of the Friends was multifaceted. Meeting three times annually, they organized themselves into myriad subcommittees, reflecting the many aspects of their work, which they wanted to go far beyond fundraising. By 1948, the Friends were operating The Brigham Shop, a gift shop, and a coffee shop, now known as Pat's Place. They also hired an executive secretary that same year. In other developments, they noted: "Miss Juliet Carpenter, the Director of Volunteers, went as our delegate to the Conference of Women's Hospital Auxiliaries held in conjunction with the meetings of the American Hospital Association. Here women from all over the country met to discuss their problems and it was a help to know that many of our own troubles were common to most of the auxiliaries."[78]

By this time, the Friends had a board and officers. Their concerns included Budget, Equipment, Painting, Projects, Shop, Red Cross, Surgical Dressings (chaired by Carrie Hall), the Patient Library (procuring and reviewing books before distributing them), and Nominating and Membership Committees. Beyond these, members served as liaisons to Social Service and volunteers, produced a newsletter, organized on an annual Pops concert, ran a Christmas party (at which Surgeon-in-Chief Francis Moore played accordion), worked in the coffee shop (run by Mrs. Elliott Cutler), and for years ran a "Diversional Therapy" program, consisting of educational activities and crafts for patients.[79]

The scope of their work was remarkable. In the 1950s, the Friends added to this suite of programs the comanagement (with other charitable concerns) of a thrift shop. They had several vice-presidents, one of whom represented the hospital at "the Nursing Council of the United Community Services, on which representatives of twelve Hospitals examined whether certain duties now performed by nurses could not more appropriately be done by someone less skilled."[80] Membership grew year after year, and by 1953 it numbered 640.[81] By 1963, the PBBH's fiftieth anniversary, the Friends provided a mission statement and balance sheets in the annual report and noted that they had provided about $42,000 in contributions (partly underwriting *The Fabrick of Man*, a 128-page interpretive history of the hospital written by poet David McCord), as well as an enormous amount of unpaid labor during the gala anniversary celebration.[82]

In the decades after World War II, the operations of the organization mirrored larger societal changes: they became more diverse in membership and professionalized in their work. At the same time, however, the Friends, which had a primarily female membership, were much affected by the movement of women into the paid work force. Shortly before the merger of the PBBH with the Boston Hospital for Women and the RBBH, the Sixty-Third Annual Report noted the need to reevaluate goals in the face of "changing times" and the impending new hospital. Nevertheless, they continued to be involved in efforts as diverse as the shops' management and diversional therapy and provided needed funding, including a loan program for residents.

By 1978, there was certain pathos in one of the first reports of the Affiliated Hospitals Center, in which the president of the PBBH Friends wrote of the difficulty of obtaining funds and volunteers for the many services they struggled to provide. Similarly, the head of the Boston Hospital for Women's Ladies Board noted the changes that were likely to be ahead in this much larger hospital community. However, the

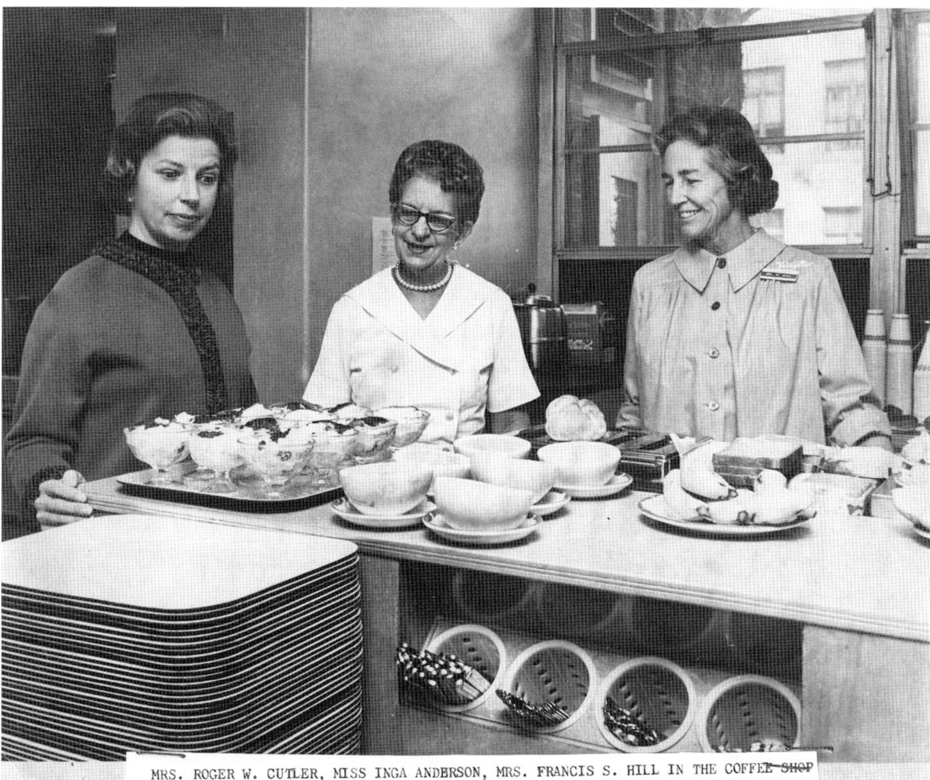
MRS. ROGER W. CUTLER, MISS INGA ANDERSON, MRS. FRANCIS S. HILL IN THE COFFEE SHOP

FIGURE 6-24 The Peter Bent Brigham coffee shop, circa 1960s.

renamed Friends of BWH survived and thrived. Today, the Friends continue to volunteer and play a leading role in fundraising for the hospital. These "efforts have resulted in more than $8 million of investment towards unmet capital needs, patient enhancements, and unfunded programs of more than two hundred fifty departments."[83]

Much of the history of the auxiliaries remains untold, although a trove of records remains at the Center for the History of Medicine at HMS's Countway Library. A debt of gratitude is owed for their financial contributions as well as their support of nursing, social work, public relations, libraries, development, patient relations, the gift and coffee shops, and other areas. In many ways, the Friends—in their work today and the enormous contributions of the past—are at the heart of the hospital.

Scientific Charity and Scientific Management

Like other teaching hospitals, the Brigham applied science to the provision of community care in terms of organization as well as therapeutics. Its staff was divided into professionalized sectors responsible for different aspects of service. At first glance it might seem that the work of "curing and caring" at the hospital was entirely divided, mostly by gender. The largely male corps of physicians and surgeons reported directly to the trustees and held most institutional power. The female-dominated professions of nursing, social work and, as they emerged, occupational therapy and dietetics were responsible for the "caring" sides of the institution. With pharmacy, they reported to the superintendent rather than the trustees.

The reality, however, was complex. Harvey Cushing, who carried on voluminous correspondence with patients to the end of his life, wrote compellingly of the PBBH's "soul," "the object for which hospitals were first established." "[As] a place for rest, for comfort of the sick, for kindly advice and counsel I know no place where, in the long run, there is less friction and more kindly feeling and consideration for patients."[84]

The hospital provided an enormous amount of "caring" as well as "curing," and not only by nurses and social workers. At the same time, however, its staff was continually aware of the balance between resources for caring and resources for the hospital's investigatory and teaching missions. However, if the hospital directed all resources to charitable patient care, it could not conduct the research potentially beneficial to a community far larger than its immediate environs. And if it did not receive outside funding—either through philanthropy or from the payments of private patients—it would not survive to do any of this work. While helping to ameliorate patients' interconnected socioeconomic and medical concerns, hospital staff also continually evaluated institutional limits created by financial constraints.

To help achieve a balance, the Brigham brought the scientific method to management systems that would ultimately benefit clinicians, clinic operations, and most of all, the patient. For instance, in the PBBH's first decade, it worked with other Boston teaching hospitals to develop a joint disease classification system. Forms, procedural manuals, and detailed record-keeping systems were part of the PBBH's earliest operations. Nevertheless, Christian, Cushing and others regularly asked for alertness when using measurement systems designed to improve efficiency, calling for watchfulness lest the PBBH begin to practice "machine medicine."[85]

Rituals and Reunions

Despite the many difficulties PBBH encountered—the tension of providing compassionate care while carrying out its scientific mission, maintaining a physical plant that seemed insufficient ten years after the hospital opened, the heartbreak of war and Depression—it was a resilient organization, in part because of its cohesive character. And sometimes, it laughed at itself.

In the early years of the PBBH, a tradition was established for the "hospital family" to come together in reunion. Staff, distinguished guests, and alumni gathered with the trustees and service committees for scientific programs and, occasionally, staff-written musicals, which provided often-farcical commentary on hospital life, world events, and even government policy. It was not only physicians who participated—nursing held a separate program to mark its achievements. Held at five-year intervals with more elaborate celebrations at the quarter century, reunions marked not only the hospital's remarkable advances, but also the challenges and differences within it. In the terminology of the anthropologist Barbara Myerhoff, they served as definitional ceremonies for the PBBH as it established and refined its identity.[86]

Creating Community: The Fifteenth Nursing Reunion

In April 1928, the hospital held its second reunion, commemorating its fifteenth anniversary. One aspect of the program focused on the students and alumni of the Peter Bent Brigham Hospital School of Nursing (PBBHSON). Three hundred eighty-one women had now graduated, and well over 115 attended the reunion. The nursing program consisted of events similar to those held for physicians. Each day there were ward rounds and then presentation of scientific papers in the amphitheater. The nurses' scientific program reflected the status of the modern profession and featured reminiscences by early faculty, thoughts on nursing in foreign countries, and papers on technical, industrial, and chronic disease nursing. An elaborate farce was also presented, written, produced, and acted by the residents and the Nurses Alumnae Association.

In her "Welcome to Graduates" at the 1928 reunion, Carrie Hall paraphrased the words of Henry Christian, saying, "You are the Brigham Hospital." Hall reflected on the essence of nursing at the PBBH, composed of "the things we do and the things we carry away from here and make good use of and apply in some other place and add to the sum total of knowledge and build up something as good or better somewhere else."[87] That spirit was evident in the entire program—the challenges of nursing education and service and the accomplishments of graduates, which included global service and participation in entirely new nursing roles, such as that of the industrial nurse. One presentation, by early faculty member Sally Johnson, who was by then superintendent of nurses at MGH, described her experiences as a member of the first PBBH nursing faculty, beginning when the hospital was just a "hodge-podge of dirt and stone." In her talk, Johnson reiterated what it had meant to go through training at the PBBH: the absorption of a code of honor, modesty, and hard work as well as a sense of purpose.

Many of the themes of early reunions were later carried over in alumni contributions to the PBBHSON *Alumnae Journal,* which demonstrate the contributions of the school as graduates took their education in hand to advance the profession. A 1928 sample of these articles includes the following:

"Nurses at X-ray Work," by Christine McDonald, head of the X-ray department at the Rockefeller Institute in New York,[41] was a clear-headed look at the status of an emerging profession. "As in most new work," she writes, "much depends upon the initiative, earnestness and care given small details, as to how far the nurse may advance." However, McDonald also noted that no matter how much knowledge she absorbs, the nurse could not advance beyond a certain level without a medical degree. McDonald also listed the various occupational health hazards, including those associated with fertility.[88]

"L'Hopital General of Port Au Prince, Haiti" described the history of the island and the hospital, as well as the challenges students encountered as they encountered American-style nursing. It also portrayed common health problems of the patients as well as the public health issues that led to them.[89]

"The Industrial Nurse," by Eva E. Gaboury, examined the origins of industrial nursing, which Gaboury linked to the reformist impulses of twenty-five years before. Gaboury saw many of the qualifications necessary for the profession as similar to those of the ideal nurse. She noted the hectic nature of the work as well as its holistic character. The personal was particularly important, she wrote, noting that attention to this had an important preventive purpose.[90]

Creating Community: The Twenty-Fifth Hospital Reunion

> *"Things were different in the good old days*
> *They would shudder at our modern ways.*
> *They did not have patients who could not pay,*
> *And they didn't have recessions or the W.P.A.*
> *They did not have insurance or state medicine,*
> *They wouldn't understand what a fog we're in."*
>
> —From the twenty-fifth anniversary play in 1938

In May 1938, the Peter Bent Brigham held its twenty-fifth reunion. The staff wrote and performed a play for the occasion: a fascinating (and funny) portrait not only of the hospital family but of the world around it. Most PBBH physicians and graduate nurses, past and present, either participated or were characters in the production. Among the cast were Hartwell Harrison and Carl Walter, who like many others would become prominent PBBH physicians. (Plays would also be produced for other reunions as a PBBH tradition.)

In the second scene and third scenes, the staff argued over the origin of the 1930s deficit and what to do about the institution's continual financial straits. Illustrious medical figures were wildly caricatured. John Homans, wearing a tweed jacket, knickers, and a high collar, rode a bicycle onto the stage, cursing loudly (for which he was famous). The next scene involved others who might not have been physicians, but nevertheless were very important in the Brigham's daily life. "Joe Front" (the nickname of a well-known staff member, Joseph McQueen, who was the PBBH night telephone operator through the 1950s) manned the general information desk of the hospital. In his scene, Joe functioned as a one-man admissions service, sorting patients into medical and surgical categories for "Dr. Choppingblock," who was in a mad rush to "cut somebody up." At rounds, "Professor Whizzbottle" (Physician Pro Tem) listened as house officer "Stuffingbox" presented: "His family were all Democrats, but there is no other history of insanity." Fitz, the attending physician, remarked of the patient, "He's a W.P.A. worker, but we haven't been able to find anything else wrong with him." In this scene, there was also (as there is throughout the play) a great deal of amusing commentary on the idiosyncrasies of Surgeon-in-Chief Elliott Cutler and Chief of Medicine Henry Christian.

A number of topical and political concerns also emerged. The concern of hospitals and organized medicine over "socialism" and "governmental control" of the profession was evidenced in a small commentary in the final scene, in which James Roosevelt was proposed as a visiting surgeon. "Wonderful boy, doing a wonderful job down there, but I hate the idea of mixing up insurance and medicine," Cutler said. In the finale, all the cast sang: "The poor Brighamitis, in a dreadful plight is, There's no other way it can be; Unless we can collar a bunch of new dollars, and continue as a charity!"[91] Thus the play ended on an enduring theme for the hospital: the absolute necessity of new sources of financial support. Although the hospital disparaged government interference, it had, after all, only survived the Depression through donations from the Community Federation, a joint fundraising effort of Boston charities.[92] And despite the lightheartedness, there was more than a hint of foreboding in the play, which showed that the hospital was not immune to pressures from the outside world.

World War I and the Peter Bent Brigham

The exigencies of war impacted every parent hospital. At the PBBH, World War I made serious inroads on the hospital staff. Many members of the medical, surgical, and nursing services all served in Europe. Of the fifty base hospitals staffed by the elite of American medicine, three were affiliated with Harvard. Base Hospital #5 was staffed largely by PBBH physicians and was directed by Harvey Cushing, a post that he held from 1917 to 1919. He also served as senior consultant in neurological surgery. Base Hospital #5 was to be a remarkably successful entity, containing more than 1,000 beds and marked by efficiency as well as multispecialist cooperation. Like the other field hospitals, it was a surgically oriented enterprise, emphasizing short-term and acute care.[93] *The Story of U.S. Army Base Hospital No. 5* by "A Member of the Unit" (Cushing) memorialized the esprit de corps of the dozens of PBBH staff affiliated with the hospital.[94] The hospital boasted a fairly low mortality rate

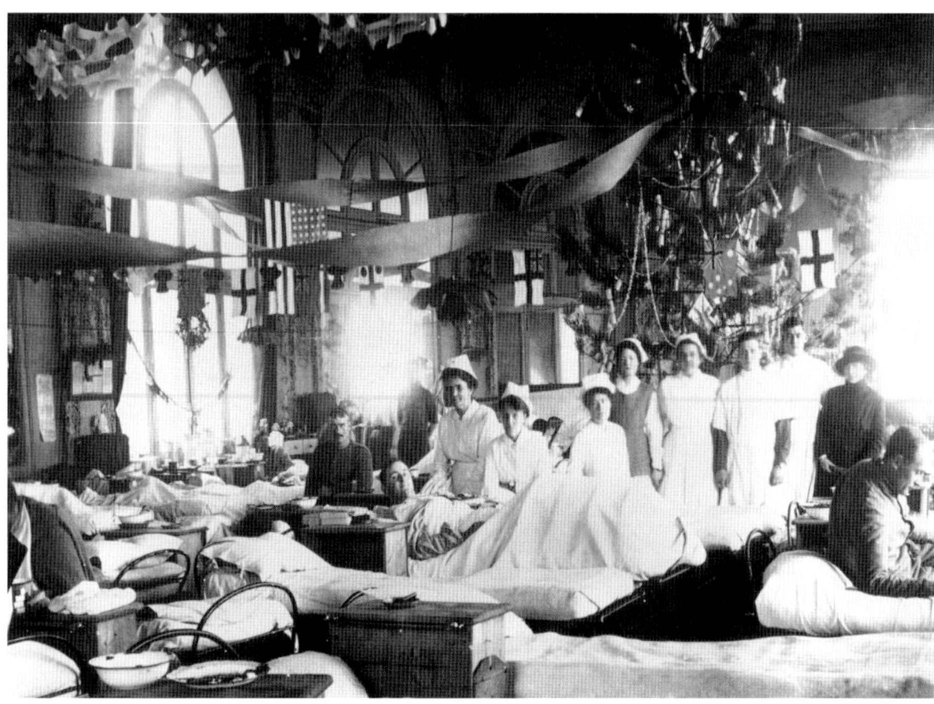

FIGURE 6-25 Christmas on the front in World War I, Base Hospital #5.

and evidenced much surgical progress, particularly in neuro- and orthopedic surgery. Carrie Hall was appointed chief nurse of the base hospital by the American Red Cross.

On the home front, wartime brought a reduction in the length of medical internships and vastly increased the workload for remaining personnel. However, more diversity came to the hospital as female physicians and retirees took on temporary roles. Similarly, the Ladies Committee took on ancillary positions wherever needed at the hospital, as would also occur during World War II. The Ladies Committee made more than a million surgical dressings for the European theater. All of this took place in a hospital that also faced, in 1918, the cataclysmic national influenza epidemic that pushed the staff to the point of collapse and claimed the lives of many patients and several staff members.

The totality of wartime commitment was later echoed in the order, discipline, and commitment evidenced in medical and nursing culture at the PBBH. After the war, Cushing even adapted a military style tunic to wear for operations. Similarly, Carrie Hall proudly wore the medals she received for her wartime service.

The Free Hospital for Women and the Robert Breck Brigham Hospital in World War I

During the war, Free Hospital for Women Chief William Graves traveled to Halifax, Nova Scotia, to assist after a munitions ship explosion. During the 1918 influenza epidemic, the hospital was turned over entirely to flu cases. Nursing shortages occurred as nurses left to take on other work, and the Free Hospital nursing school was eventually closed.[95]

The Robert Breck Brigham Hospital experienced a total closure of services during World War I. In 1917, it was taken over by the federal government for treatment of the wounded and those who had diseases resulting from war service. Patients were transferred to area nursing homes and the staff scattered.[96] Subsequently, however, the war was to prove beneficial to the institution, as leader Joel Goldthwaite chaired the committee planning orthopedic hospitals during the war and helped recruit many orthopedic personnel.[97] Goldthwaite used his war service to explore European models of the chronic disease hospital, which combined clinical care and research. After the war, this would lead to an emphasis on rehabilitation and vocational training for veterans; eventually, this positive emphasis for those previously considered "incurable" would mark both Goldthwaite's treatment of patients with rheumatic disease and the future focus of the RBBH.[98]

World War II: Mobilization

In 1942, Elliott Cutler, who had served with Cushing at Base Hospital #5 in World War I, was called into active service in the Army Medical Corps. He was named chief consultant in surgery in the European Theater of Operations. Together with the chief consultant in medicine, Cutler structured the system of care for injured and sick U.S. soldiers and drew on the experience of the PBBH blood bank, which was established in 1942 by Carl Walter. This major innovation had become the blood center serving the Boston area and was a prototype for the Red Cross blood program in World War II.[99]

On the home front, the hospital faced extreme shortages of personnel and rationing of food and supplies. The PBBH struggled to keep up the excellence of its training in spite of the shortening of house officer terms. At Harvard, 300 members of the medical school faculty served in the military. Many nurses went to war as well—as of 1944, 138 PBBHSON graduates were on duty.[100]

Both physical and medical sciences were important for wartime research. The Federal Committee on Medical Research, chaired by Alfred Newton Richards, produced numerous studies and papers on subjects as diverse as prevention of infectious and venereal disease, substitutions for quinine, wound and burn control, nerve repair, adaptations to extremes of temperature, and many other areas.[101] This would lead to an enormous postwar concentration on research, which would blossom in the 1950s through the work of returning war veterans. The Peter Bent Brigham, the

SPOTLIGHT

RESEARCH AT THE ROBERT BRECK BRIGHAM HOSPITAL AND ITS MERGER WITH THE BRIGHAM

K. Frank Austen

The Robert Breck Brigham Hospital for Incurables (RBBH), located high on Boston's Mission Hill, opened its doors in 1914, dedicated to the comprehensive care of patients with rheumatologic diseases. A formal connection with the Peter Bent Brigham Hospital through discussions between George Thorn, physician-in-chief, and J. Sidney Stillman, RBBH chief of medicine, to rotate PBBH house staff to the RBBH was established in 1944. After the discovery in 1949 of the capacity of adrenal hormones to suppress inflamed rheumatoid joints, the RBBH was the first Boston hospital to use these agents. This was possible through the support of George Thorn, whose clinical and research interests focused on the adrenal gland. Collaborative research ensued, involving John Vaughn of the PBBH and Theodore Bayles at the RBBH, the first glimpse of the RBBH's future research directions. Bayles had begun to emphasize clinical research, obtaining a training grant for rheumatic diseases research in 1956 and an award for an eight- to ten-bed Clinical Research Center in 1961. Trainees participated in studies of patients with ochronosis and gout and of optimal analgesic control of joint swelling and pain. Theodore Potter became chief of the orthopedic surgery program in 1962. Reconstructive surgery was critical, as there were no proven remission-inducing treatments, although the medical faculty did use gold therapy and aspirin. Patient care was a model of integrated rheumatologic-orthopedic management that was also dependent on nursing, physical therapy, and occupational therapy. In this setting, a Clinical Treatment Center for Juvenile Rheumatoid Arthritis was established (1963), with support from the National Foundation. In 1965, the Arthritis Foundation took responsibility for supporting the center's outpatient effort, termed "total patient care."

Despite these successes in clinical care and translational research, the Board of Directors and the hospital director (Horace Altman) were concerned about the increasing complexity of patient care that required additional resources and specialties. The requirements for additional administrative personnel imposed by Medicare and Medicaid after their enactment in 1965 and the unexpected shortage of available nurses were additional challenges. Stillman and the RBBH faculty began discussions with Robert Ebert, the dean at Harvard Medical School (HMS), that led the RBBH to become an HMS teaching hospital linked academically via the PBBH. With Stillman's consent, K. Frank Austen was appointed physician-in-chief at the RBBH in 1965. Austen had long, productive, and innovative involvement in rheumatologic diseases and immunology since his student days at HMS. Dean Ebert recruited two other rheumatologists with a laboratory immunology focus different from that of Austen to broaden the training and investigational environment: John David, who developed an in vitro assay for studies of cell-mediated immunity while at New York University, and Peter Schur, who worked in immune complex and complement pathway biology at the Rockefeller Institute. This triad settled into the supportive environment at the RBBH in 1966.

Further integration of multidisciplinary programs for the care of patients with rheumatic diseases followed. The chairs of the Board of Directors of the RBBH (George Kuehn) and the PBBH (Alan Steinert, Jr.) committed funds to Dean Ebert for a chair of a Department of Orthopedic Surgery for both hospitals, to be based at the RBBH. The position was accepted by Clement Sledge, a highly regarded clinician and investigator at the Massachusetts General Hospital and was the first recognition of a surgical subspecialty as a separate appointing department for either Brigham. Sledge's Orthopedic Surgery Department included Fred Ewald, William Thomas, Marvin Weinfeld, Richard Scott, Ed Nalebuff, and Louis Millender. This staff pioneered in total joint replacements in adults and children with rheumatoid arthritis. Superb programs in bone radiology, headed by radiologists Leland Sosman and Barbara Weissman, and in occupational and physical therapy were created. Under the leadership of Ronald J. Anderson, a former trainee who returned in 1971 to direct the clinical training programs, the Home Service Department and the Consultation Clinic were physically combined into a single Ambulatory Clinic. This unit offered opportunities for clinical training at multiple levels, the development of a clinical faculty with an academic mission, and improved care for all patients. Matthew Liang was recruited from Stanford in 1977 to lead a rheumatic disease outreach effort. His program grew to include aspects of healthcare delivery, costs, needs, and prevention as well as outstanding research in epidemiology and health services. Michael Weinblatt, a former trainee, published a seminal article in the *New England Journal of Medicine* (1985) that established methotrexate as the first treatment for rheumatoid arthritis with a disease-modifying effect. A second National Institutes of Health–funded training program was initiated in 1968 for allergic diseases. Albert L. Sheffer provided the clinical training for these fellows by expanding his private office, located outside the institution.

The discussion of a formal merger had moved through formation of a "mission group" in 1961 to a joint venture, consisting of the Boston Hospital for Women, the PBBH, and the RBBH. A committee representing each of these institutions met regularly for lunch to discuss a merger. The lunch was elegant but the progress meager. Hence the planning process shifted to individual hospital planning committees, which brought their consensus recommendations to a central planning committee. By 1975, the RBBH was ready to move to the new facility, named the Affiliated Hospitals Center, to include the three merging facilities, that could provide all the core functions needed to care for patients with complex medical problems. However, the initial Certificate of Need had been disapproved by the responsible state agency because the significant unhappiness in the contiguous neighborhood community had not been recognized. HMS Dean Ebert recruited a social scientist, Stephen J. Miller, from Brandeis University to analyze the issues, develop a remedial plan, and determine how best to implement this plan. Miller included Eugene Braunwald and K. Frank Austen in his interactions with the community during evening meetings in homes or in the local Mission Church. Community members complained that the presence of the merging institutions would drive up housing prices and rental rates and increase congestion and would not provide adequate medical services to the local community. With the participation of Harvard University and HMS, Miller hired members of the community with leadership potential to organize a decision-making process in the community so that their concerns could be addressed. In the end, these and other community concerns were met when the institutions provided resources for construction and accepted geographic limits for any future institutional expansion. The resubmitted Certificate of Need received a unanimous approval in late 1975, and the construction of the Affiliated Hospitals Center building commenced.

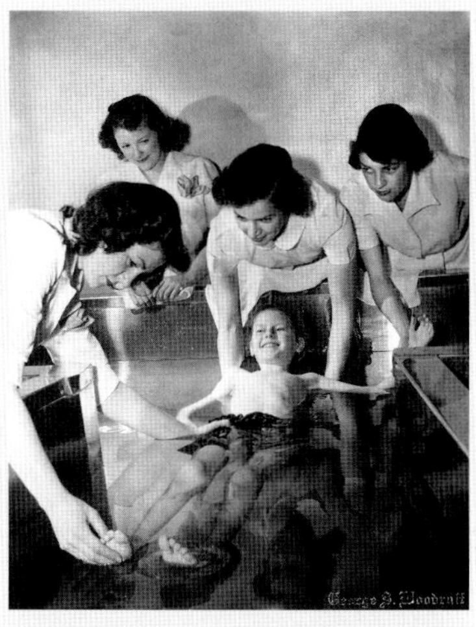

FIGURE 6-26 Robert Breck Brigham nurses with child in therapy pool, circa 1940s–1950s.

The research programs of the RBBH moved from the Parker Hill to a building at HMS (the Seeley G. Mudd Building) in 1977, prior to the opening of the new hospital. The RBBH gained outstanding campus-based laboratories at a discounted cost while contributing to the fiscal well-being of HMS. The clinical RBBH moved into the new Affiliated Hospitals Center building in 1980. It maintained some independent identity briefly by taking the top floors, which at that time included a pool for physical therapy.

Subsequently, changes within both the institution and the healthcare environment led to a fully integrated patient care system. In retrospect, the wisdom of the merger for the RBBH was seminal. The changes in healthcare reimbursement, with emphasis on short stays and ambulatory care, coupled with the astonishing advances in treatment, would have progressively reduced the inpatient census and limited the existence of the old, independent RBBH.

The RBBH Department of Medicine, a separate entity at HMS since 1966, maintained its independent appointing status until 1995, when it became a Division of Rheumatology and Immunology in the Department of Medicine at the Brigham and Women's Hospital (BWH). The Ambulatory Center, which has always partnered with Orthopedic Surgery in the care of patients with musculoskeletal disease, was overseen after Ronald Anderson by Michael Weinblatt (1985) and then Jonathan Coblyn (1999). Weinblatt also started a therapeutics unit focused on rheumatoid arthritis in 1985.

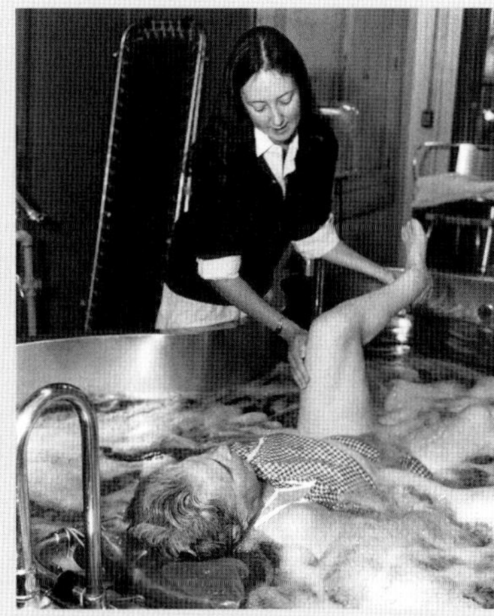

FIGURE 6-27 Robert Breck Brigham adult pool therapy, circa 1970s.

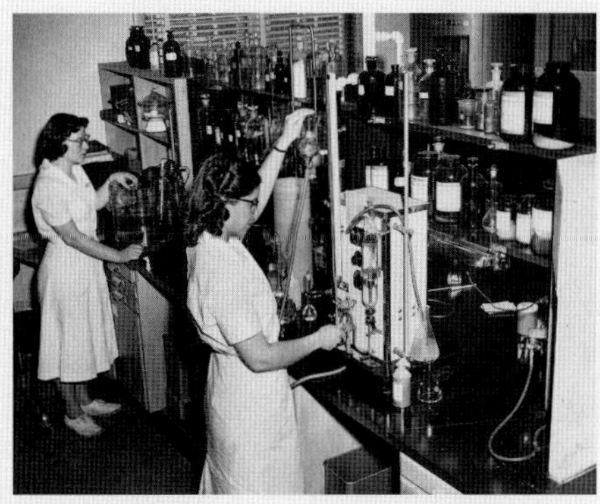

FIGURE 6-28 Robert Breck Brigham laboratory, circa 1950s.

By 1992, the staff had trained more than 173 postdoctoral fellows, of whom more than sixty-six had reached the rank of full professor or the equivalent in a research institute. In 1993, Michael Brenner, a rheumatologist who had defined a key subset of T cells while at the Dana-Farber Cancer Institute, joined the division. He replaced K. Frank Austen as chief of the division in 1995. In 1997, the research group moved from the Seeley Mudd site into two floors of BWH space designed in an open style by Brenner.

The current program in rheumatology includes specific diseases and problems: systemic lupus erythematosus (led by Bonnie Bermas, Elena Massarotti, Karen Costenbader, Peter Schur), rheumatoid arthritis (Michael Weinblatt, Jonathan Coblyn, Nancy Shadick), degenerative arthritis (Tony Aliprantis, Bill Docken), genetics of rheumatic diseases (Robert Plenge, Elizabeth Karlson), and health services research (Daniel Solomon, Jeffrey Katz). Visits expanded to 34,031 for rheumatology and 7,501 for allergy in 2011. In that year, Joshua Boyce became director of the Inflammation and Allergic Diseases Section. Boyce's basic research in the biology of the mast cell and the metabolic pathways for producing receptor-active arachidonic acid metabolites has led to clinical trials with novel interventions for asthma funded by the National Institutes of Health. The hub of the ambulatory allergy service for all age groups, located at 850 Boylston Street, has more than doubled in office suites since 1993 under the leadership of John Costa. A major advance has been the development of desensitization therapy for adverse drug reactions by Mariana Castells that has proven of great value to the oncology service. A multidisciplinary center for patients with mastocytosis under Cem Akin intersects with members of the Gastroenterology Division, the Dana-Farber Cancer Institute, and the Department of Pathology.

The RBBH persists in concept within the integrated BWH as two prime subspecialties, each in a growth mode, and as a major site of research into innate and adaptive immunity, providing a steady stream of new knowledge and talented physician scientists.

Free Hospital for Women, the Robert Breck Brigham, and the Lying-In would also make important contributions to this postwar research.

War's end brought other lasting changes to the PBBH community, including an expansion of diversity to the male physician trainees and staff, as medical school quotas were dropped for Jews and Catholics (although, ironically, female physicians who had served as substitutes generally left the staff). Brigham veterans returned with research interests they had developed during the war. In coming years Brigham researchers would examine not only the trauma of war but also psychosocial aspects of disease. This emphasis was evident in the outpatient clinics—especially

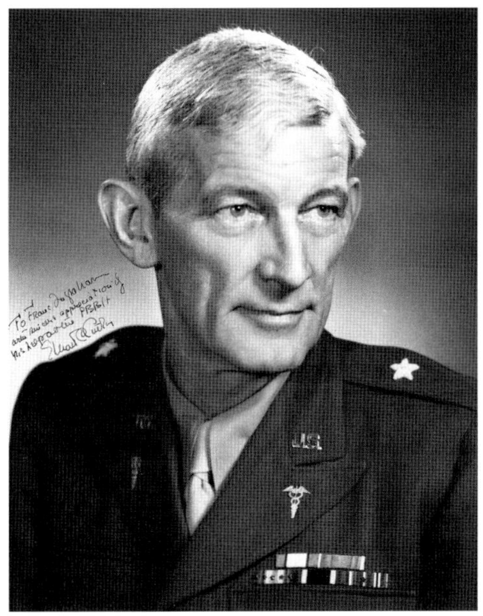

FIGURE 6-29 Brigadier General Eliot Cutler, World War II.

the alcoholism clinic and the medical psychiatric clinic—as well as research on responses to stress and other areas. Funding for research began flowing freely to academic medical centers, including the PBBH. As early as 1950, the PBBH received more than half a million in research dollars from the federal government and other sources; this would greatly increase over the years and aid facility development.[102] In part because of the influx of refugees from Europe, research and community-related interventions carried new intellectual strains.

The decades after World War II seemed to herald the triumph of American medicine. Nevertheless, as before, questions about the role of the physician—whether he or she was to be a clinician, researcher, teacher, ameliorator of community problems, or all of the above—would frequently be

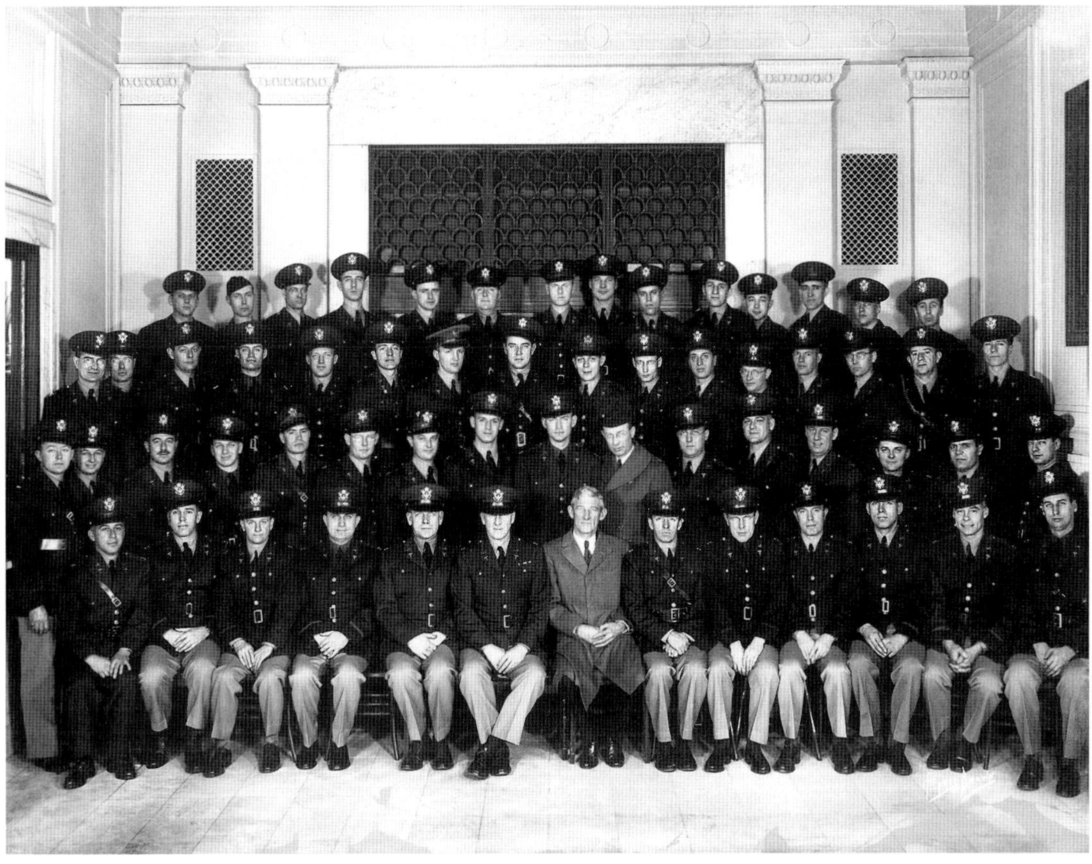

FIGURE 6-30 Fifth General Hospital, Harvard Unit, 1942.

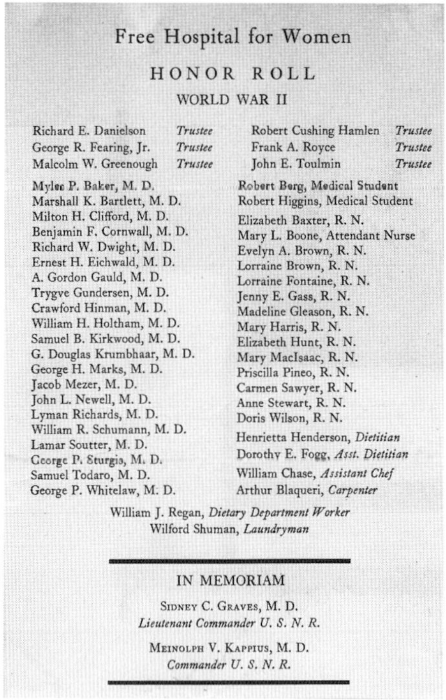

Free Hospital for Women

HONOR ROLL

WORLD WAR II

Richard E. Danielson *Trustee*
George R. Fearing, Jr. *Trustee*
Malcolm W. Greenough *Trustee*

Robert Cushing Hamlen *Trustee*
Frank A. Royce *Trustee*
John E. Toulmin *Trustee*

Myles P. Baker, M. D.
Marshall K. Bartlett, M. D.
Milton H. Clifford, M. D.
Benjamin F. Cornwall, M. D.
Richard W. Dwight, M. D.
Ernest H. Eichwald, M. D.
A. Gordon Gauld, M. D.
Trygve Gundersen, M. D.
Crawford Hinman, M. D.
William H. Holtham, M. D.
Samuel B. Kirkwood, M. D.
G. Douglas Krumbhaar, M. D.
George H. Marks, M. D.
Jacob Mezer, M. D.
John L. Newell, M. D.
Lyman Richards, M. D.
William R. Schumann, M. D.
Lamar Soutter, M. D.
George P. Sturgis, M. D.
Samuel Todaro, M. D.
George P. Whitelaw, M. D.

Robert Berg, Medical Student
Robert Higgins, Medical Student
Elizabeth Baxter, R. N.
Mary L. Boone, Attendant Nurse
Evelyn A. Brown, R. N.
Lorraine Brown, R. N.
Lorraine Fontaine, R. N.
Jenny E. Gass, R. N.
Madeline Gleason, R. N.
Mary Harris, R. N.
Elizabeth Hunt, R. N.
Mary MacIsaac, R. N.
Priscilla Pineo, R. N.
Carmen Sawyer, R. N.
Anne Stewart, R. N.
Doris Wilson, R. N.
Henrietta Henderson, *Dietitian*
Dorothy E. Fogg, *Asst. Dietitian*
William Chase, *Assistant Chef*
Arthur Blaqueri, *Carpenter*

William J. Regan, *Dietary Department Worker*
Wilford Shuman, *Laundryman*

IN MEMORIAM

Sidney C. Graves, M. D.
Lieutenant Commander U. S. N. R.

Meinolph V. Kappius, M. D.
Commander U. S. N. R.

FIGURE 6-31 Free Hospital for Women Honor Roll, 1942.

raised in the decades to come. Not long after the war was over, the hospital also experienced another round of financial challenges. Increasingly sophisticated care increased expenses, and the Brigham had always operated with, at best, a marginal surplus.

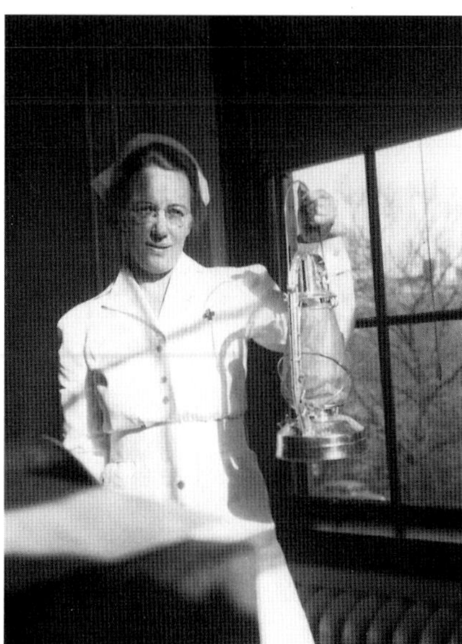

FIGURE 6-32 Free Hospital for Women nurse with blackout lantern during WWII.

Now staffing costs rapidly escalated because of competition for workers as well as changing federal wage policies. The hospital continued to give a large amount of free care—about $300,000 worth in each of the years 1945-1950, well in excess of endowment income. The hospital had largely been kept open through the Depression and war by the Community Fund (later United Community Services) of Boston, and even now, their annual contribution of $100,000 was vital to the hospital.[103]

As the PBBH began to recover from one worldwide cataclysm, another—in Korea, America's "forgotten war"—loomed. The 1950 Annual Report notes "sky high prices for everything having to do with hospital operation. The Armed Forces began to reach out for the Hospital's professional personnel...with the certainty of more serious drafts to come."[104] The PBBH staff also took the prospect of nuclear cataclysm and its potential role in provision of medical services very seriously, even developing a hospital emergency plan in the absence of one from the state or federal government.[105]

Innovation Continues

In recognition of the PBBH's financial challenges, in 1954 the hospital planned to embark on a three-year study of operations, as the hospital was now facing the challenge of preserving the traditional mission of patient care while significantly expanding research. Then, as now, cost and quality were central concerns. Even as more patients were able to use Blue Cross to fund their care, hospital leaders examined other insurance models, such as the Scandinavian system (studied by Merrill Sosman) and the British National Health Service (studied by Francis Moore).[106] The hospital also established a Public/Community Relations Department to facilitate understanding of PBBH's mission and relationships with the community. In the decades to come, Chiefs George Thorn and Francis Moore in particular would reflect on the hospital's mission, the role of the physician—"Science or Service?" as Moore put it—and responses to health problems.[107] The possibilities of a merged new facility were implicit in these reflections, especially after Congress passed the Health Research Facilities Act of 1956.

SPOTLIGHT

A BRIGHAM NURSE AT WAR

Bernice Sinclair

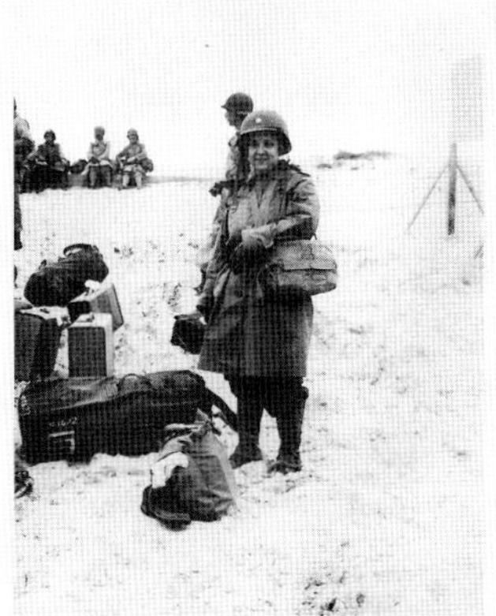

FIGURE 6-33 Bernice Sinclair in WWII uniform.

Like many other Peter Bent Brigham Hospital nurses, in World War II, Bernice Sinclair was affiliated with Base Hospital #5. She reported on her experience in the School of Nursing's Alumnae Journal, giving a flavor of her overseas service and the camaraderie of the Peter Bent Brigham community.[108]

"I shall never forget how casually we received the news of the invasion, which was to mean so much to us and for which I had been waiting in the United Kingdom for over two years.... this was the much awaited, long planned for D-Day...We went out on a small lighter to the big ship that was to take us across the Channel. When I saw the ladder over the side of the boat that we would have to climb up I thought I would never make it with all that weight hanging from me.... It was quite a job to get my short legs over the rail but with a lot of help and laughs I finally landed on the deck of the big boat...

"We rode in an open car and were showered with flowers by the wildly cheering people who seemed to be everywhere. Needless to say the appearance of a Femme Americaine created something of a sensation. Whenever we stopped children crowded to the car to take our hand. I knew how movie stars must feel when their public mobs them...

"A little later I had the fun of going to the 5th General Hospital which was in bivouac and obtaining some fifty nurses for work in the Third Army hospitals. It was grand to make my rounds and see so many old friends there, working on the wards and in the Operating Rooms...

"During the summer our hospitals were in tents, usually forty patients to a ward tent with one nurse and one or two enlisted men.... Sheets and blankets are used only for the sickest patients, pillows practically nonexistent. We have to improvise backrests, scrub-sinks and many other items. Tents are usually lighted by electricity, water has to be supplied in 5-gallon tins... Since practically all the patients are battle casualties, they arrive in a receiving tent, are sorted and then go to X-Ray, Shock or the pre-op wards. After operation they go to the Chest, Abdominal, Orthopedic or whatever ward is indicated. There are 40 nurses for 400 patients...

"There have been many times when the hospital is set up in only a shell of a building as the hospitals are usually following a division and often wait outside a town until it has been cleared by the Infantry....

"The Buzz bombs crashed a couple of times each night, but if you hear it you are alive, so why lose any sleep.... I crossed the Rhine over a pontoon bridge, but I am sure I shall be much more thrilled when I cross the Merrimac River in New Hampshire...

"We saw so many things I would like to tell you about but I will have to save—the hordes of liberated slave labor persons radiant with their new freedom, trudging along the highways with their little load of worldly goods fastened on their backs or pulled carts, walking many times in bare feet but waving frantically at the Americans...

"For an old lady of forty-four who came into the Army over-age to be with a somewhat fixed hospital set-up, I certainly have found myself in some very different situations. I trust this won't last much longer because I'm getting jeep knees and a jeep seat and I don't want to be too old and decrepit to be in a Victory parade. The rest can wait till I see you. Please forgive the mistakes of a poor typist and typewriter that has seen better days."

One of the most intriguing and prescient aspects of the PBBH's culture and outreach to community in the postwar years was its enhanced focus on the problems of a patient population with a longer lifespan. Most of the diagnoses that brought patients to the PBBH in the early years—rheumatic fever and tuberculosis among them—had been greatly ameliorated. Now routine issues were more and more those connected with chronic disease. Collaborative approaches to care emerged, highlighting the central roles of nursing and liaison with community. Among these mid-century community and preventive health efforts were the geriatrics clinics, the medical psychiatric unit, and the Psychological Metabolic Research Unit, which embarked on a comprehensive study of stress and metabolism, funded in part by the U.S. Army, using a multidisciplinary approach that included a sociologist and a psychologist.

THE TUMULTUOUS 1960s

In some ways, the 1960s may have seemed a triumphant time. Long gone were the days when the hospital had to struggle for legitimacy in a decade when hospitals were still viewed as questionable enterprises by some members of the public. Inpatient and emergency room use increased significantly, even as the hospital received funding from the government (Medicare) and other sources for clinical and community efforts. More than $1.4 million in free care was provided in 1963 alone.[109] More research funds were awarded to the Brigham each year, resulting in the formation of offices of grants and contracts and operations research. Clinic and Emergency Department visits continued to escalate, and the Outpatient Department was reorganized to render better patient care. At the same time, however, hospital staff worried not only about government control but how to best adhere to Osler's humanist as well as scientific vision in an era of specialization and amplified focus on research.[110] Further recognition was given to the critical roles of professional nursing and social work in hospital-based care. The social movements of the Sixties—civil rights, feminism, and student unrest—all affected PBBH culture, not least in relation to the community surrounding it.

The hospital's emphasis on ambulatory, prevention, and community-oriented care, however, belied "ivory tower" stereotypes. Physician-in-Chief George Thorn called for such an approach to become a fourth realm of service beyond patient care, research, and teaching, perhaps entailing a new specialty combining medicine and sociology. He was a proponent of community-based research and advocated for a strong ambulatory nursing presence. Thorn also frequently emphasized the need for a "comprehensive" approach to medical problems: "By this is meant an appreciation of the psychologic and emotional factors in the genesis and perpetuation of illness, as well as an understanding of the more specific patho-physiological causes of disease or malfunction."[111]

A Revolution in Primary Care

Early in the 1960s, the outpatient clinic at the PBBH was remodeled in a manner anticipating the future—not only that of greater general emphasis on ambulatory care, but as a template for the prospective merger hospital. The hospital reorganized all of its medical and medical subspecialty clinics so that each patient was under the care of one physician. In addition, as noted in the Forty-Ninth Annual Report, "the new medical program has made possible advances in nursing patient care, dietary consultation, and social service."[112] Physicians would work closely with a team including nurses, social workers, dietitians, and others. The new vision even incorporated sociologists to examine program outcomes.

Community-oriented programs now focused on numerous health risk behaviors, including alcoholism and sexually transmitted disease. Because of the passage of Medicare, hospital leaders understood that caring for an older population would be more and more important, and this was reflected at the Pearl Geriatric Clinic, where care followed a team-based approach.

By the 1970s, however, perhaps the most significant change in the relationship of the hospital with the community was the development of community health centers affiliated with the hospital. The first two Brigham-affiliated centers were the Brookside Community Health Center and the Southern Jamaica Plain Health Center. Brookside was originally established as the Brookside Park Family Life Center in 1970, a "grassroots" program based on community input and funded through the Model Cities Program to address the need for accessible, affordable health care that addressed families' social needs. The Brookside Community Policy Board affiliated with the PBBH in 1974 and subsequently with BWH and Partners HealthCare. Its history reflects ongoing development to meet patient and community needs: "In 1970, after initially opening for business in a school classroom, the health center moved to four house trailers and then into a renovated parish hall basement. By 1975, the health center had settled into its current location."[113]

Today, Brookside offers its more than 10,000 patients a suite of integrated services, including adult medicine, pediatrics, obstetrics, family planning, gynecology, dentistry, oral surgery, nutrition/Women, Infants, and Children (WIC), mental health, and social service. Obstetrics includes certified nurse- midwifery, a specialty sometimes considered to be the "face" of the Brigham in the community because the Brigham-based midwives also work at community health centers providing well-woman, family planning, and prenatal care, and bring their clients to BWH to give birth. Brookside also provides health promotion and community support services, including dental health, case management, a WIC program, nutrition and physical fitness youth programs, and parenting classes, as well as breast-feeding support and other services.

Founded in 1971, the Southern Jamaica Plain Health Center (SJPHC) serves almost 11,000 patients, including 7,500 adults and 3,500 children who utilize the two largest departments, Adult Medicine and Pediatrics.[114] Other services include prenatal and Ob/Gyn care for women (including midwifery as above), mental health care, and specialty care, including cardiology and podiatry. Like Brookside, SJPHC increasingly focuses on health promotion, including fitness and mind/body programming, for its diverse patient population.[115] The center participates in the Youth Health Equity Collaborative, the Violence Prevention Collaborative, and other partnerships. Working to guide youth into health careers through "pipeline" programs is also a focus. SJPHC's website "History" section notes:

> *After the Brookside and Martha Elliot Health Centers were established, mothers in the South Street area organized to get a center in the southern part of JP. Out of that effort came a two-room operation located in Curtis Hall, with Nurse Practitioner Barbara Hohman and a small staff providing services for children. Within a couple of years, the first physician was added, pediatrician Martin Leber; the affiliation with Children's Hospital was changed to a long-term affiliation with Brigham and Women's; the Center moved to its initial Centre Street storefront in 1974; it hired an Adult Medicine physician and were soon able to add a second, longtime Medical Director Michael Lambert. Eventually SJPHC was able to obtain the storefront next door for Adult Medicine.*
>
> *For the first five years after moving to our new facility, SJPHC experienced very rapid growth. By the end of 2004, the health center was providing services to over 10,000 patients. The number has been stable since 2004 because there is not adequate space in the facility for further growth.*
>
> *One part of SJPHC that continues to grow is its youth and community programming. Through a teen leadership program, Team Mita, collaboration in the South Street Initiative, and other efforts, it is working hard to address issues of youth violence, childhood obesity, asthma, and other key health issues that affect Jamaica Plain.*[116]

Today, like other components of the BWH network, SJPHC continues to provide a range of services to address the connection between health care and health promotion, using the partnership-based approach that has been a hallmark of its history. In all, there are now fourteen community practices affiliated with BWH, in Cambridge, Brookline, Norwood, and other areas; these include the Phyllis Jen Center on the Nesson Pike at BWH.

NEW OFFICE OF COMMUNITY MEDICINE CREATED AT THE BRIGHAM

Continued and consistent contacts over the past 1½ years between the administration of the Peter Bent Brigham Hospital and concerned citizens of the Jamaica Plain area of Boston have borne fruit here in the creation of the Office of Community Medicine.

Having grown more and more aware of the threatening limitations on existing health care at the community level, the Brigham, in the person of Dr. Andrew G. Jessiman, Director of Ambulatory Services, set up with the endorsement of the Hospital Executive Committee, the Staff, and the Board of Trustees this mechanism, within the administrative structure, to maintain the momentum developed in the relationship between the Hospital and the community of Jamaica Plain.

The immediate responsibilities of the Office of Community Medicine are to continue to stimulate resident interest in health care and preventive medicine, to coordinate the many institutions and agencies already involved in providing health services, and to project the Hospital's special commitment to the citizens of Jamaica Plain.

To achieve its more long-term goal, helping to provide more and better facilities in answer to the primary health requirements of community residents, this office is presently focusing its efforts on the acquisition of a planning grant from the Department of Health, Education, and Welfare. These funds will allow professional medical economists and statisticians to determine how and what should be done to ameliorate the health situation in Jamaica Plain. Having once established, rather than only speculated upon, the real needs of the community, definite plans can then be made for the extension of existing health facilities, or the development of new services.

The unique element in this approach to community medicine is in using the defined wants of a given area as a point of departure and then soliciting the assistance of a medical institution, as opposed to the traditional process of the converse: the hospital choosing a given set of services and then offering that to the population.

Miss Kathleen Ridder, former Clinic Manager of the Martha Eliot Health Center in Jamaica Plain, brings to the management of this new department her extensive knowledge of and experience with the entire makeup of Jamaica Plain, its residents, and their health needs. Her assistant, Mrs. Burch Ford, has recently returned from a community development assignment with the Peace Corps in West Africa and was previously employed in the public relations department of the Johns Hopkins Medical Institutions.

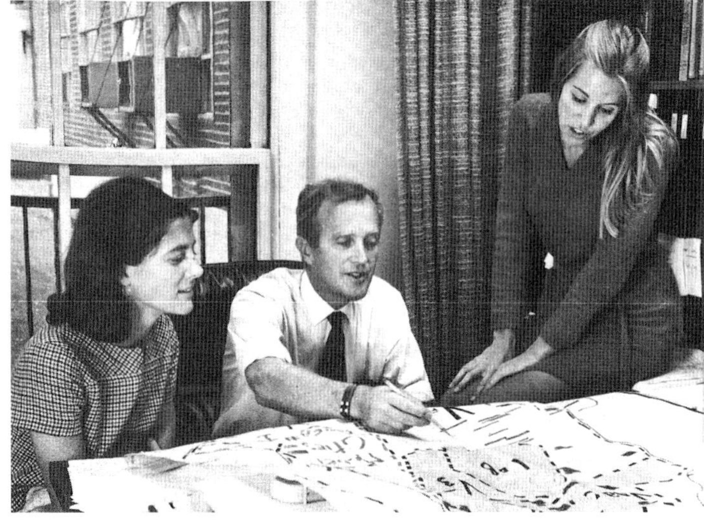

(left to right)
Mrs. Burch Ford, Dr. Andrew Jessiman, Miss Kathleen Ridder

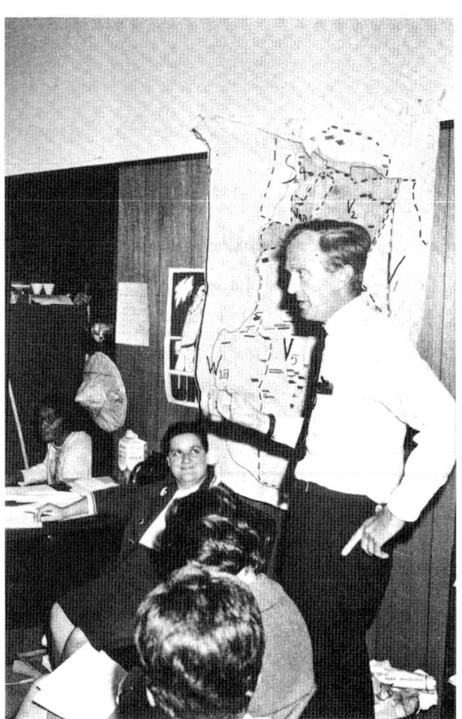

Dr. Jessiman gets down to work in the Community

FIGURE 6-34 1969 article from the Brigham Bulletin on community health.

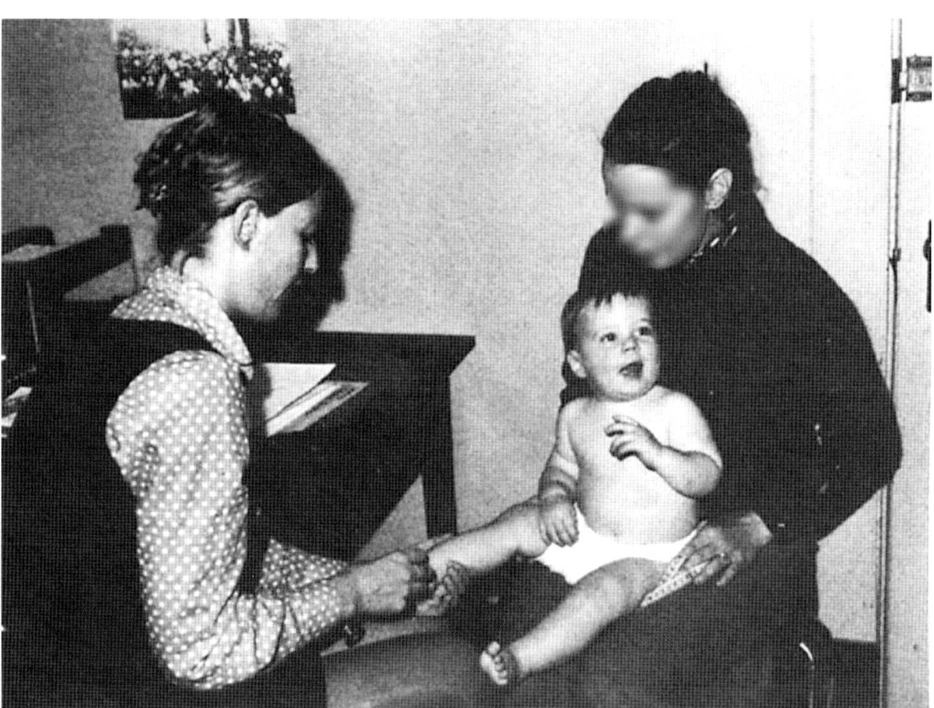

FIGURE 6-35 1971 Brigham Bulletin photo at the Southern Jamaica Plain Health Center.

SPOTLIGHT

COMMUNITY MEDICINE IN THE 1960s AND 1970s AND THE HARVARD COMMUNITY HEALTH PLAN

Andrew Jessiman

In 1965, I became the associate director and administrator for ambulatory services and the emergency room at the Peter Bent Brigham Hospital. Supported by funding from the Pearl Foundation for the care of the elderly, I established a home care program for patients discharged from the inpatient services and living in Mission Hill, adjacent to the hospital.

Learning of this outreach program, Eva J. Salber of the Childrens' Hospital and the Harvard School of Public Health contacted me. She was providing pediatric care at the Bromley Health housing project, just over the hill from the Brigham, and asked if the Brigham would provide medical care to adults. I met with the community committee of the Bromley Health Project to learn what services they wanted. Some members had concerns about the Brigham, noting the emergency room was their only source of both primary and acute medical care, and that any visit to the emergency room required long hours of waiting.

I addressed this by creating two streams of care in the emergency room, one of which was for primary care. I continued to meet with members of the committee to address additional problems, gaining trust and support in the process. In 1967, the clinic reorganized to become the Martha Eliot Health Center, a collaborative effort of Children's Hospital, the Boston Hospital for Women, and the Peter Bent Brigham Hospital. In 1970, Brigham internists commenced providing service to adults, with the enthusiastic approval by Chief of Medicine George W. Thorn.

The Model Cities Program for the city of Boston began under the leadership of Paul Parks in 1969. While creating health clinics citywide, he inquired whether the Brigham would provide adult health care to the clinics that were to be newly established in Jamaica Plain (the Brookside Park and Southern Jamaica Plain Health Centers). Although this was a compelling request, this greater involvement in community health care delivery necessitated commitment by the Brigham's clinical departments and the Board of Trustees. In the process, we confronted a general perception, of which the Jamaica Plain community was aware, that the Brigham was an "ivory tower" and not particularly interested in the health and well-being of communities. Conversely, many hospital staff believed that the Brigham was providing community care of the highest quality via the emergency room.

The Brigham clearly needed a humane commitment as well as positive communication to its neighbors. Stimulated by this reality, I recommended successfully to the trustees that members from the community committees be appointed to their board. Ultimately, the trustees approved the Brigham's commitment to these community programs and formed a Community Service Advisory Committee to promote its aims.

In 1969, to facilitate the creation of the new Brookside Park and Southern Jamaica Plain Health Centers, I formed the Brigham Office of Community Medicine. Its central task was to interact with members of the community, assist in providing means of health care to its constituents, and provide staff support for the Health Centers' development into politically active healthcare organizations. Although the communities relating to these two health centers were geographically proximate, their populations differed. Individual meetings with different approaches were necessitated during the development of the health centers. Nursing, dietary, and administrative staff met with community leaders and planned not only the physical structure but also the staffing and organization in a manner that was unique for each center.

The Brookside Park Family Life Center began operation in 1970 and in 1974 signed an affiliation agreement with the Brigham, thus operating under the hospital's license. The Southern Jamaica Plain Health Center opened and affiliated formerly with the Brigham at about the same time. As the Brigham's responsibilities increased, the administrative load of running the Office of Community Medicine required full-time leadership, which I could not assume. Harold May was appointed by Francis Moore in 1970 to be the first such director.

OUTREACH TO THE LARGER COMMUNITY

When Robert Ebert became dean of Harvard Medical School (HMS) in 1965, previously percolating plans for developing a prepaid group practice health plan came to life. I was asked by George Thorn to represent the Brigham in a working group to explore this possibility. The group, which also included physicians H. Richard Nesson (ultimately the president of the Brigham), Joseph L. Dorsey (a Brigham-trained internist, and ultimately chief of Harvard Vanguard Services at the Brigham), and economist Jerome Pollack (Harvard professor of economics and HMS associate dean for medical care planning), traveled the nation to observe the quality of care and organizational structure of other prepaid practices. We reported our very positive findings to members of the Brigham staff and its trustees.

Based on our report, the Brigham joined with HMS, other Harvard hospitals, and medical insurers to develop a facility that delivered comprehensive, high-quality services to a broad cross-section of the community, including Medicaid recipients, while at the same time effectively controlling the costs of these services. The product, The Harvard Community Health Plan, opened for business in 1969.

My tenure as the Brigham's administrator of ambulatory services was associated with a necessary and satisfying evolution of the hospital's mission. Care was being given through the two neighborhood health centers to residents of a large local community and, through the Harvard Community Health Plan, to those in other parts of New England. Through these practical actions, the hospital staff and its constituents developed a relationship of respect and trust. I had derived pleasure, learned much, and earned affection from working with fine women and men in our community. My respect for the leadership and vision of the medical staff and the Board of Trustees burgeoned.[117]

The 1970s

> *"Activities at the Brigham in 1974 ranged from the unhappy to the euphoric."*[118]

The 1970s were a time of flux at the PBBH as they were in society at large. Two intertwined themes developed: community health efforts stemming from the societal revolutions that began in the 1960s, and slow movement toward a merger that would allow the hospital to deliver better care and possibly ameliorate some of the problems of local communities contingent to the hospital. After an educational and negotiation process, the merger of the Peter Bent Brigham into the Affiliated Hospitals Center (AHC) was approved by community groups. Groundbreaking occurred in 1975.[119] Listening—by hospital leadership and hospital staff at all levels—was the key to resolving concerns, as was meaningful, inclusive representation and planning when it came to initiatives that affected the community and city, as both Andrew Jessiman and K. Frank Austen have detailed earlier in this chapter. Only a grassroots, "bottom up" approach to community-based health planning would be effective.

The hospital continued to expand and deepen the former focus as "Great Society" programs were implemented. At the same time, as barriers toward the admission of women and minorities, particularly African Americans, began to fall at medical schools, the makeup of PBBH staff started to change. As Eugene Braunwald began his Brigham career as physician-in-chief, PBBH noted his prior experience in community programs, including developing a comprehensive medical program in a community on the Mexican border. Under Braunwald's leadership, new primary care residencies would begin at both the PBBH and its affiliate, the Harvard Community Health Plan.

BIOGRAPHY

HAROLD L. MAY

Ann C. Conway

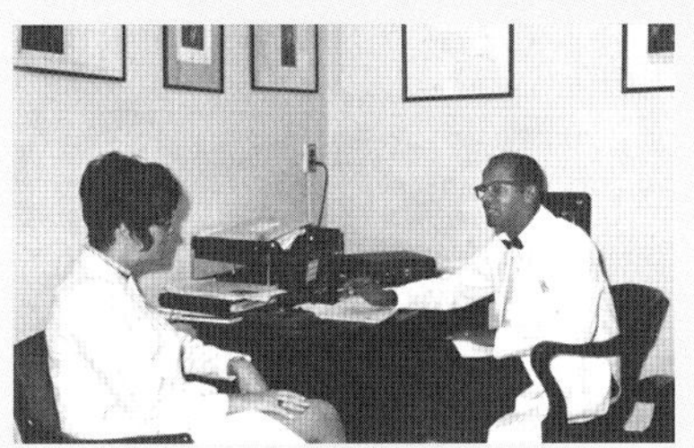

FIGURE 6-36 Harold May (right), 1971.

Harold May was a remarkable figure central to the story of expanded and inclusive Brigham-related community health programs in the 1970s. May, who was director of community health and medical care programs until 1975, graduated from Harvard Medical School in 1951 and received his MPH from the Harvard School of Public Health in 1974. The first known African American surgery resident at Massachusetts General Hospital, May was also a member of the Tuskegee Airmen, the first African American military aviators in the United States armed forces.[120]

As the Peter Bent Brigham Hospital (PBBH) Sixty-Second Annual Report in 1975 notes, prior to his Brigham appointment, May had been chief surgeon at Haiti's Albert Schweitzer Hospital, where he had spent thirteen years. "The decision that he had to make to leave his life of service, care, education, and ministry to the people of Haiti was not an easy one. It was his feeling, however, that at this time the very problems that had brought him to Haiti now existed in the large cities of the United States."[121]

Under May's directorship, both medical care and community health education were greatly strengthened. He worked closely with the neighborhood health centers and was medical director of what was then called the Brookside Family Life Center. May worked very actively with the PBBH Community Services Advisory Committee and its several subcommittees to establish trust between community members and the hospital.

May also worked to improve emergency services on several fronts, assuming a central role in addressing the concerns about care that are mentioned in Andrew Jessiman's account:

He, with others on the staff...pioneered in establishing model emergency care legislation for upgraded equipment, ambulances, disaster drills and offered at the PBBH the first Emergency Medical Technician course meeting national standards, in Boston. He (also) became chairman of the Emergency Services Subcommittee for the Regional Health Planning Council for Greater Boston.

His interests in health education were channeled into the development of a Continuing Education Program offered to neighborhood medical practitioners, the writing, organization and teaching of a course on Emergency Medical Care for fourth-year medical students at Harvard Medical School, and most importantly, the establishment of the Community Health Education Program.[122]

Although he remained on the surgical staff, after leaving the Brigham, May became director of medical services at the Wrentham Developmental Services (formerly Wrentham State School for the Retarded) for some years. He left that position in 1994 to establish FAMILY, Inc. (Fathers and Mothers, Infants, eLders, and Youth), an organization devoted to developing support services for children and families. FAMILY now offers a number of programs in Dorchester and Haiti, which are collaborative and holistic, emphasizing FAMILY's core view of humankind's interconnectedness:

> *FAMILY is more than a program; it's an organizing system—a way for people, programs, and systems to work together in harmony. It brings about societal change through systems realignment. Our mission is to develop systems of mutual support that will enhance the quality of life for all children and families, starting at the local level, thereby helping to move our society toward health and wholeness.*[123]

Mission Hill Revisited

By the mid-1970s, Mission Hill had substantially changed from the insular, still partly rural community it had been at the time of the Brigham's founding. The PBBH and surrounding neighborhood now experienced tensions similar to those of other neighborhoods and academic teaching centers in what was now termed "the inner city." The issues were multifaceted. Boston had an African American community long predating the arrival of the Irish, which was augmented during and after World War II as blacks migrated from the South. As was the case elsewhere, this migration coincided with the rapid industrial decline of Northern cities. In Boston, neighborhoods once relatively diverse in race and class increasingly became homogenous and racially segregated.

In Boston, the school busing controversy of the 1970s and 1980s exacerbated underlying socioeconomic inequality and led to extreme racial tension in Mission Hill and elsewhere in the city.[124] Violence emerging from the crisis led many parents able to do so to withdraw their children from the schools or move to the suburbs. Nevertheless, hospitals like the Brigham remained in urban areas, serving as major providers of emergency services as well as ambulatory and inpatient care—even as other social institutions fled urban locations in the face of high crime rates and the 1980s crack epidemic.

Although it did not experience the degree of white flight evidenced elsewhere in Roxbury and the city, Mission Hill was no longer the homogenous Irish community it had once been. New life came as a diverse population of blacks, Hispanics, and young people of all races gradually moved into the community. In 1969, the Mission Hill Health Movement was created to help obtain accessible health care for the community. But tensions between the Brigham and the community emerged as the result of conflicting sets of needs—the need of hospitals with aging facilities to develop the capacity for better care and that of the community to preserve itself and be a meaningful participant in collaborative decision making. Ironically, the extremely complex merger process once seen as internal to the Harvard Medical Area's institutions ultimately meant that the individuals and institutions involved learned to better understand and include the surrounding community, not only in decision making, but in multisector community services developed from the 1960s onward.

SPOTLIGHT

THE CENTER FOR COMMUNITY HEALTH AND HEALTH EQUITY

Ann C. Conway

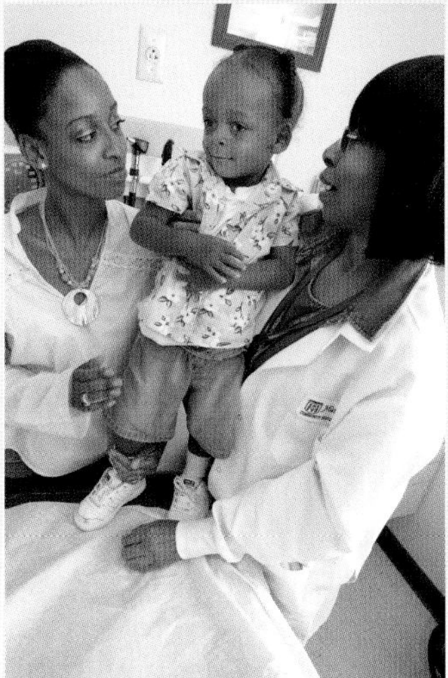

FIGURE 6-37 Clinical care in Mattapan. Shown are (left to right) mom Tristan Thomas with her son Tahkeel and case manager Beverly Jones of the Mattapan Community Health Center.

Brigham and Women's Hospital has long offered healthcare programs that take patients' social context into account. The emphasis of the Center for Community Health and Health Equity (CCHHE, formerly the Office for Women, Family and Community Programs) is on equal access, health through the lifespan, and the gap in health outcomes that disparities create. Members of the Center staff identify populations at risk and provide resources and support, not simply in prevention but in workforce development and fostering vibrant relationships between BWH and the community.[125]

In 2007, Wanda McClain became executive director of the CCHHE. Supported by physician, nursing, and administrative leadership, and based on strong relationships with community partners, CCHHE's approach is multifaceted, integrative, and research based. Its programs fall into five categories: Health Equity Programs, Violence Intervention and Prevention, Youth Programs, Health Equity Research and Intervention, and Community Programs.

HEALTH EQUITY PROGRAMS

Birth Equity Initiative

The Center for Community Health and Health Equity has developed a comprehensive Birth Equity Initiative to address low birthweight and differences in infant mortality, particularly in the African American community. The center's comprehensive approach marries the clinical, community, health system, and research sectors to address the complexity of disparities: *clinical* strategies seek to prevent preterm birth and reduce maternal psychosocial stress; *community* strategies address the social determinants of health and enhance civic engagement for this often "invisible" problem; *health system* involvement enhances women's health through a *life course* approach; and *research* determines the optimum approach for an intervention and analyzes clinical and psychosocial outcomes.

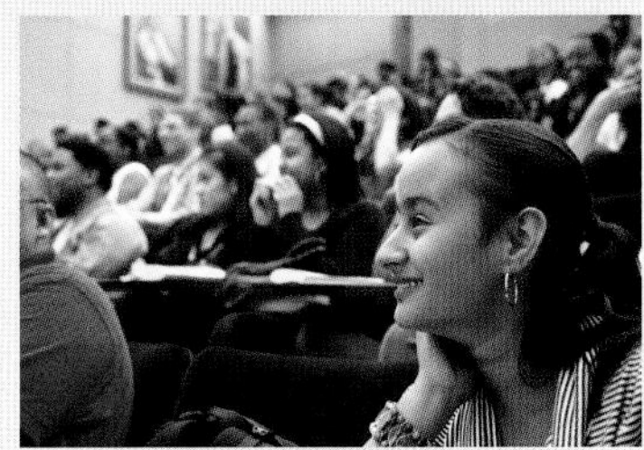

FIGURE 6-38 Student Success Jobs Program graduation, 2010.

Perinatal Case Manager Program

The Perinatal Case Manager Program began by partnering with six community health centers, providing case management services to pregnant and postpartum women. After more than two decades of service, it continues to help women with healthcare coordination, health education and access.

Connecting Hope, Assistance and Treatment (CHAT) Program

The CHAT program provides resources for low-income women with breast cancer who do not have adequate income or insurance to pay for necessary services related to their breast cancer diagnosis. These include help with the cost of medication, breast prostheses, other supplies, transportation to treatment, child care during treatment, and other expenses.

Open Doors to Health Colorectal Cancer Screening

A collaboration with Dana-Farber/Brigham and Women's Cancer Center, the three-year old "Open Doors" program strives to improve rates of colorectal cancer screening among patients served through the two BWH licensed community health centers (Southern Jamaica Plain Community Health Center and Brookside Community Health).

VIOLENCE INTERVENTION AND PREVENTION

The CCHHE provides a range of programs to address interpersonal and societal violence, experiences that bring disparities to the fore. The Passageway program provides services for patients, employees, and community members who are experiencing abuse from an intimate partner. Support services include advocacy, safety planning, counseling and support, education, and referral. Services include advocates within the hospital who identify and assist both patients and employees. More recently, Passageway has extended into the community through advocates connecting with community health centers, Faulkner Hospital, and community organizations.

The Violence Recovery Program, based on a successful Baltimore prototype, is a collaboration between the CCHHE and the Department of Surgery's Division of Trauma, Burn and Critical Care. The Violence Recovery Specialist (VRS) works as part of a multidisciplinary team to offer support and ongoing advocacy for the patient and family during the hospitalization. The goal is to reduce the burden of violence in Boston by providing nonjudgmental, comprehensive services to patients and families admitted to BWH after sustaining any violent intentional injury. After discharge, the VRS provides case management planning, advocacy, and support services as identified by the patient and VRS.

YOUTH PROGRAMS

The CCHHE continues the tradition of helping youth in the community and supporting workforce development through several programs that provide opportunities for young people interested in health careers. At the same time, its programs strengthen BWH-community bonds through volunteer programs that offer mentoring and support to community organizations and local schools. These benefit the more than 400 hospital employees who participate in addition to the youth they work with and learn from.

Among these CCHHE initiatives are the longstanding Student Success Jobs Program, featured on the NBC Nightly News and elsewhere. This introduces students from seven Boston secondary schools to medical, nursing, and science careers through a paid internship program that incorporates mentoring and hands-on experience. Recruiting begins in the tenth grade, and currently about seventy-five young people are served each year. More than 95% go on to college, most majoring in science/health related subjects.[126] The Brigham also provides scholarships to graduating seniors, with more than $100,000 awarded since 2006. Demonstrating the program's success, as of 2012, two students were attending Harvard and one, Stanford.

A second initiative, the Project TEACH Program, designed for a slightly younger audience, offers paid summer internships at BWH as well as the opportunities to participate in academic research projects. Another opportunity to learn about health and science careers is through the middle school Summer Science Academy, which provides field trips, intensive instruction, and other opportunities to explore careers in health care. Students are paid to work on research projects that demonstrate the link between scientific concepts and applications in the hospital. The Health and Science Club, for fourth and fifth graders, uses a project-based approach to teach science and investigative concepts through participatory projects led by BWH volunteers. The CCHHE's evaluations have shown that the program improves both knowledge retention and test scores.

HEALTH EQUITY RESEARCH AND INTERVENTION

Center for Community Health and Health Equity research focuses on "social determinants of health research and collaborates with individuals, institutions, and communities to contribute the best science, evidence, and resources toward eliminating inequities in health status for diverse groups."[127] This collaboration is community oriented and best practice based. In an ongoing process, research results are disseminated to partners and communities to help identify funding resources, build capacity and networks, and develop understanding of meaningful and effective research practices.

For the past thirty years, community health programs have been increasingly asked to demonstrate quantitative as well as qualitative outcomes of their efforts. The CCHHE has a strong research and evaluation cast and has demonstrated very positive outcomes for these community health and workforce development efforts. Nevertheless, it continues to examine its efforts through community needs assessment and other mechanisms, working to educate internally and externally about its efforts and their alignment with other BWH initiatives.[128] This assessment recently led to a new program in 2012 that brings community-based research alive; researchers work with the community in cosponsored projects that illuminate the research process and show how results are disseminated.

This integrative approach is overseen by BWH's twenty-nine-member Health Equity Oversight Committee, chaired by BWH's president, which meets regularly to set priorities. In this approach, BWH uses a "balanced scorecard" process to identify disparities and develop targeted interventions.[129] A measure of the success of the center's work and commitment is evident in the 2011 BW/F Strategic Plan, which identified health equity as a key commitment, complementing other strategic directions. A recent presentation shows very positive outcomes for many center programs. "98% of fourth and fifth grade students participating in Health and Science Clubs achieved a 25% increase in test scores. 94% of Project TEACH participants plan to pursue a career in health or science. 98% of SSJP high school alumni attend college; 60% have been the first in their immediate family to attend college."[130]

COMMUNITY PROGRAMS

Other longstanding CCHHE efforts include health care, employment, social programs and services, and many other quality-of-life issues facing the community. The range of organizations embraces schools (both public and private), housing developments, civic groups, youth organizations, and other service-related groups in Mission Hill. BWH support to these Mission Hill entities includes financial and technical assistance, volunteers, direct health services, and providing access to the hospital's professional staff, who contribute their time and services to assist in addressing health-related issues facing the community. Among the many groups and organizations BWH interacts with are the Alice H. Taylor Tenants Task Force, Maurice J. Tobin School, Mission Church Grammar School, Mission Hill Health Movement, Mission Hill Main Streets, Mission Hill Youth Collaborative, Parker Hill/Fenway ABCD, Mission Roxbury Tenants of Harvard, and Sociedad Latina.

Birth in the Death Zones

A community health issue of profound importance was Boston's infant mortality crisis in the 1980s. One cannot overstate how dire the crisis was. In 1985 alone, Boston experienced a 32% increase in infant mortality. Mortality among whites declined, but among African Americans, it increased by 65%. Stunned, observers attributed the numbers in part to a rise in very-low-weight prematurity, stemming from poor nutrition, worsening housing conditions, limited access to care, and other issues. Michael Weitzman of Boston's Department of Health and Hospitals noted: "The real problem is the enormous disparities between poor and non-poor women and between black and white."[131]

In September 1990, a *Boston Globe* spotlight series, "Birth in the Death Zones," focused on the human reality, noting discriminatory treatment, casual racism, and judgmental attitudes among some hospital staffs, the upcoming closure of St. Margaret's Hospital in a high crime area of Dorchester, and the diminution of the National Health Service Corps, which had once placed 1,500 physicians around the country in underserved areas similar to Roxbury but now had been cut to a total of 250 providers nationwide. One doctor noted burnout in the neighborhood health centers as a result of increasing rates of drug addiction and violence.[132]

BWH administrators and staff saw the effects of health disparities every day. At the time of the article's publication, the hospital delivered 32% of all Boston's maternity services to Medicaid and Healthy Start mothers, more than all other Boston hospitals. Nevertheless, as the *Globe* reported, in 1984 alone, seven infants had died before their first birthday in the shadow of the Longwood Medical Area.

In response to the crisis, with collaborators Beth Israel and Children's Hospitals, BWH targeted the issue, committing $4 million to the Harvard Institute for Reproductive and Child Health, whose aim was "to reduce infant mortality and improve the health status of low income Boston families."[133] BWH also established its own Center for Prenatal and Family Health, and provided $54 million in uncompensated free care during 1992 alone. But the infant mortality crisis would not begin to abate for years. Until very recently, Boston's African American infant mortality rates remained three to four times higher than those of whites.[134] In 2011, the Boston Public Health Commission reported that black infant mortality had decreased 47% from 2008 to 2009; they attributed the decline to a new approach of integrated perinatal and maternal prevention efforts. However, the rate was still much higher than that for whites.[135]

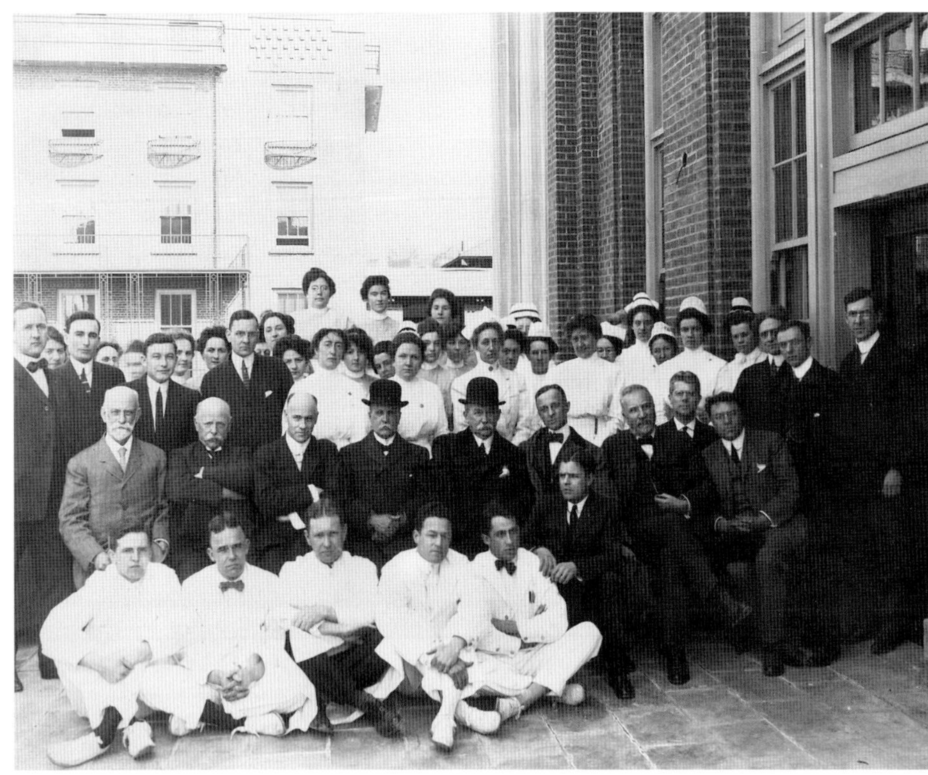

FIGURE 6-39 Osler visit with the original Peter Bent Brigham hospital staff, 1914.

Diversity, Community Engagement, and Workforce Development

By the standards of its day, the Brigham was built to be a meritocracy, looking outward from the insular world of nineteenth-century academic medicine, which had often been more based on social lineage than on native ability. PBBH physicians were recruited from the best and brightest, not just at Harvard but from other schools around the country. Those accepted for house officerships in the early years included Jews and a few women. However, elite hospital medicine was still overwhelmingly white, male, Anglo Saxon, and Protestant. In part this was attributable to the feeder system from medical schools, which retained formal and informal quotas preventing admission of too many Jewish students and others. This initial lack of diversity was also true of nursing schools, although at PBBH, Irish women appeared to join in larger numbers after the initial decade of the School of Nursing's existence.

Diversity at hospitals has always been affected by requirements to enter educational systems as well as their quality. In the early decades of the twentieth century, a high school diploma was required for admission to the new nursing schools, but only nine percent of the population possessed this in 1910.[136] Such requirements additionally affected the supply of social workers and other professions initially connected to nursing. Similarly, not only the issue of quotas but that of "pipeline"—providing newer Bostonians with the education necessary to qualify for medical school and thus to enter service at a hospital like PBBH—would not begin to be resolved until after World War II and then not for all ethnic and racial groups.

In the Brigham's early years, the patient population consisted of the commonly used categorizations of "American"—those born in the United States, including Boston's small but longstanding African American population, and "Foreigners"—immigrants from Ireland, Italy, Poland, Russia, China, and many other countries.[137] The hospital came into contact with many of these patients in the Out-Door Department and, from the beginning, noted that their physical concerns were linked to larger public health problems associated with poverty, overcrowding, family strife, and other environmental concerns.

SPOTLIGHT

WOMEN PHYSICIANS AND SCIENTISTS AT BRIGHAM AND WOMEN'S HOSPITAL

Carol C. Nadelson and Tina Gelsomino

During the early twentieth century, Harvard Medical School (HMS) and its affiliated hospitals employed women who Dean Eleanor Shore called "invisible faculty." They "conducted their research at a time when no women's names appeared in faculty directories, catalogues, or histories of HMS." A few women physicians and scientists worked at the Peter Bent Brigham Hospital in its early years. Some remained and developed their careers at the Brigham, and others went on to distinguished careers elsewhere. Until the 1970s, very few Brigham women had HMS faculty appointments.

The first woman staff physician at the Brigham was a roentgenologist and researcher named Gladys Carr, who was on the staff from 1914 to 1917. She was followed by Louise Eisenhardt, who worked at the Brigham with Harvey Cushing from 1915 to 1932 and was one of the world's foremost neuropathologists and investigators of brain tumors. Five other women professional researchers and clinicians were on staff from 1939 to 1940, and probably did not have HMS faculty appointments. Another Brigham pioneer, Olive Watkins (Smith), began her research at the Free Hospital for Women in 1929, after receiving a PhD in 1928 from HMS. She ultimately became the director of her husband's laboratory, the Fearing Lab. She made seminal contributions to understanding disseminated intravascular coagulation, toxemia of pregnancy and diethylstilbestrol, and enabling neonatal exchange transfusions for erythroblastotic infants. Despite her success, she also had no academic title until 1960, when she was appointed assistant professor of biological chemistry in the Department of Obstetrics and Gynecology at HMS.

Women had been house officers at the Brigham long before HMS first admitted women in 1946. In the Brigham's Fourth Annual Report in 1917, the acting president noted that: "the Peter Bent Brigham Hospital has been much affected by the war... Dearth of candidates and consequent difficulty in filling vacancies made it seem wise in the course of the year to abrogate the rule against nominating women as House Officers and members of the staff. This was done for the period of the war, and women have been appointed to such positions with satisfactory results."

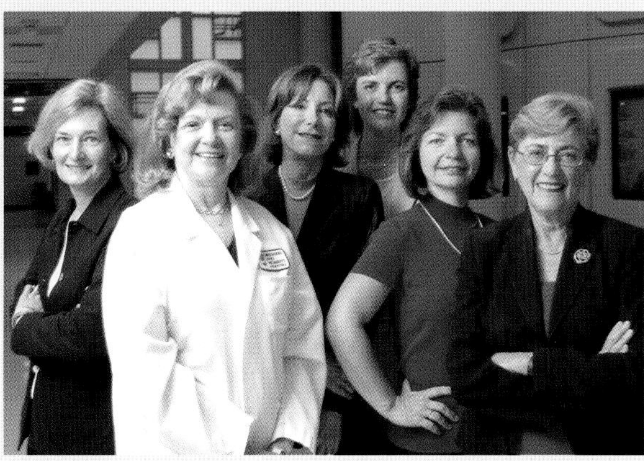

FIGURE 6-40 Cynthia Morton, Director, Partners Cytogenetics Laboratory; Director, Center for Uterine Fibroids; Director, Center for Hereditary Deafness; Program Director, Developmental Genome Anatomy Project; Julie Glowacki, Director of the Skeletal Biology Program in the Department of Orthopedic Surgery; Meryl LeBoff, Director of the Skeletal Health and Osteoporosis Center and Bone Density Unit; Nina Longtine, former Director of Molecular Diagnostics, Co-Director, Personalized Cancer Medicine Partnership; now Vice Chair of Molecular Pathology and Genetics, Mount Sinai Medical Center; Ursula Kaiser, Chief, Division of Endocrinology, Diabetes, and Hypertension; Carol Nadelson, Senior Advisor, Center for Faculty Development and Diversity.

The first HMS graduate to be appointed a house officer at the Brigham was Mary Efron, who was an intern in Medicine in 1951-1952. A handful of women house officers were appointed during the next three years. Thereafter, the flow stopped until the 1970s, when Eugene Braunwald and Marshall Wolf actively recruited women (see Chapter 2). Subsequently, the numbers increased slowly until the late 1970s and early 1980s, when the pace quickened. In the Department of Medicine alone, 20% of interns were women in the late 1980s. Women have occupied about 45% of internship positions since 2000. Appointed to leadership positions during their training, women were chief residents in medicine in 1985-1986 (Nancy Berliner, currently chief of hematology), 1989-1990 (Jane Weeks, who went on to become chief of population sciences at the Dana-Farber Cancer Institute until her untimely death in 2013), 1990-1991 (Paula Johnson, the first African American chief resident, currently chief of the Division of Women's Health in the Department of Medicine and the Connors Center for Women's Health and Gender Biology), and subsequently.

In the 1950s, a small number of women joined the Brigham as both clinicians and researchers. By the 1960s, the numbers of women on staff as physicians and scientists with HMS faculty appointments began to increase. This slow trend, which continued into the 1970s, included stellar physicians. Shirley Driscoll, the first woman chief resident in Pathology at the Brigham from 1954 to 1955 and a pathologist at the Boston Lying-In Hospital commencing in 1958, became one of the first female full professors at HMS in 1975 and chief of a service (pathology of the Boston Hospital for Women Division) at the Affiliated Hospitals Center in 1978. Nina Starr Braunwald joined the Brigham in 1972 as a distinguished cardiothoracic surgeon. She was the first woman worldwide to be certified for and perform open heart surgery and to be elected to the American Association for Thoracic Surgery. She led in surgical innovations, including developing the Braunwald-Cutter cardiac valve and the stented aortic homograft for mitral valve replacement. Her daughter, Allison Goldfine, says of her, "If Mt. Everest were in front of her, she would climb it." The characteristics of these pioneering women—determination, embracing challenge and moving forward—forged a path to success for those who followed.

During the late twentieth and early twenty-first centuries, many Brigham women received prestigious awards and honors, including election to the National Academy of Sciences and the Institute of Medicine. In 2002, when the National Library of Medicine and the National Institutes of Health (NIH) created a video program on women medical leaders entitled *Changing the Face of Medicine*, Brigham physicians Judy Ann Bigby, Nina Braunwald, Louise Eisenhardt, Paula Johnson, JoAnn Manson, Barbara McNeil, and Carol Nadelson were highlighted. (The project is now available online at www.nlm.nih.gov/changingthefaceofmedicine/.) Brigham women physicians are now leading or have led medical schools (Karen Antman and Laurie Glimcher), hospitals (BWH President Elizabeth Nabel), the Massachusetts Department of Health and Human Services (Judy Ann Bigby), and the National Heart Lung and Blood Institute of the NIH (Elizabeth Nabel, former). Barbara Bierer presently serves at the Brigham as the senior vice-president for research. In 2012, several women were division chiefs, but no woman chaired a department.

About 40% of the Brigham-based HMS faculty are women. Six of the fifty-seven currently occupied Brigham-based HMS clinical professorships are held by women: Samia J. Khoury (Sadie and David Breakstone Professor of Neurology), Meryl S. LeBoff (Brigham and Women's Hospital Distinguished Chair in Skeletal Health and Osteoporosis), JoAnn Manson (Michael and Lee Bell Professor of Women's Health), Cynthia C. Morton (William Lambert Richardson Professor of Obstetrics, Gynecology and Reproductive Biology), Susan Redline (Peter Farrell Professor of Sleep Medicine), and Christine E. Seidman (Thomas W. Smith Professor of Medicine and Genetics). Women physicians currently occupying two of the thirteen Brigham distinguished chairs are Clare Tempany-Adfhal (Feren Jolesz Distinguished Chair in Radiology Research) and Stacey E. Smith (Barbara N. Weissman, Distinguished Chair in Musculoskeletal Radiology).

The increased numbers of women entering careers in medicine and science brought with it an increased awareness of the challenges, including gender inequity in salary, promotion, visibility, and leadership opportunities. Obstacles to career advancement were often related to problems with career-family balance, inadequate mentoring, or lack of inclusion in collaborative research. In 1996, a Partners Healthcare Committee on the Advancement and Support of Women in Academic Medicine was charged to provide recommendations that would "serve to overcome the obstacles identified at Partners institutions." The committee conducted a well-designed survey of faculty at Partners institutions and identified differences in the career paths and trajectories of male and female faculty, as well as differences in job satisfaction and institutional support. The Committee thus made general and specific recommendations on promotion, support for professional development, and finances for women. It also called for the creation of Offices for Women's Careers at the Massachusetts General Hospital and the Brigham, which were charged to realize these goals, support and advance the recruitment and retention of women faculty, encourage women in research careers, and facilitate women's academic promotion and advancement. These offices were established, and the Brigham office was headed by Carol Nadelson from its inception in 1998 to 2013, when Kathryn Rexrode took over this role.

Early on, the Brigham's Office for Women's Careers created an Advisory committee, composed of women faculty from most hospital departments. The committee has undertaken many initiatives to meet the needs of women faculty, including those addressing expanded child care resources, support for the development and promulgation of workplace harassment policies, and an increase in the number of women in named chairs. The Office for Women's Careers offers programs to enhance mentoring, leadership and career skills, promotion guidelines, and many other subjects. It provides individualized career planning and advising for women faculty and collaborates with Brigham departments to facilitate women's promotion and advancement. It has worked actively to increase the number of women in named chairs. A Women's Leadership Program has been established to enhance the leadership skills of junior women faculty. Nadelson meets regularly with department chairs and division chiefs to discuss career paths and promotion and advancement possibilities for each woman faculty member. The Office for Women's Careers, represented by Nadelson, participates in many national and HMS-based groups with similar goals.

The careers of women at the Brigham have come a long way in a century, but we have not climbed to the top of Mt. Everest yet. We shall strive to reach that goal well before the next century.[138]

Regarding the employees of teaching hospitals, even after more Irish Catholics, Jews, and women in large numbers gained entrée, African Americans and other minorities remained rare. Medical and other health professional schools still did not admit many black applicants; in the 1950s and 1960s, only 2-3% of medical students were black. As the civil rights movement progressed, the American Association of Medical Colleges called for a proportionate increase to 12% by 1975-1976.[139] Relating this issue to the Brigham, parity for women physicians improved from the 1960s onward, though challenges still exist. As in the early days of the PBBH, a gap still exists between the population served by hospitals like the Brigham and its clinical workforce. Much remains to be done to have a physician population that matches the demographic makeup of Boston and other cities.

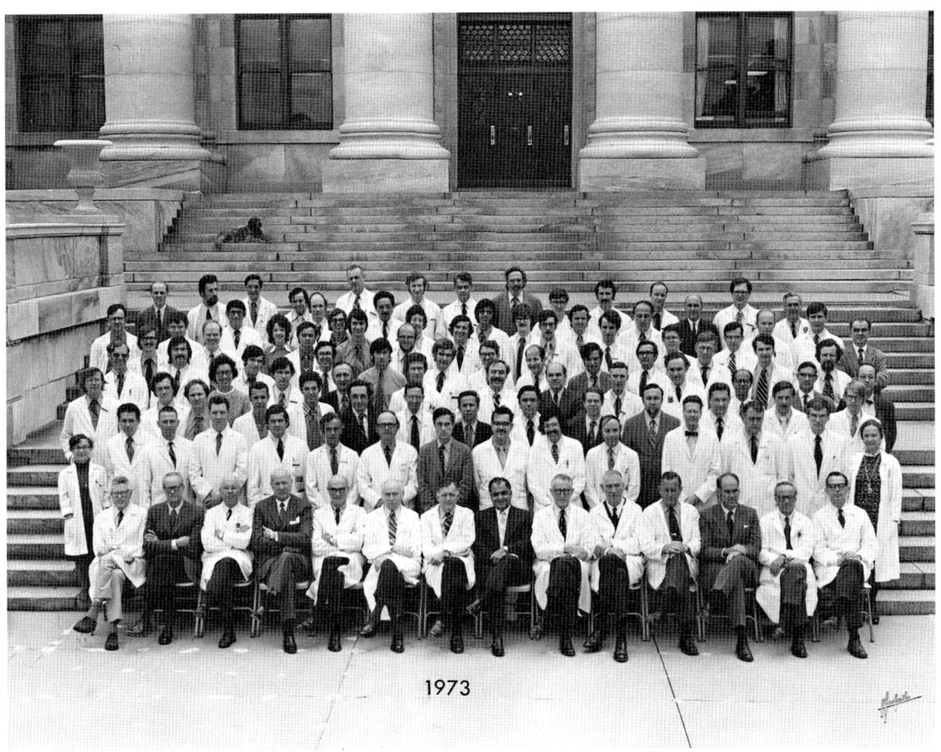

FIGURE 6-41 Peter Bent Brigham hospital staff photo, 1973.

SPOTLIGHT

THE *BRIGHAM BULLETIN* ON WOMEN IN MEDICINE, 1958

Curtis Prout

In 1958 the Brigham Bulletin ran a series on women doctors at the Peter Bent Brigham Hospital. This article was the first in the group. Author Curtis Prout was a chief resident at the Peter Bent Brigham and a primary care physician. From 1984 until 1992 he was also an assistant dean for student affairs at Harvard Medical School. He was known for his work advocating the improvement of medical care in prisons. Prout died in 2011 at the age of ninety-six.[140]

"The Bulletin is to publish a series of articles on women doctors at the Brigham. The first biographical sketch in this series on Dr. Cass, appropriately enough, is in this issue.

"At the present time [1958] it appears that of the total number of doctors at the Brigham, 275, approximately, fifteen are women. This is just under 6%. This is rather close to the proportion of women in Medicine in the country at large and also seems to be the same proportion, roughly speaking, that graduate from the Harvard Medical School each year. The selection of these percentages in each case has been arrived at independently, and without reference to any quotas, so the magic figure of 6% evidently represents that proportion of the population for whom Medicine is the chosen career and whose abilities and achievements earn them these places.

"In the early years of the Brigham Hospital women doctors were rarely seen and then principally on the laboratory services. In recent years their percentage distribution on the various services of the hospital corresponds quite closely with that on the national scene. By contrast a rival teaching institution situated farther down the Charles River Valley has under 2% women doctors on its staff and the place of women on the hospital staff is evidently a matter still of some discussion there.

"Obviously, women doctors are here to stay and in fact, only in Boston has there been much of any debate on the subject in the last ten or fifteen years. In other countries, notably Russia, the percentage of women doctors is very much higher, and their increasing numbers in Russia and in Western Europe has certainly not lowered the level of medical education and practice. Only a most die-hard feminist would expect us to demand celibacy or infertility from our women doctors. Obviously, we should not begrudge them, but rather facilitate for them, the time lost for producing and rearing a family. In short, we welcome them as doctors and as women."[141]

Workforce Development

To help find solutions to these historic problems, since the 1970s the Brigham has created programs that not only address diversity in the current workforce but also reach out to the community by providing information and support for young people interested in entering health careers. Programs for current BWH faculty and staff have also played a major role.

The Center for Faculty Development & Diversity (CFDD) was established at BWH in 2006 to provide a comprehensive and systematic approach to the professional development and career advancement of faculty and trainees across the academic continuum, thus enhancing recruitment and retention and development. Under its aegis are the Office for Women's Careers, Office for Research Careers, and the Office for Multicultural Faculty Careers.

The Office for Women's Careers (OWC) was established at Partners Healthcare in 1998, with offices at both BWH and MGH; psychiatrist Carol Nadelson was appointed the first BWH director. The Office for Research Careers became a part of the Center in 2006 and addresses the needs of trainees in the research community.

The Office of Multicultural Faculty Careers (OMC) undertakes interconnected efforts targeting recruitment, retention, and advancement of physicians, fellows, researchers, and trainees while providing

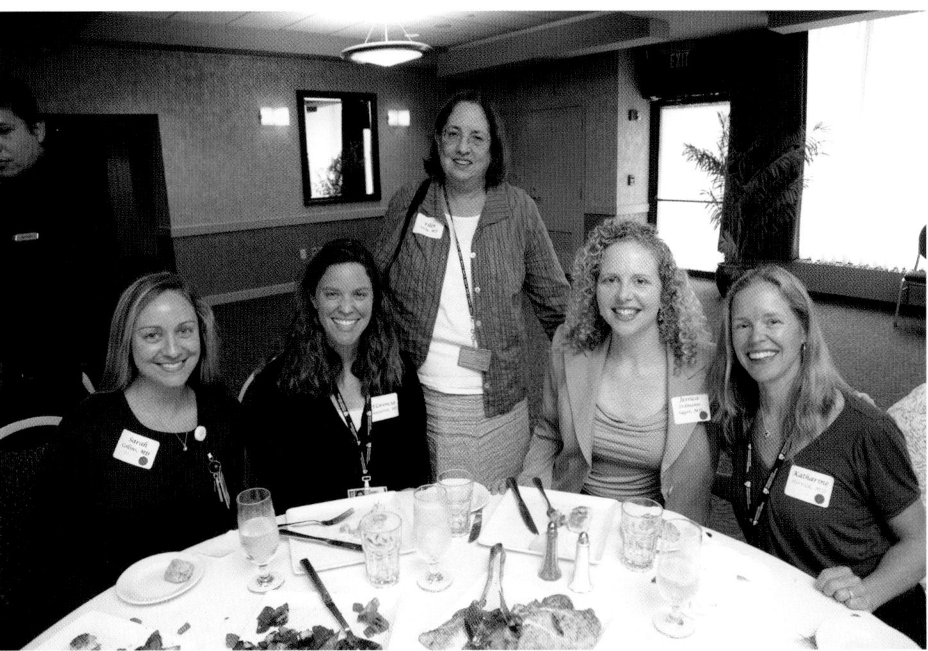

FIGURE 6-42 Standing: Vice Chair of Faculty Development Ellen Seely (Endocrinology) and new women faculty, 2012 (left to right): Sarah Collins (Nursing Informatician, Partners Healthcare); Florencia Halperin (Endocrinology); Jessica Erdman-Sager (Plastic Surgery), and Katharine Herrick (Newborn Medicine).

support for minority students interested in health careers. As the OMC notes:

In 1994, then-President Richard Nesson established the Committee on Diversity, later reorganized as the Diversity Oversight Committee (DOC), which first implemented the Minority Faculty Development Fellowship Program. Eight years later, through the leadership of Nesson's successor, President Gary Gottlieb and Marshall Wolf, the BWH Diversity Support Structure, which included the Office for Minority Career Development, was created. Led by O'Neil Britton, its focus was building and retaining a diverse community of medical students, residents and staff physicians.[142]

In 2005, Christian Arbelaez was asked by Gottlieb to represent BWH with the HMS Office for Diversity and Community Partnership and to initiate a hospital-wide diversity recruitment strategy. Concurrently, a vision for the Center for Faculty Development and Diversity began taking shape, and the Office for Multicultural Faculty Careers was established as a member office, with Arbelaez as the first Associate Director.[143]

The OMC was created to address these challenges and plays a key role in the areas of recruitment, retention and advancement of under-represented minority (URM) faculty, fellows, residents and students through advocacy, programming, research and tailored support to the URM community. In 2009, Nora Osman, who assumed leadership of the Department of Medicine's Office for Multicultural Affairs in 2004, became an Associate Director of the OMC. The need to target

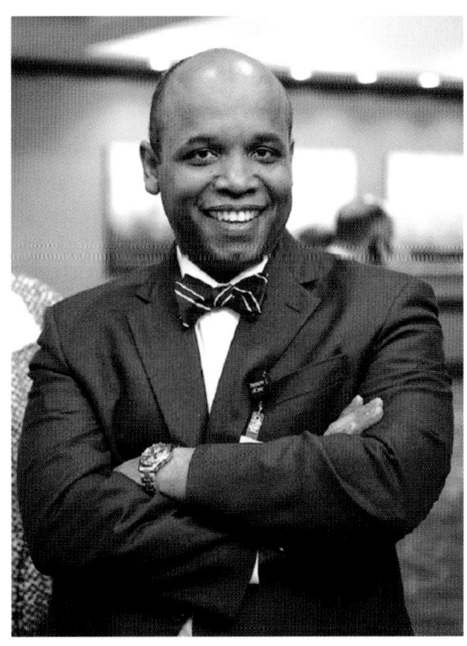

FIGURE 6-43 O'Neil Britton (Hospitalist), the first associate director of the Office of Minority Career Development at BWH before the creation of the Center of Faculty Development and Diversity. Britton is the former Chief Medical Officer at Faulkner Hospital and is now Chief Health Information Officer, Partners HealthCare Inc.

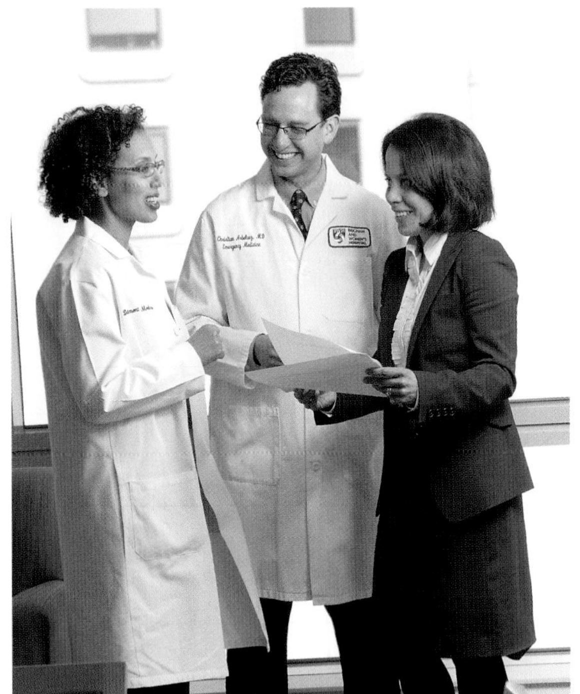

FIGURE 6-44 Left to right: Nora Osman (General Internal Medicine), and Christian Arbalez (Department of Emergency Medicine), Co-Directors of the Office for Multicultural Faculty Careers, and Ileana Jiménez García, Administrative Director of the Office for Multicultural Faculty Careers.

> *URM faculty recruitment and retention remains critical: 2010 Census data shows that minority groups comprise over thirty percent of the total population in the United States, yet they are represented by ten percent of all U.S. physicians and seven percent (URM only) of all U.S. medical school faculties.*[144]

The OMC now offers a variety of education and mentoring services as well as social and networking events for minority physicians, researchers, and students. It is also responsible for recognition, such as the Minority Faculty Career Development Award and collaborates with the HMS Office of Diversity Inclusion and Community Partnership, which addresses diversity throughout the HMS community.

Workforce Development Services for BWH Staff

Human Resources also provides a diversity and inclusion focus through its education offerings for staff, such as courses on cultural competence and leadership, valuing diversity, strategies to address the needs of older patients, and understanding disability. A major component of Workforce Development's mission is to offer skill improvement and career development courses to BWH's entry and mid level workforce, and programs include offerings such as English as a Second Language classes, high school General Equivalency Diploma (GED) preparation, work skills, online college preparation and tutoring, a citizenship course, career coaching, and financial assistance. Human Resources addresses the "pipeline" issue through its youth summer program, where more than hundred local high school students are hired to work at the hospital for seven weeks. An associated college scholarship is awarded each year, and there are two internship programs for college students as well as two work-study programs. A Teen Advisory Council helps plan student engagement events. Finally, BWH works collaboratively with Mission Hill agencies to qualify residents for employment. In 2006, another major accomplishment occurred with the opening of a satellite Human Resources office at 741 Huntington Avenue, a novel approach to offering a "front door" to members of the Mission Hill community and an example of the Brigham's commitment to its neighbors.

In recognition of the value of multilingual communication, the Brigham received a grant of more than $400,000 to develop Spanish-speaking education for members of the staff. Childcare opportunities expanded, as did programs to address social issues that might affect faculty and staff performance, such as domestic violence.[145] Employees were also publicly recognized for promoting workforce diversity internally, and diversity-related education came to the fore.[146,147]

The LBGT Resource Group

The Lesbian Bisexual Gay Transgendered (LBGT) Resource Group (a joint effort with Brigham and Women's Faulkner Hospital), provides networking and advocacy for LBGT staff and patients. The Human Rights Campaign Foundation's Healthcare Equality Index 2012 named Brigham and Women's/Faulkner as "Leaders in LGBT Healthcare Equality" in the Healthcare Equality Index 2012 report, an annual survey conducted by the educational arm of the country's largest LGBT organization. Both hospitals earned top marks for their commitment to equitable, inclusive care for LGBT patients and their families, who

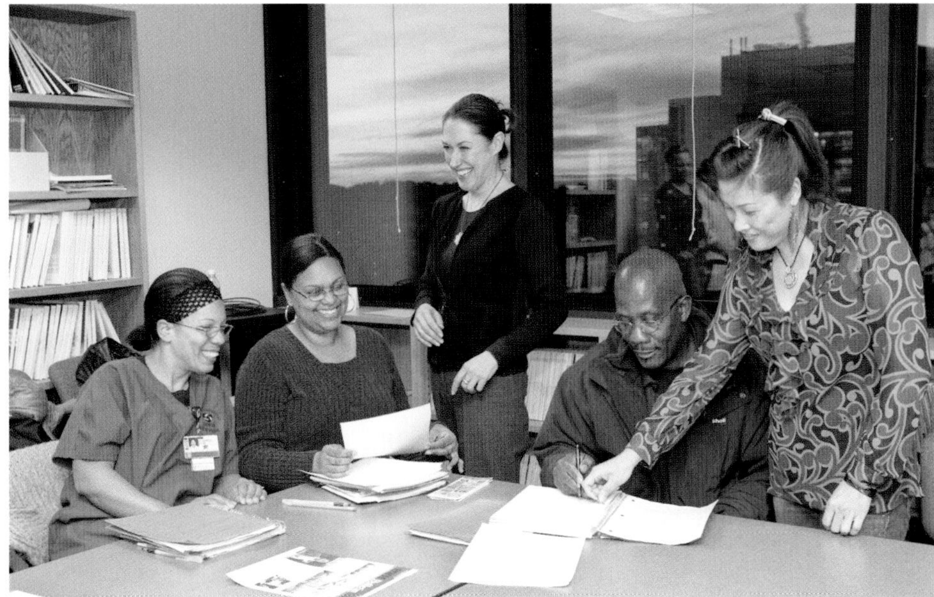

FIGURE 6-45 ESOL (English for Speakers of Other Languages) classroom at BWH. In this photo the teaching is being provided by Jewish Vocational Services. The teacher pictured is Kathleen "Kat" Brown.

can face challenges in accessing adequate health care. BW/F's inclusion policies include nondiscrimination policies for LGBT patients and employees, equal visitation for same-sex partners and parents, and LGBT health education for staff.

Youth Outreach Programs

The Center for Faculty Development and Diversity's Office for Multicultural Faculty Careers also hosts two summer programs for Native American and underrepresented minority youth interested in science and medical careers: The Four Directions Summer Research Program (FDSRP), directed by Thomas Sequist, and the Summer Training in Academic Research and Scholarship Program (STARS), directed by Chinwe Ukomadu. These give Native American and minority college juniors, seniors, and medical students an opportunity to work on basic

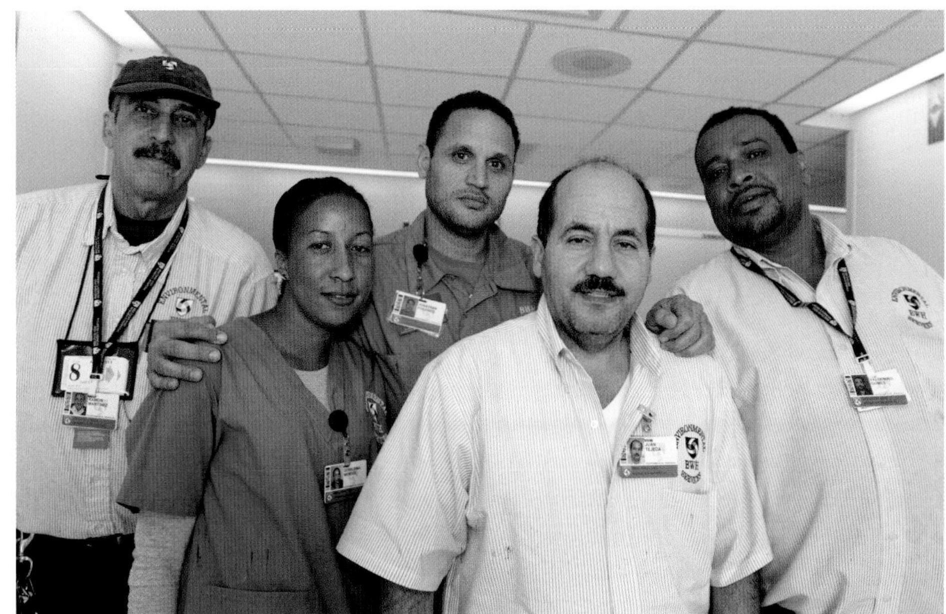

FIGURE 6-46 Workforce development programs can be used by all BWH staff. Pictured (left to right): Environmental Services staff members Ramon Martinez, Geraldina Mendes, Jonathan Polanco, Juan Tejeda, and Valdemiro Gomes.

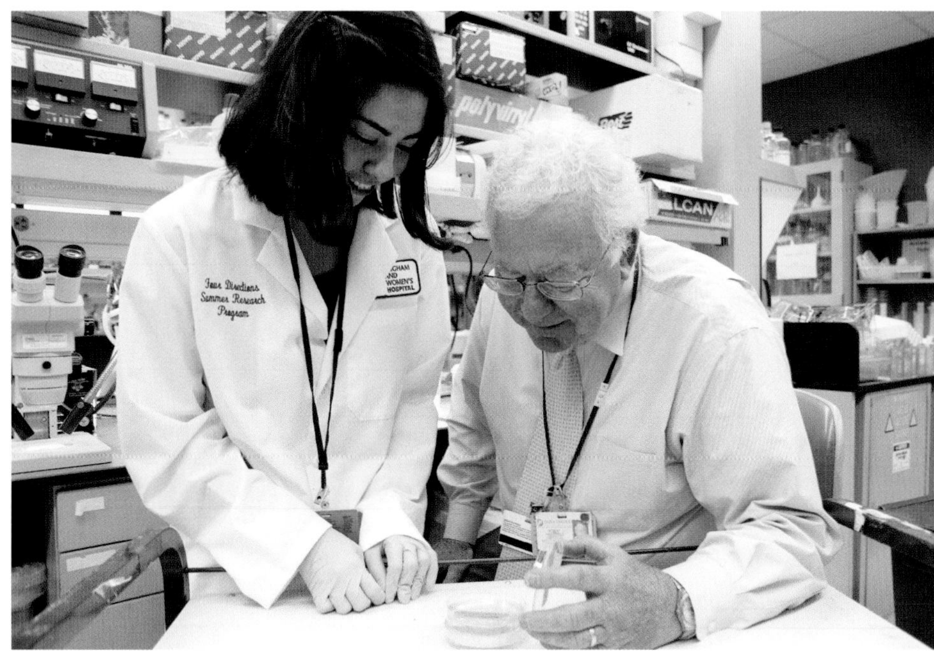

FIGURE 6-47 Robert Handin with a Four Directions Summer Research Program participant.

science research projects under the guidance of BWH faculty mentors.

A 2011 *BWH Bulletin* article noted: "The eight-week program provides the students with clinical shadowing experiences, social networking opportunities and weekly roundtables with BWH faculty representing the breadth of professional pathways in academic medicine."[148] "I was able to see the different fields in medicine and how vast it really is," said Brady Magaoay, an FDSRP participant and senior at Stanford University. "I want to return to Hawaii and become a doctor there and give back, especially since we have a shortage of doctors."[149] A STARS summer researcher noted that they'd learned about not only collaboration and networking, but about the vastness of medical and research opportunities.

STARS collaborates with the Jackson Heart Study, the largest single-site, prospective, epidemiological investigation of cardiovascular disease among African Americans. This partnership brought Curtis Haynes and other students from Tougaloo College, Jackson State University, and the University of Mississippi Medical Center to BWH to advance their research skills. "The work here has been so stimulating that I feel that I've used every single part of my brain at all times," said one STARS participant. "The faculty and everyone running the program have given me so many opportunities that I probably wouldn't have experienced otherwise."[150]

In recognition of BWH's efforts, it has been named twice to Diversity Inc.'s "25 Noteworthy Companies." The award was based on factors encompassing leadership's commitment to diversity and a workforce and management reflective of the community the hospital serves.

THRIVING IN AN ERA OF LIMITATIONS

Despite the increasing emphasis on aligning community health with clinical care, hospital costs continued their rise. In 1979, AHC Executive Vice President William Hassan noted, "Good financial management continues to keep the hospital solvent during a time when government and the public are clamoring for both reduction in services and cost containment."[151] However, signaling a new era of reining in the price of health care, Congress had passed the Health Maintenance Organization Act in 1973, calling for health maintenance organizations (HMOs) patterned after the Harvard Community Health Plan model. Even as it implemented many new services to adolescent parents and pregnant teens—including "Stress, Social Support and Primary Care," a project conducted by the Harvard School of Public Health to determine the extent of use of primary care services—and even as its neighborhood health centers received statewide awards and minority staff were recognized in the YMCA's Black Achiever Award, the AHC faced a difficult road ahead: growth in an age of limits.[152]

The Merger

> *Human nature being what it is, merger is never easily accomplished. But as the day approaches when our three divisions will be housed together, parochialism must give way to a loyalty to the medical center as a whole. Only then shall we achieve our goal of making that center second to none.*[153]

Planning for the merger of the PBBH, the Boston Hospital for Women (itself the result of the 1966 merger of the Lying-in and the Free Hospital for Women), and the RBBH took decades. Former BWH Board Chair F. Stanton Deland, Jr., along with many others, guided the long merger process, one fraught with difficulties in the realms of cost, personnel, and community relations. In his last annual report, Deland, a man of dry wit, wrote, "To the undoubted relief of many, this marks my final report as president, so perhaps I may be forgiven if I indulge in a few retrospective observations."[154] Additionally, as a member and chairperson of the Boston Lying-In Hospital Board of Trustees, Deland was an early supporter of the merger and worked with the AHC, the organizing body for what would eventually be renamed Brigham and Women's Hospital, from 1962 until his death in 1986. Original partners included Children's Hospital as well as the Massachusetts Eye and Ear Infirmary (MEEI) in addition to the PBBH, the RBBH, The Free Hospital for Women, and the Boston Lying-In Hospital. After Children's and MEEI withdrew, the others moved forward through an official merger in 1975.

Though the merger was arduous, it finally resulted in the opening of the new Brigham and Women's building in 1980. A new era of partnership began, as community representatives were brought on the board, health centers were opened, and Brigham staff worked actively with neighborhood groups to design care systems and initiatives. Inclusion was more and more the watchword. Although there would be challenges in the decades to come, the door would swing open more than ever before.

The Internal Community in the 1980s

The 1980 opening of the new BWH tower entailed not only envisioning endless administrative and operational details, with inevitable glitches (almost immediately, it was noted that there were not enough operating rooms),[155] but how to integrate cultures and philosophies of care. The question was how to create a seamless new institution made up of several elite hospitals, each with a rich and interconnected history and world-class reputation, while being responsive to external pressures of many kinds. The gaze inward and outward would need to be simultaneously incisive and inclusive.

At the decade's beginning, the new hospital faced such severe financial challenges that there was even a question of receivables and cash flow as staff moved into the new building. BWH Board Chair John H. McArthur has noted that H. Richard Nesson, president of BWH from 1982 to 1997 (whom he called "an inspired choice"), was simultaneously learning his new job and working to develop a team with the chiefs. "We were the scrappers of Brookline," he said. "The secret weapon at Brigham and Women's was the team of clinical Chiefs and Nesson, which was rapidly closing the gap with the General."[156]

The merging of staff had also meant attrition. And like other teaching hospitals, BWH was compelled to reduce length of stay and number of employees. It addressed cost containment by creating a Center for Cost Effective Care in 1981. Despite the dilemmas of providing care in an age of limits, there was still progress and optimism. Even as a new Ambulatory Services Building was opened in 1982, planning commenced for another. A Bioscience Research Building opened mid-decade. The hospital also experienced more admissions, births, and ambulatory visits each year, in part by partnering with Harvard Community Health Plan to provide health services and maintain a care continuum before and after hospitalization.

BWH was now full of remarkable people who accomplished, often in new configurations, remarkable things. In a dramatic 1983 event, a pregnant patient suffering congestive heart failure was saved, which helped pull disparate staffs together. BWH carried out New England's first heart transplant in February 1984, which was followed by four more that year as well as the 1,000th kidney transplant. There were other triumphs. Bernard Lown, with Evgeni Chazov, had founded International Physicians for the Prevention of Nuclear War, which was awarded the Nobel Peace Prize in 1985. In 1987, almost 10,000 babies were delivered at BWH, and more than $61 million in research grants, fellowships, and other sources of funding had been obtained. The hospital had greatly expanded primary care services, in part because of the leadership of hospital President H. Richard Nesson.

BIOGRAPHY

H. RICHARD NESSON, 1932-1998

Ann C. Conway

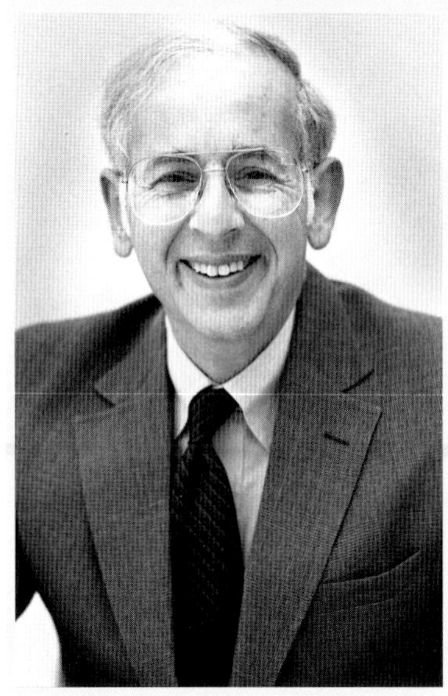

FIGURE 6-48 Richard Nesson.

H. Richard Nesson was a visionary leader who saw the possibilities inherent in individuals, communities, and a new institution. He was the president of Brigham and Women's Hospital from 1982 to 1997. During a tumultuous period, he helped build the hospital into what it is today. He understood what community entailed within a hospital, extending into the neighborhoods of Boston—his native city—as well as in national and global contexts. Skilled in communicating and developing consensus, as assistant director of the medical services at the Beth Israel Hospital, Nesson had worked to bring the private and teaching services into one unit, eliminating what he viewed as a two-class system of care. He was also the first medical director of the Harvard Community Health Plan (HCHP), one of the first HMOs, now called Harvard Pilgrim Health Care. At HCHP, he helped bring doctors from diverse communities into one unit and to reduce tensions between this emerging HMO and the outside practitioner community.

Beginning in 1977, as vice-president of Ambulatory and Community Services at the Peter Bent Brigham, Nesson worked intensively on the process that brought together the Peter Bent Brigham, the Boston Hospital for Women, and the Robert Breck Brigham. He directed a national Robert Wood Johnson Foundation–funded demonstration project to improve outpatient services. This was accomplished by disseminating the Harvard model he and others had built to other leading academic medical centers, including Johns Hopkins and Yale-New Haven. Along with Eugene Braunwald, Anthony Komaroff, and Marshall Wolf, Nesson also played a major role in developing academic primary care teaching units. Nesson became president of BWH in 1982 and later was named chief executive officer of the Partners Healthcare system.

In the BWH merger, Nesson united the clinical and administrative leadership of three disparate institutions. In 1993, he spearheaded the integration of longtime rivals Massachusetts General Hospital and BWH into

Partners' integrated delivery system, an arrangement that would be duplicated by almost all of Boston's teaching hospitals. In doing so, he "began the building of a network of over a thousand community physicians linked to academic teaching hospitals."[157]

Nesson had a strong commitment to the community. The new hospital had merged inpatient units for all patients and built on prior community outreach to create new efforts, often in collaboration with Harvard School of Public Health. During this period of financial challenge, BWH still offered more free care than any other private hospital in Boston.[158]

As policy and funding environments called for an increasing focus on quality and cost effectiveness, the new Center for Cost Effective Care examined outcomes through a clinical reporting system and ongoing feedback. In the 1980s, BWH's senior management team and trustees worked hard to develop a philanthropic base and to involve employees in suggestions for controlling costs. Nesson also initiated the development of groundbreaking health and administrative informatics systems at the Brigham, anticipating today's emphasis on effective technology in the hospital and among community-based facilities.

Resilience

Like many elite hospitals of its day, the PBBH from its inception to well after World War II was a "doctor's workshop" led by physicians and surgeons—remarkable, reflective individuals who changed the courses of their professions and those of American hospitals. But as the century progressed, the once intimate character of the American hospital altered, becoming complex and bureaucratized and led by a core of administrators to direct policy and manage operations. From the 1970s onward, historians, sociologists, and other students of the institution frequently bemoaned this "coming of the corporation" to the American hospital.

However, in the 1990s and in the new century to follow, BWH would continue to incorporate paradox, in this case developing the multifaceted complexity of an integrated health system along with other examples of the expanded vision evidenced in its diversity and community efforts. It would change the way it delivered care and how it evaluated it. In the years ahead, BWH would experience triumphs—as the 1990s began, ambulatory visits increased exponentially and research awards expanded to more than $92 million.[159] But it would also confront many challenges: cost increases, regulation, funding cuts, and competition. Space continued to be an issue, as well as Medicaid and Medicare reimbursement. The National Institutes of Health (NIH) would cut research funding and the hospital would need to build its endowment. It would need to listen and attend to patients as they developed greater consciousness of themselves as consumers, and it would need to attend to its ever-larger, further-flung, and subspecialized workforce. Those who passed through its doors—whether patients, families, or staff—would face questions of life, death, and moral choice as technology brought unprecedented possibilities as well as the need to make unprecedented decisions.

The Brigham's ability to survive and thrive had always been based on facing reality, whether it has been scientific, economic, social, or political. In the coming decades, BWH's plans would often focus on patient mix, cost reductions, revenue enhancement, length of stay, and ambulatory care.[160] But they were also concerned with innovation and building—of One Brigham Circle, "The Ledge Site" project,[161] which would hold BWH offices, and populating a new Harvard research building. New construction also includes the state-of-the-art Carl J. and Ruth Shapiro Cardiovascular Center. As an institution, BWH had never been unaware of the marketplace—it could not have fulfilled its service, educational, and research missions without comprehending it. But it had never allowed itself to be entirely defined by it. In the midst of difficulties, it was accustomed to reinventing itself with the same upstart boldness of its formation.

And, in perhaps the greatest paradox of its intricate, rich history, it would simultaneously step forward into the past. For many of the signposts ahead would herald themes evident in BWH's history—the concern for patients in their community and family context, the destruction of walls between mental and physical health, and an emphasis on health throughout the life span. The tenets of health reform, emphasizing connections between primary, secondary, and tertiary care, recalled the fluidity of boundaries evident in BWH's predecessors, as well as the humane impulse that had never left the institution.

BWH Response to the 1993 Clinton Healthcare Reform Plan

In a panel discussion almost a generation ago, a number of key BWH figures gave their perspectives on prospective federal health reform. President Bill Clinton's 1993 Health Security Act had proposed universal health care through a closely regulated HMO system, incorporating six key principles: quality, security (access), simplicity, responsibility (taking responsibility for health), choice (choice of physicians), and saving (clinical and administrative value). This was to be Clinton's fulcrum issue, so important that he had selected First Lady Hillary Clinton to run the task force responsible for the plan's implementation.

Brigham and Women's President Richard Nesson noted: "We've waited too long," and said that the overhaul was "50 years in coming." He agreed with the key principles Clinton had outlined but noted that it would be a "tough road," especially for academic health centers. Research and education, Nesson said, were vital for health systems. Echoing his PBBH forbears Christian and Cushing, Physician-in-Chief Eugene Braunwald noted that it was crucial to focus on the "soul of medicine," not only the issues of the business and style of medicine. JudyAnn Bigby, then director of Women's, Family and Community Programs (later Secretary of Health and Human Services of the Commonwealth of Massachusetts), underscored the need for a comprehensive approach to health care, entailing not simply removing cost barriers, but ameliorating the socioeconomic factors—among them poor housing, domestic violence, and addiction—which affect health status. Arnold Epstein, also of the Department of Medicine, who would serve on President Clinton's task force, followed Bigby, stating that focus on accountability, quality measurement, and performance improvement were key to the Clinton plan.[162]

The Creation of Partners Healthcare

In the 1990s, partly in response to the Clinton health reform efforts, HMS Dean Daniel Tosteson convened meetings with the leaders of HMS' five major teaching hospitals to explore greater cooperation. Eventually, and despite their historical rivalry, BWH and MGH explored the possibilities separately, with the idea of perhaps eventually having the others join them in a network. It was not an easy task. The fascinating book, *Mergers of Teaching Hospitals in Boston, New York and Northern California*, by John A. Kartor, covers the Partners merger in depth. In it, H. Richard Nesson said of BWH and MGH, "We were always jousting with one another to see who could attract the best students, the best residents, well-known surgeons, etc."[163] Nevertheless, both hospitals knew that they shared common environmental challenges as well as a vision of how to flourish while adhering to their traditional mission of patient care, research, and teaching.

The difficult task had initially involved a group of eight, including Braunwald of BWH and W. Gerald Austen of MGH. Braunwald later noted that the hospitals were coming together "with an important and totally new mission—the development of a new integrated health system....As we look down the road, the inpatient, high tech facility will be probably not even the most important component of a network, which will tilt the balance of caregiving to primary care physicians and community hospitals." H. Richard Nesson, a veteran of merger processes, noted that the formation of Partners would allow the hospitals to take a leadership role in envisioned health reform—creating a network that recognized the value of "academic teaching centers while providing care in the most cost effective settings."[164] Indeed, for BWH and MGH, a major impetus behind the Partners affiliation was to take a leading role in shaping health reform, not simply being affected by it. As Nesson envisioned it, the alliance would allow the two hospitals to create an integrated healthcare system that could be a

SPOTLIGHT

DANA-FARBER/BRIGHAM AND WOMEN'S CANCER CENTER: FOCUSED ON CANCER, FOCUSED ON LIFE

Saul E. Wisnia

The Dana-Farber Cancer Institute (DFCI) and Brigham and Women's Hospital are connected by a bright, glass-walled bridge in the Longwood Medical Area, but far more than an overpass joins these two neighboring institutions. Since 1997, they have formally partnered as Dana-Farber/Brigham and Women's Cancer Center (DF/BWCC) to provide adult patients and their families comprehensive cancer care and support. The center has specialized units for all types of cancer, each staffed with experts in all aspects of medical care. Working with a research team, these caregivers are developing new ways to prevent, detect, and treat the disease and to return patients and families to their prior lives. Volunteers who have already experienced cancer are available to offer advice or quell the fears of someone newly diagnosed, and an array of supportive resources can guide patients through their experience. "Through this kind of a partnership, we're not only improving the way we work, but we're demonstrating what the power of collaboration, and the sharing of resources and planning, can truly accomplish," says Edward J. Benz, Jr., DFCI president and director of the DF/BWCC.

WORKING IN TANDEM

The DFCI was founded as the Children's Cancer Research Foundation in 1947 by Sidney Farber, a Brigham-trained pathologist. The institution worked independently to raise survival rates for pediatric cancer, including developing aminopterin, the first chemotherapy for childhood leukemia. Treating patients of all ages since the 1960s, the DFCI was an internationally renowned fifty-bed oncology hospital by 1997.

During this same period, the Brigham was also emerging as a leader in Boston's medical oncology. Its hematology, oncology, and bone marrow transplant programs were thriving, and nationally recognized oncologic surgeons were recruited. Physicians from both the Brigham and DFCI appreciated the complementary programs and began working together informally to provide multidisciplinary consultations to adult cancer patients. This led to a decision in the mid-1990s by chief executive officers H. Richard Nesson of the Brigham and David G. Nathan of the DFCI and by Brigham Chairman of Medicine Eugene Braunwald to combine the services. Supporting this decision, David Nathan "felt, for many years . . . that cancer centers should maintain their beds in excellent general hospitals so that all the bells and whistles of modern medicine can support the oncology patients. The Dana-Farber and the Brigham's partnership represents the kind of collaboration that can take place when institutions put the patients and families first."

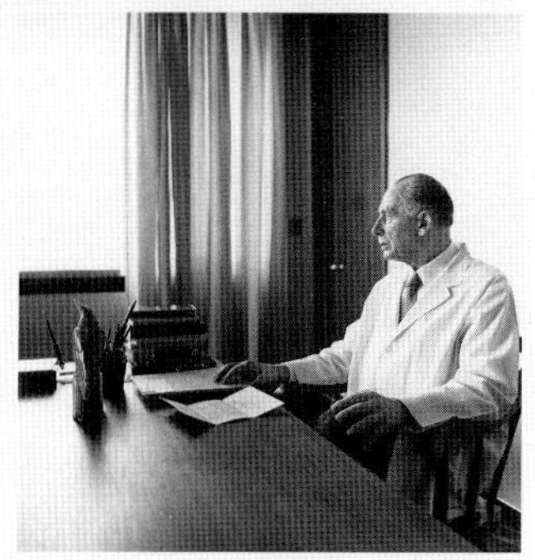

FIGURE 6-49 Sidney Farber, "the father of modern chemotherapy," watches the construction of DFCI, 1970s. In the mid-1940s, using a drug called Aminopterin, Farber achieved the first clinical remission ever reported for childhood leukemia.

In executing the merger after months of planning, the largest physical task took place on February 15, 1997, when the adult inpatients on the 12th and 14th floors of the DFCI's Charles A. Dana Cancer Center were moved through tunnels and bridges to new oncology units in the Brigham's Tower. The majority of the Brigham's outpatient cancer service was subsequently transferred to the DFCI. Many nurses and other employees shifted similarly from one institution to the other. "Before the move, we had two excellent cancer programs that were 90 feet away from each other, but not working in tandem," explains Lawrence N. Shulman, Chief Medical Officer at the DFCI. "There was really nothing to be gained by keeping them separate, and everything to be gained by bringing them together."

Addressing patient concerns about the merger, current and past DFCI and Brigham patients and relatives participated in each stage of the planning, and afterward visited their newly moved brethren. They conveyed concerns and needs to staff, and became key

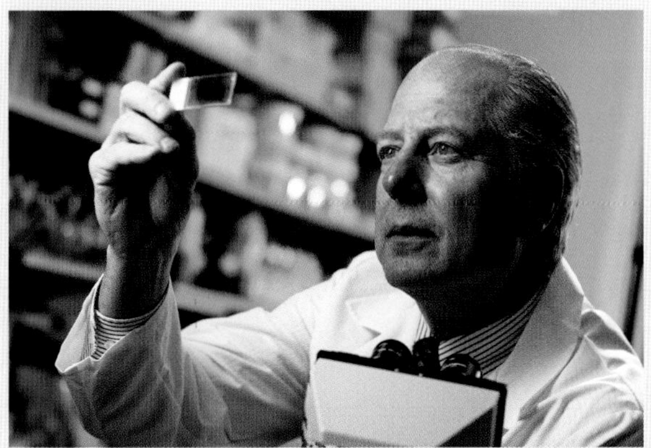

FIGURE 6-50 Christopher P. Crum, Director, Women's and Perinatal Pathology, BWH.

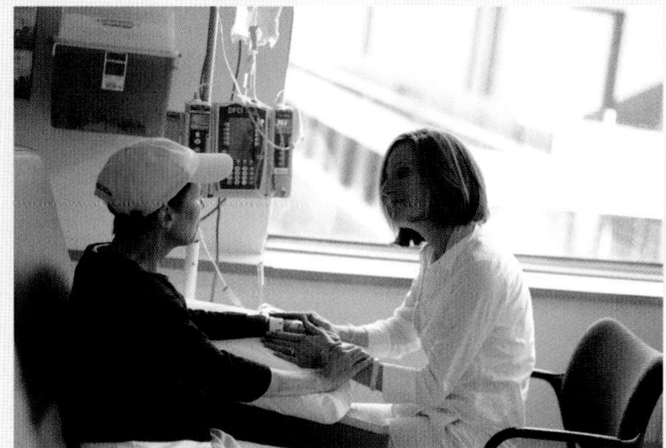

FIGURE 6-51 Nurse Colleen Chin and a patient, DFCI.

advisors worthy of their own formal group. Thus was born a DF/BWCC's valuable and continuing asset, the Adult Patient and Family Advisory Council.

CONTINUAL INTEGRATION

The new model proved successful, and leaders have continued expanding and refining it, including the following organizational changes effected in 2004:

Integrated departments, that combine the resources of a general hospital and the unique needs of a specialty center, that is, Radiation Therapy, Pathology, etc.;

A single leadership structure, including single chairs for departments at both institutions and combined medical oncology nursing;

A single clinical strategic plan, coordinated around the twelve disease centers and addressing total care (prevention, screening, diagnosis, treatment, and survivorship);

Satellite Centers in three Massachusetts sites, including the Faulkner Hospital in Jamaica Plain, where patients have access to DF/BWCC caregivers and services; and

A joint presence in the national market, in which it is ranked an outstanding U.S. cancer hospital by U.S. News & World Report.

DF/BWCC TODAY

"We are using a single set of tools and approaches, establishing single leaders and leadership forums, and devising a single set of best-practice standards to be applied through the whole cancer experience," said director Edward Benz. The DF/BWCC includes 124 inpatient medical and sixty-one surgical beds, 138 exam rooms, and 157 infusion chairs. Inpatient volume has nearly doubled since 1997, whereas outpatient volume has more than tripled. "We've evolved incredibly well in terms of our care processes and how we focus on patients and families," says Patricia Reid Ponte, senior vice-president for Patient Care Services, chief nurse at Dana-Farber, and director of Oncology Nursing and Clinical Services at the Brigham. The central facility for outpatient oncology is the Yawkey Center for Cancer Care, a new fourteen-story DFCI facility. Designed with input from leaders of both hospitals and the Adult Patient and Family Advisory Council, the Yawkey Center offers a new level of total patient care and makes the transition from inpatient to outpatient (and vice versa) smoother than ever. Inpatient surgical and medical oncology, bone marrow transplantation, and outpatient surgery are performed at the Brigham. DF/BWCC also continues to bring quality cancer care to the regional community.

Research at the DFCI is a major mission, led by nationally recognized leaders and by major funding from the National Cancer Institute (NCI). It has one of the largest clinical trials programs in the country. In 2011, the Center launched "Profile," a study of all DF/BWCC cancer patients to provide investigators with one of the world's largest databases of cancer genetic abnormalities. This resource facilitates the discovery of the genetic causes of cancers and of new, targeted therapies. The technology used for this genetic testing, OncoMap, was designed by DFCI researchers and is executed in the Brigham Department of Pathology.

Today, many patients have no idea that the Dana-Farber/Brigham and Women's Cancer Center was once two separate entities—a sure sign that all has gone as planned.

template for academic health centers and allow the hospitals to match the cost effectiveness and efficiency of other healthcare system players.

Ironically, by September 1994, the compromise Democratic bill based on the Clinton plan was declared off the table by majority leader Senator George Mitchell. Health reform had died, mainly because of opposition from conservatives, libertarians, and the health insurance industry. However, the problems would not go away, nor would, in broad terms, the proposed solutions outlined in the Clinton plan. The Balanced Budget Act of 1997 would also present challenges in a managed care milieu, projecting $115 billion in cuts to Medicare, which funded BWH's residency training.[165] The hospital responded by proposing reductions of hospital-supported residency and fellowship programs of 20%; it would merge some of these and separate research programs with MGH. Later, it would develop a common parent company structure with Jamaica Plain's well-regarded Faulkner Hospital, whose community focus would complement that of BWH. (See essay by Cara Marcus earlier in this chapter.) Demand for services in 2002 would lead to greater collaboration with Dana-Farber Cancer Institute and the eventual development of a cancer care facility at Faulkner.[166]

Nevertheless, the increasingly serious question of access for the uninsured grew, as did the ongoing question of how to link primary and secondary prevention in communities and office settings with the high-tech capacity of acute care settings like BWH. As Partners, both BWH and MGH strove together to address these issues.

SPOTLIGHT

THE BRIGHAM AND THE WEST ROXBURY VETERANS ADMINISTRATION MEDICAL CENTER

Arthur A. Sasahara and Peter V. Tishler

The Veterans Administration (VA) Hospital in West Roxbury, Massachusetts, opened in January of 1944. It became a Dean's Committee Hospital for Harvard Medical School in 1948, through the efforts of William B. Castle. The first appointments of the medical staff, made by this committee, were Thomas A. Warthin, chief of medicine (1946-1975); David Littmann, chief of cardiology (1946-1971); and Richard Warren, chief of surgery (1948 -1962). These individuals constituted the majority of the full-time staff at the VA for many years.

Formal affiliation with the Peter Bent Brigham Hospital began in academic year 1953-1954, when the VA relocated to West Roxbury after a brief sojourn to an institution on Huntington Avenue in Jamaica Plain. The VA initiated training programs in affiliation with the Departments of Surgery, Medicine, Pathology, and Radiology. To Francis D. Moore, the Brigham's chief of surgery, the staffing of the Resident Surgical Service at West Roxbury by fifteen Brigham residents at various levels of training was "an effective part of our postgraduate work."[167] George W. Thorn, the Brigham's chief of medicine, noted that the "integration of the two services will introduce major revisions in our house officer training program."[168] Brigham medical residents spent several months caring for patients on two large wards at the VA. In particular, the senior assistant residents, with many years of clinical and research experience, staffed the VA as "a junior faculty which has done much toward raising the level of patient care and teaching."[169] The full-time staff was supplemented by consultant and attending physicians not only from the Brigham (H. Richard Tyler in Neurology, John Merrill in Nephrology, Herbert Selenkow in Endocrinology, Roland Ingram in Pulmonary Medicine, Gustave Dammin in Pathology), but also from the Massachusetts General Hospital, Tufts University, and Boston University Medical Centers.

During these early years, David Littmann, "one of the finest teachers ever," trained more than a generation of Brigham house staff and Harvard Medical students to read electrocardiograms.[170] A well-rounded clinician and master of the Socratic method of teaching, he also ran the popular fellowship in cardiovascular diseases. While inventing a stethoscope, cardiac catheters, and valves, he established the first cardiac catheterization unit in the VA system, limited at the time by shortcomings in technology but successful diagnostically nonetheless. Arthur Sasahara was one of the early cardiology fellows (1957-1958). He remained at the VA, providing clinical care in cardiology, directing the cardiac catheterization laboratory, mentoring of Harvard Medical students, and carrying out research. He succeeded Littmann as chief of cardiology in 1971.

In 1975, Sasahara succeeded Warthin as chief of medicine. Over the ensuing thirteen years, Sasahara worked with Brigham physician leaders Eugene Braunwald, chief of medicine, and Marshall Wolf, director of the medical residency program, to improve the residency program in medicine. Medical interns were now added to the VA rotation. House staff rotated to the VA from both the Brigham and Beth Israel hospitals. A similar medical residency program was also established at the Brockton VA Medical Center, which was administratively integrated with West Roxbury in 1983. The size of the medical staff was increased commensurately to ensure adequate supervision, offer the modern nuances of subspecialty medicine, and improve patient care. Except for cardiology, training programs in virtually all medical subspecialty programs now offered the unique VA training experience to fellows at the Brigham. Cardiology remained a separate training and research entity, reflecting the huge prevalence of cardiovascular disease among veterans and the great demand for cardiac surgery, for which the West Roxbury was the referral center for all New England VA hospitals. Because of the expansion and the resulting complex educational mission, Peter Tishler was recruited to the new position of associate chief of staff for education at the VA. In essence, Tishler assumed the management of the complex multiple residency programs for the VA.

Similarly, the Surgical Service evolved to include both general surgery and virtually all surgical subspecialties. Perhaps the most influential surgeon, Ernest M. Barsamian, was, successively, chief of cardiothoracic surgery (1963-1971, during which he started the open heart surgery program, the first in the VA system and the third in New England), chief of surgery (1971-1978), and chief of staff (1978-1998). Working with his counterparts in surgery and the administration at the Brigham and HMS, he spread the word of the attractiveness of the VA for both medical trainees and staff physicians. He and Sasahara were largely responsible for recruiting leaders, including George E. Thibault as chief of the medical service, Sanjiv Chopra in gastroenterology, Robert Brown in pulmonary medicine, Harley A. Haynes in dermatology, Alfred F. Parisi in cardiology, John W. Rowe in geriatrics, Shukri F. Khuri in cardiac surgery (and chief of surgery from 1984 to 2004), Martin A. Samuels in neurology, Robert W. McCarley in psychiatry, and Joseph Loscalzo in cardiology.

Medical services have been exchanged between the Brigham and the West Roxbury VA Hospital over the years. The Brigham provides neuroradiology services to the VA, while the VA has provided urodynamic and electron microscopic services to the Brigham. West Roxbury provides treatment and rehabilitation to patients with spinal cord injury from both the Brigham and other VA hospitals.

The VA healthcare system is dedicated to the care of individuals who have given a significant portion of their lives to the service of this country. For them, access to an integrated, low-cost healthcare system is justified. Moreover, a significant proportion of this group is economically disenfranchised, similar to the populations cared for at various city hospitals nationwide. For them, VA health care is absolutely their privilege and necessity. Most medical care providers who trained or practice at a VA hospital are committed philosophically and practically to the provision of equally outstanding medical care to all veterans. For the West Roxbury VA, this was exemplified by many senior staff members, including Ernest Barsamian. The VA is also an important lesson in the virtues of single-payer health care: despite its shortcomings, the VA can provide fine care much of the time expeditiously, seamlessly, and at a much lower cost than insurance-based health care. Care of these individuals is further abetted by the superb VA computer system, which permits computer access to each patient's medical record at all VA facilities nationwide and provides the means for the totally computerized VA medical record system. Finally, the recent research endeavor to bank DNA from veterans for research purposes ("Million Veteran Program: A Partnership with Veterans," coordinated by the VA/Brigham's J. Michael Gaziano) promises to be an outstanding resource for genetic and genomic research on chronic disease. Although any medical care system, including the VA, has its shortcomings, we emphatically reject the printed assertion that the VA delivers exploitative, impersonal, and inappropriate health care.[171,172]

The West Roxbury VA Medical Center remains affiliated with the Brigham today, but other affiliations have come about. In the late 1990s, the Boston VA Hospital on Huntington Avenue in Boston merged with the Brockton-West Roxbury VA Medical Center. This facility, newly named the VA Boston Healthcare System, has major affiliations with both the Brigham/HMS and the Boston University Medical Center. Academic responsibility for the many clinical services at this VA are divided between these two affiliates, providing ever more clinical expertise, trainees, and indeed popularity for the VA.

New Models of Care

In the 1990s, the hospital took proactive internal steps to improve quality and reduce expenses in a competitive environment, launching a new Care Improvement Program comprised of nineteen interdisciplinary processes and care improvement teams. This involved physicians, administrators, and other caregivers working with patients and families. A Process Improvement Committee looked at ways to improve operating system efficiencies. At the same time, as it had before, in the face of constraints, BWH moved forward with new endeavors and facilities—beginning with the Longwood Medical Research Center and the Center for Women and Newborns (now part of the Mary Horrigan Connors Center for Women's Health).

BWH and other health leaders now recognized that to effectively prevent and treat the diseases that most often sickened and killed its patients, it needed to develop integrated models of care that carefully measured outcomes. It needed to target health risks throughout the life span and, along with others, help reconfigure a national system in which seemingly uncontrollable costs were centered in acute, episodic care. Reducing the rate of chronic illnesses that disabled and killed so many Americans was only possible by addressing rising rates of obesity, smoking, substance abuse, and other behaviors. This meant locating the patient in his or her family and community and embedding preventative strategies not only in the hospital and doctor's office, but within families, communities, schools, and workplaces. In the nation at large as well as in integrated health systems like BWH, the task now would be to break down the separation between preventive care and health care, particularly in the context of primary care. BWH's state-of-the-art informatics—pioneered by Nesson—could help break down some of these walls between primary, secondary, and tertiary prevention and treatment. Equally importantly, it could address ever-expanding policy emphases on quality and accountability by examining outcomes—both clinical, in terms of utilization and cost, and in the psychosocial realm. The task was to figure out how to operationalize these changes, which would be the subject of new national reforms and more BWH reinvention in the first decades of the millennium.

Global Community

Medical anthropology has meant a lot of things to different people. Some have focused on how culture impacts disease. We have been much more concerned about understanding why poor people get sick, what sicknesses they get, and how to prevent sickness. And there are applications for this right here in Boston as well.

—Paul Farmer

In its creation, the creators of the Brigham were pilgrims—traveling to Europe, analyzing and reflecting on how to develop a model based in many parts on European scientific breakthroughs and systems of education. These planners examined the best in European and innovative American hospital design. Their travels would be a feature in the decades to follow, as they examined each new clinical innovation and health policy issues, such as the development of nationalized health care. Throughout its history, the Brigham has welcomed visiting physicians, trainees, and students—and certainly, patients—from throughout the world. It also served the world through volunteerism and through sending staff and faculty to develop medical and ancillary health professions; even in the 1920s, Brigham nursing graduates provided nursing education in China, Haiti, and other settings.

In the 1990s, BWH began to embrace the global community even more comprehensively. New international efforts would begin in the United Arab Emirates, Russia, Mexico, and Pakistan—the latter two in response to emergency situations.[173] However, perhaps most transformative was BWH's collaboration with Partners In Health (PIH), as is detailed in the essay on the history of the Division of Global Health Equity later in this chapter. (See page 383.)

Health Reform Revisited: The Patient Protection and Affordable Care Act of 2010

Echoing prior calls for health system improvement, The Patient Protection and Affordable Care Act of 2010 seeks to decrease the number of uninsured Americans and reduce overall health system costs while streamlining delivery of health care and improving outcomes. It incorporates strong prevention, health promotion, and public health components, as well as an emphasis on patients and families as consumers who help direct the course of their own care.

Key components of health reform include Patient Centered Medical Homes (PCMH) and Accountable Care Organizations (ACO). These align with a national movement to provide high-quality and cost-effective health services, in part by supporting investments in better primary care. In March 2007, four leading physician membership organizations (the American Academy of Family Physicians, the American Academy of Pediatrics, the American College of Physicians, and the American Osteopathic Association) came together to support the PCMH model. They subsequently agreed on seven key model principles: (1) relationship with a personal (primary care) physician; (2) use of team-based care; (3) whole-person orientation; (4) coordination and integration of care across all settings; (5) quality and safety as hallmarks; (6) enhanced access to care; and (7) payment that appropriately recognizes the added value to patients of a patient-centered medical home.[174]

The PCMH project thus far shows strong results. A 2010 national review of efforts to improve primary care through the medical home approach concludes:

> *Investing in primary care patient centered medical homes results in improved quality of care and patient experiences, and reductions in expensive hospital and emergency department utilization. There is now even stronger evidence that investments in primary care can bend the cost curve, with several major evaluations showing that patient centered medical home initiatives have produced a net savings in total health care expenditures for the patients served by these initiatives.*[175]

Partners HealthCare and BWH have embraced the PCMH model, with a goal of 60% of primary care practices receiving PCMH recognition through the National Committee on Quality Assurance by 2013; the reminder of practices will move rapidly toward the same aim.

Brigham and Women's Advanced Primary Care Associates on South Huntington Avenue exemplifies the patient-centered medical home model. It incorporates a multidisciplinary, team-based approach including social, behavioral, and primary care integration. Also involved is nurse care coordination, pharmacy, and nutrition services, as well as a community resource specialist. These resources improve preventive care as well as post hospitalization support, thereby decreasing unnecessary Emergency Department visits and hospital admissions. The practice incorporates e-visits,[176] phone follow-up, and shared medical appointments, in addition to ongoing data feedback to facilitate quality improvement, which is provided by a population manager.[177]

In early 2012, Partners Healthcare was one of thirty-two healthcare organizations selected by the federal Centers for Medicare and Medicaid Services

(CMS) to participate in a Pioneer ACO model. ACOs are a type of payment and delivery reform that ties provider reimbursements to quality metrics and reductions in the total cost of care for an assigned population of patients. Within the model, a group of coordinated healthcare providers come together to provide care to a group of patients and agree to be "accountable" for a defined set of population outcome measures.

Pioneer ACOs are designed specifically for organizations and providers that have a track record of care coordination across care settings; CMS notes that it "allows these provider groups to move more rapidly from a shared savings payment model to a population-based payment model." In 2012, Partners Healthcare worked with 45,000 of its Medicare patients using this model, providing them with high-quality care while slowing cost growth through care coordination.[178]

In alignment with these and other internal and external developments, in 2011 BW/F released strategic planning recommendations in seven areas: seamless, high-quality patient- and family-centered care, cutting edge innovation and discovery, leadership and education, engaged workforce, health equity, affordable care for patients, and demonstrated excellence.[179] In the health equity realm, the plan detailed strategies involving providing culturally and linguistically competent care, continuing the promotion of diversity and community engagement through policies and supports, providing incentives for community engagement, expanding community-based research efforts and thereby increasing the best practice evidence base, and integrating disparate local, national and global diversity, and community-related efforts by instituting a Community Engagement Executive Committee to coordinate initiatives.[180]

Home

We shall not cease from exploration and the end of all our exploring will be to arrive where we started and know the place for the first time.

—T.S. Eliot, "Little Gidding"

In the early years of the Peter Bent Brigham Hospital, bonds among staff were familial. The chiefs had similar backgrounds and knew one another from Hopkins, trips to Europe, and the very long hours they spent at the hospital. The nursing faculty was also well-acquainted, from the professional "cream of the crop." There were deep ties between those who trained at the Brigham as students and house officers. Residents were just that—they lived at the hospital, as did nursing students—although "fraternization" was strictly regulated. Years later, other staff still lived in the building or close by. Cushing's famous technician and assistant, Adolph Watzka, had a room there; after work, he walked his dogs down Shattuck Street. Although she spent summers at her home on the Cape, Mildred Codding, Cushing's illustrator, kept an apartment near the Brigham until the end of her long life. We can imagine—although we do not know, because nonclinician employee records do not remain—that other staff had a strong sense of connection to the hospital.

The PBBH campus both fostered and reflected this intimate, domestic character. In the early years, the relatively small groups of clinicians and patients were visible to each other; the Pike was open air, the distance between buildings not long. The structures and campus were graceful: each pavilion ward had a carefully tended landscape surrounding it, perhaps the work of William Councilman, who liked to garden at the hospital. On the second floor, there were dining rooms, one for physicians and one for nurses. Physicians used the outdoor tennis courts and a squash court. Patients had their beds wheeled onto the rooftop terraces in good weather. In the heat of summer, house officers also sometimes slept on the roofs.

Many of these glimpses of hospital life are part of an informational pamphlet produced shortly after the hospital's opening. On its fragile green cover, "Peter Bent Brigham Hospital. Boston." is spelled out in simple black lettering. In one photograph, well-dressed men and women walk briskly to and from the administration building, which is reached by traversing a slight rise. Another image shows the reception area under the rotunda, where a man leans against the long, beautifully curved information desk. Other photographs show pristine laboratories, operating rooms, the pharmacy, and the roentgen department, all of which communicate the scientific ethos of the hospital—its cleanliness, modernity, and excellence. To one side of the central building was the Out-Door Department; to the other was the "Domestic" building, which included a private ward. To its left were the tennis courts. Beyond them were pavilion wards C-F. The final and panoramic photograph depicts the entire ten-acre campus. The viewer can also see the Peter Bent Brigham's neighbors, some now long vanished: the House of the Good Samaritan, Infants' Hospital, Children's Hospital, Harvard Medical School, and the Collis B. Huntington Memorial Hospital. Shifting one's gaze back to the front of the administration building, one sees an expanse of broad lawn. A horse and buggy wait at the door. The entire PBBH is surrounded by a high wrought iron and stone fence. A tiny, elegant gatehouse marks the hospital entrance.

Today, of course, the stone fence has vanished, the gatehouse long since torn down. The Brigham has grown into an entity perhaps unimaginable to its founder and even to the great men and women who gathered early in its history to mark a vision for what it was to be: "a great thing for the city and the country."

It would be disingenuous to say that the hospital community now exists in the same manner as it did at the time of the Peter Bent Brigham Hospital's founding. An institution comprised of almost 15,000 employees is a different entity than one with a staff of fewer than 200. And if one takes the broader view, if one thinks of those whose lives have been changed and made better by the PBBH and BWH—by their service, their discoveries, their education, their outreach to a city, country, and globe similarly transformed since 1913—these communities are beyond the ability to count.

Still, in this record, we see unyielding strains. To read Brigham history is to feel that nothing is entirely new—not investigations of health policy; not attempts to address poverty and racism; not learning how to listen; not care that recognizes the centrality of body, mind, and spirit; not the joy and pathos inherent in service to patients and families, often at momentous events in their lives. Nor is everyday courage new, as evidenced in the steely determination of a Harvey Cushing, a Bernice Sinclair, a young woman traveling to China to teach nurses at Peking Union Medical College, a Joseph Murray, a Dick Nesson, a Ladies Committee member winding bandages, a matron finding a job for a penniless immigrant, or anyone combating violence or raising money or watching expenses while moving forward to build what is necessary—to do what must be done. This is what the Brigham community has demonstrated hour after hour, day after day, over the years and decades, the century.

In 1963, poet David McCord, in the PBBH commemorative volume, *The Fabrick of Man,* wrote of the "220-yard brick Pike...a mark of affection amounting to what Harvard college graduates still lavish on an ancient Yard which elsewhere would be called a campus,"[181] of "hurrying east and west on rubber heels in calculated silence go the nurses, doctors, interns, residents, orderlies, lost visitors," of how the Pike "puts pedestrian yardage between the Transplanters and Pathology, between the Head Nurse and linen supply, between the Emergency Ward and the Blood Bank, between Medicine and Surgery."[182] Fifty years later, at the Brigham, "the scrapper of Brookline," everything is at once new and evocative of the past. One sees this on The Nesson Pike, a pilgrimage from the PBBH's graceful past to today. From the original rotunda at 15 Francis Street, one undertakes a journey filled with past and present: from the lobby, in front of Pat's Place, where the "Brig-o-Mat" restaurant once stood, one might look up the stairs to Administration, where so many greats have passed, or back to the Carrie Hall conference room.

Then one moves forward, past "Exit 7," past Neurology, Neurosurgery, and MRI Associates, the legacies of Cushing, Sosman, and so many more; through the Medical Research Building, Thorn's brainchild; through the blood donor center, recalling Carl Walter, Elliott Cutler, the exigencies of war; through Schuster Transplant Center and Medical Surgical Specialties, all of which evoke the past; through the Phyllis Jen Center for Primary Care and the Connors Center for Women's Health, remembering everyone from Walter Channing to Olive Smith, to the Ambulatory Building. And, of course, this is but an incomplete and paltry list of those who have contributed in myriad ways to the face of health and service at the Brigham.

When one finally emerges at the end of the journey, one has reached the Pike's terminus, the Brigham Tower. One might stand for a moment and look below, before going down the stairs to the main entrance at 75 Francis Street. The light-filled space is alive with patients, families, staff, their faces reflective of the changing century, the altered city and world beyond, as they unceasingly stream in and out—through the open door.

A GOOD PLACE TO BUILD SOMETHING NEW: GLOBAL HEALTH EQUITY IN THE DEPARTMENT OF MEDICINE

Susan R. Holman

"Engagement with practice, with delivery, has made the well-resourced hospital [one] of the most creative parts of a university—a good place to build something new."

—Paul Farmer, "The Brightest and The Best," BWH video history website, http://www.brighamandwomens.org/online/blueprint/oral-histories.aspx

The Division of Global Health Equity in the Brigham's Department of Medicine was launched in October 2001, in response to a growing interest in training physicians to address "inequalities in disease burden and in treatment outcomes, educating trainees [and] physicians ... in health disparities research and science, and providing a clinical platform for identifying underserved patients likely to benefit from more aggressive management of acute and chronic disease."[183] Today, the division numbers more than thirty core Brigham faculty with as many affiliated Brigham faculty, a specialized residency program, and faculty and trainees who work in places such as Botswana, Chile, Haiti, Lesotho, Malawi, Mexico, Peru, Roxbury, Russia, Rwanda, South Africa, and the Navajo Nation in New Mexico. Division research activities focus on HIV/AIDS, multidrug-resistant tuberculosis (MDR-TB), cholera vaccines, surgery, cardiology, chronic diseases, community health worker training, and high-tech innovations in remote rural settings. The overall motivation is a common commitment to equity in health care around the globe.[184]

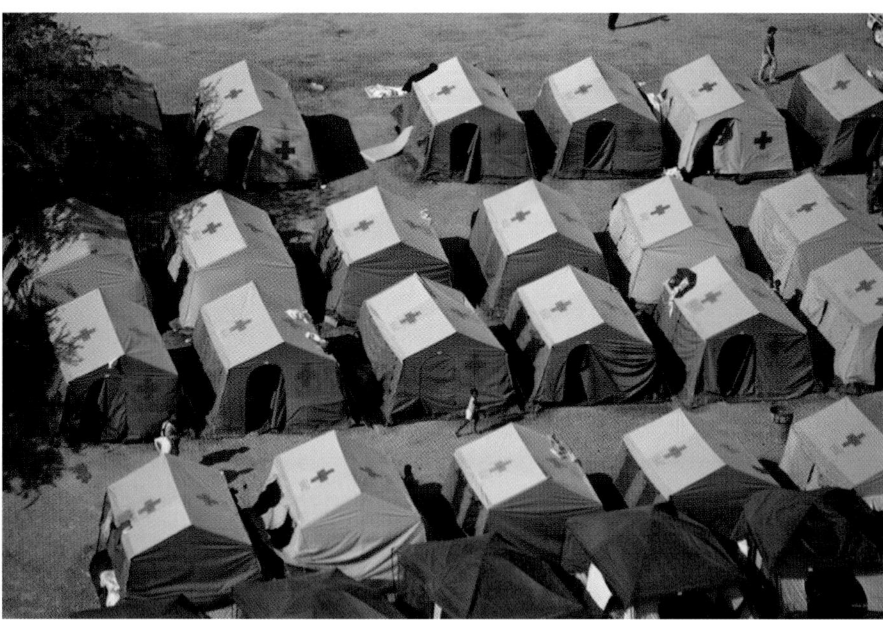

FIGURE 6-52 Hospital tents in Haiti.

Beginnings

The division's hard-won success today builds on a foundation laid by Brigham leaders willing to advance the hospital's role in what has come to be called global health, particularly Victor Dzau, chair of the Department of Medicine from 1996 to 2004; Marshall Wolf, emeritus vice-chair for medical education; Eugene Braunwald, Department of Medicine chair from 1972 to 1996; and Howard Hiatt, former dean of the Harvard School of Public Health and former chief of medicine at the Beth Israel Hospital. It was during Braunwald's tenure that Paul Farmer and Jim Yong Kim, who met during medical school, founded Partners In Health (PIH), a not-for-profit nongovernmental organization that was—and still is—legally distinct from both Brigham and Women's Hospital (BWH) and Harvard Medical School. However, PIH has been the "service arm" of the division from the start, providing many of the resources to enable medical trainees to learn firsthand what it means to practice medicine in the context of poverty and inequities. Division activities maintain close ties to PIH, its country affiliates, and the shared conviction that "health inequalities are best addressed through a movement for social justice involving a multitude of partners working on behalf of the destitute sick."[185]

In the 1990s, Marshall Wolf—called "one of the most generous, nurturing, and effective mentors in medicine"—tailored the research residency program to enable Farmer and Kim to share a single residency slot and thus divide their research and training time between Boston and Haiti to ensure continuity of care for their patients.[186] The result set a precedent for others, and by 2000, training opportunities were further enhanced by a new program at Harvard Medical School in Infectious Disease and Social Change.[187]

Victor Dzau, Braunwald's successor, took these ideas to the next step. As he recalls:

> *I was very much influenced by what [Kim and Farmer] did.... You have to remember that I was born in China, post-war, and I watched a lot of poverty and health disparities.... But most of my adult career in medicine has been around research and being a physician scientist. So when I came back to the Brigham as the Chair of Medicine and met Paul and Jim, that really rejuvenated that passion of mine.... I was watching all these young people spending their free time and elective time going to work at Haiti and elsewhere. And so I recall distinctly the day when I said, 'This is not sustainable. If you want to sustain this area, you've got to create a career path. You've got to create a place by which people can say, "I can actually make a whole livelihood out of this." So why not create a discipline out of this? And hence the idea of a division.*[188]

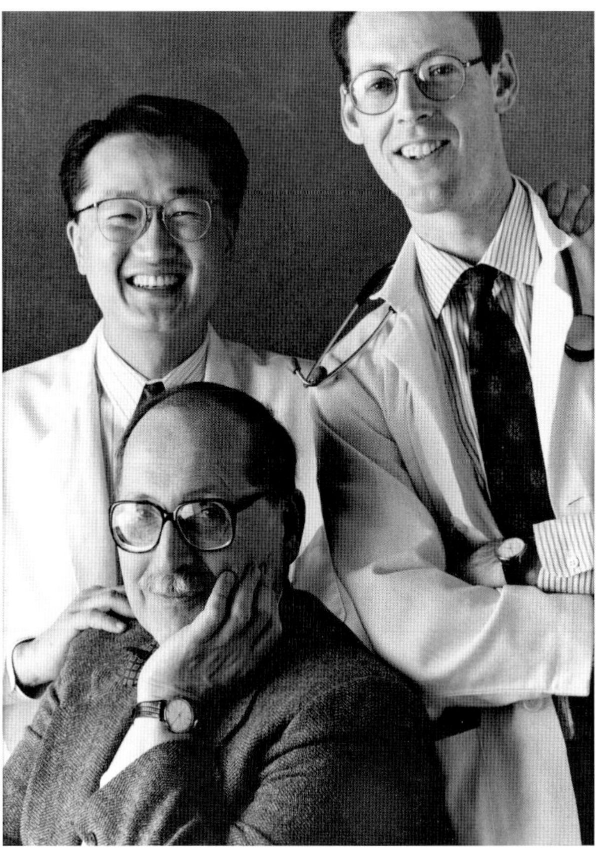

FIGURE 6-53 Clockwise from bottom: Marshall Wolf, Jim Kim, and Paul Farmer.

The new division was formally announced on October 5, 2001, with Kim as chief and Farmer and Hiatt as deputy chiefs.[189]

BIOGRAPHY

JIM YONG KIM

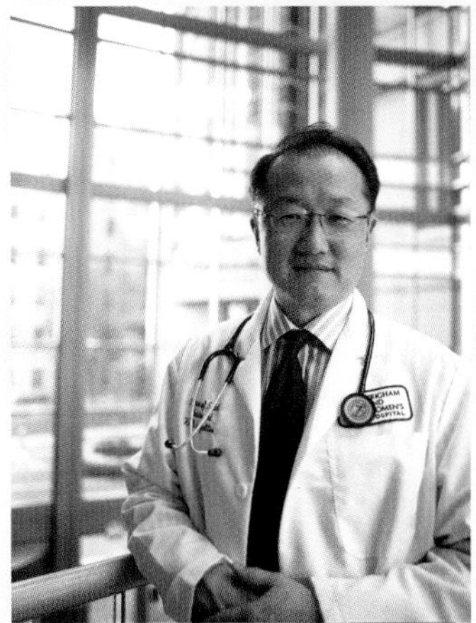

FIGURE 6-54 Jim Kim at BWH.

Born in 1959 in Seoul, South Korea, Jim Yong Kim moved with his family to the United States at the age of five and grew up in Muscatine, Iowa. Kim graduated with an AB *magna cum laude* from Brown University in 1982. He earned an MD from Harvard Medical School in 1991 and a PhD in anthropology from Harvard University in 1993.

Jim Kim became the twelfth president of the World Bank Group on July 1, 2012. A physician and anthropologist, Kim has dedicated himself to international development for more than two decades, helping to improve the lives of underserved populations worldwide. Kim came to the Bank after serving as president of Dartmouth College, a preeminent center of higher education that consistently ranks among the top academic institutions in the United States. Kim is a cofounder of Partners In Health (PIH) and a former director of the HIV/AIDS Department at the World Health Organization (WHO).

As president of Dartmouth—an institution that comprises a liberal arts college, graduate programs in the arts and sciences, and renowned professional schools of medicine, engineering, and business—Kim earned praise for reducing a financial deficit without cutting any academic programs. Kim also founded the Dartmouth Center for Health Care Delivery Science, a multidisciplinary institute dedicated to developing new models of healthcare delivery and achieving better health outcomes at lower costs.

Before assuming the Dartmouth presidency, Kim held professorships and chaired departments at Harvard Medical School, the Harvard School of Public Health, and Brigham and Women's Hospital, Boston. He also served as director of Harvard's François-Xavier Bagnoud Center for Health and Human Rights.

In 1987, Kim cofounded Partners In Health, a Boston-based nonprofit organization now working in poor communities on four continents. Challenging previous conventional wisdom that drug-resistant tuberculosis and HIV/AIDS could not be treated in developing countries, PIH successfully tackled these diseases by integrating large-scale treatment programs into community-based primary care.

As Director of the WHO's HIV/AIDS Department, Kim led the "3 by 5" initiative, the first-ever global goal for AIDS treatment, which sought to treat 3 million new HIV/AIDS patients in developing countries with antiretroviral drugs by 2005. Launched in September 2003, the program ultimately reached its goal by 2007.

Kim's work has earned him wide recognition. He was awarded a MacArthur "Genius" Fellowship (2003), was named one of America's "25 Best Leaders" by *U.S. News & World Report* (2005), and was selected as one of *TIME* magazine's "100 Most Influential People in the World" (2006).

Other faculty in the new division at its inception included Heidi Behforouz, Chi-Cheng Huang, J. Keith Joseph, Serena Koenig, Joia Mukherjee, Michael Rich, and Sonya Shin.[190] Each of these faculty continues to have a tremendous impact in the global health arena. Margaret Paternek, the division's first administrative director, created its operating systems, recruited administrative staff, and strove to get the new division on stable financial footing.

"We were a small shop in those days, a pretty flexible group," recalls Amy Judd, hired to direct program development.[191] "At my first interview with Jim, the Division title was 'Social Medicine and Health *Inequalities*.' I suggested they might consider a different, more positive name. And they still hired me." When the team moved to One Brigham Circle in the summer of 2003, it was not long before the sign on the door changed to the Division of Global Health

Equity.[192] Judd also worked closely with Hiatt to identify and court outside funding sources, soon landing a Lilly Foundation grant to fund a set of MDR-TB training, research, and advocacy initiatives in Russia. Building on PIH's successful collaboration with clinicians in Tomsk, Siberia, in which MDR-TB patients in the prison and civilian sectors were being treated and cured, the program has resulted in the scale-up of MDR-TB treatment in many regions of Russia and other former Soviet Union countries.

The publication in September 2003 of *Mountains Beyond Mountains: The Quest of Dr. Paul Farmer, A Man Who Would Cure the World*, written by Tracy Kidder, was a watershed event for the future of the division.[193] The book's publicity attracted new and experienced staff, medical trainees, and junior faculty who shared an interest in health disparities and social justice. At this transitional juncture, Kim took a leave of absence from Harvard, moving to Switzerland to work for Jong-Wook Lee, the newly elected director-general of the World Health Organization (WHO), in Geneva. Lee had invited Kim to direct WHO's "3 by 5 Initiative," an emergency effort to scale up treatment for HIV/AIDS in the world's most affected countries, with a measurable outcome of providing treatment to three million people by the end of 2005. With Kim in Geneva and Farmer frequently out of town, Hiatt invited a local Harvard-trained pediatrician, Paul Wise, to join the division to help fill the need for local mentors. Wise was a valued leader during his brief tenure, but moved to California in late 2004 to direct Stanford's Department of Pediatrics Center for Policy Outcomes and Prevention.

BIOGRAPHY

PAUL FARMER

Medical anthropologist and physician Paul Farmer is a founding director of Partners In Health (PIH), an international nonprofit organization that provides direct healthcare services and has undertaken research and advocacy activities on behalf of those who are sick and living in poverty. Farmer is the Kolokotrones University Professor and Chair of the Department of Global Health and Social Medicine at Harvard Medical School, Chief of the Division of Global Health Equity at Brigham and Women's Hospital, and the United Nations Deputy Special Envoy for Haiti.

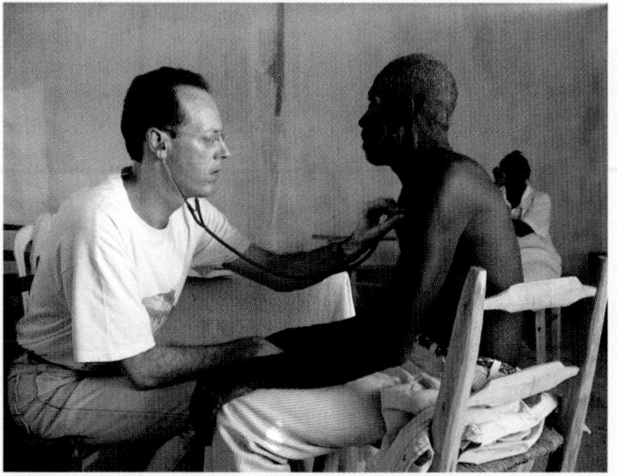

FIGURE 6-55 Paul Farmer examines a man in Haiti.

Farmer and his colleagues in the United States and in Haiti, Peru, Russia, Rwanda, Lesotho, and Malawi have pioneered novel community-based treatment strategies that demonstrate the delivery of high-quality health care in resource-poor settings. Farmer has written extensively on health, human rights, and the consequences of social inequality. His most recent book is *Haiti After the Earthquake*. Other titles include *Partner to the Poor: A Paul Farmer Reader, Pathologies of Power: Health, Human Rights, and the New War on the Poor, The Uses of Haiti, Infections and Inequalities: The Modern Plagues*, and *AIDS and Accusation: Haiti and the Geography of Blame*. Farmer is the recipient of numerous honors, including the Margaret Mead Award from the American Anthropological Association, the Outstanding International Physician (Nathan Davis) Award from the American Medical Association, a John D. and Catherine T. MacArthur Foundation Fellowship, and, with his PIH colleagues, the Hilton Humanitarian Prize. He is a member of the Institute of Medicine of the National Academy of Sciences and of the American Academy of Arts and Sciences.

Meanwhile, under Hiatt's mentoring, junior faculty were rapidly emerging as able leaders and inspiring mentors themselves, each leading initiatives that engaged trainees in clinical care, education, and research. Serena Koenig, for example, had established a research and clinical career in Haiti, where she focused on HIV/AIDS and MDR-TB. Keith Joseph led the division's collaboration with PIH in Malawi. Michael Rich took the lead in the first Africa project, in Rwanda in 2005, and was also editor-in-chief of the WHO's new standards for care and treatment of MDR-TB in 2006. And Joia Mukherjee, medical director of PIH since 2000, was one of the creators of the directly observed treatment short course (DOTS)-Plus model, an innovative strategy first implemented in Peru and today the WHO standard for the treatment of drug-resistant TB. A global leader in training residents to practice medicine founded on principles of solidarity and accompaniment, Mukherjee also directs the Institute of Health and Social Justice, PIH's research and advocacy arm. Brigham division-affiliated faculty physicians who trained under Mukherjee and are now leaders in their own right include Salmaan Keshavjee, Evan Lyon, Louise Ivers, David Walton, and Peter Drobac.

Louise Ivers is one who first joined the division during this transitional time. Her career demonstrates the extraordinary circumstances and challenges typical at these Brigham-affiliated sites. In 2003, Ivers, an infectious disease specialist, joined Mukherjee in Haiti, where her first experiences included sleeping in a tarantula-, cockroach-, and rat-infested shed next to the village church, nine-hour treks—often wading through deep streams—to visit patients at home, and working to address basic nutrition and housing needs in addition to building lab capacity and community health worker training. "You can't do this work for your career advancement, or for the justification of some principle," she says. "Patients must be the primary interest—the primary goal."[194] Quickly fluent in Creole, Ivers was in Port-au-Prince when the earthquake struck, on January 12, 2010, and, barely escaping a crumbling building, immediately began to care for injured survivors. After receiving the 2010 Thompson Compassionate Leadership Award at Brigham and Women's Hospital, she was one of the first physicians to alert the division of the cholera epidemic that struck Haiti in October 2010. Her clinical efforts and research publications on this epidemic have played a vital role in highlighting the tragedy and challenges of such a disaster and the opportunity for social media to strengthen public health alerts.[195] Ivers also led Haiti's 2012 cholera immunization program in the face of immense public media and policy resistance, delivering an effective two-dose oral cholera vaccination to 45,000 people in a community still suffering from the social disruption after the earthquake.[196]

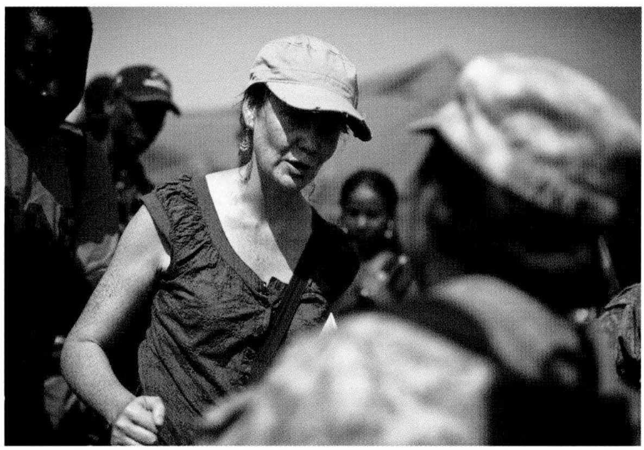

FIGURE 6-56 Louise Ivers in Haiti.

From Field Bench to Bedside: Shaping and Funding a Nontraditional Career

The division's popularity was also influencing Harvard Medical School faculty leaders responsible for shaping academic promotion criteria, as they discussed how to "push the envelope" toward new markers that would measure academic success in such nontraditional settings. Courses such as "Introduction to Social Medicine" and "Medical Ethics and Professionalism," often taught by division faculty, became required courses for first-year medical students. Division-affiliated physicians also launched a new course for Harvard undergraduates in collaboration with the Harvard Extension School, "Case Studies in Global Health: Biosocial Perspectives," that drew further on other division faculty as guest lecturers to help prepare students for "whatever it takes" to promote health equity around the world.[197]

However, not all division-supported trainees suffer the promotion pressures of an academic medical career. Some simply want to be excellent doctors for the poor. For example, a multinational global health delivery fellowship, launched in 2007, is jointly administered by the Brigham's Division of Global Health Equity, Harvard Medical School, the Haitian Ministry of Population and Public Health (MSPP), PIH, and Zanmi Lasante (PIH's partner affiliate organization in Haiti). This nontraditional collaborative three-year fellowship is the first of its kind anywhere in the world.[198] The fellows train at PIH-affiliated partner sites outside the United States, with clinical work "in-country" and medical training also offered at other locations including, in this case, Haiti. Those who have completed this training now work in PIH-affiliated hospitals and clinics at sites including Burundi, Haiti, Lesotho, Malawi, Peru, and Rwanda. In her address honoring the first graduating class in 2010, Joia Mukherjee emphasized the power of a partnership ethic in such an undertaking and affirmed these new graduates as "the backbone upon which global health will be taught in the decades to come."[199]

In all of its endeavors, the division has depended heavily on donor support. The Frank Hatch Scholars Program, for example, funded salary and benefits to allow select junior faculty the freedom they needed to shape a career devoted to treating and studying the diseases of poverty.[200] Nearly all of these private philanthropy efforts have been led by Howard Hiatt.

The Doris and Howard Hiatt Residency in Global Health Equity and Internal Medicine

Drs. Kim, Farmer and Wolf's successor, Joel Katz (Marshall A. Wolf distinguished chair in Medical Education and director of the Department of Medicine's internal medicine residency since 2000), recognized a growing interest among graduating medical students for careers that encompassed "international medicine," which at that time referred to mainly to programs delivering medicines or brief moments of care to impoverished regions without contributing to the healthcare infrastructure or sustained health or health status improvements. The growing mismatch between needs and existing teaching models inspired Kim and Farmer to task Margaret Paternek, Amy Judd, Howard Hiatt and Katz to design a new program that addressed the broad competencies required to build a career devoted to sustainable healthcare system development—from parasitology to healthcare administration and finance. Between 2002 and 2004 they designed what is now known as the Doris and Howard Hiatt Residency in Global Health Equity, and attained ABIM and ACGME approval for the novel curriculum and split sites of training between Boston and the developing world. The first residents (Nancy Lange and David Walton) matriculated in 2004. Jennifer Furin became director of the residency in the same year. This was the first board-approved internal medicine global health program in the world. Brigham residents interested in serving communities limited by poverty had until then trained in their relevant specialties of interest, usually emergency medicine or internal medicine.[201] An additional residency opportunity in global health opened the way for a dedicated focus to address issues related to economic and political effects on health, health care, and healthcare delivery. "By making global health a priority," said Hiatt, "Brigham and Women's Hospital has announced that medical care for all people independent of social status, income, and geography is part of its mission."[202] When the current Hiatt residency director, Joseph Rhatigan, reviewed alumni activities, he found that "more than 80 percent of them work full-time or most of their time in global health...a field that did not even exist ten years ago."[203] The Hiatt Residency is now "one of the most sought-after residencies in the world, attracting some of the best young minds in medicine to global health."[204]

Expansions: From Africa to New Mexico

By 2006, division faculty were actively implementing new programs. Scale-up in Russia included workshops for high-ranking officials on MDR-TB training. The inaugural venture into work in Africa followed an invitation to rebuild a hospital in Rwanda, in a collaboration with the Rwandan Ministry of Health, the Global Fund, and the Clinton HIV/AIDS Initiative.[205]

A second Africa partnership initiative in Lesotho followed in 2006, with a third launched the following year in Malawi. Other expansions included rural Kazakhstan, where a fragile health system served a rural population suffering from skyrocketing malnutrition, child mortality, and poverty-related diseases,[206] and new work in South America. In Chile, MaryCatherine Arbour directs the health component of a preschool health and education intervention in Santiago that is now planning a scale-up into public schools and public clinics.

These expanding opportunities increased the intention of both junior faculty and division staff to follow the momentum with firsthand experience developing their leadership potential in global health. For example, Hamish Fraser, a division-affiliated cardiologist with expertise in clinical decision making, cofounded the OpenMRS collaborative, an international collaboration to develop a flexible, open source medical record platform for use in developing countries that has an impact on all field sites.

In April 2007, Phyllis Jen, medical director of the Brigham Internal Medicine Associates before her tragic death in 2009, accompanied Judd and Hiatt to New Mexico on a visit that would lead the division into a new volunteer program for BWH physicians. The site visit included the Gallup Indian Medical Center, one of the largest Indian Health Service (IHS) hospitals in the United States, and its affiliate hospital in Shiprock, New Mexico, both facilities serving the Navajo nation (over a quarter of a million people). The visit exposed stark healthcare disparities for Native Americans, with conditions of healthcare services "similar to the needs of people in many developing countries."[207] Back in Boston, the team wrote a proposal that was selected by the BWH Physician Outreach Program to support "all interested BWH physicians, no matter their specialty, in volunteering for a week or two in New Mexico where they can make an impact through clinical care and teaching."[208] Although IHS facilities that serve the Navajo nation are adequately equipped, they are chronically understaffed, and patients face both socioeconomic and cultural obstacles to effective health care. The success of the visit and grant proposal led to the division's second domestic initiative, with its launch led in 2009 by Sonya Shin, a former Hatch Scholar who had worked with PIH over many years in Peru. The Community Outreach and Patient Empowerment (COPE) program, a formal collaboration between the Navajo Nation Community Health Representative Program, several IHS health service units, and the Brigham Division of Global Health Equity, follows the division's leading principles for action: partnership, fostering local skills and "solidarity assets," and building treatment efforts on accompaniment models. Drawing on existing community health workers to provide training, support, and resources, the program goal, says Shin, "is to make ourselves obsolete in the communities we help."[209]

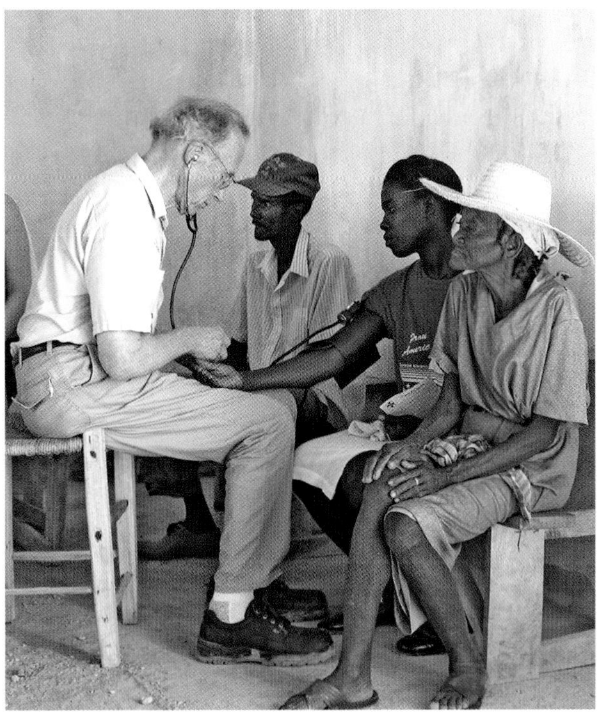

FIGURE 6-57 Howard Hiatt with patients in Haiti.

Global Health Delivery

Another Brigham-based project supported by division faculty is the Global Health Delivery Project (GHD), with the goal of working toward "nothing less than functioning healthcare systems everywhere in the world."[210] Cofounded by Kim, Farmer, and Professor Michael Porter of Harvard Business School, GHD is now led by Brigham Division faculty member Rebecca Weintraub, who is its executive director, with the support of Joseph Rhatigan, assistant professor at Harvard Medical School and the Harvard School of Public Health and director of the Hiatt Residency. Devoted to advancing value-based healthcare delivery,[211] GHD's core initiatives include education (with a focus on case studies), research, and proactive clinical care support in resource-poor settings through the creation and management of web-based "communities of practice." Since 2007, GHD has supported the development of more than twenty-five teaching case studies based on global health delivery efforts around the world, all now available online for registered users at no cost through Harvard Business Publishing.[212] This and other work associated with GHD helps to expand educational opportunities in the field of healthcare delivery across the globe.

PACT: Accompanying the Local Neighbor

In 1997, while completing her residency at the Brigham, Heidi Behforouz read in *The Boston Globe* that young black women in four Boston neighborhoods—Roxbury, Mattapan, Hyde Park, and Dorchester—faced a disproportionately high risk of developing HIV/AIDS, with a mortality rate fifteen times higher than that of the average white man with HIV in Boston. Realizing that the PIH model of "accompaniment" in Haiti would also work on a local domestic level, Behforouz applied for seed money from the Office of Minority Health (OMH) to found the Prevention and Access to Care and Treatment (PACT) Project, the Division's first local community activity.

Behforouz is another former Brigham trainee who credits Marshall Wolf for the freedom to realize her dreams during her residency. Instead of the usual six-month research stint, she says, "I told him, 'I want to keep working in the community.' And he funded my salary." Through PACT, Behforouz provides similar opportunities for other trainees, including medical students, residents, fellows, and MPH students.

PACT hires, trains, and supports community health workers who pair up with ninety to one hundred patients referred from approximately seventeen health centers in the Greater Boston area, focusing on home-based health promotion and harm reduction rather than traditional case management. PACT-trained community health workers use the DOT model that PIH first developed in Peru to provide what Behforouz describes as:

> *a very cognitive behavioral intervention...In addition to helping people navigate the system, [community health workers must] be able to be expert in terms of their medications and help them with adherence, to be able to talk with their clinicians... The community health worker is very much focused, as one of our community health workers says, on supporting people to learn to love themselves again, enough to take care of themselves.*[213]

The inequitable HIV/AIDS and related mortality risk for blacks and women, Behforouz emphasizes, "is not a technological or biomedical issue. It's really about all the structural violence and psychosocial issues that keep people from being able to utilize the services." Solving it, therefore, "takes a structural approach and an understanding of a vulnerability paradigm."

Behforouz's vision is to radically invert the way health care is currently delivered in most countries. "What we're trying to promote [is] that every patient should have a community health worker who is a *bona fide* care team member and has access to the doctor or the nurses needed," she says. Behforouz's dream is that eventually "most people get their care in the community via this team of highly qualified and well-supported

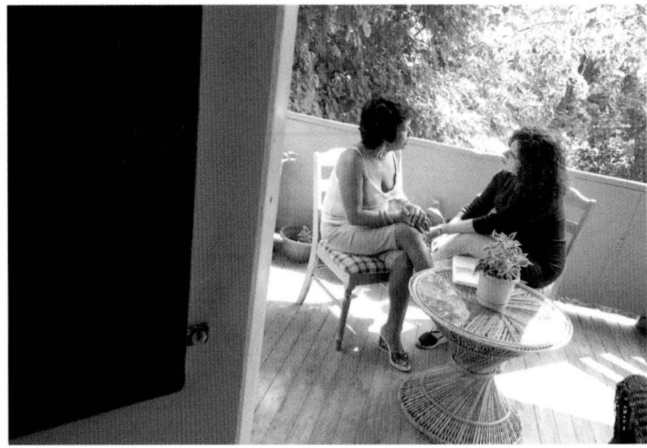

FIGURE 6-58 PACT client (left) and caregiver Maria Pia Terra.

community health workers and relegate the licensed clinicians to things that only they can contribute."

The PACT experience has proven that the community health worker model works—and is cost-effective. For example, analyzing two years of medical costs for a sample of seventy patients, Behforouz and colleagues saw a 60% reduction in hospitalizations and a 35% reduction in total medical expenses.[214] Behforouz also works closely with a number of BWH committees that share a commitment to global health equity, including the BWH Center for Community Health and Health Equity (formerly the Office for Women, Family and Community Programs), which has been one of PACT's most consistent funding sources.

The success of the Brigham's Division of Global Health Equity reflects the strong community-based commitment of a dedicated network of faculty and staff, at both the Brigham and its affiliated sites worldwide. For as long as we continue to have such leaders who can encourage risk, innovation, and hope for the cause of global health equity, BWH will indeed be a good place to build something new.

REFERENCES

1. Peter Bent Brigham Hospital, "Peter Bent Brigham Hospital Founder's Day, November 12, 1914" (pamphlet), Boston, 1914, p. 2.
2. Charles E. Rosenberg, "Inward Vision and Outward Glance: The Shaping of the American Hospital 1880-1914," *Bulletin of the History of Medicine* 53 (Fall 1979), pp. 346-91.
3. Sari Roboff, *Mission Hill: Boston 200 Neighborhood Series* (Boston: Boston Redevelopment Authority, 1976), p. 1.
4. Oscar Handlin, *Boston's Immigrants* (New York: Atheneum, 1969), p. 20.
5. Ibid., p. 22.
6. Ibid., p. 21.
7. Paul DiMaggio, "Cultural Entrepreneurship in Nineteenth-Century Boston," *Media, Culture, and Society* 4 (1982), pp. 33-50.
8. Also known as the House of Industry.
9. Channing's second wife died in childbirth, with Channing delivering the stillborn baby.
10. He also resigned as attending physician at the Massachusetts General Hospital. No reason was ever given, though one can speculate that he felt overcommitted and needed to focus on his private practice.
11. *Boston Lying-In Hospital, Admissions, 1832-1844* (Center for the History of Medicine, Countway Library, Harvard Medical School) (This manuscript covers the first twenty-four years at the hospital. Subsequent nineteenth-century records no longer exist.); M.A. DeWolfe Howe, *The Humane Society of the Commonwealth of Massachusetts: An Historical Review, 1795-1916* (Boston: Printed for the Humane Society, 1918); Frederick C. Irving, *Highlights in the History of the Boston Lying-in Hospital*, typescript (Boston: Massachusetts General Hospital, Archives and Special Collections); Frederick C. Irving, *Safe Deliverance* (Boston: Houghton Mifflin, 1942); Amalie M. Kass, *Midwifery and Medicine in Boston: Walter Channing, M.D. 1786-1876* (Boston: Northeastern University Press, 2002); Amalie M. Kass, "The Obstetrical Case Book of Walter Channing, 1811-1822," *Bulletin of the History of Medicine* 67 (1993): 494-523; *Massachusetts General Hospital, Report on a Lying-in Department* (Boston: Massachusetts General Hospital, Archives and Special Collections, October 1845); Henry R. Sprague, *A Brief History of the Massachusetts Charitable Fire Society* (Boston: Little, Brown, 1893).
12. Ibid., p. 114.
13. Ibid., p. 89.
14. Ibid., p. 115.
15. See Hasia Diner, *Erin's Daughters in America* (Baltimore: Johns Hopkins University Press, 1983).
16. Handlin, p. 184.
17. Irving, pp. 203-4.
18. Ibid., p. 200.
19. Irving, p. 191.
20. "Edward Everett Hale," Wikepedia, http://en.wikipedia.org/wiki/Edward_Everett_Hale. Accessed July 22, 2012.
21. Elmer Osgood Cappers, *History of the Free Hospital for Women 1875-1975* (Boston: Free Hospital for Women, 1975), p. 17.
22. "Gynecology could be taught to students in public clinics despite the opposition of older members of the profession who thought this immodest." Cappers, p. 19.
23. Ibid., p. 21.
24. Ibid., p. 37.
25. Ibid., p. 37.
26. Ibid., p. 44.
27. Cappers, p. 35.
28. Ibid., p. 35.
29. Ibid., p. 43.
30. Ibid., p. 49.
31. Ibid., p. 44.
32. Ibid., p. 75.
33. Nancy Anderson, "A History of the Robert Breck Brigham Hospital," p. 2.
34. Ibid., p. 6.
35. Rosenberg, "Inward Vision and Outward Glance," p. 313.
36. "J.E.M.," "Joel Ernest Goldthwaite, 1866-1961," *J Bone Joint Surg* 43A (April 1961), pp. 463-4.
37. Letter to Olga Warburton (O.W.) from Lloyd Brown (L.B.), August 25, 1954.
38. Anderson, pp. 1-6.

39. "Transfer for Hospital," *Jamaica Plain News*, January 5, 1901, 2.
40. Ellen Morse, *The Good Men Do Lives After Them,* (Boston: Faulkner Hospital, 1927).
41. *Boston Comes to Faulkner,* (Boston: Faulkner Hospital, 1931).
42. L.A. Hodgdon, "Health of the District, West Roxbury, 1903." *Genealogical and Personal Memoirs Relating to the Families of the State of Massachusetts.* Volume 2, edited by William Richard Cutter, William Frederick Adams. Lewis Historical Publishing Company, 1910, p. 1118
43. Annmarie Adams, *Medicine by Design: The Architect and the Modern Hospital, 1893-1943* (University of Minnesota Press, 2008); "West Roxbury Is to Have a $100,000 Hospital for Its Own Residents," *Boston Herald*, October 7, 1901; *American Architect and Architecture*, Volumes 75-78, 1902.
44. "The New Faulkner Hospital is Opened for an Inspection by Invited Guests," *Boston Herald*, February 26, 1903.
45. *First Annual Report of the Faulkner Hospital* (Boston: Faulkner Hospital, 1903).
46. *A Short History of Faulkner Hospital* (Boston: Faulkner Hospital, 1970).
47. "Cases," *Boston Medical and Surgical Journal* CLXIII (1910), p. 390; E.B. Benedict, et al, "Corsage Pin in Stomach," *Journal of the American Medical Associations* 175 (1961) p. 48; J.J. Putnam and G.A. Waterman, "A Contribution to the Study of Cerebellar Tumors and their Treatment," *Journal of Nervous and Mental Disease* 33 (1906): p. 297.
48. *Annual Report* (Boston: Faulkner Hospital, 1928); *Faulkner Hospital School of Nursing Announcement* (Boston: Faulkner Hospital).
49. *Trustees Records* (Boston: Faulkner Hospital, February 21, 1962).
50. *Annual Report* (Boston: Faulkner Hospital, 1935-1940).
51. *Trustees Records* (Boston: Faulkner Hospital, 1984-1986).
52. Elizabeth Loder, Dhirendra Bana, Paul Rizzoli, and Carly Lavigne, *John R. Graham and the Graham Headache Center: Pioneers in Modern Medicine* (Boston: Faulkner Hospital).
53. *Annual Report* (Boston: Faulkner Hospital, 1970).
54. *A Tradition of Caring Continues.*
55. V.W. Conner and G. Kutsuflakis, "Putting Supplies at the Bedside via the Friesen Concept," *Hosp Materials Managet Quart* 16 (1994), pp. 35-40.
56. "The Patient Unit," *Transplant*, October 2, 1975, pp. 1-2; "Getting the Message Across – More Quickly, More Quietly," *Transplant*, November 26, 1975, pp. 1-2; "The First Floor of the New Faulkner," *Faulkner Herald*, April 1974, p. 6.
57. *Report of the President of Harvard College and Reports of Departments* (Boston: Harvard University, 1973-1974).
58. A.J. Sussman, J.R. Otten, R.C. Goldszer, et al, "Integration of an Academic Medical Center and a Community Hospital: The Brigham and Women's/Faulkner Hospital Experience," *Academic Medicine* 80 (2005), pp. 253-60.
59. Roboff, p. 1.
60. Roboff, p. 3.
61. Refers to the period of September-December 1914.
62. The PBBH was the first general hospital in Boston to admit patients with either tuberculosis or syphilis. From: Twenty fifth Anniversary Meeting, Medical Service of the Peter Bent Brigham Hospital, March 31, 1938 (typescript), Twenty Fifth Anniversary Reunion, Volume 1, 180.
63. Alice M. Cheney, "Social Service," *Third Annual Report of the Peter Bent Brigham Hospital for the Year 1916* (Cambridge: The University Press, 1917), p. 35.
64. Henry A. Christian, "Report of the Physician-in-Chief," *Third Annual Report of the Peter Bent Brigham Hospital for the Year 1916* (Cambridge: The University Press, 1917), p. 129.
65. Joseph B. Howland,"Report of the Superintendent," *Eighth Annual Report of the Peter Bent Brigham Hospital for the Year 1921* (Cambridge: The University Press, 1922), p. 12.
66. Henry A. Christian, "Report of the Physician-in-Chief," *Fifteenth Annual Report Report of the Peter Bent Brigham Hospital for the Year 1928* (Boston, 1929), p. 146.
67. Alice M. Cheney, "Report of the Social Service Department," *Eighteenth Annual Report of the Peter Bent Brigham Hospital for the Year 1931* (Boston, 1932), p. 60
68. Joseph B. Howland,"Report of the Superintendent," *Twenty-First Annual Report of the Peter Bent Brigham Hospital for the Year 1934* (Boston, 1935), p. 19.
69. Alice M. Cheney, "Report of the Social Service Department," *Eighteenth Annual Report*, p. 66.
70. Henry A. Christian, "Report of the Physician-in-Chief," *Fifteenth Annual Report of the Peter Bent Brigham Hospital for the Year 1934,* (Boston, 1935) p. 53.
71. Alice M. Cheney, "Report of the Social Service Department," *Twenty-Fifth Annual Report of the Peter Bent Brigham Hospital for the Year 1938* (Boston, 1939), p. 54.
72. Norbert A. Wilhelm, "Report of the Director," *Thirty-Second Annual Report of the Peter Bent Brigham Hospital for the Year 1945* (Boston, 1946), p. 21.
73. "Gifts to the Hospital During the Year 1923," *Tenth Annual Report of the Peter Bent Brigham Hospital for the Year 1923* (Boston: Wright & Potter, 1924), pp. 4-5.
74. Alice M. Cheney, "Social Service," *Second Annual Report of the Peter Bent Brigham Hospital for the Year 1915* (Cambridge: The University Press, 1916), p. 38
75. Alice M. Cheney, "Report of the Social Service Department," *Twenty-First Annual Report of the Peter Bent Brigham Hospital for the Year 1934* (Boston, 1935), p. 39
76. Francis D. Moore, "Report of the Surgeon-in-Chief," *Fortieth Annual Report of the Peter Bent Brigham Hospital for the Fiscal Year Ended September 30, 1953* (Boston, 1954), p. 54.
77. Ibid., p. 55.
78. Linda W. Hertig, "Report of the Friends of the Peter Bent Brigham Hospital," *Thirty-Fifth Annual Report of the Peter Bent Brigham Hospital for the Year 1948* (Boston, 1949), p. 103.

79. Ibid., pp. 102-7.
80. Anita Magruder, "Report of the Friends of the Peter Bent Brigham Hospital and Volunteer Service," *Fortieth Annual Report of the Peter Bent Brigham Hospital for the Fiscal Year Ended September 30, 1953* (Boston, 1935), p. 124.
81. Ibid., p. 123.
82. Helen H. Hale, "Annual Report of the President of the Friends," *Peter Bent Brigham Hospital Fiftieth Annual Report*, 1962-1963 (Boston, 1963), p. 376.
83. Brigham and Women's Hospital, "About the Friends of BWH," http://www.brighamandwomens.org/about_bwh/friendsofBWH/AboutUs.aspx, accessed July 17, 2012.
84. Harvey Cushing, "Report of the Surgeon-in-Chief," *Ninth Annual Report of the Peter Bent Brigham Hospital for the Fiscal Year Ended September 30, 1922* (Cambridge: The University Press, 1923), p. 54.
85. Henry A. Christian, "Report of the Physician-in-Chief," *Ninth Annual Report of the Peter Bent Brigham Hospital for the Fiscal Year Ended September 30, 1922* (Cambridge: The University Press, 1923), p. 102.
86. Barbara Myerhoff, *Number Our Days* (New York: Simon and Schuster, 1978), p. 32.
87. Peter Bent Brigham Hospital School of Nursing Alumnae Association, *Alumnae Journal* (Boston, Mass.: Alumnae Association of the School of Nursing, Peter Bent Brigham Hospital, June 1920), p. 6.
88. Ibid., pp. 15-8.
89. Peter Bent Brigham Hospital School of Nursing Alumnae Association, *Alumnae Journal* 10 (Boston, Mass.: Alumnae Association of the School of Nursing, Peter Bent Brigham Hospital, June 1928), pp. 11-4.
90. Ibid., pp. 19-20.
91. "Peter Bent Brigham Hospital Silver Anniversary Program: 25th Anniversary Play. Wednesday and Thursday Evenings, May 4th and 5th, 1938, at 8 P.M." (pamphlet, unpaginated—hereafter referred to as PBBH Silver Anniversary Program).
92. Initiated in 1935, The Community Federation of Boston was a "permanent joint form of raising funds for the charities of Boston." Through subscriptions, substantial funds were raised. PBBH staff contributed to the federation and also accepted significant wage reductions to support charitable care at the hospital. (*Twenty-Second Annual Report*, p. 1).
93. Rosemary Stevens, *In Sickness and in Wealth: American Hospitals in the Twentieth Century* (New York: Basic Books, 1989), p. 91.
94. A Member of the Unit, *The Story of U.S. Army Base Hospital No.5* (Cambridge: The University Press, 1919).
95. Elmer Osgood Cappers, *History of the Free Hospital for Women*, p. 58.
96. Arnold Arluke and Glenn Gritzer, *The Making of Rehabilitation: Political Economy of Medical Specialization, 1890-1980* (Berkeley: University of California Press, 1985), p. 41.
97. Ibid, p. 41.
98. J. Sydney Stillman, "History of the Medical Service of the Robert Breck Brigham Hospital," p. 2.
99. "War Diary," Elliott Cutler, U.S. Army Medical Dept. Office of Medical History. http://history.amedd.army.mil/booksdocs/wwii/actvssurgconvol2/chapter2.1.htm. Accessed July 7, 2012.
100. Elsa E. Storm, "Report of the School of Nursing," *Thirty-First Annual Report of the Peter Bent Brigham Hospital for the Year 1944* (Boston, 1945), p. 80.
101. Kenneth Ludmerer, *A Time to Heal* (New York: Oxford University Press, 1999), pp. 132-3.
102. In the period 1940-1960, federal research funding nationally would increase 100-fold, and as a research leader, the PBBH would be an important recipient of this largesse.
103. Robert Cutler, "Report of the President," *Thirty-Seventh Annual Report of the Peter Bent Brigham Hospital for the Year 1950* (Boston, 1951), p. 8.
104. Ibid., p. 1.
105. Ibid., p. 1.
106. Francis D. Moore, "Report of the Surgeon-in-Chief," *Forty-Second Annual Report of the Peter Bent Brigham Hospital for the Fiscal Year Ended September 30, 1955* (Boston, 1955), p. 114.
107. Francis D. Moore, "Report of the Surgeon-in-Chief," *Forty-Fifth Annual Report of the Peter Bent Brigham Hospital for the Fiscal Year Ended September 30, 1958* (Boston, 1958), p. 88.
108. Marilyn King, "Letter from Bernice J. Sinclair (1924) 9 May 1945," in *The Peter Bent Brigham Hospital School of Nursing: A History 1912-1985* (Boston: Brigham and Women's Hospital, 1988), pp. 105-14 (originally published in The Peter Bent Brigham Hospital School of Nursing *Alumnae Journal* [June 1945]).
109. Charles B. Barnes and Alan Steinert, Jr., "The Joint Report of the Chairman of the Board of Trustees and the President," *Peter Bent Brigham Hospital Fiftieth Annual Report*, 1962-1963 (Boston, 1963), p. 9.
110. Ludmerer, *A Time to Heal*, pp. 180-90.
111. George W. Thorn, "Report of the Physician-in-Chief," *Forty-Third Annual Report of the Peter Bent Brigham Hospital for the Fiscal Year Ended September 30, 1956* (Boston, 1956), p. 19.
112. George W. Thorn, "Report of the Physician-in-Chief," Peter Bent Brigham Hospital *49th Annual Report 1961-1962, fiscal year ending September 30* (Boston, 1963), p. 26.
113. "The History of Brookside," http://www.brighamandwomens.org/Departments_and_Services/medicine/services/primarycare/brookside_history.aspx. Accessed July 22, 2012
114. Interview with Tom Kieffer, July 2012.
115. Kieffer interview.
116. "Mission and History, Southern Jamaica Plain Health Center." http://www.brighamandwomens.org/

Departments_and_Services/medicine/services/primary-care/sjphc/SJPHC_mishis.aspx. Accessed July 22, 2012.
117. Andrew G. Jessiman, "The Brigham and the Community," *Brigham Bulletin* (Volume 20, February 1975): 6-10.
118. Richard P. Chapman and Alan Steinert, Jr., "The Joint Report of the Chairman of the Board and of the President," *Sixty-First Annual Report, Peter Bent Brigham Hospital, 1973-1974* (Boston, 1974), p. 7.
119. "Groundbreaking Protested," *Boston Globe*, December 21, 1975, p. 2.
120. Elena Olson, Emeli Valverde, and L. Adaora Nwachukwu, "The Untold Story: URM Pioneers at MGH," Bicentennial Gala and Alumni Reunion, Multicultural Affairs Office, Massachusetts General Hospital, February 11 and 12, 2011, http://www.massgeneral.org/news/assets/urmhistoryslideshow.pdf, accessed November 8, 2012
121. Andrew G. Jessiman, "Report of the Division of Community Health," *Sixty-Second Annual Report, Peter Bent Brigham Hospital 1974-1975* (Boston, 1975), p. 13.
122. Ibid., p. 13.
123. FAMILY Inc., "FAMILY History," FAMILY (Fathers and Mothers Infants, eLders and Youth). http://www.familysystem.net/history.html. Accessed November 8, 2012.
124. Walter Haynes and David Richwine, "A Fourth Day of Turmoil in the City: 27 Injured in Roxbury Street Attacks," *Boston Globe*, August 14, 1975, p. 1; James Ayres and Manli Ho, "Streets Calm as State, MDC Police Move In," *Boston Globe*, October 11, 1974.
125. Author interview with Wanda McClain, May 3, 2012.
126. Ibid.
127. Center for Community Health and Health Equity, Brigham and Women's Hospital, " Health Equity Research and Intervention," http://www.brighamandwomens.org/about_bwh/communityprograms/our-programs/research.aspx?sub=0. Accessed May 15, 2012.
128. One objective of the 2012 Brigham and Women's/Faulkner Strategic Planning Report calls for "communication and integration across disparate local, national, and global programs by instituting a Community Engagement Executive Committee to ensure a coordinated approach to community engagement efforts." ("Discovery and Innovation: Working Together to Provide Superior Healthcare," *Brigham and Women's/Faulkner Strategic Planning Report*, (2012)p. 21.)
129. Gary Gottlieb, MD, MBA, "Improving Quality and Reducing Disparities at Partners Health Care: What We Know and What We Need to Know," PowerPoint Presentation, undated.
130. Ibid.
131. Richard A. Knox, "Hub Infant Deaths Up 32%, Blacks Bear the Brunt of 1985 Mortality Hike," *The Boston Globe*, February 9, 1987, p. 1.
132. Richard A. Knox, "Birth in the Death Zones," *Boston Sunday Globe*, September 10-12, 1990.
133. BWH "Community Health Services Report" (Boston: Brigham and Women's Hospital, 1993). BWH also contributed $400,000 to neighborhood health centers designated by the MA Department of Public Health (a one-time commitment).
134. "Center for Health Equity and Health Education Birth Equity Initiative," Brigham and Women's Hospital. http://www.brighamandwomens.org/about_bwh/community-programs/our-programs/health-equity/birth-equity.aspx. Accessed July 7, 2012.
135. "Mayor Menino, Public Health Commission Announce Drop in Black Infant Deaths in City of Boston," Press Release, City of Boston, July 25, 2011. Noting the association of infant mortality with the stresses of discrimination, poverty, and disenfranchisement, the Boston Public Health Commission had restructured their child, adolescent, and family health efforts two years before. They attributed the sharp decline in part to a combination of case management services through Boston Healthy Start Initiative, as well as a home visiting program carried out through the Healthy Baby/Healthy Child (HB/HC) program, which provided housing and social service support, involvement of fathers, and teen education.
136. Marc Joseph, "It 'Takes A Village' To Fix Our Education System." *International Business Times*, http://www.ibtimes.com/articles/370211/20120803/education-reform-policy-federal-funding-aid.htm. Accessed August 3, 2012.
137. Herbert B. Howard, "Report of the Superintendent," *First Annual Report of the Peter Bent Brigham Hospital for the Years 1913 and 1914* (Cambridge: The University Press, 1915), p. 21.
138. Sources for this essay include: Henry K. Beecher and Mark D. Altschule, *Medicine at Harvard: The First 300 Years* (Hanover, NH: University Press of New England, 1977); Elmer Osgood Cappers, *History of the Free Hospital for Women 1875-1975* (Boston: Boston Hospital for Women, 1975); Frederick C. Irving, *Highlights in the History of the Boston Lying-In Hospital* (unpublished manuscript read at the dinner of the 108th anniversary of the founding of the hospital—Walter Channing Day, October 24, 1940); John F. Jewett, "Sesquicentennium of the Boston Lying-In Hospital—150 trailblazing years," *Contemp OB/Gyn* 21 (1983), pp. 198-206; D. avid McCord, *The Fabrick of Man: Fifty Years of the Peter Bent Brigham* (Boston: Peter Bent Brigham Hospital, 1963); National Library of Medicine, National Institutes of Health, "Changing the Face of Medicine: Profiles of Achievement," www.nlm.nih.gov/changingthefaceofmedicine; Nora N. Nercessian, *"Worthy of the Honor": A Brief History of Women at Harvard Medical School* (Boston: President and Fellows of Harvard College, 1995); Eleanor Shore, "The Invisible Faculty," *Harvard Medical Alumni Bulletin* (Spring 1983), pp. 40-5.
139. Ludmerer, *A Time to Heal*, p. 250.

140. Michele Richinick, "Dr. Curtis Prout, 96, physician, advocate for prison health care," *Boston Globe*, February 6, 2012, http://www.boston.com/news/local/massachusetts/articles/2012/02/06/prison_healthcare_advocate_dr_curtis_prout_a_primary_care_physician_into_his_90s/. Accessed January 14, 2013.
141. Curtis Prout, Guest Editor, "Women in Medicine," *The Brigham Bulletin*, Peter Bent Brigham Hospital, Volume V, No. II, Winter 1958, p. 2. Archival issues of the *Brigham Bulletin* dating from 1943-1961, including the issues containing this series on women in medicine, have been digitized and are available online at http://pds.lib.harvard.edu/pds/view/42588502
142. Brigham and Women's Hospital Center for Faculty Development and Diversity, "5th Anniversary Report, 2011," p. 6.
143. Ibid.
144. Per AAMC guidelines, at BWH, underrepresented minorities (URM) are defined as African-American, Alaskan/Hawaiian Native, Latino, and Native American.
145. "Bright Horizons Center Dedicated," *Brigham Bulletin*, November 30, 2000, http://www.brighamandwomens.org/about_bwh/publicaffairs/news/publications/DisplayBulletin.aspx?issueDate=11/30/2000%2012:00:00%20AM and "BWH to Double Daycare Slots," February 28, 2000, http://www.brighamandwomens.org/about_bwh/publicaffairs/news/publications/DisplayBulletin.aspx?articleid=59. Accessed November 8, 2012; "Domestic Violence Addressed," *Brigham Bulletin*, October 13, 2000, http://www.brighamandwomens.org/about_bwh/publicaffairs/news/publications/DisplayBulletin.aspx?articleid=1076. Accessed November 8, 2012.
146. "Hispanic Heritage Event at SJPHC," *Brigham Bulletin*, September 22, 2000, http://www.brighamandwomens.org/about_bwh/publicaffairs/news/publications/DisplayBulletin.aspx?articleid=1060&issueDate=9/22/2000%2012:00:00%20AM. Accessed November 8, 2012.
147. "Black History Month Continues," *Brigham Bulletin*, February 18, 2000, http://www.brighamandwomens.org/about_bwh/publicaffairs/news/publications/DisplayBulletin.aspx?articleid=92. Accessed November 8, 2012.
148. "CFDD Summer Programs Shape Young Researchers' Futures," *BWH Bulletin*, August 18, 2011, http://www.brighamandwomens.org/about_bwh/publicaffairs/news/publications/DisplayBulletin.aspx?articleid=5323. Accessed November 8, 2012.
149. Ibid.
150. Ibid.
151. William E. Hassan, Jr., "Report of the Executive Vice President," *Affiliated Hospitals Center 1979 Annual Report* (1980), p. 13.
152. Ibid., p. 14.
153. F. Stanton Deland, "Report of the President," *Affiliated Hospitals Center 1979 Annual Report*, p. 12.
154. Ibid., p. 11.
155. "Report of the Department of Surgery," *Brigham and Women's Hospital 1980 Annual Report, October 1, 1979-September 30, 1980*, p. 313.
156. John A. Kastor, *Mergers of Teaching Hospitals in Boston, New York and Northern California* (Ann Arbor, MI: University of Michigan Press, 2003), p. 38.
157. Anthony L. Komaroff, Eugene Braunwald, Joseph L. Dorsey, David M. Eisenberg, Howard H. Hiatt, Phyllis Jen, and Beverly Woo, "Harry Richard Nesson," Medical Faculty Memorial Minute, *Harvard Gazette*, March 23, 2006. http://www.news.harvard.edu/gazette/2006/03.23/18-mm.html. Accessed November 8, 2012.
158. Ibid.
159. "1993 Banner Year for Research," *BWH*, June 7, 1994, p. 20.
160. "The BWH Strategic Plan," *Brigham Bulletin*, November 30, 2001, http://www.brighamandwomens.org/about_bwh/publicaffairs/news/publications/DisplayBulletin.aspx?issueDate=11/30/2001%2012:00:00%20AM. Accessed November 8, 2012.
161. "New Buildings Part of Plan to Meet Space Challenges," *Brigham Bulletin*, November 17, 2000, http://www.brighamandwomens.org/about_bwh/publicaffairs/news/publications/DisplayBulletin.aspx?issueDate=11/17/2000%2012:00:00%20AM. Accessed November 8, 2012.
162. "Hospitals at a Crossroads," *BWH*, November/December 1993, pp. 16-7.
163. Kastor, *Mergers of Teaching Hospitals*, p. 30.
164. "Partners," *BWH*, June/July 1994, p. 6.
165. "Preparing Physicians for Tomorrow's Challenges," *BWH*, Spring 1997, p. 6.
166. "Partners Health Care System Enters New Phase," *BWH*, Summer 1996, p. 24.
167. Francis D. Moore, "Report of the Surgeon-in-Chief," Forty-first Annual Report of the Peter Bent Brigham Hospital for the Fiscal Year Ended September 30, 1954 (1954), p. 80.
168. George W. Thorn, "Report of the Physician-in-Chief," Fortieth Annual Report of the Peter Bent Brigham Hospital for the Fiscal Year Ended September 30, 1953 (1953), p. 15.
169. George W. Thorn, "Report of the Physician-in-Chief," Forty-first Annual Report of the Peter Bent Brigham Hospital for the Fiscal Year Ended September 30, 1954 (1954), p. 55.
170. T.F. O'Brien, personal communication, 2012.
171. M. Kantor, *Uncle Sam's Shame. Inside our Broken Veterans Administration* (Westport CT: Praeger Security International, 2008).
172. S.F. Khuri, "The NSQIP: A New Frontier in Surgery," *Surgery* 137 (2005), pp. 20-7.
173. *BWH* (March 2000) notes that in late 1990s, Partners initiated an international program to provide services in other countries, including the United Arab Emirates. Other

settings included emergency assistance, such as in the Gulf of Mexico after Hurricane Katrina, Mexico after Hurricane Stan, and in Pakistan after an earthquake.
174. "Joint Principles of the Patient Centered Medical Home," Patient-Centered Primary Care Collaborative, http://www.pcpcc.net/content/joint-principles-patient-centered-medical-home. Accessed July 7, 2012.
175. Kevin Grumbach, MD, et al., "The Outcomes of Implementing Patient-Centered Medical Home Interventions: A Review of the Evidence on Quality, Access and Costs from Recent Prospective Evaluation Studies," *USCF Center for Excellence in Primary Care* (Nov. 2010), http://www.pcpcc.net/files/evidence_outcomes_in_pcmh.pdf. Accessed October 20, 2011.
176. An e-visit is a virtual/electronic visit with a physician or other qualified health professional that uses secure electronic communication for a single patient encounter.
177. "Medical Home Opens on South Huntington," *Brigham Bulletin*, September 23, 2011,http://www.brighamandwomens.org/about_bwh/publicaffairs/news/publications/DisplayBulletin.aspx?issueDate=9/23/2011%20 12:00:00%20AM. Accessed October 20, 2011
178. "Partners Selected to participate in ACO Model," *BWH Clinical and Research News*, January 20, 2012. http://www.brighamandwomens.org/about_bwh/publicaffairs/news/publications/DisplayCRN.aspx?articleid=1972. Accessed October 20, 2011
179. A *BWH Bulletin* article reports that "a seamless model of care ensures continuity and responsiveness...It's a concerted effort to make sure all the elements come together.... We want to be certain that everyone who is in contact with a patient—from the time the patient calls for an appointment right through all facets of inpatient and outpatient care—regularly meet to identify and solve problems." ("Growing DF/BWCC Provides Seamless Patient Care," *BWH Bulletin,* June 2, 2006, http://www.brighamandwomens.org/about_bwh/publicaffairs/news/publications/DisplayBulletin.aspx?articleid=2764. Accessed December 7, 2012.
180. "Nabel Outlines BW/F Strategic Planning Recommendations," *BWH Bulletin*, December 13, 2011, http://www.brighamandwomens.org/about_bwh/publicaffairs/news/publications/DisplayBulletin.aspx?issueDate=12/13/2011%2012:00:00%20AM. Accessed December 7, 2012.
181. McCord, p. 27.
182. Ibid., pp. 28, 31.
183. *BWH Clinical & Research News*, October 31, 2001, online at http://www.brighamandwomens.org/about_bwh/publicaffairs/news/publications/DisplayCRN.aspx?articleid=120. Accessed June 1, 2012.
184. "Equity is the only acceptable goal," Paul E. Farmer, as quoted in Tracy Kidder, "Profiles: The Good Doctor," *The New Yorker*, July 10, 2000, p. 44.
185. Ted Constan and Joia Mukherjee, "Note to the Reader," *Partners In Health Program Management Guide* (Boston: PIH, 2011), p. viii, online at http://www.pih.org/pmg. Accessed June 1, 2012.
186. Kristin DeJohn, "Tapping Potential: BWH Profiles in Medicine: Marshall Wolf, MD," *BWH Magazine*, Spring 2011, p. 18.
187. DGHSM was founded in 1980 as the Department of Social Medicine and Health Policy; in 1984, when HMS established a separate Department of Health Care Policy, the DSMHP became the Department of Social Medicine, until Jim Yong Kim was appointed Chair in 2006, when it became the Department of Global Health and Social Medicine. HMS DGHSM, "History of the Department," http://ghsm.hms.harvard.edu/about/history/. Accessed June 1, 2012.
188. Victor Dzau, interview by Peter Tishler, http://videocenter.brighamandwomens.org/videos/victor-dzau-md. Last updated June 18, 2013.
189. "Division of Social Medicine and Health Inequalitie[s], BWH *Clinical and Research News*, October 31, 2001, online at http://www.brighamandwomens.org/about_bwh/publicaffairs/news/publications/DisplayCRN.aspx?articleid=120. Accessed June 1, 2012.
190. Jim Yong Kim, "Social Medicine and Health Inequalities," *Brigham and Women's Hospital Department of Medicine, Annual Report, 1996–2001,* faculty roster, p. 177.
191. Amy Judd, interview, March 13, 2012.
192. My emphasis.
193. Although the book pushed Farmer to celebrity status, he was already in the national spotlight in part due to Kidder's earlier *New Yorker* profile, "The Good Doctor: Paul Farmer Set Out Twenty Years Ago to Heal the World. He Still Thinks He Can," *The New Yorker*, July 10, 2000, pp. 40-57.
194. "Lester Leung, "Pathways through medicine: Careers in medicine—Medicine in developing countries, From an interview with Louise Ivers, MD, Partners in Health," http://www.nextgenmd.org/archives/399. Accessed June 1, 2012.
195. See, e.g., Louise C. Ivers and David A. Walton, "The 'first' case of cholera in Haiti: Lessons for Global Health," *Am J Trop Med Hygiene* 86 (2012), pp. 36-8. On the effect of social media, see Rumi Chunara, Jason R. Andrews, and John S. Brownstein, "Social and News Media Enable Estimation of Epidemiological Patterns Early in the 2010 Haitian Cholera Outbreak," *American Journal of Tropical Medicine and Hygiene* 86 (2012), pp. 39-45. For a more detailed narrative of Ivers' role in the cholera epidemic, see Paul Farmer (with colleagues), *Haiti after the Earthquake* (New York: Public Affairs, 2011), pp. 188-216.
196. http://www.pih.org/news/entry/the-cholera-vaccine-campaign-an-update-from-dr.-louise-ivers/. Accessed June 1, 2012. See also Louise C. Ivers, Paul E. Farmer, and

William J. Pape, "Oral Cholera Vaccine and Integrated Cholera Control in Haiti," [Commentary] *Lancet* 379 (2012), pp. 2026-8.

197. For more information, visit the course website (where all 2011 lectures are available for viewing) at http://globalhealthdelivery.org/ghd-academic-offerings/case-studies-in-global-health-biosocial-perspectives/. Accessed June 1, 2012.

198. Partners In Health, "Global Health Delivery Fellows Honored for Accomplishments and Leadership," March 30, 2010, at http://www.pih.org/news/entry/global-health-delivery-fellows-honored-for-accompishments-and-leadersh/. Accessed June 1, 2012.

199. Joia Mukherjee, MD, MPH, quoted in idem, http://www.pih.org/news/entry/global-health-delivery-fellows-honored-for-accompishments-and-leadersh/. Accessed June 1, 2012.

200. For the Hatch Scholars Program as DGHE's "main source of financial support for its physicians working abroad in poor countries and here at home," see http://www.brighamandwomens.org/Departments_and_Services/medicine/services/socialmedicine/giving_hatch.aspx. Accessed June 1, 2012.

201. "A lasting legacy in medical education: Katz chosen as first incumbent of Wolf Chair in Medicine," *BWH Bulletin*, November 10, 2006, http://www.brighamandwomens.org/about_bwh/publicaffairs/news/publications/DisplayBulletin.aspx?articleid=3519. Accessed June 1, 2012.

202. Brigham and Women's Hospital, "What Can One Person Do? Doris and Howard Hiatt Residency in Global Health Equity," n.p. (but on p. 1), http://www.brighamandwomens.org/Departments_and_Services/medicine/services/socialmedicine/residency/Residency.pdf. Accessed June 1, 2012.

203. Paul Farmer, video interview by Peter Tishler. BWH History Videos: The Brightest and the Best. http://brw.sites.vm2.broadcastmed.net/videos/paul_farmer_mdphd. Last updated July 2013.

204. BWH, "What can one person do?"

205. Paul Farmer, "Division of Global Health Equity," Brigham and Women's Hospital Department of Medicine *Annual Report*, 2011.

206. On Kazakhstan, see, e.g., Salmaan Keshavjee, "Bleeding Babies in Badakhshan," *Medican Anthropology Quarterly* 20/1 (March 2006), pp. 72-93.

207. Phyllis Jen, quoted in *BWH Clinical and Research News*, "Volunteer opportunities available with Indian Health Service," August 1, 2008, http://www.brighamandwomens.org/about_bwh/publicaffairs/news/publications/DisplayCRN.aspx?issueDate=8/1/2008%2012:00:00%20AM. Accessed June 1, 2012.

208. Amy Judd, personal communication, July 11, 2012.

209. T. Yazzie, A. Long, M.-G. Begay, S. Cisco, H. Sehn, S. Shin, and C. Harry, on behalf of the Gallup and Shiprock Navajo Nation CHR Programs, "Community Outreach and Empowerment: Collaboration with Navajo Nation CHRs," *J Ambulat Care Manage* 34/3 (2011), p. 289.

210. Jim Yong Kim, "A proposal for the Global Health Delivery Program at Harvard University," draft, January 2008, unpublished document, p. 4. For the details in this section, I especially thank Keri Wachter, GHD Program Manager, and Julie Talbot, GHD Publications and Curriculum Development Manager. My profound thanks as well to Rebecca Weintraub, GHD executive director, for generously permitting me to participate in the 2012 Faculty Network Workshop.

211. That is, health outcomes achieved per unit of cost expended. For more on the concept of "value-based health care delivery," see, e.g., Michael E. Porter, "Value-based health care delivery," presented at the American Psychiatric Association on May 8, 2012, http://www.isc.hbs.edu/pdf/2012%205%208_EMS_APA%20Deck%20(for%20May%208th)_final.pdf; see also the GHD brief definition at http://globalhealthdelivery.org/2012/05/value-based-health-care-delivery/. Accessed June 1, 2012.

212. For more information see http://www.ghdonline.org/cases.

213. Heidi Behforouz, interview, March 27, 2012.

214. Karen Weintraub, "Personal approach to HIV," [interview with Heidi Behforouz] *The Boston Globe*, October 3, 2011. http://articles.boston.com/2011-10-03/lifestyle/30239007_1_community-health-aids-patients-hiv. Accessed June 1, 2012.

BIBLIOGRAPHY

Archival Sources

Brigham and Women's Hospital Archives in the Francis A. Countway Library of Medicine. (Includes the archives of the Boston Lying-In Hospital, the Free Hospital for Women, the Peter Bent Brigham Hospital, the Robert Breck Brigham Hospital, the Boston Hospital for Women, the Associated Hospitals Center, and Brigham and Women's Hospital.)

Faulkner Hospital Archives. Brigham and Women's Faulkner Hospital.

Henry A. Christian papers, Harvard Medical Library in the Francis A. Countway Library of Medicine.

Peter Bent Brigham Hospital School of Nursing Papers, Nursing Archives, Boston University Mugar Memorial Library.

Published and Other Sources

"1993 Banner Year for Research." *BWH*, June 7, 1994, p. 20.

A Short History of Faulkner Hospital. Boston: Faulkner Hospital, 1970.

Abrahm, Janet L. "Waiting for the Platelet Count to Rise: Negotiating Care at the End of life." *Cancer Investigation* 21, no. 5 (2003): 772–781.

Adams, Annmarie. *Medicine by Design: The Architect and the Modern Hospital, 1893-1943*. Minneapolis: University of Minnesota Press, 2008.

Addison, Thomas. *On the Constitutional and Local Effects of Disease of the Suprarenal Capsules*. London: Samuel Higley, 1855.

Affiliated Hospitals Center. "News." *Inside AHC*, June 1978, p. 11.

Ahrens, Edward H., Jr. "The Birth of Patient-Oriented Research as a Science (1911)." *Perspectives in Biology and Medicine* 38, no. 4 (1995): 548.

Alumnae Journal. Peter Bent Brigham Hospital School of Nursing. Boston: Alumnae Association of the School of Nursing, Peter Bent Brigham Hospital, 1924–1932.

American Academy of Hospice and Palliative Medicine, 2006. "Statement on Clinical Practice Guidelines for Quality Palliative Care." Accessed July 11, 2013. http:www.aahpm.org/positionsquality.html.

American College of Nurse Midwives. "A Brief History of Nurse Midwifery in the U.S." Accessed December 13, 2012. http://69.63.143.222/A-Brief-History-of-Nurse-Midwifery-in-the-U-S.

American College of Nurse-Midwives. "Differences between Nurse-Midwives, Other Midwives, and Doulas." *American College of Nurse Midwives* website. Accessed December 13, 2012. http://www.mymidwife.org/Differences-Between-Nurse-Midwives-Other-Midwives-and-Doulas.

American Hospital Association. "Chartbook: Trends Affecting Hospitals and Health Systems," 2011. Accessed April 14, 2012. www.aha.org/research/reports/tw/chartbook/index.shtml.

Anderson, Nancy. "A History of the Robert Breck Brigham Hospital." Unpublished manuscript, 1988. Typescript.

Annual Report. Affiliated Hospitals Center. Boston: The Center, 1977–1979.

Annual Report. Brigham and Women's Hospital. Boston: Brigham and Women's Hospital, 1980.

Annual Report. Faulkner Hospital. Boston: Faulkner Hospital, 1903–1970.

Annual Report of the Peter Bent Brigham Hospital, 1915–1976. Publisher varies. Cambridge, MA: The University Press, 1913–1923; Boston: Wright and Potter, 1924–1925; Cambridge, MA: The University Press, 1926.

Anversa, Piero, Jan Kajstura, Annarosa Leri, and Joseph Loscalzo. "Tissue-Specific Adult Stem Cells in the Human Lung," *Nature Medicine* 17 (2011): 1038–1039.

Apfel, Roberta J., and Susan M. Fisher. *To Do No Harm: DES and the Dilemmas of Modern Medicine*. New Haven, CT: Yale University Press, 1984.

Association of American Medical Colleges. AspiringDocs.org: An AAMC Campaign to Increase Diversity in Medicine. "America Needs a More Diverse Physician Workforce." Accessed June 15, 2012. https://www.aamc.org/download/87306/data/physiciandiversityfacts.pdf.

Austen, K. Frank, and Walter E. Brocklehurst. "Anaphylaxis in Chopped Guinea Pig Lung III. Effect of Carbon Monoxide, Cyanide, Salicylaldoxime, and

Ionic Strength." *Journal of Experimental Medicine* 114, no. 1 (1961): 29–42.

Ayres, James, and Manli Ho. "Streets Calm as State, MDC Police Move In." *Boston Globe,* Oct. 11, 1974.

Baker, Jeffrey P. *The Machine in the Nursery: Incubator Technology and the Origins of Newborn Intensive Care.* Baltimore: Johns Hopkins University Press, 1996.

Banks, Henry H. "Orthopaedic Surgery at the Peter Bent Brigham Hospital 1913-1970." Osgood Lecture, Massachusetts General Hospital, May 21, 1983.

Banks, Henry H. "Memoirs." Unpublished manuscript.

___, interview with James H. Herndon, July 14, 2009.

Barr, Sarah. "Mass. Nurse-Midwives No Longer Need Physician OK to Practice," *Capsules: The Kaiser Health News Blog,* February 9, 2012. Accessed December 14, 2012. http://capsules.kaiserhealthnews.org/index.php/2012/02/mass-nurse-midwives-no-longer-need-physician-ok-to-practice/.

Barrett, Nora A., Opu M. Rahman, James M. Fernandez, Matthew W. Parsons, Wei Xing, K. Frank Austen, and Yoshihide Kanaoka. "Dectin-2 Mediates Th2 immunity through the Generation of Cysteinyl Leukotrienes." *Journal of Experimental Medicine* 208, no. 3 (2011): 593–604.

Beecher, Henry K., and Mark D. Altschule. *Medicine at Harvard: The First 300 Years.* Hanover, NH: University Press of New England, 1977.

Benedict, E.B., Lloyd E. Hawes, Charles R. Stewart, John W. Spellman, and William F. Walsh. "Corsage Pin in Stomach." *Journal of the American Medical Association* 175 (1961): 48.

Benner, Patricia, Patricia Hooper-Kyriakidis, and Daphne Stannard. *Clinical Wisdom and Interventions in Acute and Critical Care: A Thinking-in-Action Approach.* New York: Springer Publishing Company, 2011.

Bhengu, Busisiwe R., Busisiwe P. Ncama, Patricia A. McInerney, Dean J. Wantland, Patrice K. Nicholas, Inge B. Corless, Chris A. McGibbon, Sheila M. Davis, Thomas P. Nicholas, and Ana Viamonte Ros. "Symptoms experienced by HIV-infected individuals on antiretroviral therapy in Kwazulu-Natal, South Africa." *Applied Nursing Research* 24, no. 1 (2011): 1–9.

Black, Peter McL., Matthew R. Moore, and Eugene Rossitch, Jr., eds. *Harvey Cushing at the Brigham.* Park Ridge, IL: American Association of Neurological Surgeons, 1993.

Black, Peter McL., Thomas Moriarty, Eben Alexander III, Philip Stieg, Eric J. Woodard, P. Langham Gleason, Claudia H. Martin, Ron Kikinis, Richard B. Schwartz, and Ferenc A. Jolesz. "Development and Implementation of Intraoperative Magnetic Resonance Imaging and its Neurosurgical Applications." *Neurosurgery* 41, no. 4 (1997): 831–845.

"Blanza Honored with Essence of Nursing Award." *BWH Nurse,* March/April/May 2012: 1.

Bliss, Michael. *Harvey Cushing: A Life in Surgery.* New York: Oxford University Press, 2005.

___. *William Osler: A Life in Medicine.* New York: Oxford University Press, 1999.

___, William B. Castle, James H. Means, and George W. Thorn. "Henry Asbury Christian." *Harvard University Gazette* XLVII (January 19, 1952): 117–118.

Blumenthal, David. "Employer-Sponsored Health Insurance in the United States – Origins and Implications." *New England Journal of Medicine* 355 (2006): 82–88.

Blumgart, Herman L., William B. Castle, J.H. Means, and George W. Thorn. "Memorial Minute." *Harvard University Gazette,* January 19, 1952.

Bolli, Roberto, Atul R. Chugh, Domenico D'Amario, John H. Loughran, Marcus F Stoddard, Sohail Ikram, Garth M Beache et al. "Cardiac Stem Cells in Patients with Ischaemic Cardiomyopathy (SCIPIO): Initial Results of a Randomised Phase 1 Trial." *Lancet* 378(2011): 1847–1857.

Bonner, Thomas Neville. *Iconoclast: Abraham Flexner and a Life in Learning.* Baltimore: Johns Hopkins University Press, 2002.

Bosk, Charles L. *Forgive and Remember: Managing Medical Failure.* Chicago: University of Chicago Press, 1979.

"Boston Comes to Faulkner." Boston: Faulkner Hospital, 1931.

The Boston Herald, August 5, 1911.

___, August 13, 1912: 1.

Boston Redevelopment Authority. "Briefing Book: Demographic Profile of the Foreign-Born in Boston, Boston Redevelopment Authority." Accessed July 7, 2012. http://www.cityofboston.gov/Images_Documents/BRA%20Briefing%20Book%20Demographic_tcm3-16615.pdf.

"Boston Teaching Hospitals' Response to the Kane Report." *Health Affairs* 12, no. 3 (1993): 234-237.

Brandt, Allan. *The Cigarette Century: The Rise, Fall, and Deadly Persistence of the Product That Defined America.* New York: Basic Books, 2007.

Brenner, Barry M. "In Memoriam Ramzi S. Cotran: December 7, 1932-October 23, 2000." *Journal of the American Society of Nephrology* 12, no. 4 (2001): 635.

Brigham and Women's Hospital. "About the Friends of BWH." Accessed July 17, 2012. http://www.brighamandwomens.org/about_bwh/friendsofBWH/AboutUs.aspx.

___. "Center for Health Equity and Health Education Birth Equity Initiative." Accessed July 7, 2012. http://www.brighamandwomens.org/about_bwh/communityprograms/our-programs/health-equity/birth-equity.aspx.

___. "Center for Faculty Development and Diversity 5th Year Report." Accessed May 22, 2012. http://www.brighamandwomens.org/Medical_Professionals/career/CFDD/5YearReport.aspx.

___. "Midwifery Practice: Location." Accessed December 13, 2012. http://www.brighamandwomens.org/Departments_and_Services/obgyn/Services/midwifery/mission.aspx?sub=0.

___, "Southern Jamaica Plain Health Center Mission and History." Accessed May 29, 2012. http://www.brighamandwomens.org/Departments_and_Services/medicine/services/primarycare/sjphc/SJPHC_mishis.aspx.

___. "The History of Brookside." Accessed June 20, 2012. http://www.brighamandwomens.org/Departments_and_Services/medicine/services/primarycare/brookside_history.aspx.

___, "Your Rights as a Patient." Accessed July 3, 2012. http://www.brighamandwomens.org/Patients_Visitors/patientresources/RightsPatient.aspx.

"Brigham People: Gabriel Spagnoulo." *Brigham Bulletin* II, November 1951: 2.

Brooks, David, interview with Ann Conway, May 18, 2012.

Brown, Esther Lucile. *Newer Dimensions of Patient Care, Part 3: Patients as People*. New York: Russell Sage Foundation, 1964.

___. *Nursing for the Future*. New York: Russell Sage Foundation, 1948.

Buhler-Wilkerson, Karen. *No Place Like Home: A History of Nursing and Home Care in the United States*. Baltimore: Johns Hopkins University Press, 2001.

Buresh, Bernice, and Suzanne Gordon. *From Silence to Voice: What Nurses Know and Must Communicate to the Public*. Ithaca: Cornell University Press, 2006.

Burgess, May Ayres. *Nurses, Patients, and Pocketbooks.* New York: National League of Nursing Education, 1928.

Burke, Martha Byron, interview with Ann Conway, August 14, 2012.

___. "BWH Social Work." PowerPoint presentation provided August 2012.

BWH Bulletin: For and About the People of Brigham and Women's Hospital. Archives 1999-2013. http://www.brighamandwomens.org/about_bwh/publicaffairs/news/publications/BulletinArchives.aspx.

___."A Lasting Legacy in Medical Education: Katz Chosen as First Incumbent of Wolf Chair in Medicine." November 10, 2006. Accessed June 1, 2012. http://www.brighamandwomens.org/about_bwh/publicaffairs/news/publications/DisplayBulletin.aspx?articleid=3519.

___. "Black History Month Continues." February 18, 2000. Accessed November 8, 2012. http://www.brighamandwomens.org/about_bwh/publicaffairs/news/publications/DisplayBulletin.aspx?articleid=92.

___. "BWH to Double Daycare Slots." February 18, 2000. Accessed July 10, 2013. http://www.brighamandwomens.org/about_bwh/publicaffairs/news/publications/DisplayBulletin.aspx?articleid=59.

___. "The BWH Strategic Plan." November 30, 2001. Accessed November 8. 2012. http://www.brighamandwomens.org/about_bwh/publicaffairs/news/publications/DisplayBulletin.aspx?issueDate=11/30/2001%2012:00:00%20AM.

___. "Bright Horizons Center Dedicated." November 30, 2000. Accessed November 8, 2012. http://www.brighamandwomens.org/about_bwh/publicaffairs/news/publications/DisplayBulletin.aspx?issueDate=11/30/2000%2012:00:00%20AM.

___. "Calling for Thompson Compassionate Leadership Award Nominations." January 15, 2010. Accessed December 7, 2012. http://www.brighamandwomens.org/about_bwh/publicaffairs/news/publications/DisplayBulletin.aspx?articleid=4739.

___. "CFDD Summer Programs Shape Young Researchers' Futures." August 18, 2011. Accessed July 10, 2013. http://www.brighamandwomens.org/about_bwh/publicaffairs/news/publications/DisplayBulletin.aspx?articleid=5323.

___. "Domestic Violence Addressed." October 13, 2000. Accessed November 8, 2012. http://www.brighamandwomens.org/about_bwh/publicaffairs/news/publications/DisplayBulletin.aspx?articleid=1076.

___. "Figuring Out a Year Gone By." December 21, 2001. Accessed July 10, 2013. http://www.brighamandwomens.org/about_bwh/publicaffairs/news/publications/DisplayBulletin.aspx?articleid=1619.

___. "Growing DF/BWCC Provides Seamless Patient Care." June 2, 2006. Accessed December 7, 2012. http://www.brighamandwomens.org/about_bwh/publicaffairs/news/publications/DisplayBulletin.aspx?articleid=2764.

___. "Hispanic Heritage Event at SJPHC." September 22, 2000. Accessed November 8, 2012. http://www.brighamandwomens.org/about_bwh/publicaffairs/news/publications/DisplayBulletin.aspx?articleid=1060&issueDate=9/22/2000%2012:00:00%20AM.

___. "Medical Home Opens on South Huntington." September 23, 2011. Accessed October 20, 2011. http://www.brighamandwomens.org/about_bwh/publicaffairs/news/publications/DisplayBulletin.aspx?issueDate=9/23/2011%2012:00:00%20AM.

___. "Nabel Outlines BW/F Strategic Planning Recommendations." December 13, 2011. Accessed

December 7, 2012. http://www.brighamandwomens.org/about_bwh/publicaffairs/news/publications/DisplayBulletin.aspx?issueDate=12/13/2011%20 12:00:00%20AM.

———. "New Buildings Part of Plan to Meet Space Challenges." November 17, 2000. Accessed November 8, 2012. http://www.brighamandwomens.org/about_bwh/publicaffairs/news/publications/DisplayBulletin.aspx?issueDate=11/17/2000%2012:00:00%20AM.

———. "Obituary: Kenneth John Ryan, MD, 75." *BWH Bulletin*, January 11, 2002. Accessed September 4, 2012. http://www.brighamandwomens.org/about_bwh/publicaffairs/news/publications/DisplayBulletin.aspx?articleid=1633.

———. "Survey Follow-up Continues." November 10, 2000. Accessed November 8, 2012. http://www.brighamandwomens.org/about_bwh/publicaffairs/news/publications/DisplayBulletin.aspx?issueDate=11/10/2000%2012:00:00%20AM.

———. "A Taste of Diversity at BWH." September 18, 2000. Accessed November 8, 2012. http://www.brighamandwomens.org/about_bwh/publicaffairs/news/publications/DisplayBulletin.aspx?articleid=1042.

Cabot, Richard C. "Pernicious and Secondary Anemia, Chlorosis and Leukemia." *Modern Medicine: Its Theory and Practice*, vol IV. Philadelphia: Lea & Febiger, 1908, 612–639.

Caligtan, Christine A., Diane L. Carroll, Ann C. Hurley, Ronna Gersh-Zaremski, and Patricia C. Dykes. "Bedside Information Technology to Support Patient-Centered Care." *International Journal of Medical Informatics*, 2012: 442.

Cappers, Elmer Osgood. *A History of the Free Hospital for Women 1875-1975*. Boston: Free Hospital for Women, 1975.

"Cases." *Boston Medical and Surgical Journal*, CLXIII (1910): 390.

Castle, William B. "The Conquest of Pernicious Anemia." In *Blood, Pure and Eloquent: A Story of Discovery, of People, and of Ideas*. Edited by Maxwell Wintrobe. New York: McGraw Hill, 1980.

Center for Community Health and Health Equity, Brigham and Women's Hospital. "Health Equity Research and Intervention." Accessed May 15, 2012. http://www.brighamandwomens.org/about_bwh/communityprograms/our-programs/research.aspx?sub=0.

Center for Community Health and Health Equity, Brigham and Women's Hospital. "Violence Intervention and Prevention Programs." Accessed May 15, 2012. http://www.brighamandwomens.org/about_bwh/communityprograms/our-programs/violence/default.aspx?sub=0.

Centers for Disease Control and Prevention. "Number, Rate and Average Length of Stay for Discharges from Short-Stay Hospitals by Age, Region, and Sex: United States, 2009." National Hospital Discharge Survey, Selected Tables, 2009. Accessed April 14, 2012. www.cdc.gov/nchs/nhds/nhds_products.htm.

Cheever, David. "Peter Bent Brigham Hospital 40th Anniversary: Teaching." *Brigham Bulletin*, vol 3, no. 2 (1953).

Christakis, Nicholas A. *Death Foretold: Prophecy and Prognosis in Medical Care*. Chicago: University of Chicago Press, 1999.

Chunara, Rumi, Jason R. Andrews, and John S. Brownstein. "Social and News Media Enable Estimation of Epidemiological Patterns Early in the 2010 Haitian Cholera Outbreak." *American Journal of Tropical Medicine and Hygiene* 86 (2012): 39-45.

Clauss, Roy H., William Clifford Birtwell, George Albertal, Steven Lunzer, Warren J. Taylor, Anna M. Forsberg, and Dwight E. Harken. "Assisted Circulation. I. The Arterial Counterpulsator." *Journal of Thoracic and Cardiovascular Surgery* 41 (1961): 447–458.

Cohen, Jules, and Stephanie Brown Clark. *John Romano and George Engel: Their Lives and Work*. Rochester, NY: Meliora Press/University of Rochester Press, 2010.

Cohn, Lawrence H., David H. Adams, Gregory S., Sary F. Aranki, David P. Bichell, Donna M. Rosborough, and Samuel P. Sears, "Minimally Invasive Cardiac Valve Surgery Improves Patient Satisfaction while Reducing Costs of Cardiac Valve Replacement and Repair," *Annals of Surgery* 226, no. 4 (October 1997): 421–428.

Cohn, Lawrence H., Richard Gorlin, Michael V. Herman, and John J. Collins Jr., "Surgical Treatment of Acute Coronary Occlusion," *Journal of Thoracic and Cardiovascuar Surgery* 64 (1972): 503–513.

Collins, Christine, interview with Ann Conway, April 9, 2012.

Committee on the Grading of Nursing Schools. "Nurses' Production, Education, Distribution, and Pay." New York: National League of Nursing Education, 1930.

"Community Health Services Report." Boston: Brigham and Women's Hospital, 1993.

Connor, Edward M., Rhoda S. Sperling, Richard Gelber, Pavel Kiselev, Gwendolyn Scott, Mary Jo O'Sullivan, Russell Van Dyke et al. For the Pediatric AIDS Clinical Trials Group Protocol 076 Study Group, "Reduction of Maternal-Infant Transmission of Human Immunodeficiency Virus Type 1 with Zidovudine Treatment." *New England Journal of Medicine* 331(1994): 1173–1180.

Conner, V.W., and G. Kutsuflakis. "Putting Supplies at the Bedside via the Friesen Concept." *Hospital Materials Management Quarterly* 16 (1994): 35–40.

Constan, Ted and Joia Mukherjee, "Note to the Reader." *Partners In Health Program Management Guide* (Boston: PIH, 2011), p. viii, online at http://www.pih.org/pmg, accessed June 1, 2012

Conway, Ann. "Organizational Symbolism in the Peter Bent Brigham Hospital 1913-1938: A Cultural History." PhD diss, Brandeis University, 1992.

___."A History of the Robert Breck Brigham Hospital." Unpublished manuscript, 1993.

Corless, Inge B., Dean Wantland, Busi Bhengu, Patricia McInerney, Busi Ncama, Patrice K. Nicholas, Chris McGibbon, Emily Wong, and Sheila M. Davis. "HIV and Tuberculosis in Durban, South Africa: Adherence to Two Medication Regimens." *AIDS Care* 21, no. 9 (2009): 1106–1113.

Corner, George Washington. *George Hoyt Whipple and His Friends: The Life-Story of a Nobel Prize Pathologist*. Philadelphia: J.B. Lippincott, 1963.

Cotton, Edward H. *The Life of Charles W. Eliot*. Boston: Small, Maynard and Company, 1926.

Creager, Angela. " 'What Blood Told Dr Cohn': World War II, Plasma Fractionation, and the Growth of Human Blood Research." *Studies in History and Philosophy of Science Part C: Studies in History and Philosophy of Biological and Biomedical Sciences* 30, no. 3 (1999): 377–405.

Crosby, Ranice W. and John Cody, *Max Brödel: The Man Who Put Art into Medicine*. Berlin: Springer-Verlag, 1991.

Cushing, Harvey. *The Story of U.S. Army Base Hospital No.5, by a Member of the Unit*. Cambridge, MA: The University Press, 1919.

___."The Personality of a Hospital." *Boston Medical and Surgical Journal* 185, no. 18 (1921): 529–53.

___."W.T. Councilman." *Science* 77 (1930): 613–18.

___and J.R.B. Branch. "Experimental and Clinical Notes on Chronic Valvular Lesions in the Dog and their Possible Relation to a Future Surgery of the Cardiac Valves." *Journal of Medical Research* 17 (1908):471–486.

Cutler, Elliott. "War Diary." U.S. Army Medical Dept. Office of Medical History. Accessed July 7, 2012. http://history.amedd.army.mil/booksdocs/wwii/actvssurgconvol2/chapter2.1.htm.

Dai, Guohao, Mohammad R. Kaazempur-Mofrad, Sripriya Natarajan, Yuzhi Zhang, Saran Vaughn, Brett R. Blackman, Roger D. Kamm, Guillermo García-Cardeña, and Michael A. Gimbrone. "Distinct Endothelial Phenotypes Evoked by Arterial Waveforms Derived from Atherosclerosis-Susceptible and -Resistant Regions of Human Vasculature." *Proceedings of the National Academy of Sciences of the United States of America* 101, no. 41 (2004): 14871–14876.

Danforth, William H. "A New Flexner Report?" *Journal of the American Medical Association* 209, no. 6 (1969): 930–931.

D'Antonio, Patricia. *American Nursing: A History of Knowledge, Authority, and the Meaning of Work*. Baltimore: Johns Hopkins University Press, 2010.

Day, Hughes W. "An Intensive Coronary Care Area." *Chest* 44 (1963): 423–427.

Debono, David J. "Integration of Palliative Medicine into Routine Oncological Care: What Does the Evidence Show Us?" *Journal of Oncology Practice* 7, no. 6 (2011): 350–354.

DeJohn, Kristin. "Tapping Potential." *BWH Profiles in Medicine: Marshall Wolf, MD,* Spring 2011, 18–25.

De Kruif, Paul. *Men Against Death*. New York: Harcourt, Brace and Co., 1932.

Department of Obstetrics and Gynecology, Brigham, and Women's Hospital. *Annual Reports* 1997-2011.

Dibardino, Daniel J., Andrew W. Elbardissi, R. Scott McClure, Ozwaldo A. Razo-Vasquez, Nicole E. Kelly, and Lawrence H. Cohn. "Four Decades of Experience with Mitral Valve Repair: Analysis of Differential Indications, Technical, Evolution and Long-term Outcomes." *Journal of Thoracic and Cardiovascular Surgery* 139 (2010): 76–84.

DiMaggio, Paul. "Cultural Entrepreneurship in Nineteenth-Century Boston." *Medicine, Culture and Society* 4 (1982): 33–50.

Diner, Hasia. *Erin's Daughters in America*. Baltimore: Johns Hopkins University Press, 1983.

Dinneen, Joseph F. "The Hospital Orderly They Call 'Doctor.'" *Collier's Weekly,* December 1, 1951: 27–51.

"Discovery and Innovation: Working Together to Provide Superior Healthcare." *Brigham and Women's/Faulkner Strategic Planning Report*. Boston: Brigham and Women's Hospital, 2012.

"Division of Social Medicine and Health Inequalities." *BWH Clinical & Research News*, October 31, 2001. Accessed June 1, 2012. http://www.brighamandwomens.org/about_bwh/publicaffairs/news/publications/DisplayCRN.aspx?articleid=120.

Donahue, M. Patricia. *Nursing: The Finest Art*. 3rd ed. Maryland Heights, Missouri: Mosby, 2011.

Doyne, Dermot, interview with Ann Conway, June 19, 2012.

"Dr. James Warth Discovers New Cell." *Dear Doctor*, December 15, 1995.

"Dr. Theodore Potter, 83. Taught, Practiced Orthopedics," *Boston Globe*, December 11, 1995: 25.

Drazen, Jeffrey M. "Presentation of the 2004 Kober Medal to K. Frank Austen." *Journal of Clinical Investigation* 114, no. 8 (2004): 1174–1176.

Dykes, Patricia C., Diane L. Carroll, Ann Hurley, Stuart Lipsitz, Angela Benoit, Frank Chang, Seth Meltzer, Ruslana Tsurikova, Lyubov Zuyov, and Blackford Middleton. "Fall Prevention in Acute Care Hospitals." *Journal of the American Medical Association* 304, no. 17 (2010): 1912–1918.

Dykes, Patricia C., Diane L. Carroll, Kerry McColgan, Ann C. Hurley, Stuart R. Lipsitz, Lisa Colombo, Lyubov Zuyev, and Blackford Middleton. "Scales for Assessing Self Efficacy of Nurses and Assistants for Preventing Falls," *Journal of Advanced Nursing* 67, no. 2 (2011): 438–449.

Dzau, Victor, video interview by Peter Tishler. BWH History Videos: The Brightest and the Best. http://brw.sites.vm2.broadcastmed.net/videos/victor-dzau-md. Last updated July 2013.

Easterday, Charles L., John F. Enders, John F. Jewett, Kenneth J. Ryan, George Van S. Smith, Howard Ulfelder, and Arthur T. Hertig. "Duncan Earl Reid. Memorial Minute Adopted by the Faculty of Medicine of Harvard University," February 22, 1974. *Harvard University Gazette* LXIX #29, 1974.

Egan, Shirley, interview with Marilyn King, July 1, 1985.

Ehrlich, Paul. "Ueber regeneration und degeneration rother blutscheiben bei anamien." *Berlin Klin Wochenschr* 28 (1880): 405.

Epstein, Steven. *Inclusion: The Politics of Difference in Medical Research*. Chicago: University of Chicago Press, 2007.

"The Essence of Nursing." *BWH Nurse*, March/April/May, 2011: 6.

Evaluation Studies. *USCF Center for Excellence in Primary Care* (Nov. 2010). Accessed October 20, 2011. http://www.pcpcc.net/files/evidence_outcomes_in_pcmh.pdf.

Evans, Linda A. "A Historical, Clinical, and Ethical Overview of the Emerging Science of Facial Transplantation." *Plastic Surgical Nursing* 31, no. 4 (2011): 151.

Fairman, Julie, and Joan E. Lynaugh. *Critical Care Nursing: A History*. Philadelphia: University of Pennsylvania Press, 2000.

___*Making Room in the Clinic: Nurse Practitioners and the Evolution of Modern Health Care*. New Brunswick, NJ: Rutgers University Press, 2009.

FAMILY (Fathers and Mothers Infants, eLders and Youth). "FAMILY History." Accessed July 12, 2013. http://www.familysystem.net/history.html.

___ "Society's Healing Charter – The FAMILY Worldview." Accessed July 13, 2013. http://www.familysystem.net/our_worldview.html.

Farmer, Paul. *Haiti after the Earthquake*. New York: Public Affairs, 2011.

Farmer, Paul. "Division of Global Health Equity." Brigham and Women's Hospital Department of Medicine *Annual Report*, 2011.

___, video interview by Peter Tishler. BWH History Videos: The Brightest and the Best. http://brw.sites.vm2.broadcastmed.net/videos/paul-farmer-md-phd. Last updated July 2013.

Farmer, Paul, Fernet Léandre, Joia S Mukherjee, Marie Sidonise Claude, Patrice Nevil, Mary C Smith-Fawzi, Serena P Koenig et al. "Community-Based Approaches to HIV Treatment in Resource-Poor Settings." *Lancet* 358 (2001): 404–409.

Finland, Maxwell and William B. Castle, eds. *The Harvard Medical Unit at Boston City Hospital*. Boston: Francis A. Countway Library of Medicine, 1983.

"The First Floor of the New Faulkner," *Faulkner Herald*, April 1974: 6.

Fisher, Jill A. *Medical Research for Hire: The Political Economy of Pharmaceutical Clinical Trials*. New Brunswick, NJ: Rutgers University Press, 2009.

Fisher, Mary Collier, interview with Ann Conway, May 4, 2012.

Fitz, Reginald. *At the Heart of a Great Medical Center 1913-1938*. Boston: Peter Bent Brigham Hospital, 1938.

Flexner, Abraham. *Medical Education in the United States and Canada: A Report to the Carnegie Foundation for the Advancement of Teaching*. Bulletin No. 4. New York: Carnegie Foundation for the Advancement of Teaching, 1910.

Fox, Renee. *Experiment Perilous: Physicians and Patients Facing the Unknown*. Glencoe, IL: The Free Press, 1959.

___. "From Dialysis, to Transplantation, to Palliative Care: A Trajectory." Presentation for the Care of the Renal Patient Towards the End of Life Conference. Royal Society of Medicine. October 14, 2009: 3. Accessed August 1, 2012. http://www.renal.org/pages/media/TsarFiles/EoL_141009_ReneeCFox.pdf.

Frigoletto, Fredric D., Jr., Leon Eisenberg, Steven Gabbe, Michael F. Greene, Rudolph Kass, Brian Little, Kenneth J. Ryan, Jr., Isaac Schiff, and Dennis Thompson. "Kenneth John Ryan. Faculty of Medicine—Memorial Minute." *Harvard Gazette*, October 28, 2004. Accessed September 4, 2012. http://www.news.harvard.edu/gazette/2004/10.28/27-mm.html.

Fulton, John F. *Harvey Cushing: A Biography*. Springfield, IL: Charles C. Thomas, 1946.

Furin, Jennifer Joan, Paul Farmer, Marshall Wolf, Bruce Levy, Amy Judd, Margaret Paternek, Rocio Hurtado, and Joel Katz. "A Novel Training Model to Address Health Problems in Poor and Underserved Populations." *Journal of Health Care for the Poor and Underserved* 17, no. 1 (2006): 17–24.

Gamm, Gerald. *Urban Exodus: Why the Jews Left Boston and the Catholics Stayed*. Chapter One: "Class, Crime, Homes, and Banks," *New York Times on the Web*. Accessed July 2, 2012. http://www.nytimes.com/books/first/g/gamm-exodus.html.

Garcia, Ileana, interview with Ann Conway, June 12, 2012.

"Getting the Message Across – More Quickly, More Quietly," *Transplant*, November 26, 1975: 1–2.

Gimbrone, Michael A., Ramzi S. Cotran, and Judah Folkman. "Human Vascular Endothelial Cells in

Culture Growth and DNA Synthesis." *Journal of Cell Biology* 60, no. 3 (1974): 673–684.

Glaser, Robert J. "Soma Weiss, M.D., posthumously Hersey Professor of the Theory and Practice of Medicine." Video interview with Drs. Paul B. Beeson, Richard V. Ebert, Jack D. Myers and Eugene A. Stead. http://www.alphaomegaalpha.org/leaders.html. Palo Alto: Alpha Omega Alpha, Video, 1994.

Gordon, Suzanne. *Life Support: Three Nurses on the Front Lines.* Ithaca, NY: ILR Press, an Imprint of Cornell University Press, 1997.

Gottlieb, Gary. "Improving Quality and Reducing Disparities at Partners Health Care: What We Know and What We Need to Know." PowerPoint Presentation.

Gregory, Katherine E. "Microbiome Aspects of Perinatal and Neonatal Health." *Journal of Perinatal and Neonatal Nursing* 25, no. 2 (2011): 158.

Gritzer, Glenn, and Arnold Arluke. *The Making of Rehabilitation: A Political Economy of Medical Specialization, 1890-1980.* California: University of California Press, 1985.

Groopman, Jerome E., and Michael Prichard. *How Doctors Think.* Boston, MA: Houghton Mifflin, 2007.

Groves, Anne, interview with Ann Conway, June 29, 2012.

Gruhn, John G., Hazel Gore, and Lawrence M. Roth. "History of Gynecological Pathology. IV. Dr. Arthur T. Hertig." *International Journal of Gynecological Pathology* 17, no. 2 (April 1998): 183–189.

Grumbach, Kevin, Thomas Bodenheimer, and Paul Grundy. "The Outcomes of Implementing Patient-Centered Medical Home Interventions: A Review of the Evidence on Quality, Access and Costs from Recent Prospective Evaluation Studies." Patient-Centered Primary Care Collaborative, Washington, D.C. Accessed July 27, 2009. www.pcpcc.net/files/pcmh_evidence_outcomes_2009.pdf.

Hall, Carrie. "The Teaching of Hospital Housekeeping to Pupil Nurses." In *Proceedings of the 21st Annual Convention of the National League of Nursing Education.* New York: National League of Nursing Education, 1915.

Handlin, Oscar. *Boston's Immigrants.* New York: Atheneum, 1969.

Harken, Dwight E., and Paul M. Zoll. "Foreign Bodies in and in Relation to the Thoracic Blood Vessels and Heart, III. Indications for the Removal of Intracardiac Foreign Bodies and the Behavior of the Heart During Manipulation." *American Heart Journal* 32 (1946): 1–19.

Harrington, Thomas Francis. *The Harvard Medical School: A History, Narrative and Documentary: 1782-1905.* Vol. 3. New York and Chicago: Lewis Publishing Company, 1905.

Harrison, Tinsley R. "Tribute to Dr. Levine," *New England Journal of Medicine* 275 (1966): 222-3.

Harvard Medical School Depatment of Global Health and Social Medicine. "History of the Department." Accessed June 1, 2012. http://ghsm.hms.harvard.edu/about/history/.

Harvard University. *Report of the President of Harvard College and Reports of Departments.* Cambridge, MA: Harvard University, 1973–1974.

Harvey, Abner McGehee. *Science at the Bedside: Clinical Research in American Medicine, 1905-1945.* Baltimore: Johns Hopkins University Press, 1981.

Hatcher, Charles. *All in the Timing: From Operating Room to Board Room.* Bloomington, IN: AuthorHouse, 2011.

Haynes, Walter, and David Richwine. "A Fourth Day of Turmoil in the City: 27 Injured in Roxbury Street Attacks," *Boston Globe,* Aug 14, 1975: 1.

"Health During Pregnancy." Boston: Boston Lying-in Hospital/Harvard School of Public Health, 1941.

The Henry J. Kaiser Family Foundation. "Medicare Spending and Financing, a Primer." Accessed April 14, 2012. www.kff.org/medicare/upload/7731-03.pdf.

Herbst, Arthur L., Howard Ulfelder, and David C. Poskanzer. "Adenocarcinoma of the Vagina: Association of Maternal Stilbestrol Therapy with Tumor Appearance in Young Women." *New England Journal of Medicine* 284, no. 15 (1971): 878–81.

Herndon, James H. " Chairman's Corner." *Orthopaedic Journal at Harvard Medical School* (1999, vol 1: pages 5-9; 2000, vol 2: 5-8; 2001, vol 3: 11-17; 2002, vol 4: 11-18; 2003, vol 5: 8-13).

Hertig, Arthur T. "Forty Years in the Female Pelvis: An Unusual Case of Prolonged Dystocia." *Obstetrics and Gynecology* 42 (1973): 907–909.

———. "Acceptance of the Gold Headed Cane Award." *American Journal of Pathology* 96 (1979): 368–371.

———. "Angiogenesis in the Early Human Chorion and in the Primary Placenta of the Macaque Monkey." *Contributions in Embryology* 25 (1935): 39–81.

———. *International Journal of Gynecological Pathology 17, no.2* (1998): 183–189.

———. Quoted in the *Harvard Medical Area Focus,* October 30, 1980: 6.

Hickey, Mairead, and Phyllis Beck Kritek. *Change Leadership in Nursing: How Change Occurs in a Complex Hospital System.* New York: Springer Publishing Company, 2011: 11–18.

Hine, Darlene Clark. *Black Women in White: Racial Conflict and Cooperation in the Nursing Profession, 1890-1950.* Bloomington: Indiana University Press, 1989.

Hodgdon, L. A. "Health of the District, West Roxbury," 1903. *Genealogical and Personal Memoirs Relating to the Families of the State of Massachusetts.* Edited by William Richard Cutter, William Frederick Adams. Vol. 2. Lewis Historical Publishing Company, 1910: 1118.

Hogan, Joanne, interview with Ann Conway, July 6, 2012.

Hollingsworth, William. *Taking Care: The Legacy of Soma Weiss, Eugene Stead, and Paul Beeson*. San Diego: Medical Education and Research Foundation, 1994.

"Hospitals at a Crossroads." *BWH,* November/December 1993: 16–17.

Howard Hughes Medical Foundation. "Development, 1954-1983." Accessed September 11, 2012. http://www.hhmi.org/about/development.html.

Howe, M. A. DeWolfe. *The Humane Society of the Commonwealth of Massachusetts: An Historical Review, 1795-1916*. Boston: Printed for the Humane Society, 1918.

Hui, David, Ahmed Elsayem, Maxine De La Cruz, Ann Berger, Donna S. Zhukovsky, Shana Palla, Avery Evans, Nada Fadul, J. Lynn Palmer, and Eduardo Bruera. "Availability and Integration of Palliative Care at US Cancer Centers." *Journal of the American Medical Association* 303, no. 11 (2010): 1054–1061.

Hume, David M. and John P. Merrill. "Homologous Transplantation of Human Kidneys." *Journal of Clinical Investigation* 31 (1952): 640.

Hume, David M., John P. Merrill, Benjamin F. Miller, and George W. Thorn. "Experiences with Renal Homotransplantation in the Human: Report of Nine Cases." *Journal of Clinical Investigation* 34, no. 2 (1955): 327.

Hurley, Ann C., Anne Bane, Sofronia Fotakis, Mary E. Duffy, Amanda Sevigny, Eric G. Poon, and Tejal K. Gandhi. "Nurses' Satisfaction with Medication Administration Point-of-Care Technology." *Journal of Nursing Administration* 37, no. 7/8 (2007): 343–349.

___and Ladislav Volicer. "Alzheimer Disease: 'It's okay, Mama, if you want to go, it's okay'" *JAMA: Journal of the American Medical Association* 288, no. 18 (2002): 2324–2331.

Institute of Medicine. *To Err Is Human: Building a Safer Health System*. Washington, DC: National Academies Press, 1999.

Irving, Frederick C. "Highlights in the History of the Boston Lying-In Hospital." *Canadian Medical Association Journal* 54, no. 2 (1946): 174.

___*Safe Deliverance*. Boston: Houghton Mifflin, 1942.

Ivers, Louise C. and David A. Walton, "The 'First' Case of Cholera in Haiti: Lessons for Global Health." *American Journal of Tropical Medicine and Hygiene* 86 (2012): 36-8.

Ivers, Louise C., Paul E. Farmer, and William J. Pape. "Oral Cholera Vaccine and Integrated Cholera Control in Haiti." [Commentary] *Lancet* 379 (2012): 2026-2028.

Jessiman, Andrew G. "The Brigham and the Community." *Brigham Bulletin*, February 1975: 6–10.

___ interview with Ann Conway, June 13, 2012.

Jewett, John Figgis. "Sesquicentennium of the Boston Lying-in Hospital—150 trailblazing years." In *Contemporary OB/GYN*. New Jersey: Medical Economics Company, Inc. May, 1983: 198–206.

"Joel Ernest Goldthwait, 1866-1961." *Journal of Bone and Joint Surgery* 43, no. 3 (April 1961): 463–464.

John Hopkins University School of Medicine. "Art as Applied to Medicine." Accessed August 8, 2012. http://www.hopkinsmedicine.org/about/history/history7.html.

Johnson, Sally. "The Arrangement of Subjects Taught in the School of Nursing of the Peter Bent Brigham Hospital." In *Proceedings of the 20th Annual Convention of the National League of Nursing Education*. New York: National League of Nursing Education, 1914.

Jolesz, Ferenc A. "1996 RSNA Eugene P. Pendergrass New Horizons Lecture. Image-Guided Procedures and the Operating Room of the Future." *Radiology* 204, no. 3 (1997): 601–612.

___and Peter D. Jakab. "Acoustic Pressure Wave Generation within an MR Imaging System: Potential Medical Applications." *Journal of Magnetic Resonance Imaging* 1, no. 5 (2005): 609–613.

___. Alan R. Bleier, Peter D. Jakab, Paul W. Ruenzel, Kalman Huttl, and Geza J. Jako. "MR Imaging of Laser-Tissue Interactions." *Radiology* 168, no. 1 (1988): 249–253.

Jones, Arthur. "Groundbreaking Protested," *Boston Globe,* December 21, 1975: 2.

Joseph, Marc. "It 'Takes A Village' To Fix Our Education System." *International Business Times*. Accessed August 3, 2012. http://www.ibtimes.com/articles/370211/20120803/education-reform-policy-federal-funding-aid.htm.

Joynt, Robert J. "John Romano, MD, November 20, 1908, to June 19, 1995." *Archives of General Psychiatry* 52, no. 12 (1995): 1076.

Kanaoka, Yoshihide, Akiko Maekawa, John F. Penrose, K. Frank Austen, and Bing K. Lam. "Attenuated Zymosan-induced Peritoneal Vascular Permeability and IgE-dependent Passive Cutaneous Anaphylaxis in Mice Lacking Leukotriene C4 Synthase." *Journal of Biological Chemistry* 276, no. 25 (2001): 22608–22613.

Kane, Nancy M. "Peer Review: The Financial Capacity of Nonprofit Hospitals." *Health Affairs* 12, no. 3 (1993): 234–237.

Kantor, Martin. *Uncle Sam's Shame: Inside our Broken Veterans Administration*. Westport CT: Praeger Security International, 2008.

Kass, Amalie M. *Midwifery and Medicine in Boston: Walter Channing, MD, 1786-1876*. Boston: Northeastern University Press, 2002.

___. "The Obstetrical Case Book of Walter Channing, 1811-1822." *Bulletin of the History of Medicine* 67 (1993): 494–523.

Kastor, John Alfred. *Mergers of Teaching Hospitals in Boston, New York, and Northern California*. Ann Arbor, MI: University of Michigan Press, 2003.

Kaufman, Sharon R. *The Healer's Tale: Transforming Medicine and Culture*. Madison, WI: University of Wisconsin Press, 1994.

Keating, Peter, and Alberto Cambrosio. *Biomedical Platforms: Realigning the Normal and the Pathological in Late-Twentieth-Century Medicine*. Cambridge, MA: MIT Press, 2003.

Keefer, C. S. "Soma Weiss, 1899-1942." *New England Journal of Medicine* 226 (1942): 505–506.

Keohane, Carol A., Anne D. Bane, Erica Featherstone, Judy Hayes, Seth Woolf, Ann Hurley, David W. Bates, Tejal K. Gandhi, and Eric G. Poon. "Quantifying Nursing Workflow in Medication Administration." *Journal of Nursing Administration* 38, no. 1 (2008): 19–26.

Keshavjee, Salmaan. "Bleeding Babies in Badakhshan." *Medical Anthropology Quarterly* 20/1 (March 2006): 72-93.

Kim, Jim Yong. "Social Medicine and Health Inequalities." *Brigham and Women's Hospital Department of Medicine, Annual Report, 1996–2001.*

Komaroff, Anthony L., Eugene Braunwald, Joseph L. Dorsey, David M. Eisenberg, Howard H. Hiatt, Phyllis Jen, and Beverly Woo. "Harry Richard Nesson." Medical Faculty Memorial Minute. *Harvard Gazette*, March 23, 2006. Accessed November 8, 2012. http://www.news.harvard.edu/gazette/2006/03.23/18-mm.html.

Khuri, Shukri F. "The NSQIP: A New Frontier in Surgery." *Surgery* 137 (2005): 20–27.

Kidder, Tracy. *Mountains Beyond Mountains: The Quest of Dr. Paul Farmer, a Man Who Would Cure the World*. New York: Random House, 2003.

Kidder, Tracy. "Profiles: The Good Doctor: Paul Farmer Set Out Twenty Years Ago to Heal the World. He Still Thinks he Can." *The New Yorker*, July 10, 2000: 40-57.

Kieffer, Thomas, interview with Ann Conway, June 14, 2012.

King, Marilyn. "Conflicting Interests: Professionalization and Apprenticeship in Nursing Education: A Case Study of the Peter Bent Brigham Hospital School of Nursing during the Carrie M. Hall Years, 1912-1937." DNSc diss., Boston University, 1987. *Dissertation Abstracts Int.* (48, 19388).

__ *The Peter Bent Brigham Hospital School of Nursing: A History: 1912-1985*. Boston: Brigham and Women's Hospital. 1987.

Kirkwood, Samuel B., and Madelen Pollock. "Health During Pregnancy." Boston: Department of Child Hygiene, Harvard School of Public Health and Boston Lying-In Hospital, 1941.

Knox, Richard A. "Work Begins on Huge Hospital Complex." *Boston Globe*, December 21, 1975: 1–3.

___. "Hub Infant Deaths Up 32%, Blacks Bear the Brunt of 1985 Mortality Hike." *Boston Globe*, February 9, 1987: 1.

___. "Birth in the Death Zones," *Boston Sunday Globe*, September 10–12, 1990.

___. "Are Hospitals Crying Wolf? Harvard's Nancy Kane Says Hospitals Are Profit-Poor, but Cash Rich." *Boston Sunday Globe*. February 3, 1991: 73–83.

Koch, Robert R. "Untersuchungen über Bakterien: V. Die Ätiologie der Milzbrand-Krankheit, begründet auf die Entwicklungsgeschichte des *Bacillus anthracis* [Investigations into bacteria: V. The etiology of anthrax, based on the ontogenesis of *Bacillus anthracis*]." *Cohns Beitrage zur Biologie der Pflanzen* 2, no. 2 (1876): 277–310.

Kowalczyk, Liz. "Nurses Balk at Bid to Guide Dealings with Patients." *Boston Globe*, March 21, 2012.

Kuller, Lewis, Abraham Lilienfeld, and Russell Fisher, "Epidemiological Study of Sudden and Unexpected Deaths due to Arteriosclerotic Heart Disease," *Circulation* 34 (1966): 1056–1068.

Lam, Bing K., John F. Penrose, Gordon J. Freeman, and K. Frank Austen. "Expression Cloning of a cDNA for Human Leukotriene C4 Synthase, an Integral Membrane Protein Conjugating Reduced Glutathione to Leukotriene A4." *Proceedings of the National Academy of Sciences* 91, no. 16 (1994): 7663–7667.

Lane, Victor. "Peter Bent Brigham Hospital, 1913–1963: Report on Golden Jubilee Meetings." *Irish Journal of Medical Science* (1926-1967) 39, no. 1 (1964): 37–41.

Langmuir, Alexander D. "New Environmental Factor in Congenital Disease." *New England Journal of Medicine* 284, no. 15 (1971): 912–913.

Laszlo, John, and Francis A. Neelon. *The Doctor's Doctor: A Biography of Eugene A. Stead Jr., MD*. Durham, NC: Carolina Academic Press, 2006.

Leadley, Jennifer, and Rae Anne Sloane. "Women in U.S. Academic Medicine and Science: Statistics and Benchmarking Report 2009-2010." Association of American Medical Colleges, 2011.

Lee, Thomas H., Jr., *Eugene Braunwald and the Rise of Modern Medicine*. Cambridge, MA: Harvard University Press, 2013.

Leung, Lester. "Pathways Through Medicine: Careers in Medicine—Medicine in Developing Countries. From an Interview with Louise Ivers, MD, Partners in Health." Accessed June 1, 2012. http://www.nextgenmd.org/archives/399.

Levine, Samuel A. *Coronary Thrombosis: Its Various Clinical Features*. Baltimore: Williams and Wilkins, 1929.

___and Bernard Lown. "'Armchair' Treatment of Acute Coronary Thrombosis." *Journal of the American Medical Association*, 148 (1952):1365–1369.

___and William S. Ladd. "Pernicious Anemia: A Clinical Study of One Hundred and Fifty Consecutive Cases with Special Reference to Gastric Acidity." *Bulletin of the Johns Hopkins Hospital* 32 (1921): 254.

Lockman, Shahin, Michael D Hughes, James McIntyre, Yu Zheng, Tsungai Chipato, Francesca Conradie, Fred Sawe et al. "Antiretroviral Therapies in Women after Single-Dose Nevirapine Exposure." *New England Journal of Medicine* 363 (2010): 1499–1509.

Loder, Elizabeth, Dhirendra Bana, Paul Rizzoli, and Carly Lavigne. *John R. Graham and the Graham Headache Center: Pioneers in Modern Medicine*. Boston: Faulkner Hospital.

Loeffler, Jay S., Eben Alexander III, Robert L. Siddon, William M. Saunders, C. Norman Coleman, and Ken R. Winston. "Stereotactic Radiosurgery for Intracranial Arteriovenous Malformations Using a Standard Linear Accelerator." *International Journal of Radiation Oncology Biology Physics* 17 (1989): 673–677.

Long, Sharon K., Karen Stockley, and Heather Dahlen. "Massachusetts Health Reform: Uninsurance Remains Low, Self-Reported Health Status Improves as State Prepares to Tackle Costs." *Health Affairs* 31 (2012): 444–451.

Longo, Dan L., Dennis L. Kasper, J. Larry Jameson, Anthony S. Fauci, Stephen L. Hauser, and Joseph Loscalzo, eds. *Harrison's Principles of Internal Medicine*. New York: McGraw-Hill, 2012.

Longo, Dan L., Dennis L. Kasper, J. Larry Jameson, Anthony S. Fauci, Stephen L. Hauser, and Joseph Loscalzo. "Dedication: Eugene Braunwald," In *Harrison's Principles of Internal Medicine*. New York: McGraw Hill, 18th ed., 2012.

Lown, Bernard. *The Lost Art of Healing*. New York: Ballantine Books, 1996.

——, Raghavan Amarasingham, and Jose Neuman. "New Method for Terminating Cardiac Arrhythmias." *Journal of the American Medical Association* 182 (1962): 548–555.

——, Ali M. Fakhro, William B. Hood, and George W. Thorn. "The Coronary Care Unit: New Perspectives and Directions." *Journal of the American Medical Association*, 199 (1967): 188–198.

Lown, Beth A., and Colleen F. Manning. "The Schwartz Center Rounds: Evaluation of an Interdisciplinary Approach to Enhancing Patient-Centered Communication, Teamwork, and Provider Support." *Academic Medicine* 85, no. 6 (2010): 1073–1081.

Ludmerer, Kenneth M. *Learning to Heal: The Development of American Medical Education*. New York: Basic Books, 1985.

——. "Redesigning Residency Education—Moving beyond Work Hours." *New England Journal of Medicine* 362, no. 14 (2010): 1337–1338.

——. "The Rise of the Teaching Hospital in America." *Journal of the History of Medicine and Allied Sciences* 38, no. 4 (1983): 389–414.

——. *Time to Heal: American Medical Education from the Turn of the Century to the Era of Managed Care*. New York: Oxford University Press, 1999.

Lupu, Dale. "Estimate of Current Hospice and Palliative Medicine Physician Workforce Shortage." *Journal of Pain and Symptom Management* 40, no. 6 (2010): 899–911.

Lutz, Wendell, Ken R. Winston, and Nasser Maleki. "A System for Stereotactic Radiosurgery with a Linear Accelerator." *International Journal of Radiation Oncology Biology Physics* 14(1998): 373–381.

Lynaugh, Joan E., and Barbara L. Brush. *American Nursing: From Hospitals to Health Systems*. Blackwell, 1996.

Majno, Guido, and Kurt Benirschke. "Presentation of the Gold-Headed Cane to Arthur T. Hertig." *American Journal of Pathology* 96 (1979): 365–368.

Malka, Susan Gelfand. *Daring to Care: American Nursing and Second-Wave Feminism*. Champaign: University of Illinois Press, 2007.

Mallory, Frank B. "The Present Needs of the Harvard Medical School," *Science* 24 (1906): 334–338.

Marsh, Margaret, and Wanda Ronner. *The Fertility Doctor: John Rock and the Reproductive Revolution*. Baltimore: Johns Hopkins University Press, 2008.

Massachusetts General Hospital. "Report on a Lying-in Department." Boston: Massachusetts General Hospital, Archives and Special Collections, October 1845.

Massachusetts General Hospital Patient Care Services, Social Work. "History." Accessed June 11, 2012. http://www.mghpcs.org/socialservice/History.asp.

"Mayor Menino, Public Health Commission Announce Drop in Black Infant Deaths in City of Boston." Press Release, City of Boston. July 25, 2011.

McClain, Wanda, interview with Ann Conway, May 5, 2012.

McCord, David Thompson Watson. *The Fabrick of Man: Fifty Years of the Peter Bent Brigham*. Published for the Hospital by the Fiftieth Anniversary Celebration Committee, 1963.

McGonagle, John, interview with Ann Conway, February 15, 2012.

McMahon, Graham T., Joel T. Katz, Mary E. Thorndike, Bruce D. Levy, and Joseph Loscalzo. "Evaluation of a Redesign Initiative in an Internal-Medicine Residency." *New England Journal of Medicine* 362, no. 14 (2010): 1304–1311.

"Medicine: The Pill on Trial." *Time*, January 26, 1970.

Melosh, Barbara. *The Physician's Hand: Work Culture and Conflict in American Nursing*. Philadelphia: Temple University Press, 1982.

Merrill, John P., Joseph E. Murray, J. Hartwell Harrison, and Warren R. Guild. "Successful Homotransplantation of the Human Kidney between Identical Twins." *Journal of the American Medical Association* 160, no. 4 (1956): 277–282.

___, John P., Joseph E. Murray, J. Hartwell Harrison, and Warren R. Guild. "Successful Homotransplantation of the Human Kidney between Identical Twins." *Journal of the American Medical Association* 251, no. 19 (1984): 2566–2571.

Meyers, Robert. *D.E.S.: The Bitter Pill*. New York: Seaview/Putnam, 1983.

Minot, Gerorge R., and William P. Murphy. "Treatment of Pernicious Anemia by a Special Diet." *Journal of the American Medical Association* 87, no. 7 (1926): 470–476.

___, Edwin J. Cohn, William P. Murphy, and Herman A. Lawson. "Treatment of Pernicious Anemia with Liver Extract: Effects upon the Production of Immature and Mature Red Blood Cells." *American Journal of the Medical Sciences* 175, no. 5 (1928): 599–621.

___, William P. Murphy, and Richard P. Stetson. "The Response of the Reticulocytes to Liver Therapy: Particularly in Pernicious Anemia." *American Journal of the Medical Sciences* 175, no. 5 (1928): 581.

Moore, Francis D. "Ethical Problems Special to Surgery: Surgical Teaching, Surgical Innovation, and the Surgeon in Managed Care." *Archives of Surgery* 135, no. 1 (2000): 14.

___. *Give and Take: The Development of Tissue Transplantation*. Philadelphia: Saunders, 1964.

___. "Memorial Established for Adolph." *Brigham Bulletin*, vol. IV, no. 10 (February and March, 1957): 4.

Moore, Matthew R., John Shillito, and Eugene Rossitch. "Mildred Codding: An Interview with Cushing's Medical Artist." *Surgical Neurology* 35, no. 5 (1991): 341–344.

Moore, Sally F., and Barbara G. Myerhoff. "Secular Ritual: Forms and Meaning." In *Secular Ritual*. Edited by Sally Falk Moore and Barbara G. Myerhoff. Amsterdam: Van Gorcum & Co. 1977: 3–24.

Morse, Ellen. *The Good Men Do Lives After Them*. Boston: Faulkner Hospital, 1927.

Murphy, William P. *Pernicious Anemia*. Amsterdam: Elsevier, 1965.

Murray, Joseph E. *Surgery of the Soul: Reflections on a Curious Career*. Canton, MA: Science History Publications, 2001.

___and J. Hartwell Harrison. "Surgical Management of Fifty Patients with Kidney Transplants Including Eighteen Pairs of Twins." *American Journal of Surgery* 105, no. 2 (1963): 205–218.

___, John P. Merrill, Gustave J. Dammin, James B. Dealy Jr, Carl W. Walter, M. S. Brooke, and Richard. E. Wilson. "Study on Transplantation Immunity after Total Body Irradiation: Clinical and Experimental Investigation." *Surgery* 48 (1960): 272.

___, John P. Merrill, J. Hartwell Harrison, Richard E. Wilson, and Gustave J. Dammin. "Prolonged Survival of Human-Kidney Homografts by Immunosuppressive Drug Therapy." *New England Journal of Medicine* 268, no. 24 (1963): 1315–1323.

Myerhoff, Barbara. *Number Our Days*. New York: Simon and Schuster, 1978.

Nabel, Elizabeth, Erin McDonogh, Diana Vaprin, and Gillian Buckley. *Discovery and Innovation: Working Together to Provide Superior Healthcare*. Office of Communication and Public Affairs, Brigham and Women's Hospital, 2012.

Nagourney, Eric. "Kenneth Ryan, 75, Obstetrician and Leader in Medical Ethics." *New York Times*, January 28, 2002. Accessed September 4, 2012. http://www.nytimes.com/2002/01/28/us/kenneth-ryan-75-obstetrician-and-leader-in-medical-ethics.html.

National Library of Medicine, National Institutes of Health. "Changing the Face of Medicine: Profiles of Achievement." Accessed July 13, 2013. www.nlm.nih.gov/changingthefaceofmedicine.

Ncama, Busisiwe P., Patricia A. McInerney, Busisiwe R. Bhengu, Inge B. Corless, Dean J. Wantland, Patrice K. Nicholas, Chris A. McGibbon, and Sheila M. Davis. "Social Support and Medication Adherence in HIV Disease in KwaZulu-Natal, South Africa." *International Journal of Nursing Studies* 45, no. 12 (2008): 1757.

Nercessian, Nora N. *"Worthy of the Honor": A Brief History of Women at Harvard Medical School*. Boston: President and Fellows of Harvard College, 1995.

"The New Faulkner Hospital Is Opened for an Inspection by Invited Guests," Boston Herald, February 26, 1903.

"New Techniques in Open Heart Surgery." *Brigham Bulletin*, vol 16, no. 2 (May 1972): 5.

Nightingale, Florence. *Notes on Nursing: What it Is and What it Is Not*. Mineola, NY: Dover Publications, 1860/1969.

Nutting, Mary A. "A Sound Economic Basis for Schools of Nursing and Other Addresses." *American Journal of the Medical Sciences* 173, no. 5 (1927): 723.

Olson, Elena, Emeli Valverde, and L. Adaora Nwachukwu. "The Untold Story: URM Pioneers at MGH Bicentennial Gala and Alumni Reunion, Multicultural Affairs Office at Massachusetts General Hospital, February 11 and 12, 2011." Accessed July 15, 2012. http://www.massgeneral.org/news/assets/urmhistoryslideshow.pdf.

"Opening of the New Harvard Medical School Buildings." *BMSJ* 155 (1906): 352–353.

Orange, Robert P., Robert C. Murphy, Manfred L. Karnovsky, and K. Frank Austen. "The Physicochemical Characteristics and Purification of Slow-Reacting Substance of Anaphylaxis." *Journal of Immunology* 110, no. 3 (1973): 760–770.

Pappas, Theodore N. "Adjustment Reactions and the Surgical Intern." *JAMA* 248 (1982): 31-32.

Parker, Benjamin. *Boston Evening Transcript,* October 9, 1912, p. 1.

"Partners." *BWH,* June/July 1994: 6.

"Partners Healthcare Brigham and Women's Hospital: Promoting Healthy Families." *Bay State Banner,* vol 46, no. 33, March 24, 2011.

"Partners Health Care System Enters New Phase." *BWH,* Summer 1996: 24.

Partners In Health. "Global Health Delivery Fellows Honored for Accomplishments and Leadership." March 30, 2010. Accessed June 1, 2012. http://www.pih.org/news/entry/global-health-delivery-fellows-honored-for-accompishments-and-leadersh/.

"Partners Selected to Participate in ACO Model." *BWH Clinical and Research News,* January 20, 2012. Accessed October 20, 2011. http://www.brighamandwomens.org/about_bwh/publicaffairs/news/publications/DisplayCRN.aspx?articleid=1972.

Patient-Centered Primary Care Collaborative. "Joint Principles of the Patient Centered Medical Home." Accessed July 7, 2012. http://www.pcpcc.net/content/joint-principles-patient-centered-medical-home.

"The Patient Unit," *Transplant,* October 2, 1975: 1–2.

Paul, Oglesby. *The Caring Physician: The Life of Dr. Francis W. Peabody*. Francis A. Countway Library of Medicine, 1991.

——. "*Leadership: A Short History of the Peter Bent Brigham Hospital*." Unpublished manuscript, 1999.

Peabody, Francis Weld. *The Care of the Patient*. Cambridge, MA: Harvard University Press, 1927.

Petryna, Adriana. *When Experiments Travel: Clinical Trials and the Global Search for Human Subjects*. Princeton, NJ: Princeton University Press, 2009.

Physicians for Reproductive Health. "Kenneth J. Ryan, MD." Accessed September 4, 2012. http://prh.org/provider-voices/kenneth-j-ryan-md-memorial-program/programs-kenneth-j-ryan-md/.

Poon, Eric G., Carol A. Keohane, Catherine S. Yoon, Matthew Ditmore, Anne Bane, Osnat Levtzion-Korach, Thomas Moniz et al. "Effect of Bar-Code Technology on the Safety of Medication Administration." *New England Journal of Medicine* 362, no. 18 (2010): 1698–1707.

"Preparing Physicians for Tomorrow's Challenges." *BWH,* Spring 1997: 6.

Prout, Curtis. "Women in Medicine." *The Brigham Bulletin.* Peter Bent Brigham Hospital, vol V, no. II, Winter 1958: 2.

"Public Ceremony in Celebration of the 25th Anniversary of the Peter Bent Brigham Hospital." *New England Journal of Medicine,* August 11, 1938: 183–193.

Putnam, J.J., and G.A. Waterman. "A Contribution to the Study of Cerebellar Tumors and their Treatment." *Journal of Nervous and Mental Disease* 33 (1906): 297.

Rackemann, Francis M. *The Inquisitive Physician: The Life and Times of George Richards Minot, AB, MD, D. SC.* Cambridge, MA: Harvard University Press, 1956.

Razulis, Janice, interview with Ann Conway, April 23, 2012.

"Reginald Fitz." Office of the University Marshall, Harvard University. Accessed September 2012.http://www.marshal.harvard.edu/fitz.html.

Reid, Duncan E., Kenneth J. Ryan, and Kurt Benirschke. *Principles and Management of Human Reproduction*. Philadelphia: W.B. Saunders Company, 1972.

Reverby, Susan M. *Ordered to Care: The Dilemma of American Nursing, 1850-1945*. Cambridge and New York: Cambridge University Press, 1987.

Richinick, Michele. "Dr. Curtis Prout, 96, Physician, Advocate for Prison Health Care." *Boston Globe,* February 6, 2012. Accessed January 14, 2013. http://www.boston.com/news/local/massachusetts/articles/2012/02/06/prison_healthcare_advocate_dr_curtis_prout_a_primary_care_physician_into_his_90s/.

Riley, Marcia (Lee), interview with Ann Conway, May 2, 2012.

Robb, Isabel Hampton. *Educational Standards for Nurses with Other Addresses on Nursing Subjects*. Cleveland: E.C. Koeckert, 1907.

Roboff, Sari. "Mission Hill: Boston 200 Neighborhood Series." Boston: Boston Redevelopment Authority, 1976.

Romano, John, and George L. Engel. "Delirium: I. Electroencephalographic Data." *Archives of Neurology and Psychiatry* 51, no. 4 (1944): 356.

Rosenberg, Charles E. "And Heal the Sick: The Hospital and the Patient in 19th Century America." *Journal of Social History* 10, no. 4 (1977): 428–447.

——. "Inward Vision and Outward Glance: The Shaping of the American Hospital, 1880-1914." *Bulletin of the History of Medicine* 53, no. 3 (Fall 1979): 346–391.

——. *No Other Gods: On Science and American Social Thought.* Baltimore: Johns Hopkins University Press, 1997.

——. *Our Present Complaint: American Medicine, Then and Now*. Baltimore: Johns Hopkins University Press, 2007.

——. *The Care of Strangers: The Rise of America's Hospital System*. New York: Basic Books, 1987.

——. "Social Class and Medical Care in Nineteenth-Century America: The Rise and Fall of the Dispensary." *Journal of the History of Medicine and Allied Sciences* 29, no. 1 (1974): 32–54.

Rosner, David. *A Once Charitable Enterprise: Hospitals and Health Care in Brooklyn and New York, 1885-1915*. New York: Cambridge University Press, 1982.

Rossitch, Eugene, Jr., Matthew R. Moore, and Peter McLean Black. *Harvey Cushing at the Brigham*. New York: Thieme Medical Publishers, 1993.

Russell, J. S. Risien, F. E. Batten, and James Collier. "Subacute Combined Degeneration of the Spinal Cord." *Brain* 23, no. 1 (1900): 39–110.

Salamone, Patricia, interview with Ann Conway, April 26, 2012.

Sandvick, Clinton. "Enforcing Medical Licensing in Illinois: 1877-1890." *Yale Journal of Biology and Medicine* 82, no. 2 (2009): 67.

Sandelowski, Margarete. *Devices and Desires: Gender, Technology, and American Nursing*. Chapel Hill: University of North Carolina Press, 2000.

Sanghavi, Darshak. "The Phantom Menace of Sleep-Deprived Doctors." *The New York Times Magazine,* August 5, 2011. http://www.nytimes.com/2011/08/07/magazine/the-phantom-menace-of-sleep-deprived-doctors.html?pagewanted=all&_r=0, accessed July 2012.

Sax Paul E., Camlin Tierney, Ann C. Collier, Margaret A. Fischl, Katie Mollan, Lynne Peeples, Catherine Godfrey et al. For the AIDS Clinical Trials Group Study A5202 Team, "Abacavir-Lamivudine versus Tenofovir-Emtricitabine for Initial HIV-1 Therapy." *New England Journal of Medicine* 361 (2009): 2230–2240.

Schenck, John F., Ferenc A. Jolesz, Peter B. Roemer, Harvey E. Cline, William E. Lorensen, Ronald Kikinis, Stuart G. Silverman et al. "Superconducting Open-Configuration MR Imaging System for Image-Guided Therapy." *Radiology* 195 (1995): 805–814.

Schoen, Frederick. "Education and Training in the BWH Department of Pathology." Unpublished manuscript, 2012. Microsoft Word file.

Sequist, Thomas D. "Health Careers for Native American Students: Challenges and Opportunities for Enrichment Program Design." *Journal of Interprofessional Care* 21, no. S2 (2007): 20–30.

Serhan, Charles N., "Inflammation: Novel Endogenous Anti-inflammatory and Proresolving Lipid Mediators and Pathways." *Annual Review of Immunology* 25 (2007): 101–137.

Shamlian, Heidi, interview with Ann Conway, June 15, 2012.

Shen, Helen. "Finding Healing for the Healers," *Boston Globe Magazine*, July 15, 2012.

Shore, Eleanor. "The Invisible Faculty." *Harvard Medical Alumni Bulletin*. Spring 1983: 40–45.

Silverman, Stuart G., Kemal Tuncali, Douglass F. Adams, Kelly H. Zou, Daniel F. Kacher, Paul R. Morrison, and Ferenc A. Jolesz. "MR Imaging-guided Percutaneous Cryotherapy of Liver Tumors: Initial Experiencel." *Radiology* 217, no. 3 (2000): 657–664.

Simmons, Leo. "The 'Culture of Illness' in the Home Versus the Hospital," reprinted in *Newer Dimensions of Patient Care, Part 1: The Use of the Hospital and Social Environment of the General Hospital for Therapeutic Purposes*. Edited by Esther Lucile Brown. New York: Russell Sage Foundation, 1961, 121–125.

Slepian, Florence, interview with Ann Conway, July 12, 2012.

Smith, George Van S. "Duncan Earl Reid, 1905-1973." *Harvard Medical Alumni Bulletin*, January/February 1974: 41–42.

Smith, Olive Watkins, George Van S. Smith, and David Hurwitz. "Increased Excretion of Pregnanediol in Pregnancy from Diethylstilbestrol with Special Reference to the Prevention of Late Pregnancy Accidents." *American Journal of Obstetrics and Gynecology* 51 (1946): 411–415.

Snodgrass, Phillip J. *A Life in Academic Medicine*. New York: iUniverse, 2007.

Sprague, Henry R. *A Brief History of the Massachusetts Charitable Fire Society*. Boston: Little, Brown, 1893.

Starr, Paul. *The Social Transformation of American Medicine: The Rise of a Sovereign Profession and the Making of a Vast Industry*. New York: Basic Books, 1984.

Starzl, Thomas E. "The Landmark Identical Twin Case." *Journal of the American Medical Association* 251, no. 19 (1984): 2572.

Stelfox, Henry Thomas, Stefano Palmisani, Corey Scurlock, E. John Orav, and David W. Bates. "The 'To Err Is Human' Report and the Patient Safety Literature." *Quality and Safety in Health Care* 15, no. 3 (2006): 174–178.

Stevens, Edward F. *The American Hospital of the Twentieth Century*. 3rd ed. New York: F.W. Dodge Corporation, 1928.

Stevens, Rosemary. *In Sickness and in Wealth: American Hospitals in the Twentieth Century*. Baltimore: Johns Hopkins University Press, 1999.

Sussman, Andrew L., Jeffrey R. Otten, Robert C. Goldszer, Margaret Hanson, David J. Trull, Kenneth Paulus, Monte Brown, Victor Dzau, and Troyen A. Brennan. "Integration of an Academic Medical Center and a Community Hospital: The Brigham and Women's/Faulkner Hospital Experience." *Academic Medicine* 80 (2005): 253–260.

"Text of the Proposed Leaflet on Birth Control Pills," *New York Times*, March 5, 1970: 24.

Thomas, Lewis. *The Youngest Science: Notes of a Medicine-Watcher*. New York: Viking Press, 1983.

Thornhill, T.S. "Brigham and Women's Hospital." *Orthopaedic Journal at Harvard Medical School* (1999, vol 1: 17-20; 2000, vol 2: 11-13; 2001, vol 3: 20-23; 2002,vol 4: 22-26; 2003, vol 5: 17-26).

"Three BWH Nurses Honored by NERBNA." *BWH Nurse,* March 28, 2011. Accessed November 12, 2012.

http://www.brighamandwomens.org/about_bwh/publicaffairs/news/publications/DisplayNurse.aspx?articleid=1298.

Tilney, Nicholas L. *A Perfectly Striking Departure: Surgeons and Surgery at the Peter Bent Brigham Hospital 1912-1980*. Sagamore Beach, MA: Science History Publications, 2006.

___. *Invasion of the Body: Revolutions in Surgery.* Cambridge, MA: Harvard University Press, 2011.

___. *Transplant: From Myth to Reality*. New Haven, CT: Yale University Press, 2003.

___, Terry B. Strom, Gordon C. Vineyard, and John P. Merrill. "Factors Contributing to the Declining Mortality Rate in Renal Transplantation." *New England Journal of Medicine* 299, no. 24 (1978): 1321–1325.

"To the Memory of Soma Weiss." *The Aesculapied*. Boston: Harvard Medical School, 1942: 5.

"Transfer for Hospital," *Jamaica Plain News*, January 5, 1901: 2.

Tyler, H. Richard, interview by Peter Tishler, 2012. Last updated June 18, 2013. http://videocenter.brighamandwomens.org/videos/h-richard-tyler-md.

Tyndall, John, and Louis Pasteur. *Les microbes organisés: leur rôle dans la fermentation, la putréfaction et la contagion*. Paris: Gauthier-Villars, 1878.

Unitarian Universalist History & Heritage Society. Dictionary of Unitarian and Universalist Biography. "Walter Channing." Accessed July 4, 2012. www25.uua.org/uuhs/duub/articles/walterchanning.

U.S. Department of Health and Human Services. Hospital profile. Brigham and Women's Hospital. 2012. Accessed April 14, 2012. www.hospitalcompare.hhs.gov/hospital-profile.aspx?pid=220110&lat=42.3399&lng=-71.08989&#POC.

Verderber, Stephen, and David J. Fine. *Healthcare Architecture in an Era of Radical Transformation*. New Haven, CT: Yale University Press, 2000.

Vogel, Morris J. *The Invention of the Modern Hospital, Boston, 1870-1930*. Chicago: University of Chicago Press, 1980.

___ and Charles E. Rosenberg, eds. *The Therapeutic Revolution: Essays in the Social History of American Medicine*. Philadelphia: University of Pennsylvania Press, 1979.

Volpp, Kevin G., Amy K. Rosen, Paul R. Rosenbaum, Patrick S. Romano, Orit Even-Shoshan, Yanli Wang, Lisa Bellini, Tiffany Behringer, and Jeffrey H. Silber. "Mortality Among Hospitalized Medicare Beneficiaries in the first 2 Years Following ACGME Resident Duty Hour Reform." *Journal of the American Medical Association* 298, no. 9 (2007): 975–983.

Watkins, Elizabeth Siegel. *On the Pill: A Social History of Oral Contraceptives, 1950–1970*. Baltimore: Johns Hopkins University Press, 1998.

Weinblatt, Eve, Sam Shapiro, Charles W. Frank, and Robert V. Sager. "Prognosis of Men after First Myocardial Infarction: Mortality and First Recurrence in Relation to Selected Parameters." *American Journal of Public Health* 58 (1968): 1329–1347.

Weinstein, Debra. "Partners Graduate Medical Education Annual Report," 2010.

Weinstein, Louis, S. Miguel Edelstein, James L. Madara, Kenneth R. Falchuk, Bruce M. McManus, and Jerry S. Trier. "Intestinal Cryptosporidiosis Complicated by Disseminated Cytomegalovirus Infection." *Gastroenterology* 81(1998): 584–891.

Weintraub, Karen. "Personal Approach to HIV." *The Boston Globe*, October 3, 2011. Accessed June 1, 2012. http://articles.boston.com/2011-10-03/lifestyle/30239007_1_community-health-aids-patients-hiv.

Weiss, James Woodrow, Jeffrey M. Drazen, Nancy Coles, E. R. McFadden Jr, Peter F. Weller, E. J. Corey, Robert A. Lewis, and K. Frank Austen. "Bronchoconstrictor Effects of Leukotriene C in Humans." *Science* 216, no. 4542 (1982): 196.

Weiss, Soma. "Instantaneous 'Physiologic' Death." *New England Journal of Medicine,* 1940; 223: 793-797.

___. "Self-Observations and Psychologic Reactions of Medical Student A.S.R. to the Onset and Symptoms of Subacute Bacterial Endocarditis." *Journal of the Mount Sinai Hospital New York* 8 (1942): 1079-1094.

___. "Letter to Dr. C. Sidney Burwell, March 29, 1940." Soma Weiss papers, Francis A. Countway Library of Medicine.

Weissman, David E., Diane E. Meier, and Lynn Hill Spragens. "Center to Advance Palliative Care Palliative Care Consultation Service Metrics: Consensus Recommendations." *Journal of Palliative Medicine* 11, no. 10 (2008): 1294–1298.

"West Roxbury Is to Have a $100,000 Hospital for Its Own Residents," *Boston Herald*, October 7, 1901.

Whitcomb, Michael E. "Responsive Curriculum Reform: Continuing Challenges." *The Education of Medical Students: Ten Stories of Curriculum Change. Washington, DC: Association of American Medical Colleges/Milbank Memorial Fund* (2000). Accessed August, 2012. http://www.milbank.org/reports/americanmedicalcolleges/0010medicalcolleges.html.

White, Paul Dudley. "Samuel Albert Levine." *American Heart Journal* 72, no. 2 (1966): 291-292.

"Who's Who at the Hospital." *Brigham Bulletin*, July 1943, no. 1.

Winston, Ken R., and Wendell Lutz. "Linear Accelerator as a Neurosurgical Tool for Stereotactic Radiosurgery." *Neurosurgery* 22 (1988): 454–464.

Wolf, Marshall A., video interview by Peter Tishler. BWH History Videos: The Brightest and the Best. http://brw.sites.vm2.broadcastmed.net/videos/marshall-wolf-md. Last updated July 2013.

Woloch, Nancy. *Women and the American Experience*. New York: Alfred A. Knopf, 1984.

"Women—or The Female Factor." In "About Johns Hopkins Medicine," Johns Hopkins University School of Medicine. Accessed September 2012. http://www.hopkinsmedicine.org/about/history/history6.html.

Wooley, Charles F. "Proc, Dr. Sam, Uncle Henry, and The 'Little Green Book.'" *American Heart Hospital Journal* 3 (2005): 8-13.

Yazzie, T., A. Long, M.-G. Begay, S. Cisco, H. Sehn, S. Shin, and C. Harry, on behalf of the Gallup and Shiprock Navajo Nation CHR Programs. "Community Outreach and Empowerment: Collaboration with Navajo Nation CHRs." *Journal of Ambulatory Care Management* 34/3 (2011): 288-289.

Ye, Lichuan. "Factors Influencing Daytime Sleepiness in Chinese Patients with Obstructive Sleep Apnea." *Behavioral Sleep Medicine* 9, no. 2 (2011): 117–127.

Young-Mason, Jeanne. *The Patient's Voice: Experience of Illness*. Philadelphia: F.A. Davis Co., 1997.

Zinner, Michael, video interview by Peter Tishler. BWH History Videos: The Brightest and the Best. http://brw.sites.vm2.broadcastmed.net/videos/michael-zinner-md. Last updated July 2013.

INDEX

Page numbers followed by *f* indicate figures.

I

Q

R

Y

Z